Clinical Practice in Respiratory Care

Clinical Practice in Respiratory Care

James B. Fink, MS, RRT, RCP
Administrative Analyst
Medical Services
Edward Hines, Jr. VA Hospital
Hines, Illinois
Research Associate
Department of Pulmonary and Critical Care Medicine
Loyola University Chicago, Stritch School of Medicine
Chicago, Illinois

Gerald E. Hunt, MS, LVN, RRT, RPFT, RCP
Program Chair
Director of Clinical Education
Respiratory Care Program
Butte Community College
Oroville, California

with 13 Contributors
Illustrations by Catherine M. Albert, BA, RRT

Lippincott Williams & Wilkins

Philadelphia • New York • Baltimore

Acquisitions Editor: Lawrence McGrew
Sponsoring Editor: Holly Chapman
Senior Project Editor: Erika Kors
Senior Production Manager: Helen Ewan
Production Coordinator: Patricia McCloskey
Assistant Art Director: Kathy Kelley-Luedtke

9 8 7 6 5 4 3 2 1

Library of Congress Cataloging-in-Publications Data

Clinical practice in respiratory care / [edited by] James B. Fink, Gerald
   E. Hunt ; with 13 contributors.
        p.   cm.
   Includes bibliographical references and index.
   ISBN 0-397-55093-6 (alk. paper)
   1. Respiratory therapy.   I. Fink, James B.   II. Hunt, Gerald E.
   [DNLM: 1. Respiratory Tract Diseases—therapy. 2. Respiratory
Therapy—methods. 3. Respiratory System—physiology.   WF
145C6417 1999]
RC735.I5C566 1999
616.2' 0046—dc21
DNLM/DLC
for Library of Congress   98-21741
                                                                          CIP

Care has been taken to confirm the accuracy of the information presented and to describe generally accepted practices. However, the authors, editors, and publisher are not responsible for errors or omissions or for any consequences from application of the information in this book and make no warranty, express or implied, with respect to the contents of the publication.

The authors, editors and publisher have exerted every effort to ensure that drug selection and dosage set forth in this text are in accordance with current recommendations and practice at the time of publication. However, in view of ongoing research, changes in government regulations, and the constant flow of information relating to drug therapy and drug reactions, the reader is urged to check the package insert for each drug for any change in indications and dosage and for added warnings and precautions. This is particularly important when the recommended agent is a new or infrequently employed drug.

Some drugs and medical devices presented in this publication have Food and Drug Administration (FDA) clearance for limited use in restricted research settings. It is the responsibility of the health care provider to ascertain the FDA status of each drug or device planned for use in their clinical practice.

DEDICATION

What inspired you to consider respiratory care? What motivates you to pursue it further? I'd like to take this opportunity to introduce you to a few of my personal heroes.

I was introduced to respiratory care by a family friend, Gary Shimer, who had started as an orderly in Indianapolis, and found his way into an early inhalation therapy department. With hard work and perseverance, he became a registered therapist. When I graduated from college with a degree in philosophy, and consequently an uncertain work future, Gary suggested that I drop by the hospital and see what inhalation therapy is all about. The technicians started their shift with a long list of treatments to give, and had to rush from patient to patient, setting up treatments, checking ventilators, and occasionally drawing arterial blood and analyzing it, until they could take a coffee break (often with a cigarette). At this point, a career in carpentry was looking pretty good. Suddenly a voice on the public address system announced "Code Blue—5 West." My friend sprinted down the hallway, up two flights of stairs and around a corner like a track star, to a scene of controlled chaos. There were doctors, nurses, and technicians involved in this bizarre ballet around a patient who wasn't breathing. People were starting lines, giving boluses of medication, intubating, ventilating, compressing, monitoring, assessing, and calling out their findings—and miraculously, the patient began breathing. I knew then and there that I wanted to be a player in that dance. It was my first realization of what a good interdisciplinary team could do, and I wanted to be part of it.

Fifteen years later I was working as a manager in a major university medical center, where I met Cathy Miller. She had spent some time as a manager in a downsizing institution and wanted to immerse herself in patient care. She was so good with staff and patients and coworkers that everyone wanted her to pursue supervision opportunities. "No chance!" "Not interested!" "I just want to be a staff therapist." She did find time and energy enough to become the president of the California Society of Respiratory Care (one of the few who could keep me in line at a board meeting).

Another ten years passed and I found myself in a VA hospital, working with a group of people who were tremendously dedicated to providing their patients with good care against tremendous odds. Among a number of fine therapists, Ed Belingon stood out. For years, he had worked with the physicians and nurses to do whatever it took to get the job done, even when that level of service was discouraged by the organization's leadership. His commitment to the patients and his rapport with the physicians was so great that he opened the door for his peers and innovated changes in home oxygen and sleep medicine that dramatically reduced waiting time for services, improved patient care, and saved the VA a lot of money.

Twenty-seven years after my first shift in a hospital, I was sitting at a hospital bed where my first mentor, Gary, was recovering from a round of chemotherapy. Gary had tried his hand at supervising over the years, but always seemed most content when he was up to his elbows in direct patient care. I asked him to explain what had kept him excited and motivated in respiratory care for over 30 years. His reply—"I like turning the complex textbooks into common sense that people can use. Every time I help a doctor understand how to order effective respiratory care, I make a difference in their future. I have something very important to share that they need to know to care for their patients properly. Giving good care is fun." Gary passed away two months later. He left behind many clinicians, patients, and friends who were enriched by his life.

J.B.F.

We dedicate this book to all the heroes of respiratory care—those individuals who find joy in applying and sharing their knowledge and skills; those who learn and teach a little something new every day, and look forward to going to work (almost) every day; and those who struggle against seemingly insensitive organizations to make sure that their patients don't get the short end of health care, even when they don't see the light at the end of the tunnel.

J.B.F.

G.E.H.

CONTRIBUTORS

JOYCE ANDERSON, ND, MA, RRT, RN
Instructor
Rush University College of Nursing
Chicago, Illinois
Respiratory Care Practitioner
Hines VA Medical Center
Hines, Illinois

JOHN C. BIGLER, JD, RRT
Attorney at Law
Executive Director
California Society for Respiratory Care
Lancaster, California

VIJAY M. DESHPANDE, MS, RRT
Assistant Professor
College of Health Sciences
Department of Cardiopulmonary Care Services
Georgia State University
Atlanta, Georgia

RAJIV DHAND, MD, FCCP
Associate Professor
Division of Pulmonary and Critical Care Medicine
Department of Medicine
Loyola University of Chicago
Stritch School of Medicine
Maywood, Illinois
Hines VA Hospital
Hines, Illinois

PATRICK J. FAHEY, MD, FCCP
Chairman and Professor
Department of Medicine
Loyola University Medical Center
Maywood, Illinois

JAMES B. FINK, MS, RRT, RCP
Administrative Analyst
Medical Services
Edward Hines, Jr. VA Hospital
Hines, Illinois
Research Associate
Department of Pulmonary and Critical Care Medicine
Loyola University Chicago, Stritch School of Medicine
Chicago, Illinois

EILEEN M. HAGARTY, MS, RN, CS
Pulmonary/General Medical Clinical Nurse Specialist
Edward Hines Jr. Hospital
VA Great Lakes Health Care System
Assistant Professor of Medical-Surgical Nursing
University of Illinois at Chicago, College of Nursing
Hines, Illinois

ROBERT HEIDEGGER, RRT
Corporate Respiratory Director
Integrated Health Sciences, Inc.
Owings Mills, Maryland

GERALD E. HUNT, MS, LVN, RRT, RPFT, RCP
Program Chair
Director of Clinical Education
Respiratory Care Program
Butte Community College
Oroville, California

PAIGE KELLY, MA, RRT, RCP
Manager of Clinical Education
Oridion Medical Inc.
Danville, California
Part-time Faculty Member
Respiratory Care Program
Skyline College
San Bruno, California

BRIAN LAWLOR, MS, RRT
Director of Home Medical Equipment
Visiting Nurses Association
Rockford, Illinois

ROBERT M. LEWIS, ND, RN, RRT
Family Nurse Practitioner
Healthsouth
Chicago, Illinois

MICHAEL J. MAHLMEISTER, MS, RRT, RCP
CEO
Mahlmeister & Associates
San Francisco, California

CHARLES J. VANDERWARF, BS, RRT
Clinical Resource Manager
Department of Respiratory Care
Loyola University Medical Center of Loyola University
  Chicago
Chicago, Illinois

JOHN R. WALTON, FACHE, MBA, MHA, RRT
Senior Vice President
Northern Division
Integrated Health Services, Inc.
Owings Mills, Maryland

PREFACE

The clinical practice of respiratory care has emerged as a product of modern critical care medicine. This book was undertaken to bridge the gap between the common practice of respiratory care and the empiric foundations on which such practice should be based. Over the past 30 years we have seen exponential growth in medical knowledge and technology, increasing both the quality and cost of health care. Respiratory care evolved from the early administration of oxygen therapy and has continued to expand to a broad base of both diagnostic and therapeutic interventions in a large variety of settings. The common practices that have been passed through generations of physicians and practitioners are often based more on anecdotal observation than on the more recently acquired empiric evidence. With the exponential increase in medical and technological advances supporting cardiopulmonary function, a practical understanding of the empiric foundations supporting respiratory care is essential for the physician, nurse, respiratory care practitioner, and others involved in patient care. *Clinical Practice in Respiratory Care* is designed to help this broad range of practitioners, responsible for ordering, evaluating, and providing respiratory care, to do the right things, for the right reasons.

This book is for all practitioners of respiratory care, not just RCPs. The key to effective health care in today's environment is functional interdisciplinary teams, working together to provide optimal care of the patient. An effective team has an understanding of the strengths and limitations of each of its members. In order for the health care team to derive maximum benefit, all the members (and especially the captain) need to have an appreciation of the specific knowledge, skills, tools, and techniques that the respiratory care practitioner brings to the table. *Clinical Practice in Respiratory Care* is designed in part to help the members of the team to understand the scientific basis of respiratory care, to formulate better care plans, to determine its benefit, and to analyze critically how the respiratory care is being performed.

Clinical Practice in Respiratory Care provides an exploration of the evidence supporting modern respiratory care, with exercises that allow you to apply your own experiences to challenge the assumptions that often underlie "traditional" ordering patterns to determine why we do things, when we do them, and how we do them. This book is designed to provide the practitioner with all the key information and skills required to assess a patient's needs, develop an effective care plan, and negotiate with the physician and health care team to change the care plan to best meet the needs of the patient. This text provides the practitioner with the tools to do the right thing for the right reasons.

To that end, many of the chapters in this text are not exhaustive in exploring their subject area. Rather, we focus on key elements in the topic that have direct bearing on clinical practice. We have attempted to invoke a casual style, with humor and critical thinking challenges, to spice up some typically dry topics and generate interest and enthusiasm. Our goal is to sprinkle enough tasty intellectual morsels throughout the text to stimulate a better grasp and comfort level with the information presented.

The text is organized with an exploration of the role and legal/ethical responsibilities incumbent upon practitioners of respiratory care. The next four chapters describe how the lungs function, how we measure the limits of lung function, how function changes with disease, and how we assess those changes. Physics, pharmacology, safety, and infection control complete the stage for transforming the basics into clinical practice as the six major categories of therapy are explored. We then present the considerations for applying these therapies in the pediatric patient. The text concludes with an exploration of how the practice of respiratory care changes in the rapidly expanding subacute and home care arenas.

Special Features of this Text

Several unique elements have been incorporated into the design of the text to inform the reader and promote critical thinking. Below is an explanation of these various elements along with their icons, where appropriate.

Key Terms

These words are listed in the beginning of each chapter. Additionally, the index lists in bold each key term and the page number where it is defined.

Standard Boxes

Boxes are used for listing items, describing a clinical procedure, and providing more in-depth background on some topics. There are also Medico-Legal Alert boxes that appear in the legal chapter and present legal and ethical issues that the respiratory care practitioner should be aware of. These are set off by a separate icon.

Critical Thinking Challenges

Four types of boxed features occur in the text:

1. *Case Scenarios* are case examples that put principles into action. Some will include a question and answer section to make sure that the reader truly understands the implications of the case study.

2. *Shifting Care Plans* are examples in which the respiratory care practitioner has to respond to the unique characteristics of each individual case.

3. *Challenging Assumptions* feature instances in which the presumed course of action may not be the best one, or in which a standard practice is challenged.

4. *Go Figures* can be either unanswered case scenario questions or problems that need solving.

Additionally, each chapter begins with objectives and outlines to help the user grasp the key concepts of each topic. The therapy chapters have algorithms recommending treatment plans. Bibliographies listing classic sources are used in the basic chapters such as anatomy and pathophysiology, whereas cited references listing specific journal articles and texts are employed in the therapy chapters, providing the reader with access to current, relevant clinical studies. It is our belief that all these features will help the reader synthesize the textual matter more readily and grasp the big picture of respiratory care so that he or she will be able to attain excellence in practice.

ACKNOWLEDGMENT

We would like to thank our contributors for sharing their expertise, innovation, and creativity. We also extend deep appreciation to Andrew Allen (currently at Saunders) who had the foresight to sign on this unusual project, and editor Larry McGrew and assistant Holly Chapman for the contagious enthusiasm and dedication above and beyond the call of duty that was required to bring it to fruition. The project editor, Erika Kors, and production team of Patricia McCloskey, Kathy Kelley-Luedtke and Helen Ewan, demonstrated an uncanny ability to transform our crude manuscript into an innovative and dynamic reader interface.

To our wives, Terry and Donna, and our families and friends, who patiently gave us the space and support through years of late nights, weekends, and compromised home life—we promise to be more attentive, at least until the next edition.

To our readers—you are today's reality of what respiratory care is and will be. Although we hope we exceed your expectations, when we don't we want to hear about it. Please send your comments, complaints, and suggestions to JIMFINK@AOL.COM.

CONTENTS

CHAPTER 6
ASSESSING SIGNS AND SYMPTOMS OF RESPIRATORY DYSFUNCTION   **143**
Joyce Anderson • James B. Fink

CHAPTER 7
PHYSICAL PROPERTIES OF GASES AND FLUIDS   169
Vijay Deshpande • James B. Fink

CHAPTER 8
PHARMACOLOGY ASSOCIATED WITH RESPIRATORY CARE   189
Michael Mahlmeister

CHAPTER 9
INFECTION CONTROL AND SAFETY 229
James B. Fink

CHAPTER 10
GAS THERAPY   249
Gerald E. Hunt

CHAPTER 13
BRONCHIAL HYGIENE AND LUNG EXPANSION **343**
James B. Fink

CHAPTER 16
PEDIATRIC CONSIDERATIONS 437
Robert M. Lewis

CHAPTER 17
SUBACUTE CARE   463

Robert Heidegger • John Walton

Clinical Practice
in Respiratory Care

The Role of the Respiratory Care Practitioner: From Clinical Practice Guidelines to Maintaining Your Sanity

Paige Brown Kelly • James B. Fink

> *"Everybody gets so much information all day long that they lose their common sense."*
>
> Gertrude Stein

Key Terms

advance directive
aggressive communicator
assertive communicator
clinical practice guidelines
conflict resolution
consensus conference
consensus statement
durable power of attorney
gerontology
hard negotiation
integrity
living will
medicalization
passive communicator
positional bargaining
psychoneuroimmunology
soft negotiation
value history

Objectives

- Describe the role of the respiratory care practitioner.

- Identify key requirements for the application of respiratory care by other health care practitioners.

- Discuss the impact of clinical practice guidelines on the practice of respiratory care.

- Contrast your concept of health with that of your patients and health care institution.

- Describe the value of good communication and negotiation skills in dealing with patients and staff.

- Identify the myth of aging.

- List five steps in the process of dying.

- Discuss the care provider's role in caring for patients while maintaining his or her own health.

The purpose of this chapter is to acquaint the reader with what respiratory care practitioners (RCPs) do, why they do it, and how they can benefit patients and themselves. What RCPs do extends beyond individual tasks and techniques to more complex roles in assessment, evaluation, care plan negotiation, and education. Why we apply specific techniques is defined largely within the scope and purpose of clinical practice guidelines that have been developed in the past decade by the American Association of Respiratory Care (AARC) and other professional organizations to provide a referenced empiric basis for the provision of care. How we provide these services determines whether the patient's clinical and emotional needs can be met without compromising the health and emotional stability of the practitioner.

WHO WE ARE: THE ROLE OF THE RESPIRATORY CARE PRACTITIONER

Respiratory care as an allied health specialty has evolved during the past 50 years. From the simple beginnings of providing oxygen in the hospital, often as an extension of nursing service or central supply, respiratory care now extends to the provision of a broad variety of diagnostic and therapeutic services in diverse settings, from intensive care units to subacute clinics and even to the home. The explosive evolution of technology and science in the fields of pulmonary medicine and respiratory care has required today's practitioners to receive extensive specialty training, ranging from the technical or Associate of Science level to graduate-level training. RCPs assume a variety of roles in clinical care, diagnostic testing and evaluation, education, supervision, management, and research.

WHAT WE DO: THE RESPONSIBILITIES OF THE RESPIRATORY CARE PRACTITIONER

Respiratory care practitioners have a variety of tools, maneuvers, and procedures at their disposal to diagnose, assess, monitor, treat, and educate patients. RCPs understand how these tools work, when they work best, and when another tool or strategy might work better. Because of the specificity and limitations of scope of practice, RCPs understand these tools better than almost anyone, other than the experienced physician with a subspecialty of pulmonary or intensive care medicine or anesthesiology.

This does not mean that RCPs want to "play doctor," or that RCPs are better than anyone else. It does mean that respiratory care training programs dedicate more time to a limited number of procedures specific to respiratory care, in much greater detail than any other allied health or medical training program. With medical knowledge estimated to double every 5 years, the professional RCP has a better chance of keeping up with advances in science associated with this relatively narrow field than does a physician or care provider with a much wider scope of practice.

Respiratory care practitioners provide care to the patient with the tools of the trade, based on the orders and direction of a physician. Box 1–1 lists the therapeutic interventions and diagnostic procedures that the RCP performs.

It is important to be able to perform each task properly, but the practice of respiratory care extends beyond simply performing the procedures correctly. The RCP needs to assess the need for each procedure, weighing the potential benefits against hazards and potential side effects, and to assess the outcome for each therapy to determine if the stated or implied objective has been achieved.

The RCP must understand the patient's condition, the physician's goals for therapy, and the strengths and limitations of each tool and procedure. Before administering respiratory care, the RCP must determine whether the ordered procedure has a high probability of achieving the clinical outcomes or whether another procedure or a modification of the original procedure may be more beneficial in helping the physician to meet the clinical goals of the patient. If the latter is the case, the RCP must contact the physician and negotiate a care plan that is in the best interest of the patient.

The appropriateness of therapy should be monitored and assessed with each treatment. The RCP must identify whether the patient has benefited from, no longer needs, or is negatively impacted by any procedure performed. The

Box • 1–1   TASKS OF THE RESPIRATORY CARE PRACTITIONER

THERAPEUTIC INTERVENTIONS

Oxygen therapy
Aerosol therapy
Airway care
Lung expansion
Bronchial hygiene
Invasive and noninvasive mechanical ventilation
Advanced procedures such as ECMO

DIAGNOSTIC PROCEDURES

Pulmonary function testing
Arterial blood gas analysis
Hemoximetry
Pulse oximetry
Capnography
Metabolic assessment
Sleep studies
Electrocardiography
Stress testing
Holter monitoring
Hemodynamics
Cardiac output measurement

RCP then is obliged to take appropriate action to modify the care plan based on patient condition and response.

Effective treatment plans benefit from patient cooperation. Fostering patient cooperation requires ongoing communication with patients, assuring them about what is being done, why it is being done, and how they can help themselves get better. To achieve this goal, the RCP must be a good and effective communicator.

The RCP is an educator of patients, families, staff, and physicians, sharing information about procedures; how, when, and why to do them; and what to do if the procedures do not provide the desired results.

In the United States and Canada, the RCP acts as a skilled technical extension of the pulmonary and critical care physician, at the bedside and in the diagnostic laboratory. In most states, RCPs are the only licensed care providers other than nurses at the patient's bedside on a 24-hour-a-day, 7-day-a-week basis. RCPs receive the same educational foundation as registered nurses (eg, chemistry, physics, mathematics, anatomy, physiology, pathophysiology, microbiology, and basic medical procedures) before specializing in cardiopulmonary anatomy, physiology, pathophysiology, pharmacology, monitoring, assessment, and diagnostic and therapeutic procedures.

Can any one health care professional provide respiratory care? Sure. All they need is adequate training and skills development to understand how the procedures work, what they are intended to accomplish for the patient, when the patient might benefit from one procedure over another, how to perform the procedure, and how to identify when the desired goals have been achieved.

Can registered nurses provide respiratory care? Absolutely. Even when RCPs are licensed by the state, registered nurses may perform respiratory care procedures within their scope of practice, if those procedures are within their individual ranges of demonstrated competency. Practice and demonstrated competency should be based on an individual's education and experience. Because there is so much to learn in nursing, most nursing curricula in the past 20 years have entailed minimal emphasis on and preparation in respiratory care procedures. For example, an independent review of respiratory care and nursing programs in the United States found that, in topics such as oxygen and aerosol therapy, nursing programs at the associate's, bachelor's, and master's levels provided less than 5% of the instructional and laboratory time dedicated by even the most fundamental respiratory training programs.

Respiratory care practitioners are uniquely prepared for their role in the delivery of health care in the following ways:

Teaching environment: Interns, residents, fellows, and other student practitioners in a wide variety of health-related professions present a constantly changing mix of practitioners being introduced to the tools, service strategies, and options available from the respiratory care service. The educational role of the RCP is key to cost-effective use of care alternatives.

Research environment: RCPs in university teaching hospitals and acute care facilities must interface and support clinical protocols that are an extension of research in a variety of disciplines, and they must explore issues specific to respiratory care.

Role: Much of the practice of respiratory care in the hospital setting takes place in critical care environments. Larger units have dedicated respiratory care personnel with unit-based assignments. Smaller critical care units may have RCPs assigned to more than one area. Judicious use of RCPs can provide fast response times and cost-effective coverage of changing service volumes. As increasingly complex new techniques and devices become available for diagnostics, monitoring, and treatment, institutions are faced with the need for expensive orientation and training programs to support the safe and effective use of these new technologies at the bedside. The RCP is uniquely equipped by training and experience to support these new technologies in the critical care and acute care arenas.

Respiratory care provides a relatively small, dedicated group of direct care providers with the mission of supporting high technology that may not be applied routinely at every bedside in the critical care setting. It is cost-prohibitive to train all bedside personnel throughout the hospital to provide all the desirable technologies. The costs associated with training and with the subsequent use of new technologies frequently enough to maintain skills are key to the use of RCPs.

Some examples of the current scope of respiratory care practice in the high technology arena include the following:

- Perform diagnostic procedures, including metabolic charts, bronchoscopy, cardiac output testing, point-of-care testing, arterial blood gas testing, pulmonary function testing, electrocardiography, stress testing, and sleep laboratories.
- Initiate, calibrate, maintain, and troubleshoot monitoring, including pulse oximetry, capnography, transcutaneous O_2 and CO_2, and indwelling arterial and pulmonary lines.
- Operate assistive devices, including ventilators, CPAP, BiPAP, ECMO, intraaortic balloon pumps, and ventricular assist devices.

The Role of the Respiratory Care Practitioner in the Acute Care Setting

Respiratory care practitioners provide valuable services in both the critical and acute care settings. Respiratory care developed as a profession from the need for assistive personnel responsible for oxygen and other associated therapies. As these technologies expanded, so did the complexity of RCP training and the tendency for other allied health professionals to have less respiratory care–specific training in their curricula. Each acute care site should be evaluated for the most appropriate mix of skilled personnel, but when determining options, the roles and abilities of the RCPs listed in Box 1–2 should be considered.

Some examples of strategies that reduce institutional and patient costs include the following:

• Use MDI or continuous nebulizer versus SVN every hour around the clock.
• Use PEP for CPT when postural drainage is indicated.
• Support institutional adoption of turning, coughing, and stir-up regimens in lieu of expensive RCS inter-

---

Box • 1–2 ROLE OF THE RESPIRATORY CARE PRACTITIONER IN THE ACUTE CARE SETTING

Providing direct patient care with oxygen, aerosol, bronchial hygiene, and ventilatory support in collaboration with other members of the health care team and in accordance with accepted clinical practice guidelines

Acting as consultant to physicians, nurses, and assistive personnel in developing appropriate care plans and equipment use

Assisting with assessment and evaluation of patients, both initially and throughout the course of therapy

Developing and negotiating care plans with the physician. Identifying the most effective and efficient care options for meeting the physician's identified objectives for patient management in light of the specific clinical indications and patient response to interventions

Developing and facilitating strategies that improve effectiveness of interventions and reduce resource use (reducing hospital and patient costs) with ultimate goal of reducing readmissions and length of stay

Providing orientation and education to other members of the health care team in specific services available from respiratory care, in light of specific indications and patient response to care

Identifying opportunities to improve care, and developing strategies to facilitate the realization of those opportunities

Participating in discharge evaluation and providing recommendations for home-based therapies

Developing care strategies that improve care and reduce resource use. Through assessment and evaluation of the patient, working with physician to meet clinical objectives in the most cost-effective manner

---

ventions to prevent and treat postoperative atelectasis and pneumonia.
• Educate patients in the correct use of therapy and devices, such as the MDI withholding chamber and peak flowmeters, to improve their ability to provide self-care at home.

WHY WE DO IT: THE IMPORTANCE OF CLINICAL PRACTICE GUIDELINES

Much of medicine has evolved based on anecdotal observations associating events or interventions with patient outcomes. Although medicine now is considered a science, a considerable number of medical practices are based on anecdotal reports that have not been empirically confirmed. It is fair to say that many traditional practices were adopted because there was a real need for an intervention and because something appeared to work. Once that causal relation was established, it was often expanded to a broader range of patients who might also benefit from the intervention. This was the case, for example, in the development of intermittent positive-pressure breathing therapy for the prevention and treatment of nosocomial pneumonia as well as in the evolution of postural drainage therapy. In both cases, a valuable tool was adopted, overused, and extended to a situation in which it consumed many resources with minimal therapeutic results.

In some cases, the science may exist to refute a practice, but the inertial response, "but this is how we have done things for years," allows the practice to continue, even in light of scientific evidence that another way might be superior. For this reason, many professional medical associations, including the AARC, have developed consensus statements and clinical practice guidelines.

Consensus conferences usually reflect the work of a panel of experts who research and present state-of-the-art practices applied to specific aspects of care. Although the research presented is often substantial, the outcome of a conference, the **consensus statement,** may be influenced by the bias of the panel of experts. **Clinical practice guidelines** evolve from a review of published evidence that supports a clinical practice. A panel of experts then determines what has been proved and what is speculation associated with the practice, often defining issues that require further study to understand better the implications of the clinical practice. The AARC Clinical Practice Guidelines define the procedure or practice; indications; contraindications, hazards, or complications; limitations of the methodology; assessment of need; assessment of outcome; and resources in terms of personnel and equipment. Although far from perfect, these guidelines are a major step toward identifying the empiric foundation of clinical practice. At its best, respiratory care is based on this empiric foundation, integrating the clinical practice guidelines into the rationales for what, when, and how respiratory care is delivered.

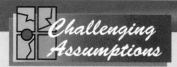

CRITICAL THINKING CHALLENGES

The postural drainage technique was developed in the 1930s, before antibiotics, when many patients who required lung to be removed because of tuberculosis also had bronchiectasis (a condition in which sacs in the lungs collect thick, foul-smelling pus-filled secretions). When surgeons took out the lung, they saw the pus-filled secretions invade the surgical field. A physiotherapist figured that **posturing** the patient to **drain** the pus out of the lung before surgery might allow for fewer complications. It worked. Today, many cardiovascular surgeons routinely order postural drainage and percussion for the treatment of postoperative coronary artery bypass surgery, in patients with or without lung disease. The surgeon's goal for ther-

apy is to reverse or prevent atelectasis. Postural drainage, done properly, takes about 1 hour of practitioner time for each treatment and does not have any therapeutic effect on patients who do not have large quantities of secretions. Turning the patient from side to side every 2 hours, however, reverses and prevents atelectasis and is a recognized component of basic nursing care (so no additional cost). Many surgical intensive care units try not to turn fresh postoperative heart patients for fear of pulling out a tube or stressing an incision. Postural drainage is interpreted in those units to mean percussion over a lung field without turning the patient, a practice shown to be of absolutely no value.

Clinical practice guidelines and consensus documents are tools that back the health care provider with documented empiric data in an effort to eliminate ineffective or suboptimal therapeutic practices. Physicians are trained as scientists, and although they practice the art of medicine when they must practice beyond the science of the situation, they generally modify their approach when presented with adequate empiric data that a long-standing practice does not work. Clinical practice guidelines are a valuable tool to support the care provider in negotiating the most effective therapy for an individual patient.

HOW WE DO IT: TAKING CARE OF THE PATIENT AND OURSELVES

To deliver optimal care in an increasingly global society, health care providers must learn to be flexible and to maintain compassion for people whose values and beliefs may differ widely from their own. Health care workers today face demands that are dramatically different from those who entered the profession just a decade ago. The economics of health care are undergoing a rapid transformation. Our citizens are demanding the best available care at the same time that our society is generally unwilling to pay for the time and resources required to support that care. As a result, health care providers are under increasing pressure to do more with less, to work "smart," and to avoid time-consuming activities that do not contribute to the bottom line. All too often, this translates into cutting corners to get the job done. It is vital that you find a balance that allows you to work within this environment, providing high-quality care in a cost-effective manner that does not interfere with properly caring for your patients, your coworkers, and yourself.

Respiratory care providers need to work closely with and to understand the community they serve. This commu-

nity is composed of people with a remarkable range of diversity in age; gender; family relationships; racial, cultural, and ethnic identities; income level; education; and occupation. This community extends beyond patients to include other customers and coworkers. Care must be delivered under tighter time constraints and stricter reimbursement directives. The challenges are obvious! How can you provide quality care and remain sane?

The following theoretical frameworks for communicating clearly and fairly in a variety of common situations (such as dealing with the aging patient, differing cultural beliefs, communicating with coworkers, and confronting issues of death and dying) emphasize maintaining boundaries in emotional and demanding situations. Each of the following topics deserves further study. This chapter also explores a sampling of techniques used for the practitioner's self-care and restoration. These topics are not meant to be inclusive of all areas of human diversity but rather to reinforce your ability to stand back before judging when faced with the challenges inherent in personal differences. Good communication, an open mind, and honorable intentions are vital ingredients for providing high-quality and fulfilling service in the health care community.

WHY DID YOU CHOOSE HEALTH CARE?

Everyone who enters a health care profession has his or her own motives and beliefs about what good health means. During the educational process, the health care provider is often asked to accept standard institutional definitions of health, and personal definitions and beliefs may become shrouded by more abstract and technical ones. What did health mean to you before you started this educational process? Why did you choose to become a member of the health care community? Was it because of a love of science, a genuine desire to serve humankind by making people feel better, or the lure of a good salary with great hours? Perhaps an experience with yourself or someone you love? Whatever your reasons, you must be prepared to reexamine your personal beliefs and be ready to explore new ones as they evolve. The challenge, as you explore your answers, is to accept the fine balance between being professional and knowing your limitations. Understanding appropriate boundaries is a new concept for many of us, especially when serving people in the health care setting. We are just now becoming aware of the unhealthy consequences of not understanding personal limitations.

The issue of personal boundaries is too often dismissed in health care. The caregiver is often viewed as having limitless resources for compassion and abilities to resolve problems, both physical and mental. Experience teaches us that this demand can leave individuals frustrated and disenchanted with their chosen profession. The ability to feel compassion for those you care for and work with is important. The ability to draw boundaries is best said in the Alcoholics Anonymous Prayer:

> God grant me
> the serenity to accept the things I cannot change,
> the courage to change the things I can,
> and the wisdom to know the difference.

Too often, care providers who start out with seemingly boundless energy and compassion become overextended and so drained that they are left with very little to give to their patients or themselves. This overextension can lead to physical and emotional exhaustion. Many respond with cynicism, bitterness, and the building of emotional barriers that shut out much of their world. Their work life may become a series of chores without the "luxury" or joy of feeling the uniqueness of each encounter. Care given in an insensitive and robotic manner deprives everyone, including the caregiver, of the dignity and joy that we all deserve.

Carefully consider your own definitions of health. They will be tested by the best and worst aspects of humanity. You will care for people whose lives are cut short by aberrant behavior such as child abuse, drunken driving, and violent responses to anger, hate, and fear. You will grow to care for people who find life's priorities changed by a terminal illness, and you will befriend the families and loved ones that these patients will leave behind. All this can leave you frustrated, confused, drained, and even angry. You will not always agree on the course of treatment or believe you did all that you were capable of doing.

Just how do people cope in these situations? It is important to reflect on these experiences and to resist the temptation to dismiss or bury them because of their painful or seemingly futile nature. Making time for discussion with others is always helpful and can allow closure in situations that, left unattended, can negatively affect your future work. No matter how technical your work seems, it operates on a foundation of human interactions.

You will be asked to provide knowledge and wisdom as a friend, counselor, teacher, and health care professional. This will challenge your own issues of authority, death and dying, cultural values, aging, and politics (to name just a few) as you grow into your chosen profession. Remaining objective and basing actions on carefully considered facts are difficult responsibilities when faced with a life-and-death situation, especially when your patient's beliefs and desires conflict with your own. Working in the health care environment is but a part of a broader whole. Nothing is created in a vacuum—neither epidemic immune disorders nor the social injustices that result in physical abuse.

As technology improves and resources become more scarce, the goals of health care should remain unchanged. The World Health Organization defines health as "a state of complete physical, mental, and social well being and not merely the absence of disease." Realizing this lofty goal requires accepting the reality that health care is not a closed, isolated system directed solely by hard science Those of us who are health care workers by profession are also products of the community in which we live and of our individual genetic blueprints. We must strive to connect ourselves and our patients to the resources that exist both inside and outside the institution of health care. We must always question what is good and what needs to be changed.

WHAT YOUR PATIENT WANTS

What expectations and rights do patients have? Too often, the person seeking help must have symptoms viewed as "illness" that are documented based on observations made by caregivers. The patient's motivation for seeking care is often quite different from your own priorities for attaining that healthy state. Your goal should be to include your patients as equal partners from the beginning. Should you treat only the symptoms or the whole person? The World Health Organization mission statement indicates that the answer is to do both. To leave someone dependent is both costly and unethical. Starhawk, a cultural anthropologist, distinguishes between two different kinds of power: "power over" and "power from within."[1] Power over is about control, authority, domination, and strength in the sense of force and annihilation. It emphasizes objectivity in the name of fairness and defines each participant in a hierarchic manner that often leaves the patient at the bottom. The health care community is seen as having authority over the patient. Power from within acknowledges and responds to interconnectedness, to relatedness, and to cooperation. It emphasizes individual contexts in the name of caring. Power from within implies a more horizontal structure of information exchange and decision-making responsibilities, in the belief that ethical decision making ultimately must rest with those most affected by the decision.[2] Power from within supports the rights and responsibilities of all the participants, giving patients a more active role in defining the goals and outcomes that will affect their lives.

To begin the process of developing inclusive goals, you must be able to elicit information about the patient. Jecker and colleagues defined an easy format for an organized approach to reaching shared goals when differing perspectives exist[3] (Box 1–3).

Identifying the goals of the parties involved simply entails trying to diagnose the situation by gathering information, organizing it, and thinking about it. The ability to listen and elicit your patient's participation is begun in this stage. Start by getting to know as much about the person you are caring for as possible. Their family members or loved ones may provide useful information. Getting to know your patient can be pursued creatively while you attend to routine procedures. The skill of paying attention to a wide variety of cues improves with experience.

Paying attention begins with active listening. Most people are anxious to tell their stories or offer their opinions. Too often, this results in individuals rehearsing their remarks internally while another is speaking.[4] The resulting tragedy is that no one really hears what the other has said. In health care, it is dangerous not to listen effectively; you can easily miss important information and bypass warnings of impending problems.

The ability to work effectively with others begins with a commitment to put aside for a moment your own predetermined beliefs and self-interests and to look carefully at another's perspective. The personal skill of communicating is extremely valuable in ensuring continuity of quality care in a busy and demanding environment. The skill is to meet each situation with a clear mind and in a composed state[4] (Box 1–4).

Unfortunately, listening to gather information often leads to listening only for specific information and ignoring everything else. For example, with coworkers, you may find that you are listening only for weak points in an argument so that you will be ready with ammunition when your turn to speak comes. If you reflect back to the four intentions, you'll find that when the desire to listen is there and equal participation is your intention, effective communication has begun.[4]

All health care providers are accountable to improve and understand better communication skills. To engage in meaningful communication, you have to ask questions and give feedback. Some techniques can help you to ensure that what you have heard is correct. Begin by paraphrasing, using lead-ins such as, "So, basically what you felt was . . . ."

Box • 1–3 INTERACTING WITH PATIENTS

1. Identify the goals of the people concerned.
2. Identify mutually agreeable strategies.
3. Meet ethical constraints.

Box • 1–4 FOUR INTENTS OF REAL LISTENING

1. Understand someone.
2. Enjoy someone.
3. Learn something.
4. Give help or solace.

---

or "Do you mean that . . .?" Then, clarify by asking questions that sharpen your understanding of what the person is trying to communicate. Once it is clear to you what the person has said, begin to talk about your reactions without being judgmental. Communication is an ongoing process; leave the door open for the other person to clarify any misperceptions you might have, to ensure that the dialogue will continue and not result in sparring or defensive posturing.

Listen actively and with empathy—simply know that everyone is trying to survive (Box 1–5). It helps to ask yourself questions such as, "What need is this (anger) coming from?," and "What is this person asking for?"

The following techniques were adapted from a publication written in the early 1960s by Samhammer and Larson entitled, *Interacting With Patients*.[5] They are suggestions for providing an environment conducive to expressing interests and concerns about the care given and the direction in which the patient would like it to go.

Offer yourself. Often, you will find yourself with a patient who is unable to speak or prefers not to. You can still convey concern and interest toward this patient by being alert to the tone of feeling communicated by the patient through posture, gesture, facial expression, voice quality, and inflection. Resist the temptation to make immediate responses or to ask questions when a prolonged verbal pause occurs. Show a desire to understand without making any demands on the patient. The patient should not feel a need "to give" in order to receive attention. "We can sit here quietly; there's no need to talk unless you want to." "I have a few minutes, I'd like to stay with you for a while to make sure you are all right." Sitting or walking with a patient who is unable or unwilling to communicate with words often helps. Elicit the help of other caregivers, and take the opportunity to move a patient outdoors, away from the hospital environment, or in view of the outdoors whenever possible. This can mean a great deal to those not able to do so on their own. It will establish trust between you and the patient.

Give broad openings and offer general leads. Try to provide an opportunity for the patient to take the initiative in introducing a topic and determining the direction of conversation. If you notice pictures of family or loved ones in the room, ask who they are. Those closest to your patient can help to stimulate the

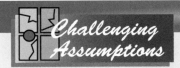

CRITICAL THINKING CHALLENGES

Twelve Blocks to Active Listening

1.	Comparing	Assessing the other while they speak
2.	Mind reading	Trying to figure out what the person really is thinking and feeling
3.	Rehearsing	Focusing attention on the preparation and crafting of your next comment
4.	Filtering	Avoiding hearing things that are threatening, negative, critical, or unpleasant
5.	Judging	Prejudging someone as stupid or unqualified before you take time to evaluate the content of what is said
6.	Dreaming	Allowing something that the person says to trigger a chain of private associations
7.	Identifying	Referring everything a person tells to your own experience
8.	Advising	Hearing no more than a few sentences before you begin searching for the right advice
9.	Sparring	Interjecting comments that disagree or put down the other before you have had time to acknowledge what you heard
10.	Being right	Going to any length to avoid being wrong
11.	Derailing	Responding by making a joke or remark to avoid seriously listening to the other person
12.	Placating	Agreeing with everything, even though you have only half-listened to what was said; you just want to appear nice, pleasant, and supportive

motivation to participate in his or her own recovery. "Is this your grandchild?" "Perhaps it will help to talk about your feelings." "And then?"

Make observations. When change is observed in the patient's efforts, try to articulate what you perceive without attaching a judgment to it. "You keep rubbing your forehead; are you in discomfort?" "It looks like you didn't need any breathing treatments last night, are you feeling better today?"

Encourage comparisons. Ask the patient to describe similarities and differences about thoughts, feelings, and situations and to comment on how they affected him or her. "You said you were upset when you came to the hospital. How do you feel now?" "I read on your chart that you use a different machine for your breathing treatments than the one we use here. Do you think ours works as well?"

Encourage descriptions. Give the patient the opportunity to verbalize his or her perceptions, in hope that the patient will describe how he or she feels or views a situation. "How do you believe it should be done?" "What's your opinion?" "How do you feel about going home?"

Voice doubt. Express uncertainty about the reality of a patient's perception, but be careful not to contradict or belittle the patient's view. Try to encourage honest feedback. "I see no other person in the room." "Are you sure you understood what the nurse meant?" "You say you are not upset, but you give the impression that all is not well."

Provide information. Give the patient facts or specific information that is needed. Questions should be answered simply and directly, but if you do not know the answer, handle the question carefully and honestly. "This medication should help you breath more easily." "No, it's not unusual to have a headache after this treatment." "I don't know, but I will let your doctor know about your concern."

Rephrase the preceding suggestions in a manner you are comfortable with. No one wants a robotic caretaker. Be yourself, and carefully monitor the effects you have on your patients so that you can adjust when needed. You should try to create an environment in which your patients can participate and exercise choice.

It is not up to you to solve every problem that comes your way or to perfect the patient's world to your standards

---

Box • 1–5   PRACTICE ACTIVE LISTENING

1. Maintain good eye contact.
2. Lean slightly forward.
3. Reinforce the speaker by nodding or paraphrasing.
4. Clarify by asking questions.
5. Actively move away from distractions.
6. Be committed to understanding what was said, even if you are angry or upset.

of healthy living. The burden in health care is carried by a team, and it behooves you to seek out specialists so that you can report clearly to the correct person. Engaging patients effectively is an art, and confronting your listening skills can provide more options for communicating.

MUTUALLY AGREEABLE STRATEGIES

Once you understand the patient's expectations and desires for health care, you are ready to advocate for a collective strategy. This section deals with how we present ideas and how we can structure a more effective presentation. This planning stage entails both generating ideas and deciding what to do. How do you propose to handle this patient's problem? What are the most important concerns, and how can they be resolved objectively?

During the discussion stage, the parties communicate back and forth, looking toward agreement. Differences in perception, feelings of frustration and anger, and difficulties in communication can be acknowledged and addressed. At this time, note any options already present, and identify any criteria already suggested as a basis for agreement. Each side should come to understand the interests of the other. Both can then generate options that are mutually advantageous and seek agreement on objective standards for resolving conflicting interests.

Pay close attention to your tone of voice, apart from the verbal content, including pitch, resonance, articulation, tempo, volume, and rhythm. Your tone of voice unintentionally may betray your moods and attitudes. No matter what you say, the sound of how you say it will reveal a great deal about who you are and what you feel.

MEETING ETHICAL CONSTRAINTS

How should you deal with situations in which disagreements, misunderstandings, and differing perspectives get in the way of providing care? This subject is often found under the heading of **conflict resolution**. Conflict resolution begins with stable individuals who are able to see a purpose for being in a given situation that goes beyond their individual motivations and desires. Drawing from the Eastern tradition of being part of a group works for harmony for all involved. The single most important aspect of Eastern culture is the notion of operating instinctively on the principle of group consensus; individuals who achieve self-gratification at the expense of the collective welfare are regarded as unspeakably reprehensible, and individual self-assertion in almost any form is rigorously discouraged.[6] This is a difficult concept in the Western tradition, which cherishes individual identity over group identity. Yet health care involves, by all standards, a team approach. The ability to work effectively with a group is enhanced by a more inclusive style of decision making.

Many care providers' ambitions have faltered when their perceptions of what is appropriate health care clash with others' priorities. Good communication seems to vanish when people feel personally challenged and are unprepared to participate in resolving conflict. The ability to express feelings, thoughts, and wishes while not violating or intimidating others is an art. The concept of teamwork demands, for the sake of good care, your being aware of how you present your ideas. Learning to be assertive does not mean behaving aggressively but rather knowing when and where to assert yourself. You will often find yourself in situations that require a clear presentation of your ideas for a particular plan of care. The physician and patient must trust you before they will legitimately include or accept your ideas.

McKay and associates, the authors of *Messages: The Communication Skills Book,* refer to recognizing three styles of communication: assertive, aggressive, and passive.[4] **Passive communicators** do not express their feelings, thoughts, and wishes directly, but may communicate them indirectly by frowning, mumbling, or whispering something under the breath, or they may withhold their feelings and wishes completely. Passive communicators may smile a lot and subordinate their needs to those of others, may find themselves at a loss for words, or may begin rambling and using phrases that are vague. Their posture may slump, and they may use indirect eye contact while they fidget, using phrases like, "I mean" and "you know"—implying that you can read their thoughts. Passive communicators give the impression that they don't know what they mean; for this reason, their opinions and feelings are often dismissed.

Aggressive communicators are quite capable of stating how they feel, what they think, and what they want, but often at the expense of others' feelings and rights. They tend to humiliate others by using sarcasm or humorous putdowns. They are likely to go on the attack when they don't get their way, and they stir up guilt and resentment in others by pointing a finger of blame. Their sentences begin with "You . . .," followed by an attack or negative label. They use absolute terms, such as "always" and "never," and describe things in a way that implies that they are always right and superior.

Assertive communicators make direct statements regarding their feelings, thoughts, and wishes. They stand up for their rights and take into account the rights and feelings of others. They listen attentively and let others know that they have heard them. They are open to negotiation and compromise, but not at the expense of their rights and dignity. Good communicators make direct requests and direct refusals. It is imperative in dialogue to give and receive compliments, learning to communicate effectively with criticism without becoming hostile or defensive.

Once you take responsibility for how you say things and are open to discussing changes in a manner respectful of yourself and others, positive changes will occur in your communication style.

Negotiation is a basic process of communication designed to reach an agreement. It is a way to handle differences. Resorting to old strategies or avoiding a probable confrontation often leaves those involved feeling dissatisfied, worn out, or alienated. In the book, *Getting to Yes*, the authors differentiate between hard and soft negotiation.[7] **Soft negotiation** avoids personal conflict and makes concessions easy, whereas **hard negotiation** is a contest of wills in which only one side must win. The hard bargainer often "beats" the soft bargainer. Standard negotiating strategies fall between these two. **Positional bargaining**, in which each side takes a position, argues for it, and then makes concessions to reach a compromise, often concludes with a decision that is inefficient and may produce unwanted effects. An alternative strategy is based on principles of negotiation and helps the parties to make fair decisions based on the individual merits of both sides, without taking advantage of any of the people involved.

Some reasons that health care workers back off from asserting their knowledge and end up going along with care plans with which they don't agree are cited in Box 1–6 and were adapted from *Messages: The Communication Skills Book*.[4] Many people find one or more of these reasons sufficient to back off when given an opportunity to advocate for a patient or just to present ideas. A few feeble attempts accompanied by failure leave many care providers without the courage to persevere.

We offer instead a healthier way of talking to yourself before negotiating for your patient's safety and well-being.[4] By practicing some of the following tips, you might discover that you are a good negotiator and that people will then seek your advice more frequently. In addition to becoming aware that you are there for the patient's safety, you may find that, through healthy dialogue, you also learn a tremendous amount. This process is very rewarding and will continue to provide you with benefits throughout your career as you gain experience and sharpen your skills.

Box • 1–6   REASONS FOR NOT ASSERTING YOURSELF

1. You are afraid you will be wrong, and there is an unspoken belief that to be trusted, you must know everything. To make a mistake is to prove yourself unworthy.
2. Physicians deserve respect, and you should always keep your opinions to yourself.
3. You should be flexible and adjust. Others have good reasons for their actions, and it's not polite to question them.
4. You could make the situation worse, so why risk your reputation?
5. People don't like show-offs or overly confident people; it's better to just go along. You might be seen as antisocial if you disagree.
6. No one ever listens to you anyway.

Once you are ready to discuss a problem or conflict, you should address it at two levels. At one level, negotiation addresses the substance; at another, it focuses on the procedure for dealing with the substance. The following four points define a straightforward method of negotiation that can be used under most circumstances. Each point deals with a basic element of negotiation and suggests what you should do about it.[7]

People: Separate the people from the problem.
Interests: Focus on interests, not positions.
Options: Generate a variety of possibilities before deciding what to do.
Criteria: Insist that the result be based on some objective standard.

The first point addresses emotions that can easily become entangled with the objective merits of a problem. People tend to identify their egos with their positions. Hence, before working on the substantive problem, the "people" problem should be disentangled from it and dealt with separately. The participants should come to see themselves as working side by side, attacking the problem, not each other.

The second point is designed to overcome the drawbacks of focusing on a person's stated position when the goal of negotiation is to satisfy the underlying interests of the patient. Compromising is not likely to produce an agreement that will effectively take care of the human needs that led the negotiators to adopt these positions in the first place. Define your interests, not your position.

The third point addresses the difficulty of designing an optimal solution while under pressure. Trying to decide in the presence of adversity narrows your vision. Having a lot at stake and searching for the one right solution inhibits creativity. You can offset these constraints by setting aside a designated time within which to consider a range of possible solutions that advance shared interests and creatively reconcile differing interests. Before trying to reach an agreement, invent options for mutual gain.

The final point, insisting on using objective criteria, is extremely important in the clinical setting. Rather than relying on phrases such as, "because I said so," the opposing parties are asked to produce objective criteria to substantiate their position. Insisting on criteria based on expert opinion or standard of practice is a better way to resolve differences and to help produce a workable solution for all involved. It is also a reminder that being a good clinician entails continuing your education so that you can advocate wisely for your patient.

In the scenarios presented in the accompanying *Go Figure!* display, organize the issues using the format discussed to resolve the problems in an efficient and caring manner. Then divide the problem into the following three stages:

1. Identify the goals of the people concerned.
2. Identify mutually agreeable strategies.
3. Meet ethical constraints.

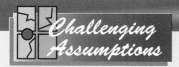

CRITICAL THINKING CHALLENGES

Passive	Assertive
1. I'll embarrass myself by being wrong.	1. I can always learn from my mistakes.
2. The physician deserves respect. I should keep my opinion to myself.	2. I have a right to my opinion and convictions.
3. I should be polite, flexible, and adjust to what they request.	3. I have a right to protest any treatment for my patient that I believe is inappropriate or when I believe another is better.
4. What if I make the situation worse for my patient?	4. I have a right to discuss and negotiate a change; it's an opportunity to learn.
5. They'll think I'm showing off.	5. I have a right to receive recognition for my work and knowledge.
6. No one ever listens to me anyway.	6. I have a right to be the final judge of my feelings and decide whether they are legitimate or not.

CROSS-CULTURAL CONSIDERATIONS

We cross cultural lines every day of our lives. We robe as we go to work as the professional and disrobe when we return home as a member of a household. We change our vocabulary as we address those in our different environments. Within each culture, we find a subculture and look for rules that establish an equal playing field. Medicine, which is supported by a strong allegiance to science, is too often seen as "value free" and not guided by emotion. Ethical challenges are too often overshadowed by the myth that our decisions are made objectively and with a socially neutral veil of universality. We must look closely at our choices and be careful not to undermine the connections that people have established in their lives. How we strive for balance and stability for those involved in the delivery

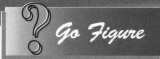

CRITICAL THINKING CHALLENGES

What Would You Do . . . ?

1. You enter the room of a patient whom you have been asked to assess and recommend therapy for. The patient appears anxious and is in obvious respiratory distress. When you introduce yourself, she reacts in a hostile manner by accusing you of being just one more person out to make money off her. How do you proceed?

2. You have been taking care of this patient in the intensive care unit for the past 3 weeks. She was extubated almost 24 hours ago, is progressing very well, and probably will be discharged from the hospital soon. This will be your first encounter with her in a situation in which she is able to verbalize directly to you. You have a standard protocol for continuing the patient's regimen of care, but you realize that her cooperation is crucial for success. You would like to include the patient in the treatment course. The patient seems at a loss when asked how she feels about what has happened and what she expects in terms of an outcome. What are some ways you could engage this patient and help her to participate in her care?

3. John is coming to the end of his shift and is working diligently to organize his shift's activities by finishing his charting clearly, noting the significant changes that occurred in the patient so that he can report directly to the provider who follows him. He leaves his work area neat and organized. When the next provider arrives, she seems unconcerned about the diligent care John has given and, at times, appears not to listen to his report. When he arrives at work the next day, he finds that the patient's progress has waned and that the provider who followed him made few efforts to continue care as John had done the night before. She also failed to contact the physician to suggest changes in therapy when it was necessary. John also finds the patient in a sloppy and disorganized environment. How can he effectively voice his feelings about this situation and not alienate this coworker?

and receivership of health care depends on how honestly we are able to look at our own underlying beliefs about what constitutes a healthy existence.

Our learning is based on the Western model, which often omits discussion of existing opposing values. How do we formulate a strategy for resolving these differences? Let's take a deeper look at our criteria for developing an ethical solution that considers all of the participants equally.[3]

Identifying Goals

We become more knowledgeable of other cultural practices when we practice a systematic method of exploring beliefs held by people who may be foreign to us but whose differences we come to appreciate and to engage humanly. A part of us continues to experiment, while another part struggles to sustain certain beliefs or principles. We continue to practice listening skills while identifying individual goals, but now we are faced with the incredible influences of separate cultures.

Often, truly listening to a person while putting aside your own perceptions and biases allows you to discover what you share, although each goal is achieved on a slightly different path. There is no single ethical "core" for all of us; some find it in religion, or in work, or in various personal attachments or connections. Your purpose is to identify, by listening to the patient, the family, or loved ones, the motivation that brought the patient to you.

Mutually Agreeable Strategies

Once the provider in a cross-cultural encounter has clarified provider and patient goals, the next step is to identify alternative mutually agreeable strategies to meet those goals. In the hospital environment, a ritual of agreement may be signing informed consent forms, or postponing signing until the patient has had time to discuss the strategy with the family and develops trust in the care providers. Most hospitals try to provide consultants familiar with the patient's cultural circumstances who are fluent in the patient's native language and trained in medical interpreting. New tools have become available for hospitals, such as the AT&T Language Line, with 24-hour service that guarantees access to interpreters who speak 147 different languages. Hospitals also have language "banks" that store the names of staff members who are bilingual. Using flash cards that contain common phrases written in the patient's language can also be helpful.

Meeting Ethical Constraints

The final step engages the health professional in ethical deliberation about the acceptability of alternative means of realizing goals. Once again, you are engaged in the process of dealing fairly with your own beliefs while searching for a single absolute truth that will embrace all participants' values. The work of Taylor and Gaita can help to organize this process.[8]

First Level of Ethical Analysis

- The means chosen to achieve the goals of the medical encounter should be compatible with the health care provider's own values as well as with the ethics of the health care profession to which the provider belongs. As the American College of Physicians notes, "the physician (in a cross-cultural setting) cannot be required to violate fundamental personal values, standards of scientific or ethical practice, or the law."
- The means should also be compatible with the patient's values and the values of the culture with which the patient identifies. This safeguards patients against the abuses of power and authority by health professionals.
- At this level of analysis, the constraints are justified by the integrity of the health care professional. Here, **integrity** refers to the inclination to act in accordance with your own moral beliefs and character.[8] In this context, you are able, within the limits set by integrity, to resolve culturally based conflicts. Integrity is a higher-order virtue that does not presuppose specific lower-order virtues (ie, societal norms) to which a person's actions must conform; an example would be participating or not participating in an assisted suicide.

Second Level of Ethical Analysis

The second level of analysis involves examining more basic ethical goals. Again, personal integrity furnishes guidance, but at this level, convictions and principles are reached after carefully examining and questioning the facts. Rather than blindly and stubbornly holding fast to principles for their own sake, you agree to expand your viewpoint to include those of others. A person of integrity shows the qualities of a reasonable person, including "a deposition to find reasons for and against the possible lines of conduct . . . open to him . . . to consider [viewpoints] . . . in the light of further evidence and reasons which may be presented . . . [and] to know his/her own emotional, intellectual, and moral predilection."[8]

Health care professionals should examine critically what is brought to each medical encounter and consider, after thorough deliberation, alternative viewpoints about treatment. This does not require a betrayal of personal beliefs but may result in a change in some of those beliefs in light of new evidence and circumstances. In the health care setting, the force of ethical principles depends on circumstances of context, such as the values of patients, family members, and relevant social groups; personal and professional values of health care providers; and the institutional setting in which the ethical situations arise.[8] Context is key here because it shapes the actual meaning of ethical principles. In health care, the generality of bioethical principles to "do good" and "avoid harm" renders varying interpretations inescapable, and health professionals cannot function effectively on predetermined general principles alone.

The following case scenario presents a situation, taken from the work of Jecker and colleagues,[3] involving a Western physician and a Navajo patient, who have different moral vocabularies and cultural frameworks. The cultural differences make the resolution of even a relatively straightforward ethical conflict more challenging.

After a sincere effort has been made to establish links between different cultures, we need to explore the basic differences between health care providers and consumers, which also intersect with issues of culture and subcultures. The ideas and attitudes of "professionals" can be viewed as the product of the "culture" of health care itself. In her book, *Cultural Diversity in Health and Illness*, Spector illustrates the following models of consumers' (patients') perceptions and providers' viewpoints.[9]

Individual perceptions are defined by the following motivational factors:

Perceived susceptibility: What is the known family history of this person to a given disease, and does the provider agree with the risk factors?

Perceived seriousness: This varies from person to person and is related to how much the patient believes that this problem will alter his or her life. The provider perceives this alteration from a background of pathophysiology as well as from trying to estimate the lifestyle changes that the patient will experience.

Perceived benefits: What will the patient do when he or she feels vulnerable, and what barriers exist that would prevent the patient from taking action? These barriers may relate to ability to pay for help, to availability of resources, or to problems in scheduling time for medical intervention (such as difficulty in taking time from work). The provider tends to set definitions of who should be consulted, when help should be sought, and what therapy should be recommended.

Modifying Factors

Modifying factors are areas of conflict between patient and health care provider.

CRITICAL THINKING CHALLENGES

Case Scenario

A 55-year-old Navajo man with hypertension is being evaluated for one of many routine clinical visits. As at each previous visit, his blood pressure remains elevated. He has been educated about high blood pressure, its cause, and its natural progression if left untreated. He is taught measures to control it, including nonpharmacologic measures, such as proper nutrition, moderate alcohol intake, exercise, and losing weight. He has not followed any of the advice, nor has he consistently taken his medication. He is being treated with two drugs.

Practitioners of Western medicine often disclose the risks associated with a disorder to motivate better patient compliance. Traditional Navajo culture believes that healing is a process of moving the patient from a negative state of illness or "imbalance" to a positive state of harmony and health. Negative thinking is regarded as deleterious. According to traditional Navajo beliefs, people acquire disease through a process of "witching." In this case, divulging the negative consequences of hypertension could be seen as witching.

The physician understands this, so how can he work effectively with this patient?

First, the physician must identify goals consistent with both the patient and himself. He learns from the patient by engaging others who know him, that he *does* want to stay healthy, exist in a harmonious way with nature, think in a positive and hopeful way, and live long enough to see his grandchildren's children. The physician identifies his own goals of minimizing the patient's risk of morbidity and mortality, convincing him to adhere to his prescribed treatment, and ensuring that he be informed about the purpose and importance of the treatments.

The second step leads the physician to determine mutually acceptable means to realize the goals of both the patient and the provider. Stating the goals in this situation shows that achieving health is a shared goal, but the understanding of how this will be achieved is different. The physician's means involve educating; the patient's is avoiding witching but thinking in positive and hopeful terms. One approach could consist of reframing the medical regimen in a way that focuses on the positive benefits that the patient will gain if he abides by the treatment. The physician might begin by affirming the goal that his patient stay healthy and by telling the patient that the medication will facilitate this mean. The physician could also make the case that this will further the patient's aim to see his grandchildren's children. The goals of motivation and education are reached in a manner that is more compatible with the patient's traditional belief system.

Demographic variables: Race and ethnicity are often cited as variables when the provider and consumer are from differing backgrounds. Here, the individual's perceptions of health and illness must be clarified.

Sociopsychological variables: These include social class, peer group, and reference group pressures that vary between the provider and patient. Traditional beliefs regarding how illness is cared for may differ from the health care provider's "modern" approaches.

Structural variables: These apply when different terms are used to explain the problem. The consequence of this is poor communication, in which neither participant truly understands the other.

In order not to impose foreign values on either patient or provider, both parties should refrain from assuming that their own ethical standards and cultural traditions represent universally valid truths. One foundation that should always be upheld is the premise that diverse cultures possess worth and dignity. By deliberating fairly with representation from both viewpoints, further information should be revealed about the patient's and provider's cultures and way of life. The specific details of the case then guide the process toward a resolution.

DEALING WITH THE ELDERLY

> Though we have begun to examine the socially taboo subjects of dying and death, we have leaped over that long period of time preceding death known as old age.
> Robert Butler

Life expectancy is rising along with an increase in our aging population. One hundred years ago, 2.4 million Americans were older than 65 years—less than 4% of the population. Today, that number has risen to over 30 million people, or 12% of the population according to the Census Bureau. These figures have stimulated much speculation and research, not to mention an economy based on services directed at meeting needs specific to aging.

Our culture comprises many viewpoints on aging that lead to inappropriate expectations and patronizing care. In a culture that is obsessed with youth, old age is too often seen as a pathologic clinical problem with physical and mental suffering. Many people reaching this time of life slide into these expectations, feeling disenfranchised, with a loss of power and social value. A more cultivated awareness would honor old age as a time for individual growth through service, for renewal, and for spiritual growth.[10]

Gerontology, the study of aging, is challenging dysfunctional myths and providing information about the physiologic realities of the aging body. This information offers much-needed emotional support for our aging population. Gerontologists no longer regard physical deterioration as an inevitable part of growing older, "but the result

of a sedentary lifestyle reinforced by aging stereotypes that condition us to expect physical and mental decline in our later years."[11] The health care practitioner encounters these stereotypes daily. Once again, the challenge is to draw back before reacting and reaching conclusions.

As home care continues to grow (see Chap. 18), health care providers are asked to help make the transition from "acute care" to the home less traumatic for the patient and family. This begins with educating patients from the moment they enter the hospital, which requires knowing what resources are available and what written information is available in nonmedical language.

Moving to a model of participatory care, away from dependency, requires teaching simple care, such as grooming, as well as more complex skills, such as cleaning tracheostomy tubes. It helps to remember your own process of learning as you provide information to others.

In *Having Our Say: The Delany Sisters' First 100 Years,* one sister, at the age of 100, states, "I'd say one of the most important qualities to have is the ability to create joy in your life. Of course, at my age, it's a joy even to be breathing! Sometimes I joke with Sadie [her sister], 'I sure am lucky that I'm so good at the things I enjoy the most, eating, sleeping and talking!'"[12] We need to discover what brings joy to our patients and what motivates them to stay healthy and participate in life.

Restoration of health provides patients with the ability to bring joy back into their lives. Sharing creates an environment in which the older person is not a useless member, but a storyteller with wisdom and insights precious to us all. It also provides insights for you when you seek motivating behavior and interests that will help ensure your patient's cooperation with rehabilitation programs. When you take the time to explore the interests of your elderly patients, you will find some of the reasons that you sought to be a caregiver. You also will gain insight into your own process of aging and a deeper understanding of others who are aging around you.

"Old age is neither inherently miserable nor inheritably sublime, like every stage of life it has problems, joy, fears and potentials."[13] The old must clarify and find use for what they have attained in a lifetime of learning and adapting; they must conserve strength and resources when necessary and adjust creatively to those changes and losses that occur as part of the aging experience. The elderly have the capacity for human reflection and observation that only comes from having lived a long time. For too many of our elderly, poverty or the insensitivity and ignorance of our society make the aging process unnecessarily painful, humiliating, debilitating, and isolating. A classic example is portrayed in the accompanying case scenario.

The older get sick more often and more severely than the young. It is estimated that about 86% have chronic health problems. Medicare and Medicaid pay less than half of the elderly's medical expenses, and a serious illness can lead to instant poverty. Too often, elderly patients afflicted with

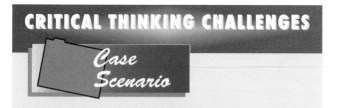

CRITICAL THINKING CHALLENGES

Case Scenario

Seventy-three year old Emil Pines was picked up by the police wandering along Market Street in San Francisco. He was mentally confused and unable to remember his name and address. After a medical examination, it was determined that he had not eaten for several days and was dehydrated. Food and liquids were prescribed immediately, and shortly therefore, Emil's mind cleared. He remembered that he had used his pension check to pay for emergency house repairs and had not enough left for food that month.

treatable conditions are diagnosed as senile and sent to institutions for the rest of their lives. Older women fare worse then men in these situations because their average life expectancy is 7 years longer than that of men. They often end up widows, with income levels gravely inadequate for meeting basic living needs.

In addition to dealing with the problems of physical and economic hardship, the elderly are affected by stereotypic myths that are based on fear and prejudice rather than on insight and knowledge. Determining a patient's abilities based on chronologic aging is inappropriate. There are great differences in the rates of physiologic, chronologic, psychological, and social aging within each person and from person to person.[13] Older people actually become more different rather than more alike with advancing age. Experience with elderly patients will reveal many "young" 80-year-olds as well as "old" 80-year-olds.

Many believe that the elderly are unproductive, yet history points to many people who have remained active and involved in life well beyond the age of 65. Considerable numbers of people become creative for the first time in old age. It is extremely important to remember that the elderly patients you care for are probably very able to help plan as well as participate in their health care.

Forgetfulness, confusion, and reduced attention span are widely accepted as part of the normal process of aging. The term *senility* is an overused and is a highly stigmatizing label. Some behavior categorized as senile is the result of brain damage, but more often it is not. Depression and anxiety are often viewed as regressive signs, pointing to declining mental abilities. Yet with the challenges presented in old age, it is easy to forget that depression and anxiety are an appropriate emotional response and that the patient is still capable of a full range of other emotions.

Drug tranquilization is often misdiagnosed, and its correction can reverse so-called senility. Malnutrition and unrecognized physical illnesses, such as congestive heart failure, may produce senile-like behavior by reducing the supply of blood, oxygen, and food to the brain. Depression, anxiety, psychosomatic illnesses, paranoia, and irritability are some of the internal reactions to external stresses. All these emotional states manifest themselves in many forms, including rigid patterns of thinking, helplessness, manipulative behavior, and often anger and rage. Again, the challenge is to see beyond the stereotype and to pursue detailed information about your patient. Often, the elderly person you care for will be more prejudiced against aging than you are. Older people are not always victims, passive and controlled by their environment; they too initiate direct actions and stimulate responses. Manipulation by older people is best recognized for what it is, a valuable clue that there is energy available that should be redirected toward greater benefit for themselves and others. The problem arises when this good feeling is called "youth" rather than "health," thus tying it to chronologic age instead of to physical and mental well-being.[13]

The increasing **medicalization** (the process by which problems and behaviors become reinterpreted as illnesses) of both normal and deviant behavior is finally receiving considerable attention. Caring appropriately for elderly patients entails clarifying the complex, interconnected elements of our communities that support physical and mental health up to the very end of life. Offering dignity in health care requires looking closely at the health care system's preoccupation with "curing" all illnesses. Life is a continuing process from birth until death, and it seems strange that it so seldom occurs to us to study life as a whole.

DEATH AND DYING

Health care providers are often naive about the harsh realities of health care. There is still too much fragmentation and lack of continuity between the hospital and the home. Too often, people leave the decision about their last days alive to those who know them the least. The only way we can hope to bridge this gap is by trying to understand the community we serve and by being more sensitive to the unique challenges confronting us. This section explores death and dying in an attempt to help the practitioner provide paths for the patient to make decisions and participate in this final passage.

The discussion of how a patient wishes to die, which may include choosing among several possible scenarios, should be undertaken long before the patient's last week of life. Too often, death is seen as a disease to be conquered, and the subject is denied by a society that focuses on progressing forward and remaining youthful. A patient's final days are often left to the hospital to arrange. Families and loved ones spend time during visiting hours, then wait at home for a call to tell them it's over. But the fact remains that we all die, it's only a matter of time. Death and dying should be embraced as a natural and honorary passage of one's life.

"Growing is the human way of living, and death is the final stage in the development of human beings."[13] The challenge facing us as health care workers is not only to become aware of our own feelings and emotional reactions to death but also to stop and relate those feelings to the people we are serving during the final stage of living. The crisis of dying can be met in a dignified way by striving to open channels of communication between patients and those who care for them.

Kübler-Ross divided the experience of dying into five stages:[14]

1. Denial ("No, not me . . . .")
2. Rage and anger ("Why me?")
3. Bargaining ("Yes me, but . . . .")
4. Depression ("Yes me.")
5. Acceptance ("My time is very close, and it's all right.")

These stages are helpful but not absolute. People do not necessarily follow this order or experience each stage. Further information on death and dying and on stages of dying developed by other researchers is available and should be consulted. Kübler-Ross was one of the first pioneers in the study of death and dying, and her stages have remained extremely useful in understanding the dying person's emotional state.

Working with a dying patient can leave you wondering about your own mortality. A psychiatrist at a hospital I once worked at told us, "People outside health care experience death only a few times during their life; you will face it weekly, and it will often lead you to question your own life and its importance." Don't underestimate its effect on you or distance yourself from all the emotions it will bring. The following story is an extreme example of what can result from neglecting this experience.

The setting of the hospital and the relationship between hospital workers and dying patients has been the subject of many publications. The comments and criticism often highlight the persistence of human vulnerability despite technologic advances. Those of us who enter the health care

CRITICAL THINKING CHALLENGES

Case Scenario

I finished a night shift and went to the reporting area, where the next-shift therapist would be waiting for the day's assignment. I was early, and I found a man, the therapist who was scheduled to work that day, sitting alone, clearly agitated, and looking like he had spent the whole night awake. His appearance was unkempt, and he had not bothered to shave or comb his hair. As he fidgeted in his chair and mumbled phrases I could not understand, I attempted to communicate with him. He was unable to communicate clearly, and I found most of his comments inappropriate and lacking any clear meaning. When the day-shift supervisor arrived, she proceeded to make the assignments while the phone began to ring and the environment began to change from a quiet one to a chaotic, frantic one. The morning was unveiling on a potentially busy shift. Consequently, this man was overlooked. People were too busy to notice or try to evaluate his behavior. Finally, when he began to make louder and more bizarre comments, a few of us took him aside. He then began to say, "I didn't kill him." Fortunately, at this hospital, there was a psychiatric unit, and the physician I called was compassionate and asked to see him right away. As I walked him over to the unit, which took about 10 minutes, he began to speak more clearly and to talk about a cardiac resuscitation that had occurred about a week before. The patient he was referring to had been a long-time resident of the ICU and before that had several stays on the medical floors for treatment involving a chronic lung condition. He was well known and loved by most of the staff. During his final days in the ICU, it was clear that this patient was never going to go home and

was never going to survive without the mechanical ventilator. Yet little discussion had formally occurred between all the different health care specialists who had taken care of him during the past couple of years. There was no consensus about how to proceed realistically with his care. Most staff felt extremely frustrated and helpless about what they were doing. On the day that the patient's heart arrested, a full code issued. The resuscitation bag that the therapist used temporarily disconnected from the piece that attached directly to the patient's tracheostomy. While the therapist frantically sought to find the piece to reconnect it, a physician "called the code." This means that all resuscitation efforts were to end and the patient was pronounced dead. The other members, without pausing, started to clean the patient area and remove all evidence of life support. It was done in a silent and methodical way. No one expressed sadness or relief but quickly moved to clear the area and prepare the patient for transfer to the morgue. The therapist was left feeling extremely guilty about the patient's death, although no one accused or asked about the faulty equipment. The therapist silently went on to care for his other patients and continued to stay on schedule with his busy assignment. There would be no formal discussion about this code, and no one made an attempt to say any words of respect to this patient that the staff had cared for during a 5-year period.

On the day that the therapist broke down, he was admitted to the psychiatric hospital on a residential status, where he stayed for 2 weeks. He never returned to hospital work again.

profession to help people recover from illness are often left, within the context of the hospital culture, with a feeling of failure when our patient dies, and with a desire to search for anything that could have been done to prevent that death. As the previous case scenario showed, an inability to face the inevitability of death leaves some with a haunting belief that it was a mistake and that someone should bear the burden of blame. This does not mean that mistakes are always acceptable, but only illustrates the damage done to the whole process of care by avoiding meaningful discussions about feelings and actions that occur during this process.

How can we bridge the gap between technology and emotion and avoid isolation of these ideally complementary facets of patient care? How do we broaden the role of professional behavior to include a genuine concern not only for the patient but also for ourselves as human beings? Let's draw from the earlier discussion of communication and diversity to add the human condition of vulnerability. The reality is that of an institutional culture that often makes people wholly dependent on strangers for critical decisions and appropriate care. The human resources within the institution are already burdened with so many responsibilities that often a patient's anger is perceived as violating acceptable behavior and may lead to further neglect. The role of mentor, counselor, and friend is transprofessional; no one member of the health care team is always going to be the appropriate one to handle each situation. By better communication and use of the team approach, however, those best suited to supporting the dying patient and the grieving health care worker can be sought and engaged. When caring for people is seen as a privilege unique to all involved, the need to commit to ongoing communication and discussion of everyone's role and feelings, case by case, will be understood.

My experience in working with terminally ill people has been neither morbid nor debilitating but rather the richest of all my memories. At times, it meant allowing the process of grief to dictate my mood and to slow my activity for a while. To participate with one experiencing this final passage is truly an honor and an invitation for personal growth. In an early work, Sudnow distinguished between two ways of looking at death. There are those deaths that are expected and those that could not have been predicted. The following scenario from his book, *Passing On,* shows how staff on a busy ward where death is common deal with severely ill patients and death.[15]

This case reveals a need to routinize and organize activities. The exchange does not reveal to what degree the staff were involved with the patients or what they did to protect themselves, but it gives a clear sense that death is a routine part of these people's work.

A death on the obstetric ward, where deaths normally do not occur, is a very different experience. When an unexpected death occurs rapidly, there is often confusion and anxiety. This can be further complicated by the venting of frustration through angry, accusatory words. When there is no commitment to discussing the event, team members

CRITICAL THINKING CHALLENGES
Case Scenario

A: Hi Sue, bet you're ready to go home.
B: You ain't just kiddin'—it's been a busy one.
A: What's new?
B: Nothin' much. Oh yes, Mrs. Wilkins, poor soul, died this morning.
A: I didn't think she'd make it that long. Do we have a full house?
B: I think so, let me see (looks at the charts). Guess so (turns to other nurse). Did Mrs. Jones die today?
A: She was dead before I got into work this morning, must have died during the night.
B: Poor dear. I hardly knew her, but she looked like such a nice old lady.
A: You look tired.
B: I am. Lucky you, it's all yours.
A: I hope it's a quiet night. I'm not too enthusiastic.
B: They all died during the day today, lucky us, so you'll probably have it nice and easy.
A: So I saw. Looks like three, four, and five are empty.
B: Can you believe it, we had five deaths in the last 12 hours.
A: How lovely.
B: Well, see you tomorrow night. Have fun.

leave who feel they are to blame, and trust is diminished among those who participated in the resuscitative efforts.

We have to believe that our ability to advance technology would also enable us to meet the challenge of adequately addressing needs of people in these stressful situations. Respect for all human beings begins by turning from procedure-oriented care to patient-oriented care. The therapist in the previous scenario was providing procedure-oriented care, often referred to as "factory health care." The concept of human beings as precious resources is lost in both the giving and receiving.

Let's look at the current model of managed care to see how it "strips" the patient's identity, autonomy, status, and role. On admittance to the hospital, the patient first sheds his or her personal clothes in exchange for a hospital gown. The ritual continues as the patient is given separate sterile plastic pans to wash, brush, expectorate, and urinate into. Often unable to form relationships with other patients, the patient becomes dependent on the staff to meet all of his or her needs. To cope with this, many patients determine which behaviors are rewarded and which isolate them further. The call button is the link between responsive care and fulfillment of needs. When patients are discouraged from participating in simple things, such as taking their own medication, this call button or lifeline becomes even more imperative and anxiety producing. Psychological literature indicates that illness frequently is accompanied by regressive behavior. The ritual of separation can only exacerbate this tendency.

Dealing with a child with a terminal disease presents another set of challenges. Although it is seen as an outrage any time we lose a loved one, somehow the death of a child seems more tragic and an even greater waste. How do we encourage communication and engage the dying child with dignity and honesty? Adults often think they are concealing the truth about imminent death from the child, only to learn later that the child had communicated the true reality to someone else. Some children are not mature enough to cope with information about their state of health, but others are. Because discussing the subject in their presence is often forbidden, they resort to symbolic and often nonverbal language.[14] An example is the story of an 8-year-old boy with an inoperable brain tumor who was very frightened of death. When given crayons and paper in a counseling session, he drew a picture of a huge tank with a small boy holding a stop sign in front of its barrel. The tank signified death, the destructive and unstoppable force, and the boy with the stop sign signified his fruitless attempts to halt it. The counselor drew another picture similar to his but with a larger boy standing next to the small boy. The larger boy had his hand on the smaller boy's shoulder. After more counseling sessions, the 8-year-old was able to come to terms with his impending death. He drew, in black crayon, a large bird with a small touch of bright yellow on one of its wings. He described it as "a bird of peace flying up to the sky with a little bit of sunshine on my wing." It was the last picture the boy drew, and he died shortly thereafter.

When a child is terminally ill, the emotional strain on the family is tremendous. The family may go through Kübler-Ross's five stages of dying: denial, anger, bargaining, depression, and acceptance. The discussion with a child about a fatal disease can be an extremely difficult ordeal. Whether such discussions should take place at all is a matter of individual choice. But again, communication between the family and health care team must be open. When a child asks a question, it should be answered in a way that he or she can understand. Dr. Stanford Friedman of the University of Rochester suggests that when a child asks, "What do I have?" he or she may be trying to find out whether doctors and parents are available and in control of the situation. Dr. Friedman advises, "A simple explanation, such as you are having trouble with your blood, may suffice with the younger child, but then he should be assured that medicine is available when he or she is uncomfortable, that his or her parents can easily reach the doctor, and that his or her problem is understood and being treated."

THE LIVING WILL AND POWER OF ATTORNEY

In a time in which ethical dilemmas are seriously discussed and legal liabilities acknowledged, we need to seek resources that will help patients receive care appropriate to their values and that will decrease their vulnerability.

The living will and the durable power of attorney for health care can address the issue of personal preference. They can enhance the autonomy of the patient and can clarify for the health care team, family, and loved ones the patient's values and what decisions should be carried out when the patient is debilitated. This information gathering is the goal of **advance directives**—the identification of the value-based preferences of the patient before the time when the patient is no longer able to speak for himself or herself. **Value history** is another term used for identifying an instrument that allows a systematic evaluation of advance health care decisions. In 1990, Medicare and Medicaid mandated The Patient Self-Determination Act to provide information about patient's right to refuse medical therapy.

The **living will** documents the decision to withhold or withdraw mechanical and other artificial means of health care when the patient is terminally ill and is no longer able to make decisions regarding such intervention. It's strength is that it is a written declaration conveying treatment refusal to the health care team. The instrument cannot be challenged by third parties so long as it has been executed according to the mandates defined in the state in which the patient is receiving care. It's shortcoming is a vagueness regarding what medical procedures should be refused, which can lead to misinterpretation on either too broad or too narrow a basis.

The **durable power of attorney** for health care legally empowers an agent to make health care decisions for a person when that patient is incapacitated. *Durable* is the key term, stipulating an appointed agent who then becomes a surrogate decision maker when the patient has lost decision-making powers. In contrast to the living will, the patient does not have to be terminally ill for the durable power of attorney to take effect. The designated agent considers the medical options available to the patient that closely adhere to previously stated or written preferences. The durable power of attorney allows a more precise adherence to the patient's preferences than the living will by reducing vagueness and enhancing flexibility.

The most publicized "death with dignity" case in the recent past centered around Karen Ann Quinlan. In 1975, Karen lapsed into a coma and was kept alive thereafter by a mechanical ventilator. When her parents signed a form authorizing the attending physician to turn the machine off, the medical authorities refused. The Quinlans went to court and petitioned for the right to make Karen's father the legal guardian so that he could give the order to have the respirator turned off. Again, the courts refused. Almost a year, later the New Jersey Supreme Court unanimously ruled that the mechanical ventilator might be disconnected if Karen's attending physicians and a panel of hospital officials agreed that there was "no reasonable possibility" she would recover. The court also ruled that there would be no civil or criminal liability if the mechanical ventilator was removed following the above-mentioned guidelines.

The decision to terminate a life is extremely difficult. The physician begins by evaluating his or her primary responsibility of minimizing the patient's risks of morbidity and mortality. By doing so, the physician may realize that he or she also subscribes to values other than the preservation of life and avoidance of harm; these may include respect for patient autonomy and self-determination. Western ethics pays homage to the idea that all people possess a right to liberty and to freedom from interference by outside parties. Evaluating these commitments in the context of each individual case may lead the physician to place greater weight on the value of freedom from outside interference. The physician does not sever his or her attachment to prior values, but rather casts these values in a different light by considering them in the context of other values that apply in this case.

Do the benefits of competent diagnosis and treatment from the physician's perspective fit into what the patient conceives of as a good quality of life? Understood in this light, the subject of medicine becomes the suffering patient and the direction of patient care does not necessarily require producing certain physiologic effects on the body but instead requires caring for the patient and producing outcomes that the patient appreciates.

Other subjects receiving media coverage today are organ donations and transplantations. More than 95% of the organs and tissues used to restore sight, functions, and life are obtained from less than 10% of our hospitals. Ethical considerations become a highly debated arena as we search for a fair way to match willing donors with potential recipients. The questions are difficult as we face the high cost of technology and make decisions about who should receive what care from limited resources. Can we determine in advance which patient will benefit from medical efforts and which will suffer more? Future research should help us to make better decisions in these areas.

TAKING CARE OF YOURSELF

The myth of the health care worker as having limitless, even "other-wordly," stamina and abilities is buried deep in our culture and is nurtured by the public, who generally yield personal responsibility for good health to the institution of medicine. As you strive to make health care an equal partnership, it helps to model healthy behavior. When working in a physically and mentally challenging environment, it helps to take care of yourself. Although a perfect state of mental and physical health is an unrealistic expectation, a sense of direction or movement toward increasing wellness is essential. When you are focused, disciplined, and flexible, it becomes more possible. This must begin with a respect for your own body. Learn to release emotional tension, clear the mind of clutter, and connect with your spiritual essence on a daily basis. Each of us has a unique belief and special idea of what this means. These qualities allow people with high ideals to maintain their visions without succumbing to stress, apathy, and organizational pressures. It has been documented that the health care field is filled with people who are overly concerned

with pleasing and helping others, often to their own detriment. In addition, institutions such as hospitals appear to generate addictive patterns, causing many health care professionals to get bogged down in the mire of bureaucracy and impassable expectations.[14,16]

Physiologically, we differ little from our ancestors, whose survival depended on quick, durable responses when aggressively pursued by hungry animals. The same adrenal glands that pumped their bodies with catecholamine hormones to support quick, durable responses supply our bodies with the same chemicals that make us ready to fight or run. Our stresses have changed, however, and our bodies are often left to deal with this surge of stimulating chemicals while remaining still. The effects of this stress on the body include feelings of restlessness, impatience, frustration, irritation, or anger; muscle tension; headaches; indigestion; and poor elimination. The more we ignore these compounding effects, however, the more likely it is that this chronic stress will lead to disease. How can we honestly advocate better health if we have chosen to ignore nature's signals ourselves? The only antidotes to stress are exercise, relaxation, and proper nutrition.

Psychoneuroimmunology, or the study of the connections among the body, mind (or psyche), nervous system, and immune system, is revealing new information about the interconnectedness of the body's systems. When viewed carefully, each individual system is influenced by the other and can be seen as one working system.

Your challenge is to reflect good health to your patients by truly paying attention and being committed to caring for yourself. Everyone is busy, but taking 10 minutes a day to reflect on your intentions and thoughtfully plan your day is an easy way to start. Whether or not you can actually see your plans through to completion, quietly reviewing what you hope to accomplish will help you stay focused and present in your day's activities. Too often, we never pay full attention to each task because we are already reviewing what we will be doing later or reliving some past event. Honest self-evaluation is also important. Be realistic when setting goals. Make sure the people and things in your life that matter the most, such as family, friends, and your good health are not neglected.

Another antidote to stress is to try participating in a meaningful ritual each morning, even if it requires getting up 15 minutes earlier. Start with a simple breathing exercise, and learn some positive aspects of proper breathing. Take a gentle, deep breath, pause, and then exhale slowly as you consciously let go of muscle tension and random thoughts. Repeat this 10 times each morning. As simplistic as this seems, it works well and costs nothing. You'll notice that it helps you view your day more calmly, instead of madly rushing out to conquer who knows what.

Stress is a fact of life, and we need to understand the effects of all the chemicals flooding our system each day and learn to minimize the damaging effects of overstimulation. In a recent study done at the University of Pittsburgh, investigators compared a group who performed several 10-

minute workouts a day with a group who averaged the same workout in just one daily session. More health benefits were seen in the group practicing in shorter sessions, and not surprisingly, these individuals were more apt to stick with their programs. See if there is place to walk or to do some easy exercises at work. Start a program for others who are interested, and find a space available at your work site. Find a place to park your car that allows a nice brisk 10- to 15-minute walk each way—that would be 30 minutes of exercise completed each work day. It will improve your outlook and endurance in this strenuous profession and world. At the end of each day, take a few minutes to restore yourself—what Judith Laster, a prominent physical therapist and yoga instructor, refers to as "taking a short holiday in your bedroom or living room."[17]

The next important step you could attempt is the creation of a support group at work; some ideas are groups for professional knowledge, emotional support, political reform, encouraging a healthy environment at work, or companionship during cardiovascular exercise. Patterns are created at work that are unique to that environment. These support groups can be nonthreatening if they do not impose absolutes but rather allow people to create helpful solutions. Sometimes, the problems you encounter are misunderstood by family and friends working in a different environment. Just as you train yourself to be a better clinician by carefully observing changes and then charting trends, you must do the same for yourself. The prize is a work experience that benefits the spirit as well as the pocketbook. Preservation of the soul means preservation of your humanity and sanity. I wish you the best in your new endeavor.

References

1. Starhawk. *Truth or Dare*. San Francisco: Harper-Collins; 1987.
2. Lind, SJ. Power from within: Feminism and the ethical decision making process in nursing. *Nursing Administration Quarterly.* Spring 1986; (11)1142–1149.
3. Jecker NS, Carrese JA, Perlman RA. *Caring for Patients in Cross Cultural Settings*. Hong Kong: Hasting Center Report, January and February 1995.
4. McKay, M et al. *Messages: The Communication Skills Book*. Oakland: New Harbinger; 1983.
5. Samhammer J, Larson K. *Interacting With Patients*. New York: Macmillan; 1963:7–37.
6. Christopher, R. *The Japanese Mind*. New York: Charles E. Tuttle; 1983.
7. Fisher R, Ury W. *Getting to Yes*. New York: Penguin; 1991:114–115.
8. Taylor G, Gaita R. *Integrity*. Proceeding of the Aristotelian Society. *American Journal of Ethics,* 1987.
9. Spector R. *Cultural Diversity in Health and Illness*. Norwalk, CT: Appleton & Lange; 1991.
10. Dass R. Be old now. *Yoga Journal*. October 1995; (24)66.
11. Schacter Z. *Age-Ing to Sage-Ing: A Profound New Vision of Growing Older*. New York: Warner Books; 1995.
12. Delany S, Delany A. *Having Our Say: The Delany Sisters' First 100 Years*. New York: Dell; 1994.
13. Butler R. *The Tragedy of Old Age in America*. New York: Harper & Row; 1975.
14. Kübler-Ross E. *On Death and Dying*. New York: Macmillan; 1974.
15. Sudnow D. *Passing On*. Englewood Cliffs, NJ: Prentice Hall; 1967.
16. Schiff AW, Fassel D. *The Addictive Organization*. San Francisco: Harper & Row; 1988.
17. Laster J. *Relax and Renew*. Berkeley: Rodmell Press; 1995.

Legal and Ethical Considerations

Michael Mahlmeister • John Bigler

Key Terms

agreement
assault
at-will employee
battery
breach of contract
causation
consideration
contract
damages
defamation
duty
false imprisonment
intentional tort
invasion of privacy
libel
malpractice
negligence
privilege
scope of practice
slander
specific performance
tort

Objectives

- Review the elements of professional negligence as they relate to respiratory care practitioners.

- Identify risk-reduction behaviors that respiratory care practitioners can engage in to reduce their risk of liability.

- Discuss issues of professional ethics in respiratory care.

The respiratory care practitioner (RCP) serves as a valuable member of the health care team, rendering diagnostic and therapeutic care and providing health maintenance and health promotion services. RCPs function along the entire continuum of care, from acute care to long-term skilled nursing facilities to home care. They may work as part of a cardiopulmonary department that staffs more than 100 RCPs or as a single practitioner in a rural hospital, physician office, clinic, or home care setting. Many RCPs provide technologically complex care using sophisticated equipment; others function autonomously in the outpatient clinic, physician office, or home. RCPs are employed as educators, researchers, business managers, administrators, consultants, and corporate officers.

Respiratory care is continually evolving to meet the demands of a changing patient population. The evolution of health care in America translates into an ever-changing scope of practice for the RCP. As health care delivery models change, RCPs find themselves continually modifying and expanding their roles and responsibilities. An important component of RCPs' preparation for practice in any health care delivery setting is an understanding of the legal and ethical issues attendant with the care they provide.

Awareness of the legal and ethical principles that govern legal liability in the health care setting can help the RCP minimize the risk of litigation and focus energy on patient support, healing, and health promotion. Understanding legal-ethical principles as they apply to an RCP's conduct also contributes towards enhancing the professional status of the RCP as a valuable member of the health care team.

Multiple factors influence the care provided by respiratory care practitioners. A major force shaping practice is new scientific information and evolving technologic and professional developments. This is well illustrated by the impact of the American Association for Respiratory Care (AARC) Clinical Practice Guidelines, introduced in the early 1990s, and of the National Institutes of Health (NIH) Asthma Guidelines, first published in 1991. These publications dramatically changed both the quality and quantity of care provided by RCPs because many respiratory care departments incorporated the scientific information contained in the AARC guidelines and NIH publication into departmental protocols of care. Standards, guidelines, and consensus statements promulgated by professional organizations such as the American College of Chest Physicians (ACCP) and American Thoracic Society (ATS) also contribute to shape the care rendered by RCPs. Federal and state laws, state licensure and title protection acts, and Joint Commission on Accreditation of Health Care Organizations (JCAHO) accreditation standards also impact on the professional actions of RCPs.

Respiratory care practitioners should be aware of potential legal and ethical problems inherent in their particular employment settings. Every ethical dilemma has legal ramifications, and every legal concern has ethical dimensions. The RCP's duty to patient, family, and colleagues requires

that they provide safe, appropriate care in a professional manner. Failure to do so places the RCP at risk of involvement in malpractice litigation. RCPs are expected to adhere to professional standards of care and to exercise professional judgment in all their interactions in the professional and clinical setting. The AARC Code of Ethics delineates the professional demeanor of an RCP. In those states with licensure or title protection for respiratory therapists, additional standards may define the professional conduct of RCPs.

PRINCIPLES OF LEGAL LIABILITY FOR THE RESPIRATORY CARE PRACTITIONER

A 1995 article estimated that 180,000 patients die each year as a result of negligence on the part of health care professionals. That is equivalent to *three* 747 jumbo-jet crashes every 2 days! Patients die because of medication errors, ventilator disconnection (unrecognized because no one reset the disconnect alarm after suctioning), and esophageal intubation undetected in a timely manner. When an RCP fails to meet the standard of care and a negative patient outcome occurs, the RCP is at risk of involvement in civil litigation and a claim of **negligence.** Although no RCP would want to provide substandard care deliberately or act in an unprofessional manner, the *potential* for practicing in a manner that contributes to patient injury or death exists every day. Failure to question inappropriate orders, failure to obtain a timely consultation when the patient deteriorates, and failure to follow established assess-and-treat protocols all represent potential opportunities for negative patient outcomes.

There is no doubt that errors such as the one described in the case scenario can be avoided and prevented. How can RCPs protect themselves from rendering substandard care or acting in an unprofessional manner that might lead to a claim of professional negligence? An understanding of the concepts of negligence and malpractice and of general health care law represents the first step. The adoption of risk-reduction behaviors represents a second step that can help ensure that an RCP meets and exceeds applicable standards of care. Box 2–1 lists a number of proactive risk-avoidance behaviors that should be adopted by all RCPs, irrespective of whether they work in an acute or subacute care setting, in a skilled nursing facility (SNF), or provide home care. Incorporating these behaviors into daily practice helps increase the likelihood of being viewed as a skilled, competent professional who provides acceptable and even superior care. Each of the proactive risk-avoidance behaviors listed in Box 2–1 is described in detail in this chapter after a discussion of the general concepts of malpractice law.

Contracts and Torts

Civil liability differs from criminal law in that, in a criminal case, the conduct is deemed so serious that the state steps in to prosecute the offending person. Civil cases are

CRITICAL THINKING CHALLENGES

Case Scenario

A 33-year-old woman with a history of asthma is seen by the RCP in the emergency room. Vital signs are as follows: heart rate, 102 beats/minute; respiratory rate, 22 breaths/minute; temperature, 98.4°F; breath sounds; inspiratory and expiratory wheezes. The RCP receives an order for a series of three MDI treatments given every 20 minutes with 4 puffs of abuterol. The patient is discharged about 90 minutes after entering the emergency room, with a lower heart rate and respiratory rate and fewer wheezes on auscultation. The patient states, "I feel a lot better, my chest doesn't feel as tight."

Three hours after discharge, the patient experiences a severe asthma attack at home and arrests. The emergency medical technicians resuscitate successfully, but she suffers significant anoxic brain damage and exists in a vegetative state.

Is there potential for a claim of negligence?

YES

Appropriate assessment was not performed to document: (1) severity of the asthma attack, (2) response to therapy, and (3) return to an acceptable discharge baseline.

According to the 1991 and 1997 National Institutes of Health Asthma Guidelines, patients presenting with an asthma attack should receive objective measurement of pulmonary function, such as FEV_1 or PEFR. If a lawsuit were initiated, the expert witnesses retained by attorneys on behalf of the patient (plaintiff) would state that the emergency room staff and facility failed to meet the standard of care in this case (ie, obtaining spirometry data).

It could be claimed that the RCP was negligent, even though he competently carried out the physician's MDI orders.

RCPs are expected to be knowledgeable about standards of care, serve as patient advocates, and question orders that do not conform to acceptable medical practice. An RCP has an independent duty to provide safe, appropriate care and does not merely carry out the orders of the physician. The RCP should have questioned the order and obtained spirometry data.

---

almost always brought by one private individual against another and fall into two general categories: contracts and torts. A **contract** is private law created by two or more people that governs a set of promises. If someone fails to perform as promised, they can be sued by the person who received less than expected under the contract. A lawsuit involving a contract is often called an action for **breach of contract**. **Torts** are civil wrongs committed by someone against the person or property of another.

Contracts

A contract can be defined as a promise or set of promises. If a party to the contract fails to meet the expectations of the contract, the law provides a remedy to the damaged party. Contracts can be written, oral, or implied by the circumstances of the people involved. For the contract to be enforced by a court, there must be an **agreement** by the parties and **consideration.** An agreement merely requires both parties to agree on the terms required by the contract. Consideration refers to the bargained-for exchange of promises. The consideration for an employment contract would be the payment of money in exchange for the employee's services to the employer.

INTERPRETATION OF CONTRACTS

When courts hear a dispute involving a written contract, often they do not allow oral testimony to supplement the agreement between the parties. Written contracts often contain a merger clause, which states that the written contract is the entire agreement between the parties and that no oral testimony, past negotiations, or subsequent oral modifications can be introduced to change the meaning of the written terms of the contract. Also, when one party has the benefit of drafting the contract, the court generally construes any ambiguity or uncertainties against the party who wrote the contract.

REMEDIES AND DAMAGES

When a party breaches a promise contained within a contract, the damaged party may either give the person an opportunity to correct the deficient performance or immediately sue for **damages.** If the contract provides for special or unique goods, the party may seek an order compelling the party in breach to fulfill the promises in the

---

Box • 2–1 PROACTIVE RISK-REDUCTION BEHAVIORS

- Know your scope of practice.
- Maintain current knowledge and competencies.
- Use chain of command.
- Operate equipment safely.
- Maintain rapport with patients and family members.
- Document completely and accurately.

contract. When the damaged party seeks a court order forcing a party to adhere to the promises contained within the contract, instead of requesting money damages, the remedy is called **specific performance.** Parties may fix the amount of damages in advance, and in the event they either party fails to live up to the terms of the agreement, they owe the amount specified in the contract. When terms of the contract provide for damages as a fixed amount, attorneys refer to these provisions as liquidated damages clauses. These clauses must provide for a reasonable amount of damages based on some logical relation to the damages actually incurred by the parties, otherwise the courts can conclude that the clause is a type of penalty and refuse to enforce it.

Torts

A tort is a type of wrongful behavior that is not based on a breach of contract. Tort liability is almost always based on fault. For example, in a negligence lawsuit, the person who seeks damages (the plaintiff) must prove that the other person (the defendant) was careless. In contrast, when a party fails to perform under the terms of a contract, the court usually imposes liability regardless of whether the party was capable of living up to the promises of the contract. Although the parties to a contract have the opportunity to define what constitutes failure to perform as promised, in a lawsuit for a tort, wrongful behavior is defined by the jury according to standards set by statutes, existing case law, and community standards. Torts fall into two general categories: intentional torts and negligence.

INTENTIONAL TORTS

Intentional torts in the respiratory care context stem from willful behavior by the RCP against the patient, family member, or professional colleague. Although relatively infrequent in health care litigation, intentional torts include assault and battery, false imprisonment, invasion of privacy, intentional infliction of emotional distress, and defamation.

Assault and Battery. Battery is defined as a harmful or offensive touching of another person. **Assault** is causing an apprehension of an immediate battery. In the patient care setting, battery typically occurs when an RCP fails to obtain the proper approval for a procedure or restrains a patient without proper legal authority. If the patient withholds approval and becomes apprehensive about the expected procedure, the practitioner could also be liable for assault. When a patient decides to sue the provider, the court looks at whether the RCP had the patient's consent to treatment, rather than at the ultimate result of the procedure. Thus, improving the patient's health would not excuse the offensive touching during the procedure to which the patient refused approval. An RCP who fails to obtain

approval from an alert, cooperative patient when obtaining an arterial blood sample or performing a mask continuous positive airway pressure (CPAP) treatment could be accused of assault and battery.

False Imprisonment. False imprisonment occurs when the defendant confines or restrains the plaintiff to a bounded area. The confinement must be intentional. In the respiratory care arena, false imprisonment could occur if the RCP restrained a patient without the proper legal authority. Hospitals have common law authority to restrain patients when they become disoriented. RCPs should avoid restraining alert and oriented patients unless there is an express written policy by the hospital conferring authority for the restraint.

Many federal and state statutes define circumstances under which restraints may and may not be used. For example, restraining patients merely because there are not enough staff to watch them *is illegal.* A medical necessity must exist for restraining any patient. The use of restraints is one of the most legally contentious areas. Any RCP working in an environment in which they are asked to apply restraints *must* know not only the facility's policy on use of restraints but also whether that policy complies with current state and federal statutes on restraint use. Ignorance is no defense.

Invasion of Privacy. The right to be free from interference with one's personal solitude is well established. An **invasion of privacy** occurs when a person's name, likeness, or private affairs are made public despite their objection or without their consent. An RCP could be found liable for invading a patient's privacy by disclosing information from the patient's medical record without the patient's consent. Some states provide immunity to hospitals so they may disclose minimal information about the patient to the general public, without the patient's consent, such as the patient's admission to the hospital and health status. A clear understanding of the laws in effect where an RCP practices can help clarify issues of invasion of privacy. Many states require health care professionals to report suspected child abuse, domestic violence, and communicable diseases to government entities; however, this does not confer on the RCP immunity for disclosing the same information to the public at large.

Intentional Infliction of Emotional Distress. When a person's intentional conduct becomes so outrageous that it leads to the emotional shock of another, the court compensates the plaintiff for his or her injuries. In the health care arena, this tort could occur if the RCP fails to treat patients and family members in a civilized fashion. Intentional infliction of emotional distress could occur when a provider insensitively exposes family to the body of the deceased patient or communicates that a patient had expired. Remember, the insensitivity must rise to the level of shocking the conscience of the community for the patient or family members to have a strong likelihood of recovering financial damages.

Defamation. A person's right to be free from attacks on his or her reputation is protected by the tort actions called **libel** and **slander.** Collectively, these actions are referred to as **defamation**. Libel is the injury to a person's reputation caused by the written word. Slander refers to an injury to a person's reputation caused by the spoken word. In the health care setting, defamation could occur from unauthorized or inaccurate release of the patient's information to third parties. The classic example concerns conversations between health care professionals overheard in the elevator or cafeteria by a third party. The defenses to defamation are consent, truth, or privilege.

A true statement, although damaging to one's reputation, is not defamatory because the injury to the reputation is caused by the actor, not the speaker. Informing another employee about an RCP who had been the object of a disciplinary proceeding by the state licensing board would not be defamatory because the damage to the RCPs reputation stemmed from the RCPs actions, not from a false statement by the speaker. **Privilege** falls into two categories: absolute privilege and qualified privilege. Speech and writings within legislative and judicial proceedings are examples of communications subject to absolute privilege, which means that even a false statement within those proceedings is not actionable. Reports of public proceedings are an example of qualified privilege; that is, false statements within the reports are excused, whereas inaccuracy in the reporting of statements is not excused.

DAMAGES IN INTENTIONAL TORT CASES

Because the provider's conduct is intentional, once the patient proves the underlying elements of the intentional tort, damages are presumed. Most states allow punitive damages to be awarded when the defendant's conduct is malicious. Intentional infliction of emotional distress, unlike most intentional torts, requires actual emotional injury for the plaintiff to recover financial damages. It is not necessary to prove *physical injuries* to recover financial damages. It is, however, necessary to establish severe emotional distress (ie, more than a reasonable person would be expected to endure without suffering some type of emotional distress).

Negligence

The most common cause of civil liability for health care providers is negligence. Used in its everyday sense, negligence means *carelessness.* Unlike intentional torts, the plaintiff must prove an actual injury to recover damages. For the plaintiff to establish liability for negligence, he or she must prove four elements: (1) duty, (2) breach, (3) causation, and (4) harm or injury. For a jury to conclude that a defendant was negligent, the defendant's conduct must

have created a risk of harm to another that outweighed the benefits to society created by the activity. Conduct becomes *unreasonable* when the risk of harm is greater than the potential benefits.

Malpractice

Malpractice is negligence applied to a defendant with a higher degree of knowledge, skill, or expertise than the average person. Physicians, attorneys, accountants, engineers, and respiratory care practitioners must perform with the same level of skill and learning commonly possessed by other members of their profession in good standing. Those whose conduct falls below that of other competent members of the profession run the risk of being sued for malpractice, should a negative patient outcome occur. Before the concept of malpractice can become meaningful, however, one needs to understand the elements of a negligence action. As mentioned earlier, four elements must be proved to establish negligent behavior.

Duty

Duty means there is a legal obligation requiring the defendant to conform his or her conduct to a standard, so as to avoid unreasonable risks to others. Another way to look at legal duty is to consider the relationship between the plaintiff (patient) and defendant (RCP). Based on the *relationship* between the parties, was the defendant's behavior reasonable? If there is no logical relationship between the plaintiff and defendant, it is likely that no duty will be imposed on the defendant. Typically, the scope of legal duty imposed depends on statutes, case law, community standards, contracts, and industry standards. Some duties touch virtually all society's citizens, such as the requirement of driving a car with reasonable care. Other duties apply only to specific people and entities. Duty rarely is a concern in an RCP malpractice case because of the context. For RCPs, a duty is imposed as a consequence of the RCP's professional relationship with the patient. As an RCP, expect a legal duty to be created based on your relationship with the patient.

When could a malpractice case turn on the element of duty? Suppose that a patient with chronic obstructive pulmonary disease experiencing respiratory distress obtains the name and telephone number of an RCP from a friend. The patient calls the RCP at home, and although the call was unsolicited, the RCP advises the patient to continue with his metered dose inhaler, rather than proceeding to the nearest emergency room for evaluation. Here, the duty that the RCP owes the patient is unclear. The RCP would argue that no patient–practitioner relationship existed and that, consequently, the RCP owes the patient no duty. On the other hand, the patient would argue that once the RCP accepted the responsibility of providing advice, the RCP must act as would other competent RCPs. Ultimately, liability would turn on the extent of the conversation and advice and whether any previous relationship existed between the parties.

Good Samaritan statutes advance the public policy of assisting others and turn on the concept of legal duty. At common law, there was no duty to assist a stranger in need; however, once a person stopped at an accident scene, courts began to impose the duty of reasonable care to ensure that Good Samaritans really are "good." Without such a duty, one could stop to "help" a stranger, provide grossly negligent care, and raise the lack of duty as a defense; for example, "Since, I wasn't *required* to help, it doesn't matter that I blew up the car with my lit cigarette." The courts imposed a duty to encourage careless people to keep driving. Unfortunately, the fear of liability caused careful people to keep on driving too. Many states thought the policy of imposing liability for negligent care on Good Samaritans was unjust. Consequently, state legislatures passed Good Samaritan statues, which exempt those who provide roadside assistance from a lawsuit as long as the care was merely negligent. Many states have also passed statutes exempting people who render basic cardiac life support from liability, provided they have attended an approved cardiopulmonary resuscitation course. Grossly negligent care is *not* excused under many Good Samaritan statutes.

Breach

A **breach** occurs when a defendant fails to conform his or her conduct to the standard of care. This aspect of the lawsuit can be thought of as carelessness. In a simple negligence case, the standard of care becomes how the reasonable person would act under a set of similar circumstances. The element of breach (whether a person's conduct fell below the standard of care) is usually one of the most heated issues in a malpractice case, for several reasons. First, there can be a dispute about which standard of care applies (see the discussion that follows on multi-skilling). Second, statutes enacted by the legislature directly impact the standard of care. When more than one statute, community standard, or hospital policy is relevant to the case at hand, considerable legal argument will be raised by both sides to ensure that the most favorable standard is the barometer for the standard of care. There will almost *always* be a dispute about whether the defendant met the standard of care. There may be extensive legal arguments, with both sides attempting to persuade the jury to adopt their version of the standard of care. The plaintiff's lawyer will argue for a higher standard of care; the defendant's lawyer will argue for a lower standard of care. Frequently, both sides will offer experts who will attempt to articulate the appropriate standard of care to the jury.

When a dispute ensues over whether the defendant met the standard of care, the medical record is often the deciding factor concerning the quality of care. Often a case waits 5 years or longer to proceed to trial. Consequently, what actually happened on a particular day will not be decided by what the RCP remembers about the case, but rather by those actions or events that were recorded accurately in the patient's chart. Because courts, and most importantly, juries, readily embrace the concept of fading memories, expect the following rule to apply: If the RCP fails to chart the procedure or observation, in the eyes of the jury, it *never occurred.* Consequently, the RCP should recognize the opportunity to reduce his or her liability significantly not only by delivering safe care but also by completely documenting that care in the patient's medical record. Strategies for creating a complete written record are developed later in this chapter.

STANDARD OF CARE FOR RESPIRATORY CARE PRACTITIONERS

In an RCP malpractice case, the standard of care reflects the RCP's higher degree of skill and expertise. The practitioner's acts or omissions are measured against that higher degree of skill possessed by the average RCP in good standing. A plaintiff's attorney will always seek to have the highest standard of care imposed on the health care professional. If successful, the attorney will force the jury to evaluate the acts of the medical professional against a heightened standard. Determining the applicable standard of care is always a question of fact (ie, the jury decides), as is the question of whether the defendant met, fell below, or exceeded the standard of care. Some examples of standards of care that apply to RCPs include conducting an Allen's test before performing radial artery puncture, setting a high pressure limit on a volume ventilator, and assessing breath sounds for tube placement after an endotracheal intubation. As mentioned previously, evolving scientific information and technology create a constant evolution of standards of care. Measurements of auto-PEEP, for example, did not exist before the discovery of this phenomenon in the late 1980s. Box 2–2 lists a number of sources from which standards of care are derived.

THE CONCEPT OF AFFIRMATIVE DUTY

The courts judge the actions of RCPs based on their own professional training and expertise, holding them accountable for patient outcomes to the extent that an action or a failure to act contributed to patient injury or death. The principle of affirmative duty goes beyond the concept of merely rendering care that does good. Affirmative duty mandates that an RCP act in a manner that *prevents patient harm.* This is the concept of patient advocacy. One of the founding principles on which Florence Nightingale established the profession of nursing was the concept of doing no harm.

Interactions with patients must occur in a manner that protects the patient by ensuring that the care they receive is in their best interest. Actions such as clarifying an illegible written order, contacting the physician when patient deterioration is seen, and requesting additional staff when patient care needs cannot be met all represent patient advocacy. Orders that are inappropriate (not only harmful but of no value) must be questioned. The Board of Regis-

Box • 2-2 STANDARDS OF CARE IN RESPIRATORY CARE PRACTITIONER MALPRACTICE ACTIONS

- Statutes and regulations
- National and state standards promoted by professional societies
- Hospital accreditation requirements
- Clinical practice guidelines or critical pathways
- Hospital policies and procedures
- Community standards
- Expert witness testimony
- Journal articles
- Books (learned treatises)
- Contracts

tered Nursing in California, for example, has language in their Practice Act that states that nurses must question, clarify, and change inappropriate orders. This implies communicating with the physician regarding orders and ultimately refusing to carry out those orders judged as potentially harmful to the patient. We believe that the same standard of care should apply to RCPs. Orders that are of no value or that are potentially harmful to the patient must be questioned, clarified, discussed, and changed.

The 1993 American Medical Association Code of Medical Ethics for physicians supports this concept of questioning orders. It states in part (you can substitute RCP for nurse) that:

> Where orders appear to the nurse to be in error or contrary to customary medical and nursing practice, the physician has an ethical obligation to hear the nurse's concern and explain those orders to the nurse involved. The ethical physician should neither expect or insist that nurses follow orders contrary to standards of good medical and nursing practice. In emergencies, when prompt action is necessary and the physician is not immediately available, a nurse may be justified in acting contrary to the physician's standing orders for the safety of the patient.

Concepts of professional scope of practice and affirmative duty contribute to an enhanced professional status for RCPs, but they also carry an added measure of legal liability if they are violated. All RCPs must recognize that their actions will be judged on the basis of their own profession's standards. The era of merely acting as a servant of the physician is gone and will never return.

MULTISKILLING AND STANDARDS OF CARE

Suppose a multiskilled RCP performs tasks traditionally within the nursing scope of practice, such as inserting an intravenous line. When an RCP inserts an intravenous line, should the standard of care be that of the skill, experience, and training of the reasonable registered nurse? When a

registered nurse undertakes the ventilator care of a critically ill patient, should the nurse's performance be measured against the specialized training that RCPs possess? These questions will remain unanswered until a consensus of legal opinion and case law has evolved; however, there is a strong public policy argument in favor of imputing the skill, experience, education, and training of RCPs when nurses undertake tasks included within traditional RCP scope of practice. Conversely, the same rationale applies when RCPs add duties traditionally included within the nursing scope of practice. Patients deserve to receive the same high standard of expertise no matter which licensed professional assumes responsibility for their care.

Hospitals and insurance companies argue for more control over employee job descriptions and less government regulation restricting employer choices to allocate tasks that cross traditional scope of practice. If the managed care providers enjoy increased flexibility in supplying the most cost-effective worker for a particular job, they should be held legally accountable for their choice. The alternative is asking patients and their families to shoulder the consequences of a choice based solely on economic factors. This may translate into receiving care rendered by health care providers cross-trained in-house with a minimal number of hours (to save the institution money) and with little or no assessment of bedside competency. Because juries may find this public policy argument persuasive, RCPs should be prepared to answer to the highest degree of skill and training that could be imputed to them, given the task they are performing and the category of professional that traditionally performed it. This concept is particularly important for RCPs who participate in patient-focused care models or other models that allow for an expanded scope of practice. It is not enough to rely on the minimal training the facility decides to provide to the RCP to perform new duties. RCPs must identify what constitutes an appropriate level of training to achieve competency and request that their employer provide that training. To do less compromises the quality of patient care and increases RCP legal liability.

To provide the best care and avoid liability, the RCP must ensure that services rendered to patients meet or exceed the highest applicable standard of care that could be imposed. Remember the general rule that the amount of training the RCP received is wholly irrelevant as evidence of adequate care. The determining factor is whether the care was discharged competently. Consequently, training that does not increase RCP competency but merely creates a paper trail of continuing education credits will not shield the RCP from liability. Simply stated, competent care is more important than the number of plaques, credentials, and CEU certificates on the RCP's wall.

Causation

The third element that must be established to support a claim of negligence is **causation.** After the plaintiff proves that the defendant behaved carelessly, he or she must prove

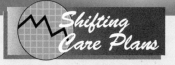

CRITICAL THINKING CHALLENGES

Shifting Care Plans

How does the RCP determine whether he or she is competent to perform a nontraditional task or is in possession of the requisite knowledge and skill to meet the standard of care? As a starting point, consider the policy and procedure (P&P) drafted by the employer for the particular task. Does the P&P call for skills and expertise typically rendered by RCPs? Was the training for the task consistent with that of other professionals previously responsible for the task? Is the P&P for the task similar to the P&P in other hospitals in the community? Has the RCP had an opportunity to execute the task competently under supervised conditions? If the answer to any of these questions is "no," the RCP should investigate further and request additional educational support and competency training.

that the defendant's behavior caused the injuries the plaintiff suffered. The plaintiff must prove two components to claim that the defendant caused the injuries: factual cause (the "but for" test) and legal cause (proximate cause).

FACTUAL CAUSE

The but for test is legal shorthand for saying, "but for the defendant's careless behavior, the plaintiff would not have been damaged." Consider the example presented next.

LEGAL CAUSE

In addition to being the factual cause of the plaintiff's injuries, the defendant's conduct must also be a proximate cause of the injury. Not all injuries factually caused by the defendant will be deemed to have been proximately caused by the defendant's acts. Proximate cause is a public policy that places a *limitation* on liability. Through the doctrine of proximate cause, society attempts to recognize those unique situations in which the relation between the harm and defendant's carelessness is so unexpected that it would be unfair to hold the defendant responsible for the injuries.

As an example, here are the facts from one of the most famous proximate cause cases in legal history: Plaintiff was standing on a platform of defendant's railroad after buying a ticket to go to Rockaway Beach. A train stopped at the station, bound for another place. Two men ran forward to catch it. One of the men reached the platform of the car without mishap, though the train was already moving. The other man, carrying a package, jumped aboard the car, but seemed unsteady as if about to fall. A guard on the car, who had held the door open, reached forward to help him in, and another guard on the platform pushed him from behind. In this act, the package was dislodged and fell on the rails. It was a package of small size, about 15 inches long, and was covered by a newspaper. In fact, it contained fireworks, but there was nothing in its appearance to give notice of its contents. When they fell, the fireworks exploded. The shock of the explosion threw down some scales at the other end of the platform, many feet away. The scales struck the plaintiff, causing injuries for which she sued. *(Palsgraf v. Long Island R.R. [1928]).*

CRITICAL THINKING CHALLENGES

Case Scenario

The plaintiff has just undergone 6 hours of thoracic surgery to have his aortic valve replaced. At 4:00 PM, he is admitted to the intensive care unit and placed on a mechanical ventilator. He remains stable until about 6:00 PM, when his blood pressure drops to 80/40 mmHg, and he has multiple premature ventricular contractions, resulting in cardiac arrest. A code blue is called, and two rounds of medications are administered. The plaintiff expires at 6:20 PM. Later, the resident who ordered the code medications realizes that he miscalculated and ordered 10 times the recommended dose of sodium bicarbonate. Several days later, the hospital pathologist performs an autopsy and opines that the cause of death was total cardiac failure secondary to an improperly sutured and dislodged aortic valve: *Question:* Is the resident who ordered 10 times the recommended dose of sodium bicarbonate negligent: *Answer:* Analyze the facts under the elements of negligence.

1. Did the resident owe a duty to the patient? Yes, a doctor–patient relationship exists between the resident and the plaintiff.

2. Did the resident fail to meet the standard of care? Yes, a reasonable physician with like skill, experience, and training would have administered the proper dose of sodium bicarbonate.

3. But for the resident administering 10 times the recommended dose of sodium bicarbonate, would the patient be alive? No, because the pathologist's report stated that the cause of death was the improperly sutured aortic valve.

Thus, even though the resident was careless, he is not negligent because his failure to order the correct dose of sodium bicarbonate was not the factual cause of the plaintiff's death.

The court found that the employee's acts rendered in an effort to help the passenger on the train were too far removed from the scales falling and injuring Mrs. Palsgraf. The outcome after the fireworks exploded was so unexpected that the court concluded it was against public policy to hold the defendant railroad responsible for Mrs. Palsgraf's injuries. Note that the factual cause of Mrs. Palsgraf's injuries was the railroad employees helping the passenger carrying fireworks on the train (*but for* the employees pushing the passenger on the train, the plaintiff would not have been injured). Thus, in this case, the court used the doctrine of proximate cause to place a limitation on the railroad's exposure to liability.

Injury or Harm

The final element in proving a case of negligence is that the plaintiff must show that he or she suffered actual damage. Further, in the usual negligence case, the plaintiff must show that he or she suffered some sort of physical injury or harm, for example, nerve damage from an improperly performed radial artery puncture. In addition, it has always been accepted that, when the defendant causes a physical impact to the plaintiff's person, the defendant is liable not only for the physical consequences of that impact but also for all of the emotional or mental suffering that flows naturally from it. The case scenario that follows is based on an actual malpractice case.

Patient Rapport

The "fifth element" in a negligence lawsuit, although not discussed in court, is finding a patient who wants to file a lawsuit. Why do patients sue? More important, are there recurring deficiencies in our patient relationships which increase patients' predisposition to sue if adverse events occur? Several studies have attempted to provide answers to these complex questions. One study reviewed 3787 pages of transcripts from plaintiffs' depositions in settled medical malpractice cases and identified faulty doctor–patient relationships in 71% of the cases. The primary relational deficiencies identified in the study were as follows:

Deserting the patient (32%)
Devaluing patient views (29%)
Delivering information poorly (26%)
Failing to understand the patient (13%)

The authors of this study concluded that a patient's decision to sue a physician is often driven by a perceived lack of caring or collaboration in the delivery of health care. Also, the investigators found that particular attention should be paid to the clinician–patient relationship after an adverse event has occurred.

Elevating the importance of patient relationships does more than encourage patients to reconsider the decision to sue. As healers, the quality of the care we provide turns on the relationships we share with our patients. We cannot ignore the patient and proclaim the role of care provider at

CRITICAL THINKING CHALLENGES

Case Scenario

The plaintiff is scheduled in surgery for a cardiac arterial bypass graft. At 6:00 AM, the plaintiff is taken to the operating room, scrubbed, and prepped for surgery. The anesthesiologist explains that she will be inducing the anesthesia by administering a combination of anesthesia gases and intravenous barbiturates. At about 7:30 AM, the plaintiff receives halothane and oxygen by mask. While under light anesthesia, the plaintiff is intubated and placed on mechanical ventilation. The anesthesiologist then administers a loading dose of vecuronium bromide and begins administration of the intravenous barbiturates. The surgery proceeds without incident. After the patient is extubated in the intensive care unit, he begins complaining that he was not under anesthesia during the operation. He begins to recall conversations that occurred between the surgeons and nursing staff during the surgery. (One conversation was particularly embarrassing to the chief thoracic surgeon, who queried the operating room staff as to why they thought the patient's attractive girlfriend was interested in such an "old guy."). As it turned out, the intravenous line that was infusing the barbiturates infiltrated, and no halothane was delivered by the anesthesia machine. Consequently, the patient received no anesthesia and no barbiturates. Since the intravenous line containing the vecuronium bromide was patent, the patient remained paralyzed but fully conscious for the entire surgery.

The plaintiff recovered fully from the operation and suffered no residual effects other than the memory of undergoing thoracic surgery without anesthesia. What are the plaintiff's damages? Clearly, there are no physical injuries for which the plaintiff can recover, but what about pain and suffering? Assuming the plaintiff can recover for pain and suffering, how much financial compensation should he recover for undergoing 6 hours of surgery with no anesthesia? Under normal circumstances, the amount of pain and suffering would be left to the discretion of the jury.

the same time. Managed care providers, insurance companies, and health maintenance organizations may exert pressure to minimize the importance of the relationship with the patient and look to the financial bottom line. Patients, however, expect a quality relationship with their health care providers. The study described earlier illustrates that if the RCP fails to meet the patient's relational expectations, there is a higher likelihood that the patient will bring lawsuit if there is an adverse event.

What can RCPs do to develop better relationships with their patients? Introduce yourself to the patient and his or her family with a first and last name. Explain your role and responsibilities in their care. Involve chronic pulmonary patients in their care by working to fine-tune the treatment regimen prescribed by the physician. Offer a beeper number or department telephone number where you can be reached if the patient or a family member has questions. Although most patients never call, simply making the offer demonstrates your openness and availability. Will following these simple guidelines guarantee that you won't be sued? Perhaps not, but fostering rapport with your patient will strengthen your relationship with that patient (and their family members). You probably *will* enhance the quality of the patient's health care experience. In the unlikely event that the patient does decide to sue, the patient will be forced to weigh losing their relationship with you against the possible financial gains from naming you in a malpractice lawsuit.

PROACTIVE RISK-AVOIDANCE BEHAVIORS

The concept of establishing patient rapport represents an example of a proactive risk-avoidance behavior. These behaviors constitute a set of guidelines for professional behavior, which if incorporated into practice, significantly reduce the likelihood of the RCP acting in a negligent manner. Health care providers who adopt these behaviors are more likely to be viewed as skilled, competent professionals by their patients, colleagues, and the legal system. Box 2–1 lists several of these risk-avoidance behaviors. Irrespective of a health care provider's employment setting, attention to these behaviors goes a long way toward reversing the downward trajectory of those jumbo jets discussed earlier in the chapter.

Know Your Scope of Practice and Standards of Care

Scope of practice refers to the range of care an RCP is authorized to perform within a particular employment setting. A state licensure or title protection act constitutes a primary legal document for defining an RCP's scope of practice. Federal and state health care regulations may also affect the *legal* scope of practice of an RCP. *Professional* scope of practice constitutes care that an RCP is trained and competent to perform, that is part of the job descrip-

tion as defined by the employer, and that meets guidelines and recommendations of professional societies and organizations. Box 2–3 lists sources that contribute to defining RCP scope of practice and standards of care.

Most states have passed licensure or title protection acts that contain language defining the scope of care that may be rendered by an RCP in that state. All RCPs should be aware of the content of their state's licensure or title protection acts. In an era of health care restructuring, scope of practice for many disciplines is continually redefined and challenged, and an awareness of current guidelines is essential. RCPs are legally bound to practice within the boundaries of their state's scope of practice guidelines. Failure to adhere to the legal scope of practice may result in a finding of negligence in a civil lawsuit, with attendant financial claims against the RCP. It may also lead to disciplinary action by the state licensing board, which has the power to impose fines or suspend or revoke an RCP's license to practice in that state. In some cases, the circumstances surrounding the act may lead to a ruling of criminal negligence and imprisonment! For example, nowhere in the California RCP Licensure Act does it say that an RCP can cut tissue. No amount of reading, observation, or training would legally allow an RCP to perform a tracheostomy!

Health care standards and laws promulgated by federal and state agencies further delineate care within the purview of an RCP. Aspects of care ranging from storage of cylinders to ECMO to patient confidentiality have standards associated with them. Organizations such as The National Institute of Occupational Safety and Health and the Centers for Disease Control and Prevention develop standards to which health care providers are accountable. It is a nationally established standard of care that gloves must be worn when obtaining a blood sample. Failure to adhere to that standard constitutes violation of federal law. This example would also logically represent a violation of your institutional and department policy and procedure on blood draws.

Professional factors further define an RCP's scope of practice and standard of care. The basic education and training one receives constitutes the foundation for one's professional care. An RCP never trained to perform an endotracheal intubation logically would avoid performing that procedure until proper training and competency development had occurred. A prerequisite for rendering safe, ap-

---

Box • 2–3 SCOPE OF PRACTICE SOURCES

- State licensure or title protection acts
- Federal and state standards
- Professional organization standards and guidelines
- Generic training
- Current competencies
- Job description

propriate care is that one possesses the *necessary, current* requisite skills and knowledge. Because respiratory care is a dynamic, evolving profession, RCPs must continually upgrade their knowledge and competency. It is not enough that one received training at some point of time in the distant past. Rather, RCPs are expected to continue to maintain their competency through periodic retraining programs and competency testing, adhering to the principle of adult lifelong learning.

In addition to training and competency, an RCP's job description may further restrict their scope of practice. A job description represents a statement from an employer concerning what an RCP can (and cannot do) at the site of employment. Rendering care outside of one's job description would constitute a violation of the employer–employee contract, compromising the RCP's credibility in the eyes of the jury. All RCPs should familiarize themselves with their job descriptions. This is particularly important for new employees, graduates, casual employees, and those who float between different work sites. The legal system will never accept the statement, "I didn't know that I wasn't allowed to do . . . at this SNF." As a professional, an RCP is expected to take the initiative to know his or her job description and job duties.

Guidelines from professional organizations serve as another consideration in defining standards of care. The AARC Clinical Practice Guidelines represent professionally established, scientifically based publications on a wide range of respiratory care procedures. Although they do not constitute standards to which one is legally bound, adhering to the recommendations contained in the guidelines significantly reduces an individual RCP's liability by (1) rendering care in a manner consistent with the best available scientific evidence, and (2) rendering care consistent with the guidelines set forth by one's own professional organization. In many cases, juries have adopted guidelines from professional societies as representative standards of care. RCPs who are cross-trained to other duties and responsibilities not commonly performed by RCPs (such as gavage feeding or chest tube insertion) should know of any existing standards of care promulgated for that procedure or duty, so that, at the least, they meet the usual and customary standards. RCPs should request appropriate supervised training and competency demonstration as well as documentation of that competency in their employee files. Once you undertake the task, you will be expected to meet the standard of care. Again, the legal system does not accept the answer, "They didn't have the (choose one: *time, money, personnel*) to train me in this task."

Document Completely and Accurately

As mentioned earlier, breach of the standard of care is the element of negligence most commonly found at the center of a malpractice lawsuit. Were established policies and

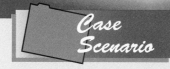

CRITICAL THINKING CHALLENGES
Case Scenario

You are working for a temporary agency (Registry) at a local hospital. On your first day there, you are called to the medical-surgical floor and asked to obtain an arterial blood gas (ABG) sample per physician order. You have done hundreds of arterial punctures in your career and perform them regularly at your other full-time job site. The licensure act in your state clearly includes ABG draws within your scope of practice. How would you proceed?

Ask the following questions:

1. What is the policy at the facility regarding RCPs performing blood draws?
   a. Training program and competency assessment requirements
   b. Authorization of registry staff to perform ABGs
   c. Duty of RCPs compared with those other staff to perform the blood draw

2. What is the location of the policy and procedure manual to help answer questions 1a to 1c?

3. What are the immediate needs and stability of the patient for whom ABGs were ordered, and what is the availability of other in-house staff to do the blood draw?

4. What policy does the Registry have regarding performance of blood draws.

This case scenario is a true story; it happened to one of the authors of this chapter! This RCP deferred the ABG to the house physician; had he performed the blood draw, he would have clearly been in violation of the department's written policy on what constituted institutional authorization for any RCP to perform a blood draw. If patient injury had occurred, there would have been major legal liability.

protocols followed? Was the patient assessed in an accurate, comprehensive manner, and was the proper care rendered in a timely, appropriate manner? Was the equipment operated safely, per the manufacturer's guidelines? What communication took place regarding the need for nursing or physician intervention?

Given that malpractice lawsuits may arise years after the actual events, the medical record becomes the central focus for determining whether the RCP met the standard of care. The entries in the medical record, or the lack of entries, represent the means by which one's care is evaluated. Thus, what is charted in the patient's medical record *today* is of critical importance *tomorrow,* when an attorney or expert

CRITICAL THINKING CHALLENGES

Case Scenario

Mary Doe is a licensed RCP in State X. She graduated from an Associate Degree program, where she was trained on a mannequin to perform oral intubations. Seven years later, she takes a position at Hospital B and is trained to serve on the code blue team and to perform oral intubations. She attends a code blue several weeks after training and performs an intubation. After intubation, she immediately assists with taping the endotracheal tube in place. Events occur as a result of improper tube placement and thus ineffective hand ventilation. The patient suffers another cardiac arrest and dies. The family sues, and attorneys note that "Respiratory Therapist Mary Doe" performed the intubation. They find no documentation that breath sounds were auscultated immediately after intubation, nor was there a measurement of end-tidal CO_2, which is a policy at this facility.

Is there potential for a claim of negligence?
YES

1. Multiple standards of care exist that clearly stipulate that breath sounds must be auscultated to confirm tube placement immediately after intubation.

2. This particular facility had a written policy of measuring CO_2 after intubation to help confirm tube placement. In deposition, it is unclear why CO_2 measurements were not done. This event occurred right at the change of shift, and there is some recollection by Mary Doe that she was paged during the intubation and that a colleague also came to relieve her (and receive report) at the end of the intubation.

Electronic Charting

Evolving information systems and data management programs are moving health care documentation practices toward electronic charting systems. Computerized, paperless charting presents several unique points of departure from traditional pen-on-paper charting. Electronic charting provides a real-time record of when an entry is made. In other words, if care was provided at 0800, and the electronic entry occurs at 1500, that 7-hour gap in time is documented electronically, for everyone to discover. Electronic charting commonly involves "menu" charting, which reduces the RCP's inclination to write a comprehensive freehand entry about an adverse event or unusual occurrence, finding, or action. Electronic charting may also place the RCP at (or absent from) the scene of the adverse event, for example, if the charting terminal and the time of charting conflict with the RCP's stated presence at the bedside. Security issues also arise related to the access others may have to an RCP's entry code or electronic device, confiden-

---

Box • 2–4 CHARTING RECOMMENDATIONS

The following are general tips for appropriate charting:

- Make sure your entries are *factual.* Describe events as they occurred, avoiding any subjective comments about the behaviors of others.
- Make sure your entries are *accurate.* List accurate times, events, dosages, personnel present, and the events in their proper chronologic sequence.
- Make sure your entries are *complete.* Provide sufficient assessment data and a full description of your actions, your communications, and the patient's status.
- Make sure your entries are *timely.* Engage in practice that involves charting immediately after the care was provided, or use appropriate mechanisms for entering a "late entry" into the medical record.
- Make sure your entries are *legible.* Illegible or sloppy charting fails to show that you rendered proper care. Sloppy charting equals sloppy care in the jurors' mind.
- Make sure your entries are *legal.* Avoid any documentation practice that falsifies the medical record, such as using white-out, modifying your original entry, or making untrue statements. Consult your superiors or your institution's risk manager if you are ever asked to falsify, omit, or alter an entry.
- Use proper mechanisms for documenting adverse events, such as incident reports.

---

witness (or jury) reads the account of the patient care rendered by the RCP. A common maxim is, "Chart your care with the jury in mind" (see Box 2–4 and the following case scenario).

Do make sure that you *always* take the time to document the care you provide, any adverse events, requests for assistance or support, and the status of your patient. A second common maxim states, "If it wasn't charted, it wasn't done." This is particularly important when adverse patient events occur or conflicts in the patient care plan arise. Remember, *the medical record is your best witness* in a lawsuit. Three particular areas of documentation bear special attention, given the evolving nature of health care delivery: electronic charting, charting protocol-driven care, and charting by exception (CBE).

CRITICAL THINKING CHALLENGES

Case Scenario

An RCP is assigned to work a 12-hour shift in the intensive care unit. A particular patient on ventilatory support develops a pneumothorax 1 hour before the end of the shift, arrests, and is not successfully resuscitated. On reviewing the medical record, it is noted that there is no documentation of auto–positive end-expiratory pressure (PEEP) measurements for the entire shift, although the department policy stipulated that they be done every 4 hours. Additionally, the ventilator record shows that peak pressures had been consistently rising over the past 24 hours and that the patient had become more agitated and tachypneic, with increased levels of sedation administered by nursing personnel. There was no entry by the RCP indicating any discussion with the medical staff concerning the rising pressures, increased agitation, and tachypnea.

Is there potential for a claim of negligence?

YES

The RCP failed to document auto-PEEP levels, as required by policy. Although the RCP claimed in deposition that they were obtained but not recorded (he was very busy that day), their absence on the ventilator flowsheet can be interpreted only in the following manner: *the RCP failed to follow policy and obtain auto-PEEP measurements every 4 hours.* The presence of a deteriorating condition, as demonstrated by rising peak pressures and tachypnea, represents assessment findings that merit communication, further assessment, and possible change in the care plan. The absence of any documentation by the RCP that the abnormal findings were discussed with a physician, and the care plan modified, implies that nothing was done for a deteriorating patient. The RCP may plead that he specifically remembers that particular patient (consider the fact that the case occurred 4 years ago!) and that he spent 15 minutes on the phone with intensive care unit staff trying to obtain order changes. The absence of any documentation of that conversation in the medical record implies *that conversation never took place.*

---

tiality of entries, and mechanisms for "read only" of past entries and for charting of "late entries."

Electronic charting can help promote complete charting when programs are used that require that certain fields of data be completed before the computer will accept the entry or upload the information. Electronic charting also standardizes entries, cuing RCPs to document comparable data with every patient. RCPs who work in an environment in which computerized charting is used should obtain complete orientation to the system. Finally, departments pursuing electronic charting must address the issue of timeliness with which electronic entries by the RCPs reach the paper medical record for access by other health care team members and for collaborative patient management. For example, even if, for 12 hours, the RCP electronically documents downward migration of an endotracheal tube, this information may be unavailable to the physician, who is trying to explain a deteriorating chest radiograph and clinical condition.

Charting Protocol-Driven Care

The growing use of therapist driven protocols (TDPs) presents several unique legal issues (see Bunch, 1994). In the area of documentation, protocol care requires RCPs to document decision-making processes clearly and to communicate any abnormal findings or reasons for deviating from established protocol algorithms. The use of written and verbal communication with nursing and medical staff will ensure that these individuals receive timely communication regarding the status of the patient. Failure to record all assessment findings and decision-making actions, as required in the protocol, increases the RCP's liability for failing to follow the established protocol should an adverse event occur and a lawsuit ensue. RCPs who provide protocol care must ensure that they receive proper training in the implementation of the protocols. Departments using protocol care should ensure that the protocols are scientifically based, formally approved within the organization, and consistently applied to all patients.

Charting By Exception

Charting by exception is relatively new to the respiratory care profession. Nurses have developed CBE systems over the years in response to studies showing that, in some situations, nurses spend more than 30% of their work time engaged in charting. As health care redesign and restructuring evolves, respiratory care professionals are beginning to look at ways to reduce charting time and duplication of documented patient data. One basic principle of CBE is the reduction of unnecessary charting. The definition of what is unnecessary, however, is elusive and institution specific. For example, is it necessary to chart peak flow, humidifier temperature setting, or ventilator mode with each every-4-hour patient and ventilator system check? What is deemed necessary charting at one facility, such as ventilator compressible volume loss, may not even be documented at another.

Each health care organization pursuing CBE policies needs to describe clearly how the system will work as well as the *what, when,* and *where* of documenting patient care information. Any RCP working in a CBE environment should receive a comprehensive orientation to CBE policies. CBE systems are not an excuse to engage in incomplete, sloppy documentation practices. Whenever an RCP is presented with a situation in which abnormalities exist or a potential or real adverse patient event occurs, the use of the usual CBE check box charting practice becomes inadequate. The rule should always be to default to complete, accurate, comprehensive freehand documentation when adverse events occur. This will ensure all parties involved (including attorneys) that you engaged in proper assessment, communication, and action in the best interest of the patient—that you adhered to the principles of affirmative duty and patient advocacy and met the standard of care.

Communicate by Chain of Command

One of the most common findings in medical malpractice litigation is an issue related to failed communication or lack of communication. In the old days of respiratory care, it was easy to know who to contact concerning a clinical problem. There were supervisors, managers, and biomedical and education staff available to provide the RCP with guidance. Health care redesign can lead to the elimination of middle management, departmental administration by non-RCP managers, and pursuit of unit-based care, all of which raise questions regarding chain of command.

Chain of command refers to that system by which an RCP has access to clinical and administrative resources available for information and conflict resolution. Resolving a situation in which an inappropriate order is received, additional help is needed, or a personnel conflict arises necessitates activation of the chain of command. All RCPs working today *must* know their chain of command. Who do they turn to for guidance and information? How do they activate the chain of command and document their efforts to seek support? Who is their expert clinical resource if the department manager is a nurse or lab manager? What are the names, telephone numbers, and beeper numbers of people in the chain of command 24 hours a day, 7 days a week? The legal system does not accept an attitude of helplessness. claiming in deposition, "I didn't know who to call," or "I was too busy to get help," or "No one told me how to use the beeper to contact the supervisor." As a health care professional, you are expected to know your chain of command for both clinical and departmental problems and to activate it in a timely manner to resolve problems. Again, the RCP is applying the principle of affirmative duty.

When activating the chain of command to resolve a problem, it is appropriate and necessary that you document those actions in the medical record. This will demonstrate clearly that you acted in a professional, timely manner when presented with a clinical or administrative problem, enhancing your legal accountability. When documenting a

CRITICAL THINKING CHALLENGES

Case Scenario

You arrive at the home of your new patient, an infant with bronchopulmonary dysplasia recently discharged from the hospital. The infant has tachypnea, bibasilar crackles, a few expiratory wheezes, and an SpO_2 that is 2% lower than it was at discharge. You attempt to contact your supervisor, who is unavailable. Your attempt to contact a particular physician at the discharge hospital is also unsuccessful. You note the abnormal findings in your record, tell the mother to keep an eye on her child, keep trying to call the doctor, and move on to the next patient. Four hours later, the infant is transported to the emergency room by emergency medical services, unconscious and intubated.

Is there potential for a claim of negligence?

YES

The RCP's duty to the patient (and family) does not end with placing phone calls. If there is a lack of response with the activation of the chain of command, the RCP must continue up the line of authority until the patient situation is resolved. Could the RCP have discussed the infant's status with a higher-level manager or supervisor at the home health agency, even if that person were not an RCP? In the situation described, the RCP had a duty to continue to attempt to communicate the abnormal findings until there was appropriate resolution of the problem. If that was not possible, the RCP should have called emergency medical services and ensured the transport of the patient to the hospital.

request for assistance, it is insufficient to merely write "doctor called" or "nurse notified"; rather, efforts should be made to document the elements listed in Box 2–5.

A variety of situations can arise that necessitate contacting a person of higher authority in the chain of command. You are serving as charge therapist, and one of your staff arrives at work reeking of alcohol. How do you proceed? You report to your critical care unit for shift report, only to inherit a new ventilator on a patient. You received no inservice on this machine and have never worked with it before. What should you do? While conducting a home visit of a new client, you note that the medical equipment is plugged into a nongrounded, multiplug outlet, which is all that is available in the house. What should you do? Box 2–6 lists common clinical situations that suggest a potential clinical or administrative problem. In all of these situations, the RCP should proceed according to the principles of affirmative duty and activate the chain of command.

Chain of command principles also apply to RCPs who find themselves in positions of authority or responsibility, such as serving as supervisor, charge, or lead therapist. An

---

Box • 2–5 DOCUMENTING A REQUEST FOR ASSISTANCE

Record...

- the exact time you called for assistance or help
- the name of the person you contacted, and his or her title if applicable
- what you have reported (clinical findings)
- what you are requesting
- their response
- the status of the patient (or situation) when you leave the bedside

---

RCP who accepts responsibility for serving as shift charge automatically inherits additional professional and legal accountability. Charge staff are often viewed by the legal system as expected to serve as the following:

- Expert resources in clinical operations
- Arbiters of disputes or conflicts between staff
- Experts in equipment and personnel triage
- Consultants for clinical problems

Respiratory care practitioners who accept charge should ensure that they receive a formal, documented orientation to charge duties and responsibilities. *Do not* accept charge responsibility unless you are competent to carry out the duties. Failure to do so places you at tremendous legal risk should any event occur that compromises the department's ability to provide safe, competent, timely care. The range of such events can run the gamut, from knowing where to get more computer printer paper to print charges, to renting a ventilator that is needed because of an increased census,

---

Box • 2–6 ACTIVATING THE CHAIN OF COMMAND

The chain of command should be activated in the following situations:

- Unexpected patient deterioration
- Inappropriate or unclear order
- Adverse response to medication or intervention
- Lack of desired response
- Significant changes in workload
- Potential for missed therapy
- Disagreements between health care providers about the patient's care plan
- Conflicts between staff and patient or family members
- Unprofessional or unethical conduct of coworkers
- Equipment performance problems

---

to implementing the disaster plan when an earthquake or tornado hits.

Operate Equipment Safely

The operation of equipment represents a major area of legal risk for the RCP. Most care rendered by RCPs involves the use of equipment, the complexity of which ranges from

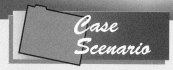

CRITICAL THINKING CHALLENGES

Case Scenario

You are house-charge RCP. A fellow RCP pages you to inform you that she is "swamped." She indicates that she will not be able to do a mask BiPAP treatment, which is due in 15 minutes, for at least 1 to 2 hours. Your response to her is: "Do the best you can, there is no one to help you. I have one nonclinical day a week, and I have to get next month's schedule." You return to completing next month's work schedule. The patient deteriorates, has a respiratory arrest, and suffers anoxic brain damage. After her call, the staff therapist wrote the following note in this patient's medical record: "Charge therapist J. Smith contacted regarding order to perform BiPAP treatment. Requested that he assign another RCP to complete 10:00 PM therapy."

Is there potential for a claim of negligence? Against whom?

YES

As charge RCP, you have a duty to ensure that patient care is not compromised. When a subordinate calls to ask for help, you have a professional and legal duty to do one or more of the following:

1. Determine the clinical needs

2. Activate the communication chain to obtain help

3. Assist directly yourself

4. Help the subordinate appropriately prioritize care

Charge and supervisory staff are responsible for the care provided by their subordinates to the extent that they are able to provide guidance and resources. Accountability for clinical operations moves up the chain of command to the charge RCP once that subordinate places a call asking for help.

If the charge RCP determines that the primary problem in this case is an employee who cannot adequately triage or prioritize patient needs, formal counseling or disciplinary action may be indicated. If the supervisor confirms that staffing is indeed inadequate, management's duty is to obtain qualified RCP staff to perform ordered therapy.

simple metered dose inhaler devices to sophisticated mechanical ventilators. The potential for improper use of equipment, with resultant patient injury, is extremely high. A review of case law regarding malpractice litigation involving RCPs showed that more than 70% of cases involved some element of equipment application. Safe, appropriate equipment operation requires three elements: knowledge about how the equipment works, competency in operating the equipment, and judgment in applying the equipment.

Knowledge concerning equipment operation requires that the RCP receive the necessary printed materials and didactic training in the proper equipment set-up, operation, and troubleshooting. Awareness of the operational specifications (and limitations) of a device is necessary to understanding under what circumstances the device should be implemented, how to monitor its operation, and how to know whether the device is operating properly. RCPs should ensure that comprehensive policies and procedures exist and that the manufacturer's product literature is available before accepting an assignment involving a piece of equipment for which they may be unfamiliar. No RCP should accept an assignment involving equipment for which they lack knowledge and training. Once again, if you accept a patient care assignment, you create a duty to meet the applicable standards of care.

Knowledge concerning equipment can come from a variety of sources. Professional journals, such as *Respiratory Care,* frequently publish articles describing equipment operation and clinical application. *ECRI* is an industry publication that presents articles on operational characteristics of respiratory equipment and product alerts. Manufacturers also serve as a source for product literature, product upgrades, and product alerts and recalls. The federal government has set up a system for reporting equipment malfunctions, called MEDWATCH. This is a voluntary reporting system by which clinicians can document and communicate equipment malfunction or failures that have the potential to cause or have caused patient harm. Through this system, potential flaws in equipment can be recognized, communicated, and corrected, reducing the risks to the public who depend on the medical equipment.

Competency refers not only to intellectual knowledge about equipment but also to possession of the psychomotor skills necessary to operate that equipment properly. Respiratory care equipment represents sophisticated technology, requiring that RCPs possess knowledge in physics, math, and computers. Clinicians must develop and maintain the skills needed to apply respiratory care devices in a manner that is safe and therapeutic. Every RCP should request hands-on training in the operation of complex monitoring and life support devices. The era of "learning" how to operate a ventilator by attending a 1-hour lecture in the respiratory care department is coming to an end. Equipment is so technologically complex that it is imperative that each RCP receive individualized hands-on training with the equipment before it is placed into clinical use. The legal risk is too great to do otherwise. New instructional models are evolving to help educate professionals. These include interactive audiovisual, three-dimensional, computer-assisted instruction and even virtual reality programs. The legal system does not accept the response, "They didn't give me the proper training to operate this equipment." As a professional, you are expected to possess the requisite knowledge and skills before accepting a patient care assignment involving equipment.

A second issue in the area of competency revolves around maintaining competency. It is recognized that technology is continually changing, as evidenced in the respiratory care profession by the frequent model and upgrade changes that occur in a particular manufacturer's ventilator. This change has led JCAHO and other organizations to require that health care providers undergo competency reassessment at periodic intervals to ensure that they are aware of the latest technologic developments and continue to possess the necessary skills to operate equipment. Respiratory care departments should establish formal schedules and programs to ensure that all staff maintain current skills in equipment operation and diagnostic and therapeutic interventions. Initial competency training and retraining should be formal, should be documented, and should find its way into the employee's file. This practice reduces the legal liability of the RCP as well as that of the department and institution or agency employing that RCP.

Judgment represents the third area that ensures that equipment is operated in a safe, therapeutic manner. A simplified version of judgment is often referred to as *common sense.* Clinical judgment, however, involves elements of knowledge, clinical experience, and critical thinking. Judgment is exercised when an RCP discontinues a ventilator that is displaying erratic readings or not operating properly. Judgment is exercised when an RCP refuses to use a monitoring device that has a frayed electrical cord or a cracked electrical plug. Judgment is exercised when an RCP chooses a particular device because it will provide the necessary support as dictated by the physician order or clinical protocol. A common question regarding equipment operation is, "Can judgment be taught?" The best that can be done is to provide the clinician with the necessary knowledge, skills, and resources on which to base clinical decisions. Engaging in simulated clinical scenarios that include troubleshooting problems can also help foster a better understanding of how RCPs engage in decision-making processes. Attention to these elements will minimize the risks of improper equipment operation leading to patient injury or death, involvement in a malpractice lawsuit, and a claim of negligence.

A second aspect of judgment that requires special discussion involves the modification of equipment, so that it is configured, operated, or applied in a manner that deviates from that stated in the manufacturer's product literature. The ability of RCPs to modify equipment is a double-edged sword. On the one hand, RCP creativity can produce a device or system that meets the immediate clinical needs. On the other hand, modification of equipment so that it performs differently from or in contrast to the manufacturer's specifications places considerable liability on the shoulders of the RCP and the respiratory care department. "Popping the hood" of the ventilator and adjusting its pneumatic or electronic controls so that it exceeds specifications is an invitation to a lawsuit. Combining adapters and one-way valves in a system that proves heavy, leading to an undetected endotracheal tube disconnect, likewise is a risk. Should any adverse patient event occur, leading to litigation, the manufacturer would claim that the device was being operated improperly and would argue for shifting the liability to the RCP, respiratory care department, and institution. Before modifying equipment so that it performs differently from what is described in the product literature, it would be prudent to consult with your superior.

The operation of equipment must occur in a manner that ensures the safety and well-being of patients and staff. Although emergency situations do arise that require the creative use of equipment, several questions must be asked before equipment is placed into clinical use. Is this necessary? What are the potential benefits? What are the potential risks? What resources are available to help guide me? Does it make sense to my colleagues? Can I demonstrate safe, appropriate use before actually applying it to the patient? Is my charge therapist (or supervisor) aware of my plan? Answering these questions will help guide the RCP and will contribute to reducing the legal risks related to equipment operation.

MANAGEMENT RESPONSIBILITIES AND THE LAW

In addition to ensuring that staff provide competent care, the respiratory care manager must exercise reasonable care when selecting, training, supervising, disciplining, and dismissing employees. Personnel who operate in the capacity of educator, supervisor, or charge therapist incur additional legal responsibilities related to their positions and duties within the health care delivery system. State licensure laws are in place to protect the public and ensure that duly licensed RCPs render safe, appropriate care. Managers who fail to meet this mandate when hiring, training, or supervising staff face the risk of involvement in malpractice litigation and disciplinary action by the licensing board if adverse events occur.

Selection

When respiratory care managers select employees, they must ensure that the employees meet the expectations of the department. Also, to protect hospital patients and staff, the manager must verify the RCP's license, credentials, and work experience listed on the job application. If the

state has a licensing board, the manager must verify that the RCP has a valid license and that the RCP is in good standing (eg, not on probation). If the RCP lists National Board for Respiratory Care credentials, they should be verified. Because it would be possible to create a fraudulent certificate, the manager is charged with a duty to investigate beyond relying on copies or purported actual certificates supplied by the prospective employee. Finally, the manager must contact the references and former employers listed on the RCP's job application or resumé to ensure that the RCP has represented his or her qualifications and work experience properly.

Training and Supervision

Managers must support employees with adequate supervision. The failure to exercise reasonable care in supervision could result in liability for both the manager, supervisor, and hospital. An employee who repeatedly fails to meet the standard of care or who engages in unprofessional conduct and is allowed to continue to work with patients would confer increased liability on the supervisor.

A continually expanding RCP scope of practice requires a training commitment from the hospital. If the new responsibility is a nontraditional task, the manager must ensure proper competency training of staff. The amount of training is not determinative as long as the training leads to competent care. Hallmarks to consider for proper training are whether the RCP has had an opportunity to execute the procedure under supervised conditions, whether RCPs generally are trained in school to perform the procedure, and whether the procedure is commonly performed in a similar fashion at other hospitals in the community. RCPs who engage in new clinical practices should request appropriate training from their superiors and ensure that documentation of that training is placed in their employee files.

Managers should check with the state licensing board for annual training requirements regarding continuing education. The manager should encourage staff to attend continuing education activities, but generally there is no requirement that the manager provide education units or compensate RCPs for attending such activities. Despite the lack of strict legal requirements for assistance with continuing education, however, the utility of providing in-house continuing education activities should be calculated in terms of the added value of employee development rather than merely strict legal requirements.

Disciplinary Actions and Termination of Employment

Usually, employees are considered **at-will employees**, meaning the employer may terminate the employee at any time, unless the employee's contract specifies a definite term, there is hospital policy to the contrary, or there is a state statute that provides requirements for termination.

Table • 2–1   EQUAL EMPLOYMENT OPPORTUNITY LAWS

Law	Provisions
Title VII of the Civil Rights Act of 1964	Prohibits unfair treatment based on race, color, religion, sex, national origin, or pregnancy
Equal Pay Act of 1963	Prohibits discriminatory compensation policies based on sex; requires equal pay for equal work, which it defines as work requiring equal skill, effort, and responsibility within similar work environments
Age Discrimination in Employment Act	Prohibits discriminatory treatment of persons 40 to 69 years of age for all employment-related purposes
Americans With Disabilities Act of 1991	Prohibits employment discrimination on the basis of physical and mental disabilities
Fair Labor Standard Act	Provides for minimum wages and maximum hours of employment
Federal Wage Garnishment Law	Garnishment is a means of enforcing a court judgment against another person by a court order to an employer to withhold a portion of the debtor's wages and forward said amount to the creditor until the debt is paid in full. This law and other state laws place limits on the maximum amounts that may be withheld. Limits on garnishment do not apply to some types of court orders, including child and spousal support.
Employee Retirement Income Security Act	This law governs nearly all pension plans for employees and applies to all employers except government agencies.

Most courts require employers to follow their own internal policies for disciplinary actions and terminations. Many states condition unemployment payments on termination by the employer without just cause. When an employer terminates an RCP for misconduct, the employee forfeits the right to receive unemployment payments. Consequently, in addition to making a complete personnel file to avoid litigation for wrongful termination, the employer must provide valid reasons for termination to limit their unemployment policy from paying an employee unemployment benefits.

Most employers have written policies for employee counseling and disciplinary action. RCPs who function in any position that involves responsibilities for corrective action and performance evaluation should be informed about all relevant policies. Management personnel must request proper training in all federal and state laws and statutes related to employment law. A basic knowledge of these laws will help managers, supervisors, and charge therapists avoid engaging in behaviors that could be interpreted as violations of the law, leading to employee grievance and or lawsuit (see the following case scenario). Table 2–1 illustrates several employment laws that should be familiar to any RCP who has a supervisory role.

ETHICS AND THE RESPIRATORY CARE PRACTITIONER

Webster's Dictionary defines ethical as "conforming to moral standards," "conforming to the standards of conduct of a given profession. . . ." As members of the health care profession, RCPs are expected to behave in an ethical manner, adhering to the AARC Code of Ethics (see Appendix A). Examples of ethical dilemmas encountered by RCPs include discovering that a patient care error was committed by a colleague and friend, and providing labor-intensive "comfort measure" care to a patient with end-stage chronic obstructive pulmonary disease. As mentioned earlier, legal and ethical considerations are irrevocably intertwined in

clinical practice. It is important that every RCP possess a basic understanding of ethical decision making in the clinical setting and of the legal implications attendant to ethical issues. A comprehensive discussion of legal-ethical issues is beyond the scope of this chapter. RCPs may wish to consult a seminal book on this topic (see Carroll, 1996) for an extensive overview of ethical theory and its implications for respiratory care professionals.

Two basic models of ethical decision making commonly are used in the health care arena. The first is based on the important concept known as *beneficence*. This ideal man-

CRITICAL THINKING CHALLENGES

Case Scenario

An RCP reports directly to the critical care unit where he has been assigned, to begin his shift. Twenty minutes into the shift, you (the house-charge RCP) receive a page from the charge intensive care unit nurse informing you that your staff RCP "reeks of alcohol" and that she is concerned for the patients.

What are your rights as an "employer" to deal with the RCP? What are the employee's rights? These questions can only be answered within the context of each state's laws and statutes, coupled with the policies in place at the particular facility where the event occurs.

While providing verbal counseling to this employee, he becomes defensive of his behavior and verbally abusive of you. He starts to walk away from you, and you grab him by the arm to continue the conversation. "I'm not finished counseling you!"

Have you violated any laws by physically touching the RCP? Refer back to the previous discussion on assault and battery!

dates that licensed professionals act in a manner that maximizes the benefits of treatment and minimizes the potential harm. The RCP achieves the ideal of beneficence through basic education and continuing development of competence. This ideal is inherent in the principle of affirmative duty, as described earlier in this chapter. When receiving an order for therapy, for example, the RCP asks, "Will my actions benefit the patient?" and "Do I possess the skills to safely, competently carry out this order so that it will benefit the patient?" To illustrate the connection between law and ethics, another question the therapist must ask is, "Am I lawfully permitted to carry out this procedure per my state practice act?"

A second ethical ideal that guides the RCP is based on the principle of patient autonomy. The RCP is morally obligated to recognize and respect the patient's rights to self-determination. A competent adult has the freedom to determine the course of treatment and to refuse treatment, even when that decision is not beneficial to his or her well-being. This legal consideration of patient control over medical treatment contributed to the development of the law known as the Patient Self-Determination Act. This act mandates, among other things, that health care facilities and agencies provide written information to patients about their rights under state law to make decisions regarding their medical care. Decisions that patients make about their care, called *advance directives*, must then be placed in their medical records. Appendix B illustrates an example of an advance directive. All RCPs must be familiar with the concept of patient autonomy and aware of advance directive policies and documents used at their employment site. A failure to adhere to the advance directives stipulated in a patient's medical record not only violates ethical principles but could also have dire legal consequences for the RCP.

In addition to professional liability issues and concerns about malpractice, RCPs must recognize that federal or state laws affect ethical decision making. Violation of laws and statutes, including the RCP Practice Act, would have legal consequences for all health care providers involved. If an emergency department refused to provide appropriate treatment to an unstable patient and attempted to transfer that patient because of inadequate or no health insurance, that action would be considered more than unethical; it would constitute a violation of the Emergency Medical Treatment and Active Labor Act, commonly referred to as the "anti-dumping" law. This law stipulates that discharge or transfer of a patient cannot be made solely on the basis of financial status until (1) a medical screening examination has been performed and (2) a medical doctor or nurse practitioner verifies that the patient is stable. The stabilized patient or guardian must provide informed consent for transfer, and the patient must be conveyed in a medical transport vehicle with trained staff.

A violation of this law rendered by the Health Care Financing Administration (HCFA) against a medical facility that receives any federal funding for Medicare patients

CRITICAL THINKING CHALLENGES

Go Figure

You are assigned to care for an adult with end-stage cystic fibrosis. The patient has decided that he does not want any heroic measures in the event that he develops acute respiratory failure, based on written advance directives. The patient decompensates on your shift; this occurs in the presence of the patient's sister, who also happens to be an attorney. She says to you, "You had better do everything you can to save my brother's life. I'm an attorney, and if you don't, I'll sue you for everything you've got!"

This scenario presents the RCP with multiple ethical dilemmas and legal considerations. A set of general questions can be used to help guide RCPs when presented with real or perceived ethical dilemmas.

1. With whom should I consult and communicate regarding this situation? The answer to this question may include physicians, nurses, risk management personnel, ethics committees, respiratory therapy manager, or pastoral care.

2. What are the written wishes of the patient (advance directive)?

3. What are the legal consequences of the options I have for taking action? Are there any federal or state laws or statutes involved in this scenario?

brings with it a $50,000 out-of-pocket fine. In addition, HCFA may elect to withdraw permission for the facility's participation in Medicare. Loss of Medicare reimbursement could result in closure of the facility. RCPs who participate in the emergency room management and discharge of patients should be aware of current federal and state anti-dumping laws.

In 1996, JCAHO introduced a preliminary Sentinel Event policy, which subsequently underwent revisions in 1997 and 1998. The Sentinel Event policy stemmed in part from a series of highly publicized cases in 1994 and 1995, in which patients either died or suffered permanent loss of function in what appeared to be avoidable circumstances. The Sentinel Event policy is an attempt to ensure that hospitals and health care agencies self-report the following cases and conduct a root cause analysis of the problem:

- Infant abduction
- Infant discharge to wrong family
- Hemolytic transfusion reaction
- Patient rape
- Suicide in a 24-hour setting
- Surgery on wrong patient or body part

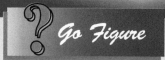

CRITICAL THINKING CHALLENGES

Go Figure

Consider the following dilemma:
You are treating an asthmatic patient who has had multiple hospital admissions during the past year. She asks you if you can keep a secret. You agree, and affirm to her that you will keep what she tells you confidential. She tells you that she routinely does not take her medication at home because it gives her a headache and shakiness. You have acknowledged the patient's rights to confidentiality, but this patient's noncompliant behavior may be contributing to her illness.

What ethical dilemma do you face, and how will you proceed?

• Unanticipated death
• Unanticipated major permanent loss of function

Adherence to the JCAHO Sentinel Event process is aimed at insuring that institutions correct systems problems which predispose them to repeat serious negative patient care outcomes. Failure to adhere to the program can influence the accreditation status of that institution. RCPs should educate themselves to the JCAHO Sentinel Event program, and also to the specific Sentinel Event policies established at their particular employment site.

JCAHO has established standards related to ethical behavior of health care organizations. JCAHO recommends that the organization establish a method for dealing with ethical dilemmas. JCAHO does not require but recommends that the organization have a formal ethics committee. An ethics committee can serve as a resource for the RCP and should be consulted when legal-ethical issues arise. Many RCPs have found that ethics rounds have helped clarify and resolve ethical dilemmas and improved patient and family satisfaction. Legal-ethical scenarios commonly faced by RCPs warrant the development of multidisciplinary collaborative policies on resolving these problems. Humane discontinuation of life support, compassionate care for the terminally ill, and chronic understaffing leading to unmet patient needs all represent ethical challenges. RCPs who work in an environment where staffing levels are such that ordered patient care is not implemented have an ethical (and legal) duty to resolve this dilemma. Adopting the attitude that it's not your problem does not serve the rights of the patient or fulfill your professional duty as a patient advocate.

Box 2–7 is a list of several areas in which legal-ethical problems may arise. As stated earlier, it is imperative that all RCPs have a basic understanding of the legal-ethical principles, examine their personal belief systems related to

Box • 2–7   AREAS IN WHICH LEGAL-ETHICAL DILEMMAS ARISE

• Confidentiality of patient records
• Do-not-resuscitate orders
• Advance directives
• Incompetent or impaired colleagues
• Staffing limitations on providing care
• Allocation of limited resources
• Financial limitations

health care, and recognize their decision-making processes when faced with ethical dilemmas. Engage your colleagues in legal-ethical discussions and examine how you feel and think about various legal-ethical situations. Values clarification can provide RCPs with insight into their ethical decision-making processes, fostering a more effective approach to the resolution of ethical dilemmas.

SUMMARY

This chapter provides an overview of legal and ethical issues related to the practice of respiratory care by an RCP. The information contained in this chapter is by no means comprehensive, nor can it substitute for formal legal and ethical advice obtained from legal professionals. Rather, this chapter serves as a foundation that will help empower every RCP to develop a sound, professional practice. RCPs are encouraged to develop their understanding of legal-ethical principles by pursuing further resources in this area, such as those listed in the bibliography. Attention to the information contained in this chapter can help RCPs to render safe, quality care and act in a professional manner which in turn can reduce the legal risks of RCPs and raise their value in the eyes of their patients, colleagues, and the public.

One final comment should be made regarding whether RCPs should purchase their own professional liability insurance. It is a common belief that an RCP will be covered by their employer's malpractice insurance if named in a lawsuit. It is interesting to note that the American Nurses Association recommends that every nurse have personal malpractice insurance. We are not aware of any position statement from the AARC on personal liability insurance.

Because malpractice insurance policies vary from carrier to carrier and malpractice laws vary among states, we suggest that every RCP do the following:

1. Check with your employer to determine whether RCPs are named on the policy, what level of legal support the employer offers, and what coverage is available once the RCP has left that employment site.
2. Consider the stability of the facility or company for which you are employed to determine the likelihood

of their being present 5 years down the road when that letter arrives from the legal firm.

3. Examine the clinical setting in which you provide care. Certain employment activities represent high-risk areas for malpractice litigation.

4. Consider personal liability insurance if you are self-employed and have contact with professional clients or patients.

Respiratory care practitioners can obtain information on inexpensive liability insurance from a variety of sources. RCPs can contact the AARC at 972–243–2272 for information on obtaining professional liability insurance through Maginnis & Associates. You can also call Maginnis & Associates directly at 800–621–3008 to obtain information on the merits of personal liability insurance.

Bibliography

American Association for Respiratory Care. *AARC Code of Ethics and Professional Conduct*. Dallas: AARC; 1998.

Bigler J. Avoiding respiratory care liability, Part I. *Pneumogram*. 1995; 20(1):6.

Bigler J, Mahlmeister M. Avoiding respiratory care liability, Part 2. *Pneumogram*. 1995; 21(2):4.

Bunch D. TDPs and legal liability. *AARCTimes*. 1994; 18(3):46.

Carroll C. *Legal Issues and Ethical Dilemmas in Respiratory Care*. Philadelphia: FA Davis; 1996.

Cullen DL. Should I tell? Reporting incompetent behavior in respiratory care. *AARCTimes*. 1988;12(12):22.

Durbin CG Jr. First do no harm: Balancing the risks and benefits of medical procedures. (Editorial) *Respiratory Care*. 1995; 40(11): 1118.

Fiesta J. Failing to act like a professional. *Nursing Management*. 1994; 25(7):15.

Healthcare Standards—1996: Official Directory. Plymouth Meeting, PA: ECRI; 1996.

JCAHO, *Comprehensive Accreditation Manual for Hospitals*. Oakbrook Terrace, IL: Joint Commission for Accreditation of Health Care Organizations; 1996.

Leape LL. Error in medicine. *JAMA*. 1994; 272(23):1851.

Mahlmeister M, Mahlmeister L. Professional accountability and the RCP. *AARCTimes*. 1991; 15(11):26.

Maginnis & Associates. *Myth and Facts about Professional Liability Insurance*. Chicago: Maginnis & Associates; 1995.

Rubenfeld GD. Do-not-resuscitate orders: A critical review of the literature. *Respiratory Care*. 1995;20(5):528.

Rushton CH, Hogue EE. Confronting unsafe practice: Ethical and legal issues. *Pediatric Nursing*. 1993; 19(3):284.

Watson ME. Median nerve damage from brachial artery puncture: A case report. *Respiratory Care*. 1995;Nov:1141.

APPENDIX A

AMERICAN ASSOCIATION FOR RESPIRATORY CARE STATEMENT OF ETHICS AND PROFESSIONAL CONDUCT

In the conduct of their professional activities, respiratory care practitioners shall be bound by the following ethical and professional principles. Respiratory care practitioners shall:

- Demonstrate behavior that reflects integrity, supports objectivity, and fosters trust in the profession and its professionals

- Actively maintain and continually improve their professional competence, and represent it accurately

- Perform only those procedures or functions in which they are individually competent and that are within the scope of accepted and responsible practice

- Respect and protect the legal and personal rights of patients they treat, including the right to informed consent and refusal of treatment

- Divulge no confidential information regarding any patient or family unless disclosure is required for responsible performance of duty, or is required by law

- Provide care without discrimination on any basis, with respect for the rights and dignity of all individuals

- Promote disease prevention and wellness

- Refuse to participate in illegal or unethical acts, and refuse to conceal illegal, unethical, or incompetent acts of others

- Follow sound scientific procedures and ethical principles in research

- Comply with state or federal laws that govern and relate to their practice

- Avoid any form of conduct that creates a conflict of interest, and follow the principles of ethical business behavior

- Promote the positive evolution of the profession, and of health care in general, through improvement of the access, efficacy, and cost of patient care

- Refrain from indiscriminate and unnecessary use of resources, both economic and natural, in their practice

Revised 12/94.

EXAMPLE OF AN ADVANCE DIRECTIVE

ADVANCE HEALTH CARE DIRECTIVE

If I, _____ , of

_____

_____

am not able to make an informed decision regarding my health care, I direct that my instructions and wishes as stated in this document be followed.

1. Effectivity. This document shall become effective immediately. The authority conveyed by this document shall not be affected by my subsequent disability or incapacity. I expect to be fully informed about and allowed to participate in any health care decision for me, to the extent that I am able.

2. Terminal Condition. If I have a "terminal condition," I direct that my life not be extended by life sustaining procedures; such procedures shall be withheld or withdrawn.

3. Coma. If I am in a "permanent coma," I direct that my life not be extended by life-sustaining procedures; such procedures shall be withheld or withdrawn.

4. Life-sustaining Procedures. By the use of the term "life-sustaining procedures," I mean any procedure, treatment, intervention, or other measure that has the primary effect of prolonging my life and is not necessary to provide for my comfort or freedom from pain.

5. Artificial Nutrition and Hydration. I authorize my agent to determine whether artificial nutrition or hydration should be withheld or withdrawn.

6. Hold Harmless. All persons or entities who in good faith endeavor to carry out the terms and provision of this document shall not be liable to me, my estate, or my heirs for any damages or claims arising because of their action or inaction based on this document, and my estate shall defend and indemnify them, except for willful misconduct or gross negligence.

7. Severability. If any provision in this document is held to be invalid, such invalidity shall not affect the other provisions that can be given effect without the invalid provision, and thus the directions in this document are severable.

I have read and understand the contents of this document. I am emotionally and mentally competent to make this declaration.

Note: Each state has developed its own specific advance directive language and documents.

Respiratory Anatomy and Physiology

James B. Fink

Key Terms

alveolar macrophages
anatomic dead space
anatomic shunt
Bohr effect
bronchioles
carina
Clara cells
collateral ventilation
dead space
gel
laryngopharynx
met Hb
nasopharynx
oropharynx
physiologic dead space
pulmonary endothelial cells
respiratory central
    controller
shunt
sol
transit time
turbinates

Objectives

- Describe the structure and function of the upper and lower airways.

- Identify features of the thoracic pump and the effect of different muscles groups during active and passive ventilation. Describe how respiratory muscles move air in and out of the lungs.

- Describe simultaneous changes in pressure among the pleura, alveoli, and airway as a function of time during relaxation and exercise breathing.

- Trace the path of oxygen from air to the tissues and the path of carbon dioxide from the tissues to air.

- Identify factors affecting ventilation and perfusion relationships and their impact on gas exchange.

- Define compliance, and show how pulmonary and chest wall compliance can differ.

- List factors that affect airway resistance in central and peripheral airways.

- List and explain four causes of arterial hypoxemia.

- Discuss how information flows to and from the central nervous system in regulating breathing.

Effective therapeutic interventions require the practitioner to understand the structure and function of the respiratory tract in both health and disease. Respiratory care is focused primarily on maintaining and restoring normal function of the respiratory tract. Understanding normal function in health is essential to directing such therapy.

This chapter discussion begins with the upper airway and follows the route of inhaled gas into the lungs to participation in gas exchange.

UPPER AIRWAY

The upper airway consists of those structures extending from the ambient air to the tracheobronchial tree, including the nose, mouth, pharynx, and larynx.

Nose

The external nose surrounds the nostrils and one third of the nasal cavity. The nasal cavity is composed of two chambers about 5 cm high × 10 cm long, with a surface area of 150 cm^2 and a total volume of 15 mL. The narrowest part of the entire airway is the nasal valve (internal ostium) located 1.5 cm from the nares, with a cross-sectional area of 0.3 cm^2 on each side (Fig. 3–1).

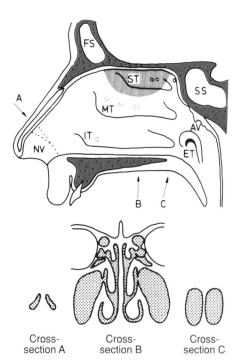

Cross-section A   Cross-section B   Cross-section C

FIGURE 3–1 • Lateral wall of the nasal cavity and cross-sections of the internal ostium (*A*), the middle of the nasal cavity (*B*), and the choanae (*C*). Hatched area in the upper figure, olfactory region; NV, nasal vestibule; IT, inferior turbinate and orifice of the nasolacrimal duct; MT, middle turbinate and orifices of frontal sinus, anterior ethmoidal sinuses, and maxillary sinus; ST, superior turbinate and orifices of posterior ethmoidal sinuses; FS, frontal sinus; SS, sphenoidal sinus; AV, adenoid vegetations; ET, orifice of eustachian tube. (Mygind N. *Nasal Allergy*, 2nd ed. Cambridge, MA: Blackwell Scientific, Inc; 1979.)

The nasal cavity is divided by a septum, whose lateral wall has bony projections on each side forming the superior, medial, and inferior turbinates, or conchae (Fig. 3–2). The nostrils are covered by skin; inside, the anterior one third of the nasal cavity is covered by a squamous and transitional epithelium overlying a rich capillary complex. The upper part of the nasal cavity is covered with olfactory epithelium, and the remainder is typical airway epithelium, composed of ciliated, pseudostratified columnar epithelium (Fig. 3–3).

Mucosa

The lateral wall of the nose has bony projections covered with mucosa, forming the superior, middle, and inferior turbinates, or conchae. This epithelium is composed of four major cell types (Fig. 3–4). The dominating cell type is the ciliated cell (Box 3–1). The cilia are found behind the front edge of the inferior turbinate, the posterior part of the nasal cavity, and lining the paranasal sinus.

The cilia have a typical ultrastructure: each cell contains about 100 cilia, 0.3 μm wide and 5 μm long. These cells move in repetitive patterns and assist in propelling debris and secretions toward the larynx, where they can be expectorated.

GOBLET CELLS

Goblet cells are secretory cells interspersed among the pseudostratified columnar epithelium (see Fig. 3–4). The concentration of goblet cells is similar in the nose to that found in the trachea and main bronchi (4000 − 7000 cells/mm^2). The goblet cell secretes less fluid than do the submucosal glands. Unlike the glands, the goblet cells are not innervated by the parasympathetic nervous system.

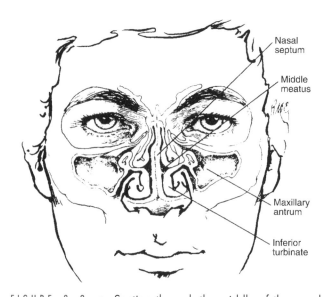

Nasal septum

Middle meatus

Maxillary antrum

Inferior turbinate

FIGURE 3–2 • Section through the middle of the nasal cavity showing the slit-like nature of the nasal passage and its relation to structures in the face. (Fishman AP. *Pulmonary Diseases and Disorders*, 2nd ed. New York: McGraw-Hill; 1988:209–223. Reproduced with permission of The McGraw-Hill Companies.)

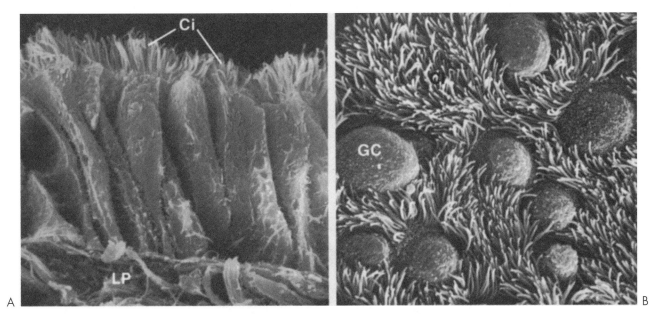

FIGURE 3-3 • Scanning electron micrographs of the mucosal epithelium. (*A*) Cross-sectional view: columnar epithelial cells with cilia (Ci) and lamina propia (LP). (*B*) Cilia and goblet cells (Gc) seen from above, at lower magnification. (Kessel RG, Karoon RH. *Tissues and Organs: A Text-Atlas of Scanning Electron Microscopy*, San Francisco: WH Freeman & Co; 1979:210.)

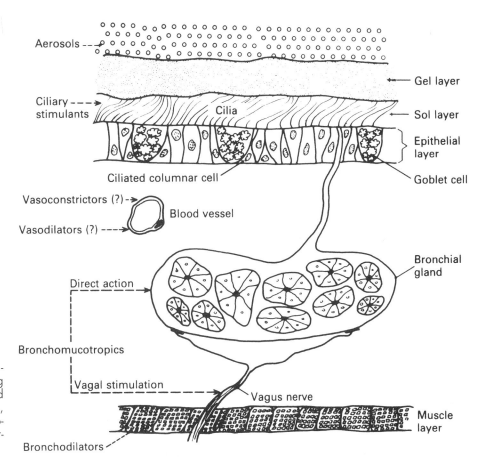

FIGURE 3-4 • Schematic diagram of the airway showing key structures within the wall and lumina of the respiratory tract, with key to types of pharmacologic agents that may affect different sites of action.

The pattern of cilia in the nose corresponds with a map of nasal airflow. There are less cilia in the upper part of the nasal cavity than along the floor. Low temperature, low humidity, and air contamination appear to contribute to a reduced number of ciliated cells. To emphasize this effect, both newborns and patients with laryngectomies have an even distribution of ciliated cells throughout the entire nasal cavity.

Full goblet cells are associated with fragmentation of the normally tight junctions, which may affect absorption of aerosolized drugs.

SUBMUCOSAL GLANDS

The two types of submucosal glands are anterior serous and seromucous.

Most of the 150 anterior serous glands on each side of the nose have long excretory ducts opening to the upper part of the internal ostium. They appear to play a role in watery rhinorrhea. The seromucous glands have a larger secretory capacity, with about 100,000 in the human nose. This number appears to be consistent through life, indicating that infants have the same secretory capacity as adults. An eight-fold greater concentration of seromucous glands occurs in the nose than in the trachea, although the glands are smaller in the nose. Afferent nerve fibers provide trigeminal parasympathetic innervation of the submucosal glands. The blood vessels are controlled primarily by sympathetic innervation. Continuous release of noradrenaline keeps the sinusoids partly contracted. In the nose, stimula-

tion of the α-adrenergic receptors provides more marked response than does the vasodilation effect from stimulation of the β$_2$-adrenergic receptors.

Most nasal secretions come from the nasal glands rather than from goblet cells. Goblet cells produce a small amount of viscous mucus and are associated with plasma exudation during inflammation. Accumulation of the secretions in the nose may be due to hypersecretion, dehydration, or reduced mucociliary clearance rate.

The epithelium rests on a basement membrane, which is composed of a layer of collagen fibers. In the nose, this membrane is thicker in patients with rhinitis and in a number of symptom-free subjects. This membrane in the bronchi is thicker in patients with asthma. This thickening in the nose is probably secondary to constant exposure to dry, unconditioned, and polluted air.

MUCOCILIARY ESCALATOR

Secretions from the submucosal glands cover the ciliated epithelium of the airway (Fig. 3–5). These relatively thin secretions form the watery **sol** layer, through which the cilia normally beat. As water evaporates from the sol layer and more viscous secretions are secreted by the goblet cells, the thicker **gel** layer forms. This thicker gel layer floats on the layer of thin secretions that continue to be secreted from the glands, replenishing the sol layer. This gel layer traps and holds dust, pollens, contaminants, and microorganisms (Box 3–2). The cilia beat in a coordinated, wave-like motion through the sol layer, with the tips of the cilia extending to the gel layer, propelling it toward the pharynx, where it is swallowed or expectorated (Fig. 3–6). The normal respiratory mucosa produces about 100 mL/day, which is commonly expelled from the respiratory tract and swallowed, often without notice.

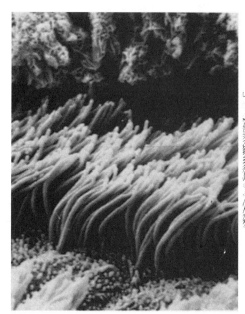

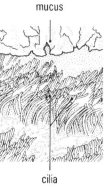

mucus

cilia

FIGURE 3–5 • Scanning electron micrograph of bronchial cilia with mucus resting on their tips. (Clinical Atlas of Respiratory Disease. St. Louis: Gower, F1.22)

The more proximally that inhaled particles are deposited, the more quickly they are removed. The deeper that particles are deposited, the longer is the time required for the lungs to clear the particle.

SITE OF DEPOSITION	TIME TO REMOVAL
Nose	<30 minutes
Bronchi	Hours
Alveoli	Days to weeks

The submucosa (lamina propria) is rich in blood vessels. Arterioles lack internal elastic membrane so that endothelial basement membrane is continuous with the basement membrane of the smooth muscle cells. There is also increased porosity of the endothelial basement membrane, so that subendothelial musculature of vessels may be more readily influenced by mediators, hormones, and drugs circulating in the bloodstream than other blood vessels. Capillaries below the surface epithelium and glands are fenestrated, allowing rapid movement of fluid through the vascular wall.

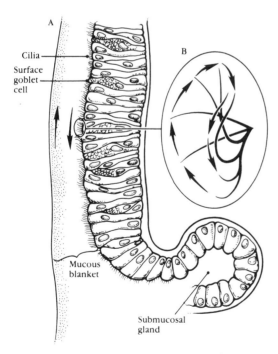

F I G U R E 3–6 • (A) The mucocilliary escalator consisting of pseudostratified columnar epithelial cells with goblet cells, submucosal glands, and cilia, covered by a mucous blanket consisting of the sater sol and the more viscous gel layer (*shaded area*). (B) The conceptual scheme of ciliary motion that allows the tips of the cilia to reach up and propel the gel layer toward the oropharynx.

Large venous cavernous sinusoids, mostly localized to the inferior turbinates, are specialized vessels adapted to support the heating and humidification demands of the nose in conditioning inhaled air. They are normally in a semicontracted condition because of sympathetic nerve-mediated smooth muscle tone.

Arteriovenous anastomoses, such as those in fingertips, toes, nail beds, and lips, allow at least half of the blood flow in the nasal mucosa to be shunted, permitting a greater total blood flow per cubic centimeter in the upper airway mucosa than in the muscle, brain, or liver.

Function of the Nose

The preferred route of ambient air to the pulmonary blood–gas interface is through the nose, providing the most efficient combination of air filtration and conditioning. The nose serves a variety of functions, including conditioning of inspired air with heat and humidity, deconditioning of exhaled air, filtration, airway protection, olfaction (smell), and phonation.

The normal nose has slit-like passages that provide for efficient exchange of heat and moisture. The width of the nasal passages is actively regulated by the sympathetic innervation and tone in the venous sinusoids. Changes in nasal passage width result in changes in airflow patterns through the nose, affecting all of the normal functions. There is a normal nasal cycle of changing passage width, with changes from one side to the other at 2- to 4-hour intervals. The nasal cycle is usually not noticed except in patients with rhinitis or deviated septa (Box 3–3).

The nose does a remarkable job of conditioning and deconditioning air, transforming even cold air (0°C) to 31°C and 98% relative humidity by the time it reaches the trachea. The nose is much more efficient than the mouth in heat and humidity regulation.

Conditioning of gas is a function of several features of the nose:

- The slit-like shape of the nasal cavity provides close contact between inhaled gas and the mucosa.
- The mucous glands and goblet cells have a high secretory capacity to provide water to the air.
- Rich vascular beds in the submucosa, with arteriovenous anastomoses, supply a large volume of blood to heat the air.
- Sinusoid contractions provide changes in passage width in response to system needs.

The function of the nose in conditioning gas is described in greater detail in Chapter 11.

FILTRATION AND PROTECTION OF THE AIRWAY
The nose is an effective filter of airborne particles larger than 10 μm, such as pollen grains and dust. Particles smaller than 2 μm, such as mold spores, tend to pass

With rhinitis, inflammation of the nose and sinuses results in vasodilation and engorgement of the venous sinusoids, narrowing the airway. A quick-onset, short-acting solution is the application of an α-adrenergic receptor nasal spray, which causes local vasoconstriction, reducing vascular engorgement and opening up the airway. The problem with this approach is that after a few hours, the effects of the drug subsides, and a rebound effect leads to even greater vascular engorgement and congestion.

through the nose into the lungs. The filtering function of the nose is caused by inertial impaction of particles as they pass through the tortuous path of air through narrow passageways. The **turbinates** create turbulence as air passes through the nose. As the path of air changes, the inertia of the larger particles carries them into the surface of the airway, where they impact and adhere (deposit). Impaction of particles increases with turbulence. The greater the turbulence, the more changes in air path direction, and the greater the impaction of particles. Less turbulence, less im-

paction. With mouth breathing, there is less turbulence and less filtration.

Once particles impact on the mucosa, they are propelled by the mucociliary blanket toward the pharynx, where they can be swallowed and expectorated.

The nose also protects the airway from irritating, tissue-damaging, water-soluble gases such as sulfur dioxide and formaldehyde, retaining most of the gas in the nose.

Mouth

Unlike the nose, the mouth serves a dual function between the digestive and respiratory tracts, passing both food and air. The structure of the mouth permits large volumes of air to flow in and out of the airway with minimal resistance. This reduction in airway resistance is at the cost of reduced efficiency in gas conditioning and filtration.

Pharynx

The pharynx is a fibromuscular, funnel-shaped cavity about 5 inches long extending from the base of the skull to the esophagus (Fig. 3–7). The pharynx is divided into three parts:

The **nasopharynx** lies behind the nasal cavities, with its roof formed by bones of the skull, and above the soft

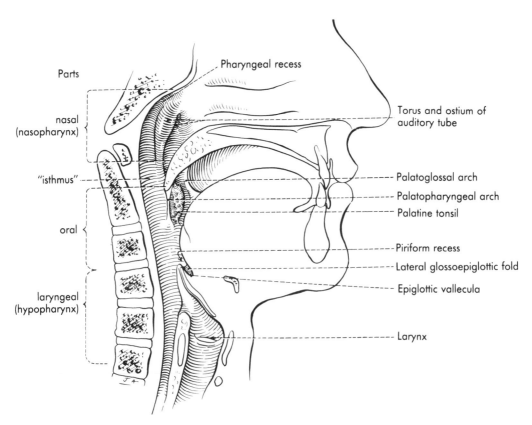

FIGURE 3–7 • Cross-sectional view showing major structures of the pharynx. (Rosse C. *Hollinshead's Textbook of Anatomy,* 5th ed. Philadelphia: Lippincott-Raven Publishers, 1997.)

palate, which divides it from the other parts of the pharynx during swallowing. The eustachian tubes open into the nasopharynx, connecting the tympanic cavities to the atmosphere, equalizing pressure across the ear drum.

The **oropharynx** lies behind the mouth and below the soft palate, extending back to the larynx. The tonsils are lymphatic tissue on the lateral walls of the oropharynx that act as part of a circular band of lymphoid tissue and as a filter to protect the respiratory tract against infection.

The **laryngopharynx** lies below the hyoid bone and behind the larynx. The larynx connects the pharynx and the trachea. Its opening is at the base of the tongue. It is broad superiorly and shaped like a triangular box. Its chief function is phonation.

Larynx

The larynx consists of nine cartilages connected with intrinsic and extrinsic muscles and ligaments. Its shape is maintained by the thyroid and cricoid cartilage. The thyroid cartilage, or Adam's apple, is the largest of the structures in the larynx and consists of two laminae fused together anteriorly. The cricoid forms a complete ring of cartilage, forming two synovial joints with the thyroid. The epiglottis is attached to the superior border of the thyroid cartilage and acts as a hinged lid to protect the airway from aspiration during swallowing. The arytenoid, cuneiform, and corniculate cartilages are paired cartilages. These cartilages are connected with ligaments and muscles.

Internally, the larynx forms two pairs of folds: the true and false vocal chords (Fig. 3–8). Both are involved in coughing and sneezing. Two sets of muscles are found in

---

Box • 3–4 HOARSENESS

Hoarseness can be caused by partial or complete paralysis of the vocal chords as well as by fixed airway obstructions, such as tumors, in the larynx.

Partial paralysis of the vocal cords can be caused by damage to the nerves. Because the left recurrent laryngeal nerve descends into the mediastinum, it may be affected or interrupted by cancer in the lymph nodes (near the left hilum) or by aortic aneurisms, granulomas, and lymphomas.

Two types of extrathoracic airway obstruction are associated with the larynx, and both are associated with hoarseness and stridor. Paralysis of the vocal chords can cause a variable airway obstruction. Flow volume loops typically show reduced inspiratory flow rates, with near-normal expiratory flows. Fixed obstructions, such as those associated with tumors in the larynx, tend to show reductions in both inspiratory and expiratory flows. Occasionally, after thoracic surgery, partial paralysis of the vocal cords is noted secondary to compression or damage of the recurrent laryngeal nerve during surgery. This is readily differentiated from hoarseness after extubation.

---

the larynx, innervated by the vagus, which open and close the glottis during inspiration and expiration, close the laryngeal aperture and glottis during swallowing, and change tension of the vocal folds during production of sound (Box 3–4). Failure of these muscles to maintain tone when a person is sleeping or obtunded may be associated with partial or complete airway obstruction.

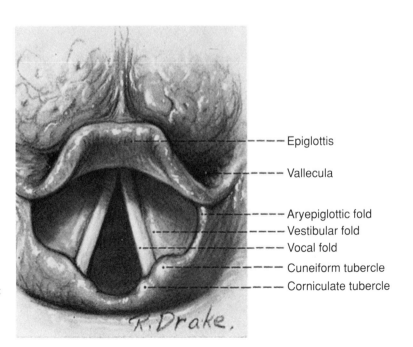

FIGURE 3–8 • The intubationist's view of the larynx with the vocal cords abducted. (Rosse C. *Hollinshead's Textbook of Anatomy,* 5th ed. Philadelphia: Lippincott-Raven Publishers, 1997.)

— Epiglottis
— Vallecula
— Aryepiglottic fold
— Vestibular fold
— Vocal fold
— Cuneiform tubercle
— Corniculate tubercle

Box • 3–5 AIRWAY PROTECTION AND INTUBATION

The protective function of the epiglottis and larynx against invasion of particulate matter becomes an issue during insertion of artificial airways, such as endotracheal tubes. The epiglottis cannot differentiate between life-threatening particulates and the life-saving attempts to secure the airway with intubation. When a straight laryngoscope blade is used to lift the epiglottis to view the vocal chords, the nerves respond with coughing and reflex laryngospasm. Consequently, when performing intubation in semialert patients, a key landmark is the vallecula, a relatively insensitive and avascular point located between the epiglottis and the base of the tongue. A curved laryngoscope blade inserted into the vallecula permits exposure of the larynx for direct visual observation of the cords with minimal reflex laryngospasm.

The larynx is the primary point of protection that differentiates the respiratory and digestive tracts. The larynx is key in three ways:

1. The epiglottis and larynx interact to protect the airway during swallowing (Box 3–5).
2. The vocal cords are key to an effective cough.
3. The larynx responds to foreign matter in the airway with laryngospasm to keep the inhaled matter from going further into the airway.

LOWER AIRWAY

Trachea

The trachea is a cylindrical tube about 2.5 cm wide and 12 cm in length that extends from the cricoid cartilage (C.6) to the sternal angle (T.5 posteriorly, articulation of the second rib with the sternum anteriorly), where it bifurcates at the carina to form the right and left mainstem bronchi (Fig. 3–9). The trachea has a framework of 16 to 20 C-shaped cartilages separated by fibrous and muscular tissue, providing considerable anterior strength to resist compression, with smooth muscle on the posterior side between the trachea and esophagus.

The **carina,** or point of bifurcation between the trachea and mainstem bronchi, is supported by overlapping C-shaped rings, providing structural strength from both front and back.

Branching of the Airways

The trachea divides into two main bronchi (Figs. 3–10 and 3–11). The left main bronchus is longer than the right, coming off at a greater angle (because of the position of the heart). The right main bronchus is shorter, wider, and more in line with the trachea (Box 3–6).

The main bronchi divide into lobar and then segmental bronchi. Each airway branches into two or more airways, with a smaller individual internal diameter than the parent airway, but with a larger combined cross-sectional area (Fig. 3–12). As air passes through to smaller airways with diameters of less than 1 mm, the resistance is reduced through the respiratory system, resulting in a cross-sec-

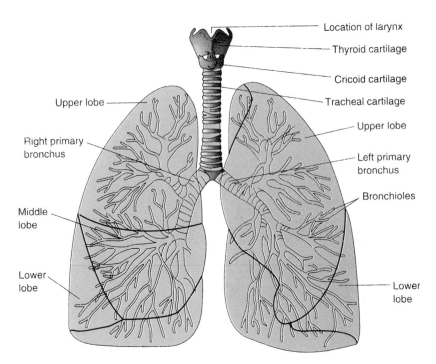

FIGURE 3–9 • Anterior view of major structures of the lower airway.

Location of larynx
Thyroid cartilage
Cricoid cartilage
Tracheal cartilage
Upper lobe
Left primary bronchus
Bronchioles
Lower lobe

Upper lobe
Right primary bronchus
Middle lobe
Lower lobe

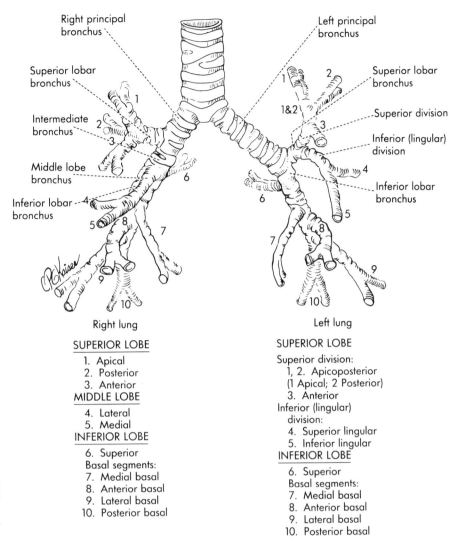

Right principal bronchus

Left principal bronchus

Superior lobar bronchus

Superior lobar bronchus

Intermediate bronchus

Superior division

Inferior (lingular) division

Middle lobe bronchus

Inferior lobar bronchus

Inferior lobar bronchus

Right lung

Left lung

SUPERIOR LOBE

1. Apical
2. Posterior
3. Anterior

MIDDLE LOBE

4. Lateral
5. Medial

INFERIOR LOBE

6. Superior
Basal segments:
7. Medial basal
8. Anterior basal
9. Lateral basal
10. Posterior basal

SUPERIOR LOBE

Superior division:
1, 2. Apicoposterior
(1 Apical; 2 Posterior)
3. Anterior
Inferior (lingular) division:
4. Superior lingular
5. Inferior lingular

INFERIOR LOBE

6. Superior
Basal segments:
7. Medial basal
8. Anterior basal
9. Lateral basal
10. Posterior basal

FIGURE 3–10 • The tracheo-bronchial tree with segmental bronchi and associated lobes identified. (Rosse C. *Hollinshead's Textbook of Anatomy*, 5th ed. Philadelphia: Lippincott-Raven Publishers, 1997.)

tional area of 1000 cm^2 at the level of the terminal bronchioles. With mouth breathing, about 80% (1.6 cm H$_2$O/L) of the total airway resistance (2 cm H$_2$O/L) is attributed to the large central airways.

The large bronchi are lined with pseudostratified columnar epithelium with a large number of mucous glands and are innervated by both the parasympathetic and the sympathetic nervous systems, connected to the brain by the vagus nerve. Irritant receptors in these airways can generate a cough reflex, with vagal stimulation resulting in bronchospasm and mucous secretion.

There are about 10 divisions of bronchi from the trachea, each with cartilage in its wall. In the main bronchi, the cartilage is less ring shaped and more irregular (providing greater flexibility) than that in the trachea. Each subsequent generation of the bronchi contains less cartilage (less structural support, but more flexibility). These branch into smaller airways without cartilage called **bronchioles**. A network of connective tissue extends from the alveoli to the hilum.

The epithelial lining in the airways changes from the larger central to smaller distal airways. In the trachea and

Box • 3–6   THE RIGHT STUFF

Because the right mainstem bronchus is more in line with the trachea than the left, there is an increased possibility that any "stuff" entering the lungs in an upright or supine position will preferentially go into the right lung. Endotracheal tubes that are extended too far, inhaled foreign bodies, and aspirated food or gastric contents tend to enter the right lung more often than the left. Thus, it makes sense when you suspect aspiration or obstruction of an inhaled foreign object to check the right lung first. Similarly, when placing an endotracheal tube, if the tube is in the lungs but extended beyond the carina, it is probably in the right bronchus, meaning no or minimal breath sounds over the left lung. Breath sounds on the right, but not on the left, indicate that the tube is extended too far and should be withdrawn a few centimeters at a time until breath sounds improve bilaterally.

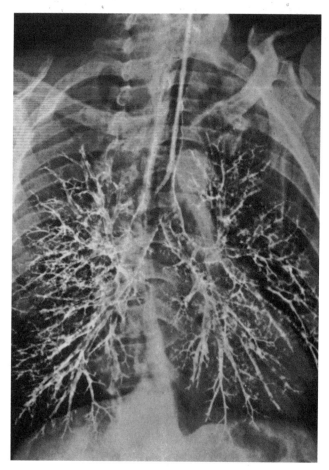

FIGURE 3-11 • A bronchogram in which both principal bronchi and most of the segmental bronchi are visualized. (Rosse C. *Hollinshead's Textbook of Anatomy,* 5th ed. Philadelphia: Lippincott-Raven Publishers, 1997.)

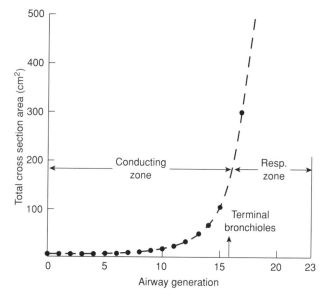

FIGURE 3-12 • Cross-sectional area of the airways increases exponentially with generations of the area, whereas forward airflow decreases. (West. *Respiratory Physiology: The Essentials,* 5th ed. Baltimore: Williams & Wilkins, 1995.)

main bronchi, the pseudostratified columnar epithelium is much like that found in the nose. The ciliated cells have cilia that beat in a coordinated movement, propelling the mucous layer toward the mouth. The goblet cells are interspersed among the ciliated cells and secrete mucus. Brush cells have microvilli (like the basal cells in the gut) and are thought to play a role in controlling fluid balance in the airway. Mucous glands are found in large and medium airways (Box 3–7).

As the airways get smaller, the columnar cells become shorter, with fewer basal cells, goblet cells, and mucous glands. The thickness of the epithelium is smaller as the columnar ciliated cells become more cuboidal. By the terminal bronchioles, there are no goblet cells or glands and fewer cilia. **Clara cells** are scattered between the ciliated cells and are thought to contribute to the surface lining layer of the bronchioles (like alveolar type II cells). They may also be progenitors of other epithelial cells (ciliated, brush, and goblet).

Throughout the lower airway, from the trachea to the terminal bronchioles, is a layer of bronchial smooth muscle that surrounds the airway and that acts like a sphincter to

constrict the airway when activated to contract (Fig. 3–14). Strands of smooth muscle can be found down to the alveolar ducts. These muscles play a major role in maintaining airway tone, helping to change caliber of airways, and shifting flow of gas to different areas of the lung (Box 3–8). The bands of smooth muscle are innervated by the vagus nerve. A large number of substances (eg, endogenous neurotransmitters, hormones, mediators, and drugs) cause airway smooth muscle to contract or to relax. When stimulated, the smooth muscle contracts, reducing the internal diameter of the airway and increasing local airway resistance, causing bronchoconstriction. Relaxation of smooth muscle leads to an open airway with minimal resistance to airflow. These muscles are also a part of the nat-

Box • 3–7 MUCOUS GLAND HYPERTROPHY

When the airway is irritated, it responds by producing additional secretions to bathe the airways and remove the irritants. When the irritation is chronic, such as with cigarette smoking over a number of years, the glands that produce the secretions become hypertrophied. Hypertrophy of the mucous glands is common in chronic bronchitis and is quantified by the Reid index (a ratio of the thickness of the gland to the thickness of the bronchial wall). Normal airways have a ratio less than 0.3. A Reid index of more than 0.36 is diagnostic of chronic bronchitis (Fig. 3-13)

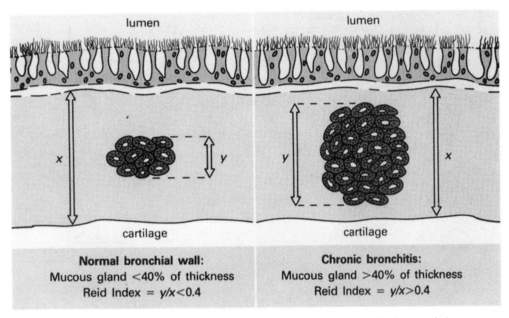

FIGURE 3–13 • The Reid index, demonstrating the ratio of the thickness of the mucous gland to the thickness of the total airway wall. (Color Atlas of Respiratory Disease. St. Louis: Gower. F9.13.)

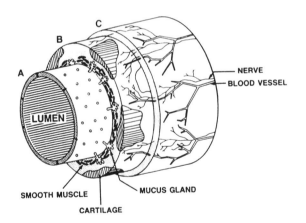

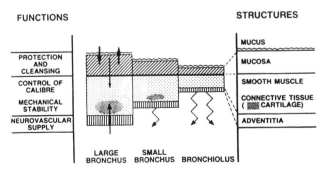

FIGURE 3–14 • Upper panel shows a schematic diagram of the three layers of a large bronchus: mucosa (*A*), smooth muscle and connective tissue (*B*), and adventitia neurovascular (*C*). Lower panel shows a longitudinal schematic diagram of the layered structure and function of airways from bronchus to bronchiole, with *extrabronchial mechanical interactions indicated by zig-zag arrows.* (Forrest and Lee)

ural defenses of the lung, constricting to keep particulates and irritants from reaching deeper into the lung.

Lung Structural Units

The lungs are divided into five lobes (upper, middle, and lower on the right with upper and lower on the left; see Fig. 3–9, Box 3–9). Each lobe is served by its own lobar bronchus, covered with two layers of visceral pleura and separated by fissures.

Each lobe is further divided into bronchopulmonary segments (Fig. 3–16). These segments are the smallest ana-

---

Box • 3–8 SMOOTH MUSCLE AND BRONCHOSPASM

Although the bronchial smooth muscles are "good guys" in normal lung function, hypersensitivity of the airway can result in airway inflammation and severe constriction of the airway, drastically increasing the work of breathing to the point of being life-threatening. This swollen mucosa and smooth muscle contraction are two key elements in the transient airway obstruction associated with exacerbations of bronchial asthma. Short-term relief therapy is oriented to relaxation of the smooth muscle with administration of bronchodilators, whereas control of the inflammation is attempted with administration of slower-acting antiinflammatory drugs.

CRITICAL THINKING CHALLENGES

Go Figure

Smooth muscles surround the airway from the bronchi to the terminal bronchioles. For the same level of smooth muscle contraction, which airways have the greater increase in airway resistance: the main bronchi or the terminal bronchioles?

tomic units capable of being removed from the lung intact. Each of the bronchopulmonary segments (10 in the left lung, 9 in the right) is supplied by its own segmental bronchus artery and vein. The segments are described in terms of their relative positions within the lobe. These segments are separated by connective tissue but not by fissures (Fig. 3–17).

Bronchopulmonary segments contain lobules that are about 1 cm in diameter. The lobules are generally pyramidal in shape, with the apex toward the connecting bronchiole that supplies them. Each lobule contains three to five acini (Fig. 3–18). The acinus is the area of lung parenchyma that is fed by a single respiratory bronchiole. The acinus is composed of alveolar ducts, alveolar sacs, alveoli, and alveoli pores. The difference between terminal and respiratory bronchioles is the presence of individual alveoli budding out from walls of the airway. Because the alveoli are more prevalent in the airway, they are described as alveolar ducts, which connect the airway to sacs composed of alveoli (Fig. 3–19). These terminal airways pass through areas of lung parenchyma that are supplied by other terminal airways (Fig. 3–20).

Pores of Kohn and canals of Lambert connect alveoli both within and across the terminal respiratory units (Fig.

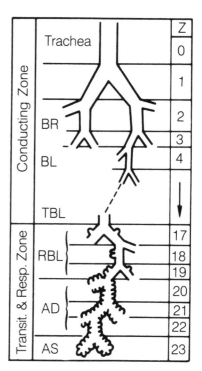

FIGURE 3–15 • Idealization of the human airways with the first 16 generations of the airway, composed of bronchus (BR), bronchiole (BL), and terminal bronchiole (TBL) and identified as the conducting zone. The last 7 generations, composed of the respiratory bronchiole (RBL), alveolar duct (AD), and alveolar sac (AC), constitute the transitional and respiratory zones. (Weibel ER. *Morphometry of the Human Lung.* Berlin: Springer-Verlag; 1962.)

3–21). The pores of Kohn are holes in the alveolar walls (less than 13 µm in diameter) that provide channels for gas movement between contiguous alveoli. The canals of Lambert connect alveoli supplied by different terminal airways. These passageways allow for **collateral ventilation** between alveoli that are fed from the same and different bronchioles. Should one feeding airway become obstructed or diseased, collateral ventilation allows the dependent alveoli to be ventilated from a secondary (unobstructed) bronchiole.

The alveoli are composed of several distinct types of cells (Fig. 3–22). The *type I pneumocyte* (or alveolar cell) is a squamous epithelial cell with a thin (0.1- to 0.5-µm) cell wall and relatively large surface area that forms 95% of the alveolar surface and is the primary conducting interface for gas transport. The type I cells have been likened to an egg on a skillet, with a small nucleus (yolk) surrounded with a wide thin cell body (egg white).

The *type II pneumocytes* are granulated cuboidal cells, rich in microvilli and osmophilic inclusion bodies. They are more numerous than the type I cells but constitute only 5% of the alveolar surface area. The type II cells have been identified as the production source for surfactant in the alveoli.

Box • 3–9   THREE LUNG ZONES

Conducting zone: Bulk movement of air and blood through bronchi and bronchioles and a parallel system of lobar and lobular branches of the pulmonary circulation (Fig. 3-15)

Transitional zone: Airways containing occasional alveoli, with a limited role in overall gas exchange; transition between conducting and respiratory zones

Respiratory zone: The air passages are lined by gas exchange membrane, within which most gas exchange occurs. Blood vessels are mainly capillaries with feeder vessels (alveolar arterioles and venules) to the most distal parts of the acinus

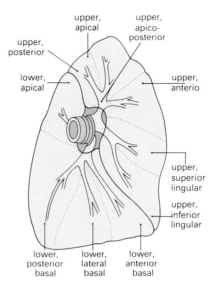

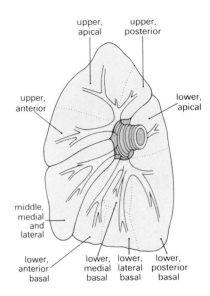

FIGURE 3–16 • Medial aspect of the left and right lungs showing the nomenclature and arrangement of the lobes and their segments. (Color Atlas of Respiratory Disease. St. Louis: Gower. F1.5, 1.6.)

The **pulmonary endothelial cells** account for 30% of the cells in the lung parenchyma, forming the capillaries that interface blood to air space. Interstitial cells provide support for the structures in the alveolar walls.

Type III pneumocytes are the **alveolar macrophages,** which provide the primary protection of the alveoli against pollutants, particulates, and bacteria. Macrophages are the primary phagocytes of the alveoli. Type III cells can phagocytose surfactant and are probably involved in the metabolic turnover of many of the extracellular components of the alveoli. These cells also phagocytose bacteria and particulates and have the ability to traverse the alveolar endothelium, probably at the connective tissue at the alveolar septum, to enter the lymphatics or the pulmonary capillaries.

Macrophages with large amounts of foreign particles are frequently found in lung lymph nodes, where they may remain permanently. Speed of transport in the lymphatic system can vary from days to months or even years.

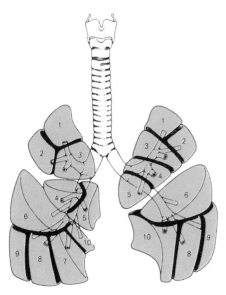

FIGURE 3–17 • Bronchopulmonary segments of the human lung. Left and right upper lobes: (1) apical, (2) posterior, (3) anterior, (4) superior lingular, and (5) inferior lingular segments. Right middle lobe: (4) lateral and (5) medial segments. Lower lobes: (6) superior (apical), (7) medial-basal, (8) anterior-basal, (9) lateral-basal, and (1) posterior-basal segments. The medial-basal segment (7) is absent in the left lung. (Fishman AP. *Assessment of Pulmonary Function.* New York: McGraw-Hill; 1980. Reprinted with permission of The McGraw-Hill Companies)

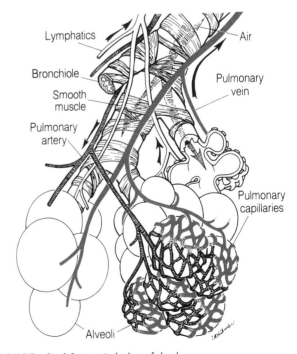

FIGURE 3–18 • Lobules of the lung.

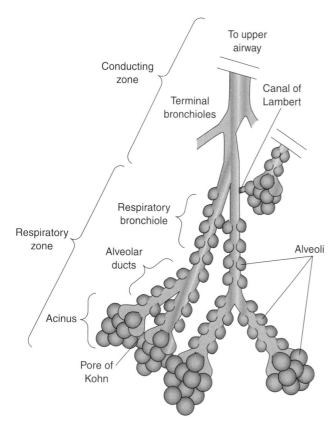

FIGURE 3–19 • Diagram of the major structures of the acinus.

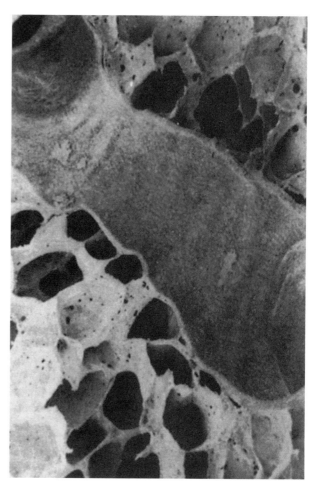

FIGURE 3–20 • Cross-section of a small bronchus and surrounding alveoli. (Courtesy of Janice A. Nowell, University of California, Santa Cruz.)

Lymphatics

The lymphatic system maintains lung water balance and serves as a pulmonary defense mechanism. The lymphatics control hydration by collecting the proteins and water that have left the pulmonary vascular space, and returning it to the circulation, as well as by aiding in removal of particulate matter from the lungs. Lymphatic vessels and aggregates of lymph tissue near major airways contribute to the immune response.

Lymphatic vessels flow alongside the blood vessels in the loose connective tissue of the bronchovascular spaces and pleura. Lymphatic capillaries consist of irregular epithelial cells without a basement membrane, presenting some large gaps that allow direct communication with the interstitial spaces. Larger vessels have smooth muscle in their walls that undergoes rhythmic contraction and funnel-shaped monocuspid valves that permit unilateral flow of lymph (Box 3–10).

VENTILATION AND PERFUSION

Respiration is dependent on the interface of air (ventilation) and blood (perfusion). To match ventilation with pulmonary blood flow, blood must perfuse ventilated regions of the lung, and air must ventilate perfused regions of the

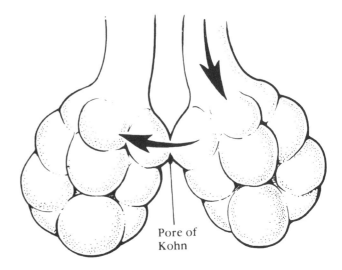

FIGURE 3–21 • Schematic of communication between the alveoli through the pore of Kohn.

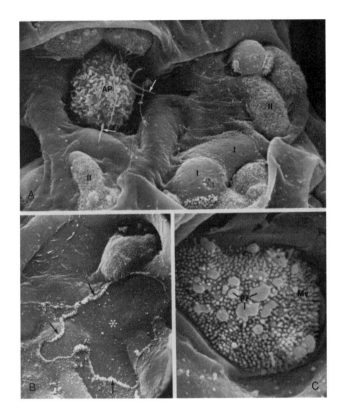

FIGURE 3–22 • Scanning electron micrographs of alveoli at high magnification. (*A*) Type I alveolar cells (I) can be easily distinguished from type II cells (II). (*B*) Intracellular type J junctions are shown as ridges (arrows). (*C*) A detailed view of a type II cell showing microvilli (Mv) and projections (Pr) believed to relate to surfactant release. (Kessel RG, Karoon RH. Tissues and organs. In: *A Text-Atlas of Scanning Electron Microscopy.* San Francisco: WH Freeman & Sons; 1979.)

lung. Mismatching of ventilation and perfusion is the most common cause of arterial hypoxemia (too little oxygen in the arterial blood).

Pulmonary Circulation

The two circulatory systems supplying blood to the lung are the bronchial and pulmonary circulations. The bronchial arteries arise from the thoracic aorta and upper intercostal ar-

---

Box • 3–10   PATHOPHYSIOLOGIC PERSPECTIVE

Lymph nodes may become enlarged in a number of inflammatory lung diseases, both noninfectious (silicosis) and infectious (granulomas). These nodes are also collection points of cancerous cells metastasized from the lungs. Many more lymph nodes occur on the left lung than on the right, and a bilateral effusion usually manifests first on the right lung.

Box • 3–11   PATHOPHYSIOLOGIC PERSPECTIVE

HEMOPTYSIS

Under normal conditions, only 1% to 2% of cardiac output goes to the bronchial arteries. With chronic infection, these vessels may hypertrophy, and blood flow may increase more than 10-fold. This is clinically important in that virtually all hemoptysis originates from the bronchial vessels.

---

teries (Box 3–11). This is the systemic circulation that serves the trachea and bronchi, down to the level of the respiratory bronchioles, supporting lung tissue, nerves, the outer layers of the pulmonary vessels, lymph nodes, and most of the visceral pleura. After bronchial arterioles form capillary plexuses, blood returns through either (1) the bronchial veins terminating in the azygos vein, emptying into the superior vena cava; or (2) a pulmonary vein terminating in the left atrium (one third of bronchial circulation). The systemic venous blood from the bronchial circulation returning through the pulmonary circulation is shunted from venous to arterial vessels without passing through the pulmonary circulation and participating in gas exchange, and is a part of the anatomic or normal built-in structural shunt (Box 3–12). Although bronchial circulation does not normally supply respiratory bronchioles and alveolar structures, it may do so in response to interruption of pulmonary circulation, supplying metabolic needs of the tissue and avoiding necrosis, but not sustaining or participating in gas exchange. Both bronchial and pulmonary arteries branch with the bronchial tree. Supernumerary arteries, however, do not travel with the airways but directly supply the gas exchange units and actually outnumber the conventional arteries, supplying about one third of the pulmonary capillaries (Table 3–1).

The pulmonary circulation generates from the right ventricle, pumping its entire stroke volume of 70 to 80 mL into the pulmonary artery, bifurcating into the right and left lungs. The pulmonary arteries branch dichotomously, following the branchings of the airways, down to the point of capillaries, with 5 to 11 capillaries coming into intimate

---

Box • 3–12 PaO_2 VERSUS PAO_2

Why is the PaO_2 less than the PAO_2? The bronchial circulation that is shunted from venous blood vessels into the pulmonary circulation returning from the lungs to the heart is the main reason that partial pressure of oxygen in arterial blood (PaO_2) is less than the partial pressure of oxygen in the alveoli (PAO_2).

Table • 3–1 DIFFERENCES BETWEEN PULMONARY AND SYSTEMIC CIRCULATIONS

Factor	Pulmonary	Systemic
Pressures	Low (pulmonary artery mean 14 mmHg)	High (aortic mean, 100 mmHg)
Pressure changes	Symmetric and of low magnitude within lungs	Asymmetric and of great magnitude depending on system supplied (eg, renal arteriole pressure much higher than hepatic circulation)
Pressure determined by	Arteriolar/alveolar gradient and/or arteriolar/venular gradient	Arteriolar/venular gradient
Vascular resistance	One-tenth of that of systemic circulation; can decrease resistance as pulmonary pressure rises	Resistance 10 times that of pulmonary circulation; less ability to lower resistance when pressure rises
Capillary support	Capillaries surrounded by gas-filled alveoli; collapse or distend depending on pressure in and around	Capillaries surrounded by tissue; less tendency to collapse or distend
Directing blood flow	System rarely directs blood between regions	Regulates and distributes blood to specific areas throughout body

contact with each alveoli. The concentration of capillaries is so dense that it should be viewed as a sheet of blood with supporting structures spreading the 80 mL of blood over the 70 to 80 m² surface area of the lung. The pulmonary veins provide a large reservoir for blood, helping to maintain consistent left-sided heart output (Table 3–2).

The pulmonary arteries are described as elastic, muscular, partially muscular, or nonmuscular, based on histology and size. The elastic pulmonary arteries (larger than 1000 μm) have elastic fibers embedded in their muscular tunica media, whereas the smaller muscular arteries (100 to 150 μm) have a circular layer of smooth muscle between the internal and external elastic laminae. As arteries decrease in size, only a spiral of muscle remains, until there is no muscle at all in vessels that are larger than the capillaries they serve. The endothelium of the pulmonary vascular system is continuous and nonfenestrated, with individual cells on a basement membrane separated by narrow gaps. The gaps allow small plasma proteins and water (less than 40 μm in radius) to pass through, normally at a rate of 10 to 20 mL/h for the entire pulmonary vascular bed.

Ventilation and Perfusion Relationships

The normal lung does a good job of matching ventilation to perfusion (Fig. 3–23). In the bases of the lungs, high blood flow matches ventilation as gravity helps direct pulmonary circulation to the dependent areas of the lung, whereas compression of tissue makes alveoli smaller, more compliant, and easier to ventilate; however, perfusion is greater than ventilation (ventilation/perfusion ratio [$\dot{V}/\dot{Q}$] < 1). At the apices of the lung, the alveoli are stretched to a larger size, reducing their compliance and resulting in reduced ventilation, but the low-pressure pulmonary circulation has a limited ability to pump blood against gravity and reduces perfusion by a greater factor, so that ventilation is greater than perfusion ($\dot{V}/\dot{Q}$ > 1). $\dot{V}/\dot{Q}$ ratios change throughout the lungs (Fig. 3–24). In the middle of the lung, at the level of the third rib, ventilation and perfusion are perfectly matched ($\dot{V}/\dot{Q}$ = 1).

- Dead space is wasted ventilation: $\dot{V} > \dot{Q} = \dot{V}/\dot{Q} > 1 =$ dead space ($\dot{V}D$)
  Absolute $\dot{V}D$, $\dot{V}/\dot{Q}$ approaches infinity ($PaO_2 = 150$ mmHg, $PaCO_2 = 0$ mmHg)
- Shunt is wasted perfusion: $\dot{Q} > \dot{V} = \dot{V}/\dot{Q} < 1 =$ shunt
  Absolute shunt, $\dot{V}/\dot{Q}$ approaches 0 ($PaO_2 = 40$ mmHg, $PaCO_2 = 46$ mmHg)

Table • 3–2 APPROXIMATE NORMAL PRESSURES IN THE HEART AND PULMONARY CIRCUIT

LOCATION	PRESSURE (mmHg)		
	Systolic	Diastolic	Mean
Superior vena cava			6–10
Inferior vena cava			6–10
Right atrium			2–5
Right ventricle	25	0–5	
Pulmonary artery	25	10	
Pulmonary capillary bed			8–12
Left atrium			5–10
Left ventricle	120	0–10	
Aorta	120	80	
Systemic arteriole			30

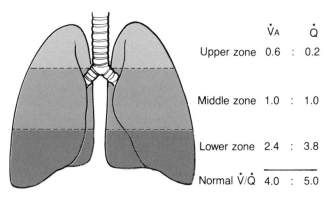

	$\dot{V}A$		$\dot{Q}$
Upper zone	0.6	:	0.2
Middle zone	1.0	:	1.0
Lower zone	2.4	:	3.8
Normal $\dot{V}/\dot{Q}$	4.0	:	5.0

FIGURE 3–23 • $\dot{V}/\dot{Q}$ in different zones of the upright lung showing marked variation in values in different areas. In the upright subject, upper segments are relatively hypoperfused, and $\dot{V}/\dot{Q}$ is high. Lower segments are relatively hypoventilated, and $\dot{V}/\dot{Q}$ is low. (Braun HA, Cheney FW, Loehn CP. *Introduction to Respiratory Physiology,* 2nd ed. Boston: Little, Brown; 1980.)

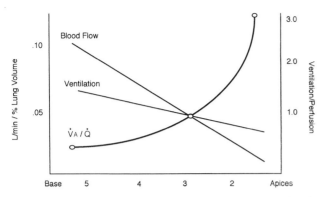

FIGURE 3-24 • Relationship of ventilation and perfusion as well as flow to percentage of lung volume from the base of the lungs to the apices.

- Ideal unit is perfect match of ventilation and perfusion.
- Silent units exist when there is no $\dot{V}$ and no $\dot{Q}$.

The blood leaving the right ventricle of the heart passes through the pulmonary artery and circulates through the lung. The cardiac output, or amount of blood pumped from the heart over time, is expressed in liters per minute. Cardiac output equals the heart's stroke volume times the heart rate.

Not all air entering the airway reaches the respiratory units of the lung and participates in gas exchange. Minute volume is the tidal volume times respiratory frequency per minute. Ventilation without perfusion is called **dead space**. When a breath is taken, a part of the breath reaches the bronchioles. Gas filling the upper airway and conducting airways that does not reach the alveoli and does not participate in gas exchange is called **anatomic dead space**. It is anatomic because it is a normal part of the structure of the airway. Dead space that is secondary to a pathologic process combined with the anatomic dead space is called **physiologic dead space**.

Compensation for Ventilation–Perfusion Mismatching

In the case of dead space, ventilation exceeds perfusion and the level of CO_2 in the airway is decreased. The decreased level of CO_2 (alveolar hypocapnia) increases smooth muscle response, resulting in bronchoconstriction, reducing airway caliber and regional ventilation, and better matching ventilation to the reduced perfusion (Box 3–13).

With shunt, the lack of ventilation results in alveolar hypoxia, stimulating pulmonary vasoconstriction and reducing perfusion (to better match the reduced ventilation; Fig. 3–25).

Diffusion and Gas Transport

Both O_2 and CO_2 move down their pressure gradients: O_2 travels from alveolar air space to pulmonary capillaries, whereas CO_2 moves from the pulmonary blood space to alveolar air spaces. At the tissue level, the direction of gas movement is reversed (Fig. 3–26). Figure 3–27 illustrates

---

Box • 3-13 PATHOPHYSIOLOGIC PERSPECTIVE

$\dot{V}/\dot{Q}$ compensatory mechanisms are so efficient that when there is an acute change in the ventilation–perfusion relationship, the system can adjust to provide normal arterial blood gas values within a few hours. Consequently, when there is a small emboli or blood clot, which reduces blood flow to ventilated areas of the lung (dead space), measures of oxygenation are not effective to quantify the effect of the emboli.

---

the relative gas tension of O_2 and CO_2 in the circulatory system.

Factors Affecting Gas Diffusion

The following factors can affect gas diffusion ($D_{L\,gas}$):

Gas phase: Diffusion of gas through gas ($1/mol$ $weight_{gas}$). Diffusion of gas is affected by low molecular weight of gas and by the relatively short diffusion path from the point of transition from tidal to diffusive ventilation, occurring at the level of the terminal bronchioles.

Membrane phase: Diffusion of gas through the alveolar epithelium and the capillary endothelium membrane ($area_{mem}/thickness_{mem}$). The area of the lung available for gas exchange is about 70 m² (750 ft²), whereas the alveolar epithelium is only 0.1- to 1.0-µm thick.

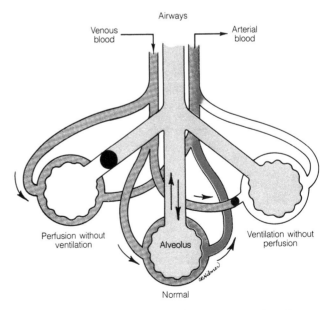

FIGURE 3-25 • Matching of ventilation and perfusion. (*Center*) Normal matching of ventilation and perfusion. (*Left*) Perfusion without ventilation (shunt). (*Right*) Ventilation without perfusion (dead air space).

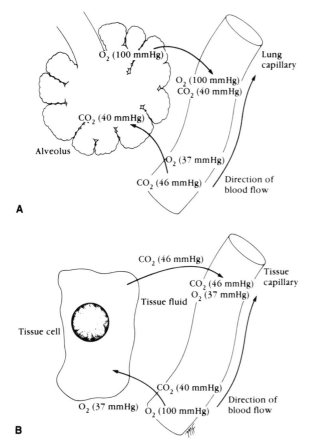

A

B

FIGURE 3-26 • Schematic of gas exchanges at the alveoli (*A*) and at the tissue level (*B*). (Snell RS. *Clinical Histology for Medical Students.* Boston: Little, Brown; 1984.)

Aqueous phase: Interstitial fluid, plasma, and erythrocyte (solubility gas). CO_2 has a higher fluid solubility than O_2; thus, larger volumes of CO_2 can diffuse through fluid with a lower pressure gradient. CO_2 also has a fast reaction with hemoglobin (Hb), allowing large volumes of gas to load and unload at both lung and tissue levels.

Pulmonary capillaries have a typical diameter of 8 μm, whereas red blood cells range in diameter from 5 to 8 μm. Consequently, red blood cells travel single file through the pulmonary capillaries, with little room to spare.

The time required for blood to transit (or cross) the pulmonary circulation is called **transit time** ($T_{transit}$; Fig. 3–28). Normally, the transit time equals pulmonary capillary volume (75 mL) divided by cardiac output (100 mL/s), or 0.75 second.

As short a time as this seems, only 0.25 second is required for gas equilibrium under normal conditions, providing a safety net of an additional 0.5 second for equilibrium to take place. Transit time can decrease with increased cardiac output or with decreased pulmonary volume. Anything that affects diffusion of gas through the respiratory membrane, such as increased thickness, can affect the time required for gas equilibrium. When the time required for gas equilibrium is greater than transit time, hypoxemia results. Hypoxemia is seen well before hypercarbia because of the faster movement of CO_2 across the alveolar capillary membrane (Box 3–14).

Shunt

Shunt occurs when perfusion is greater than ventilation. **Anatomic shunt** is the normal venous admixture that occurs because of the structure of the system. A prime exam-

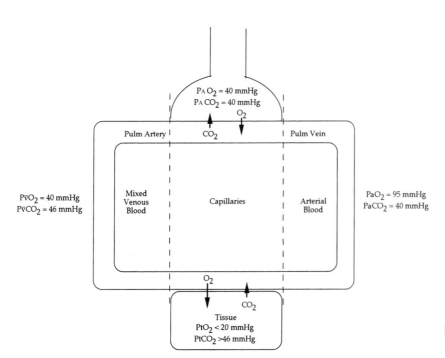

FIGURE 3-27 • The cascade of O_2 and CO_2 across the circulatory system.

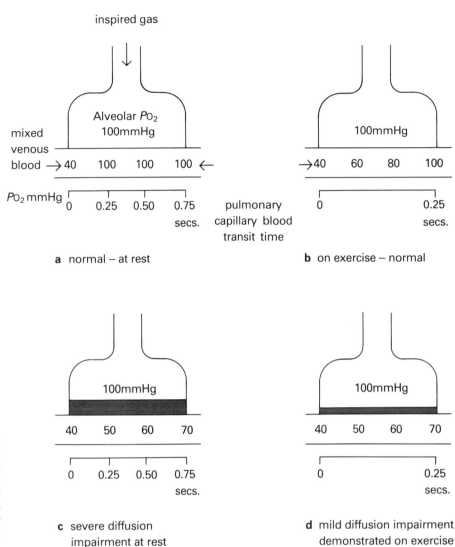

inspired gas

Alveolar P_{O_2}
100mmHg

mixed venous blood → 40   100   100   100 ←

P_{O_2} mmHg   0   0.25   0.50   0.75
secs.

pulmonary capillary blood transit time

100mmHg

→40   60   80   100 ←

0   0.25
secs.

a normal – at rest

b on exercise – normal

100mmHg

40   50   60   70

0   0.25   0.50   0.75
secs.

100mmHg

40   50   60   70

0   0.25
secs.

c severe diffusion impairment at rest

d mild diffusion impairment demonstrated on exercise

⎯⎯ thickened alveolar capillary membrane

FIGURE 3–28 • Gas diffusion across the alveolar–capillary membrane and the effect of transit time across the pulmonary capillaries in a healthy subject at rest (*A*) and with exercise (*B*), in a patient with a severe diffusion defect at rest (*C*), and in a patient with a mild defect with exercise (*D*). (*Color Atlas of Respiratory Disease*. St. Louis: Gower. F10.5.)

ple of shunt is venous blood from the thebesian and bronchial circulation bypassing the lung and mixing in with the oxygenated blood returning from the lung to the heart (Box 3–15). In addition, a small quantity of the venous blood returning from the coronary circulation mixes directly with the arterialized blood. This anatomic shunt is normally 2% to 4% of the cardiac output.

Gas Transport in the Blood

OXYGEN TRANSPORT

Only a small quantity of O_2 is capable of being dissolved directly in blood plasma. Oxygen has relatively low solubility in blood, so that O_2 content dissolved in plasma is low. In fact, only 0.003 mL/dL of oxygen can dissolve in plasma for each 1 mmHg of PO_2. Consequently, with a PaO_2 of 100 mmHg, there is only 0.3 mL of O_2 in each 100 mL of plasma.

The major mechanism of transporting oxygen in the blood is as HbO_2. Hb is the respiratory pigment turning red when bound with O_2. Oxygen binds covalently and reversibly with Hb contained within the red blood cells. A maximum of four molecules of oxygen can bind to the four Fe^{2+} sites on an Hb molecule. The Hb generally transports oxygen without oxidizing the ferrous Fe^{2+} sites to the ferric Fe^{3+} state. Oxidized Hb, or **met Hb**, does not effectively transport oxygen.

The oxygen capacity of Hb is 1.34 mL O_2/g of Hb. With a normal 15 g of Hb/dL$_{blood}$, the oxygen capacity is 1.34 mL O_2/g of Hb × 15 g of Hb/dL$_{blood}$ = 20.1 mL O_2/dL$_{blood}$. Oxygen content is the sum of the O_2 carried by the Hb and the O_2 dissolved in the plasma.

The amount of oxygen carried by Hb is a curvilinear function of PO_2 described by the oxyhemoglobin dissociation curve (Fig. 3–29). The P_{50} is the PO_2 corresponding to 50% saturation of Hb (normally for adults at 27 mmHg).

Box • 3–14   PATHOPHYSIOLOGIC PERSPECTIVE

ARTERIAL HYPOXEMIA

Hypoventilation

Decreased alveolar ventilation leads to decreased PaO_2 and oxygen content (CaO_2), with no change in the alveolar–arterial gradient. This is often associated with nervous system defects (central nervous system and neuromuscular junction) and with toxic drug effects suppressing ventilation. Treatment options include respiratory stimulants and mechanical ventilation.

Diffusion Impairment

Decreased DLO_2 leads to decreased PaO_2 and CaO_2, with an increased alveolar–arterial gradient. This is associated with interstitial diseases, such as fibrosis and pneumonia, and with increasing thickness of the alveolar capillary membrane. Another process is alveolar flooding with pulmonary edema, which reduces the surface area available for gas diffusion. Treatment of diffusion impairment includes increasing the alveolar oxygen levels with administration of oxygen. Ironically, the administration of high concentrations of oxygen with FIO_2 levels of greater than 60%, for more than 24 hours, has been associated with increased pulmonary capillary permeability, alveolar edema, and even interstitial fibrosis and decreased lung compliance.

The oxyhemoglobin dissociation curve shifts to the left or right in response to changes in the body. A shift to the right can be caused by increases in PCO_2 (called the **Bohr effect**); H^+; temperature; and 2,3-diphosphoglycerate (2,3-DPG), with chronic hypoxia. A shift to the right means a decrease in affinity for oxygen and an increase in P_{50}. This shift means that the Hb will unload greater amounts of oxygen at sites at which the tissue needs oxygen the most. The more the tissue uses O_2, the more CO_2 and H^+ that is produced, and the more O_2 that is released from the Hb. This shift is the mechanism to ensure that the oxygen is easier to deliver where it is needed the most (Fig. 3–30).

A shift to the left is caused by decreases in PCO_2; H^+; temperature; 2,3-DPG, with chronic hypoxia; carboxyhe-

Box • 3–15   VENTILATION AND PERFUSION INEQUALITY

Decreased $\dot{V}/\dot{Q}$ ratio results in decreased PaO_2 and decreased CaO_2. These inequities are found acutely with pulmonary embolism and chronically with emphysema and chronic bronchitis.

CRITICAL THINKING CHALLENGES

Go Figure

A patient has an Hb content of 22 g, PaO_2 of 58 mmHg, SaO_2 of 89%, $P\overline{v}O_2$ of 40 mmHg, and $S\overline{v}O_2$ of 74%. What is the minute oxygen consumption?

---

moglobin; and fetal Hb. The shift to the left improves loading of oxygen by Hb while reducing delivery of oxygen to tissue, often in response to reduced metabolic requirements.

Oxygen content (CaO_2) is the Hb saturation (%) times the O_2 capacity.

CaO_2 minus $C\overline{v}O_2$ (mL O_2/dL_{blood}) represents the oxygen consumption of the body.

CARBON DIOXIDE TRANSPORT

Carbon dioxide is transported by the blood in three forms (Fig. 3–31), as follows:

- *Dissolved* (10%): As described by Henry's law, there is a linear relationship between PCO_2 and CO_2 dissolved in blood. The solubility of CO_2 (0.06 mL CO_2/dL_{blood} per mmHg) is 20 times greater than O_2 solubility.
- *Carbamino compounds* (22%): CO_2 joins reversibly with nonionized terminal amino groups (NH_2^-) of blood-borne proteins and Hb.
- *Bicarbonate ion formation* (68%): Most CO_2 is transported as bicarbonate ion, formed from the CO_2 hy-

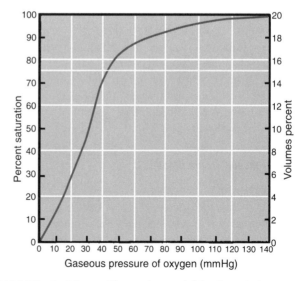

FIGURE 3–29 • The oxyhemoglobin dissociation curve.

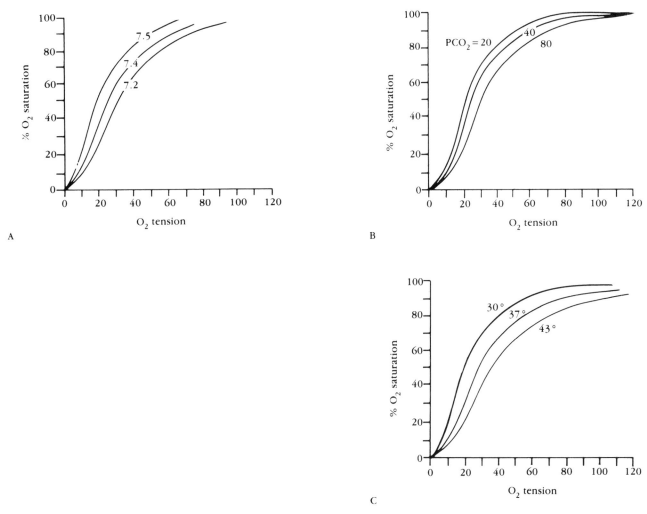

FIGURE 3-30 • Effects of (*A*) pH, (*B*) PCO_2, and (*C*) temperature on the oxyhemoglobin dissociation curve.

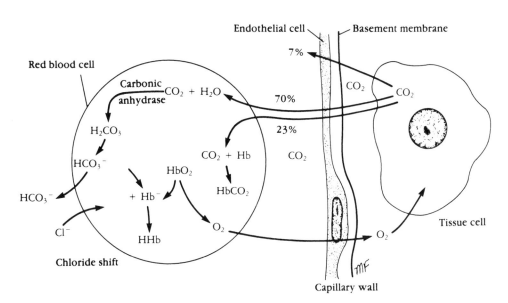

FIGURE 3-31 • Methods of CO_2 transport in the blood. (Snell RS. *Clinical Histology for Medical Students.* Boston: Little, Brown; 1984.)

dration reaction accelerated by carbonic anhydrase, found in the red blood cell:

$$CO_2 + H_2O \rightarrow H_2CO_3 \rightarrow H^+ + HCO_3^-$$

Plasma reactions are only 10% owing to the lack of carbonic anhydrase, which is found primarily in the red blood cells.

Carbon dioxide is produced by tissue metabolism and travels from tissue space to capillary blood by following the pressure gradient. A rapid hydration of CO_2 produces a high concentration of HCO_3 in the red blood cells, which then follows its concentration gradient to the plasma. The movement of HCO_3 creates a net positive charge in red blood cells. H^+ cannot move across the membrane (cation barrier), so Cl^- moves into the red blood cells. Not entirely buffered, H^+ ions accumulate in the red blood cells, creating a fall in pH below plasma level. The reaction leads to increased red blood cell osmolarity, with water moving into red blood cells, causing them to swell on the venous side of the circulation.

Partial intracellular buffering of H^+ drives O_2 from the Hb, allowing O_2 to move down its pressure gradient from blood to tissue.

Alveolar ventilation $[\dot{V}_A = f \times (\dot{V}_T - \dot{V}_D)]$ is the amount of ventilation that reaches the respiratory zone each minute. PaO_2 is directly related to $\dot{V}_A$, whereas mean $PaCO_2$ inversely relates $(1/\dot{V}_A)$ to alveolar ventilation. Hyperventilation occurs when $\dot{V}_A$ is increased above metabolic demand, resulting in increased PaO_2 and decreased $PaCO_2$. Hypoventilation occurs when $\dot{V}_A$ decreases below metabolic demand, resulting in reduced PaO_2 and increased $PaCO_2$.

It is possible to make changes in blood CO_2 without making large changes in oxygen content of the blood. This is important for acid and base regulation in both health and disease states.

Dissociation Curve for Carbon Dioxide. The presence of O_2 decreases the affinity of Hb for CO_2 (Haldane effect), shifting the CO_2 dissociation curve to the right (Fig. 3–32). At oxygen levels of normal arterial blood, the CO_2 curve is shifted down and to the right, whereas normal venous oxygen tensions shift the CO_2 curve up and to the left.

NEURAL CONTROL OF BREATHING

In normal awake humans at rest, respiration is governed by automatic control structures in the brainstem and voluntary control structures in the cerebral cortex (Fig. 3–33). One of the great factors in breathing is being awake.

The **respiratory central controller** in the brainstem determines basic rhythm generation (frequency of breathing) and pattern generation (volume of breathing). Unlike the heart, respiratory muscles have no automaticity.

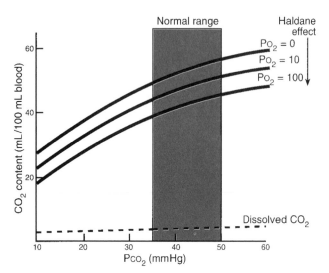

FIGURE 3-32 • CO_2 dissociation curve. (Rhoades RA, Tanner GA. *Medical Physiology*. Boston: Little, Brown; 1995.)

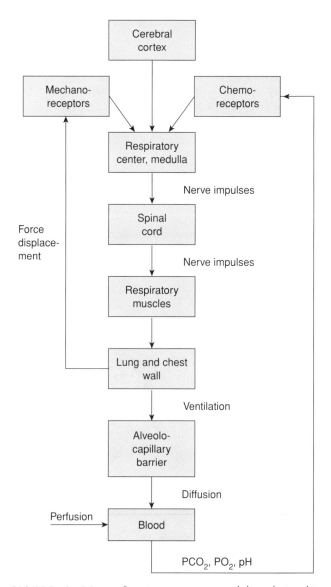

FIGURE 3-33 • Respiratory center and the relationship of key elements in neural control of breathing. (Berne. *Principles of Physiology*, 2nd ed. St. Louis: Mosby, 1996.)

Two major groups of respiratory neurons are found in the medullary center. The dorsal respiratory group includes the nucleus tractus solitarius and is located dorsomedially in the medulla. The phasic I_A alpha activated phrenic motoneurons set tidal volume, whereas phasic I_B beta neurons integrate vagal afferents from the lungs.

The ventral respiratory group is located ventrolaterally on the medulla and contains inspiratory and expiratory neurons whose output transmits to the spinal respiratory motor neurons for intercostal, abdominal, and phrenic innervation.

Cortical Modulation

Afferent sensory stimulation (being awake) overrides many of the automatic respiratory centers. Voluntary control of breathing is seen with maneuvers such as talking, coughing, singing, hyperventilation, hyperinflation, and breath holding (Box 3–16). During sleep, the automatic centers take over, controlling respiratory rate and volume.

Respiratory Effectors

Nerve impulses in efferent pathways elicit respiratory muscle contractions and changes in volume. Respiratory outputs are determined in terms of total ventilation ($V_T \times f$) and alveolar ventilation ($V_T - V_D$) $\times$ f. We also monitor $PaCO_2$, normally regulated at 40 mmHg, and PaO_2, regulated at about 95 mmHg.

Respiratory sensors include mechanoreceptors and chemoreceptors. Mechanoreceptors include lung volume and airflow, airway and muscle stretch, and motion of joints. Chemoreceptors monitor low PaO_2 (less than 70 mmHg) in the carotid arch and high $PaCO_2$ (more than 35 mmHg) in the lateral walls of the medulla, monitoring cerebral spinal fluid.

Mechanoreflexes

Vagal Reflexes From the Lungs

The lung's vagal reflexes include the following:

Pulmonary stretch receptors: Slow-adapting receptors found in nerve filaments in smooth muscles of the trachea and bronchi. These receptors act as a static volume detector stimulated by lung inflation, terminating inspiration (Hering-Breuer reflex).

Irritant receptors: Rapidly adapting receptors found in the epithelium of the larynx, trachea, and extrapulmonary bronchi. These receptors are stimulated by noxious irritants, distortion of larynx, large lung inflations, and deflations and with pneumothorax, resulting in cough, hyperventilation, and bronchoconstriction.

C-fiber pulmonary receptors are located in the unmyelinated fibers in the alveolar wall and are stimulated by vascular engorgement and interstitial edema fluid formation, with reflex responses of rapid shallow breathing, large airway constriction and bradycardia. C-fiber bronchial receptors located in the blood vessel walls of the bronchial circulation are also stimulated by vascular congestion, chemical injury, and microemboli. Reflex responses are similar to the pulmonary C-fiber with a sensation of dyspnea.

Reflexes From the Upper Airways

Nasal passage receptors are located in the nose, innervated by the trigeminal nerve. These receptors are stimulated by mechanical or chemical irritation, causing sneezing and bradycardia.

Larynx and tracheobronchial receptors are located in the upper airways, innervated by the vagus and superior laryngeal nerve. Mechanical or chemical irritation stimulates cough and wide swings in blood pressure (such as those found with the Valsalva maneuver) .

Pharynx receptors are found in the walls of the common food-carrying areas, innervated by the vagus and glossopharyngeal nerves. These receptors are stimulated by the peristaltic wave associated with swallowing, which results in the closure of the glottis.

Other reflexes that have not been identified with a point of origin include reflexes responsible for sighing, yawning, and hiccuping.

Spinal Cord Reflexes

Muscle spindle receptors found in the intercostal musculature are innervated by the somatic afferents to thoracic spinal cord. They are stimulated by low total compliance, resulting in compensatory increase in respiratory muscle activation (to overcome the low compliance).

Pain receptors are located in bare nerve endings in the viscera, muscles, and bone, innervated by visceral and somatic afferents. The stimulation of pain receptors by ischemia and bodily injury results in gasping, excited breathing, hypoventilation, and even apnea.

Joint receptors located in the legs, arms, and feet are stimulated by joint motion in exercise and result in increased frequency and volume of breathing.

Box • 3–16 RESPIRATORY CORTICAL INFLUENCES

Cortical modulation of respiration includes the following effects:

Phonation and articulation
Maximum voluntary ventilation
Voluntary breath holding
Central hypoventilation syndrome (Ondine's curse)

Chemoreflexes and Breathing

Location of Chemoreceptors

Chemoreceptors are located on the arterial side of the circulation and respond to either oxygen, carbon dioxide, or pH. Chemoreceptors do not sense the venous blood or the airway. Chemoreceptor afferents project to respiratory neurons of the dorsal and ventral respiratory groups. Peripheral chemoreceptors are located in aortic and carotid bodies, sensing decreases in PaO_2 and, secondarily, increases in $PaCO_2$. Central chemoreceptors found in the ventrolateral medulla sense increases in $PaCO_2$.

Carbon Dioxide Response Curve

Carbon dioxide response is typically seen as a change in minute volume. Minute volume will change in response to inspired $PiCO_2$. When breathing between 5% and 8% carbon dioxide in inspired gas, there is an increase of 6 L/min per 1% CO_2. Sensitivity to CO_2 decreases in sleep and in the presence of drugs. Maximum response to CO_2 is about 60% of maximum voluntary ventilation.

Oxygen Response Curve

Minute volume is a hyperbolic function of inspired PiO_2 (mmHg). When the PaO_2 is less than 70 mmHg (O_2 response threshold), minute volume response is more sensitive. Hypoxic response is accentuated by increases in $PaCO_2$.

Breathing Patterns

Apneustic Breathing

Sustained inspiratory breath holds, punctuated by brief expirations, are often attributed to brain-stem pathology or trauma. This is an ominous breathing pattern associated with terminal patients.

Cheyne-Stokes Breathing

Waxing and waning of ventilation, with periods of apnea between cycles, result in alternating phases of hyperventilation and hypoventilation and are attributed to brain-stem pathology or trauma or to low cardiac output.

Sleep-Related Breathing Disorders

CENTRAL SLEEP APNEA
Central respiratory controller problems are associated with effort to breath during sleep (also referred to as Ondine's curse).

Obstructive sleep apnea is caused by transient obstruction of the airway during sleep. Unlike central apnea, there is a strong or undiminished respiratory effort, seen as changes in pleural pressure (Fig. 3–34).

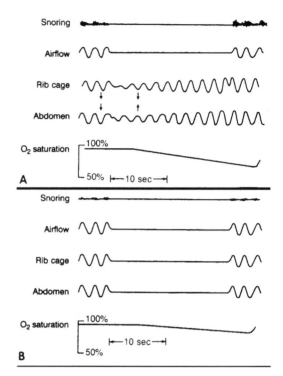

FIGURE 3–34 • Types of sleep apnea. (*A*) Obstructive apnea. This is characterized by loud intermittent snoring, complete cessation of airflow, paradoxical movement of the chest and abdomen, and moderate to severe oxygen desaturation. (*B*) Central apnea. The features are simultaneous cessation of airflow and respiratory effort and mild to moderate oxygen desaturation.

MECHANICS OF THE LUNG

The lung is an elastic structure that changes shape and volume during the respiratory cycle, creating a mechanical pump, allowing for movement of air. The lung also surrounds and protects the heart (something like "bubble wrap" used for packing valuables).

The alveoli are the functional units of the lung, where gas exchange occurs between air and blood spaces. The alveoli are the most flexible structures in the lungs. The larger the airway in the lung, the stiffer and less flexible the tissue. Cyclical changes in lung volume flush gas in and out of the lungs, bringing gas to the level of the terminal bronchioles, from which the gas moves to and from the alveoli by diffusion.

Thoracic Cage

The thoracic rib cage, consisting of the spine, ribs, and sternum, provides a relatively stiff structure that not only determines the shape and volume of the lung but also helps to protect the lung from injury (Figs. 3–35 and 3–36). The thorax has been described as a truncated cone with ends inclined anteriorly so that the posterior (spine) portion is longer than the anterior (sternum). The curved shape of the ribs provides great structural strength to resist external

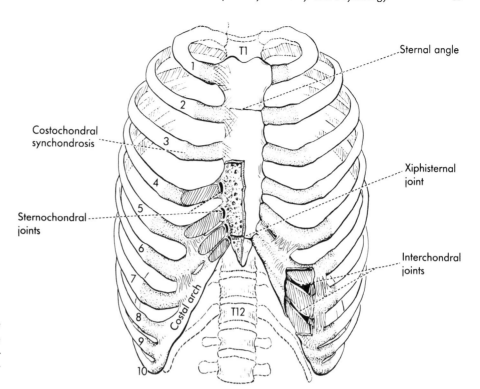

FIGURE 3–35 • Anterior view of the skeleton of the thorax. (Rosse C. *Hollinshead's Textbook of Anatomy,* 5th ed. Philadelphia: Lippincott-Raven Publishers, 1997.)

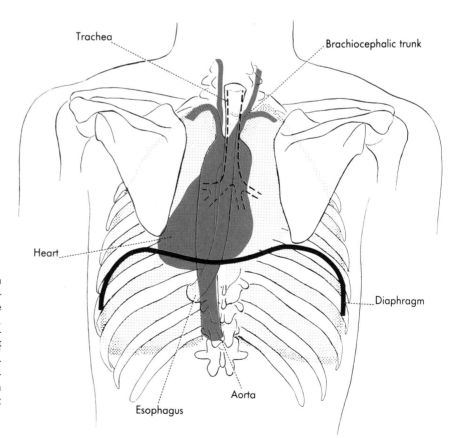

FIGURE 3–36 • The thorax seen from behind. The bulky shoulders obscure a relatively small rib cage; the diaphragm rises high up into the chest. The pleural cavities, which extend over the posterior surface of the domes of the diaphragm, are indicated by stippled areas; the heart and great arteries in the mediastinum are shown in pink. (Rosse C. *Hollinshead's Textbook of Anatomy,* 5th ed. Philadelphia: Lippincott-Raven Publishers, 1997.)

compression of the thorax. The ribs also have a limited range of movement from their insertion points at the spine and sternum, to which they are connected by cartilage and ligaments. This movement has been described as "bucket handles." The ribs move up and out on inspiration, expanding the volume of the thorax, and down and in on expiration, reducing lung volume.

In addition to providing structural strength and protection of the thoracic contents, the chest wall has an elastic component that is a function of the shape of the chest wall structures and their composition (calcification, elastin, and collagen of the ribs). The connective tissue in the chest wall stores mechanical energy, allowing the thorax to spring back into position.

The expansion of the chest wall by respiratory muscles reduces the pressure of air in the lungs, creating a pressure differential that draws air into the lungs until the pressures are equalized. With relaxation of the respiratory muscles, the elastic recoil of the lung and chest wall compresses the air in the lung, creating a pressure that is higher than atmospheric pressure and pushing air out of the lungs.

Muscles of Respiration

The muscles of breathing determine the shape of the thoracic cage through cyclical contraction and relaxation. Inspiration requires active work, whereas expiration, under normal quiet conditions, is passive. These skeletal muscles have no autorhythmicity and no basal tone.

Inspiratory muscles include the diaphragm, the external intercostals, the scalenes, and the sternomastoids (Fig. 3–37). Expiratory muscles, which include the internal intercostals and the muscles of the abdominal wall, are called into play under stress, in response to increased metabolic needs, and to compensate for disease.

The diaphragm is the primary muscle of inspiration, causing active increases in lung volume. The diaphragm is a dome-shaped muscle composed of two hemidiaphragms attached at midline and separating the thorax from the abdomen. When the diaphragm contracts, it flattens, decreasing the intrapleural pressure, decreasing the intrapulmonary pressure, and activating the thoracic pump to draw ambient air into the lungs. To contract, the flattening diaphragm displaces abdominal contents, pushing them down, and distending the abdomen outward; this, in turn, elevates and increases the diameter of the lower ribs (Fig. 3–38).

The secondary muscles of inspiration are used with high levels of ventilatory demands or with diseases that hyperinflate the lungs (such as emphysema). The external intercostals, the sternocleidomastoids, and scalenes contract to pull ribs up and out, increase the anteroposterior diameter of the thorax, and increase thoracic volume.

Respiratory muscles can voluntarily increase minute volume from normal levels of 6 L/min up to 100 L/min for short periods of time. Minute volumes of 30 to 40 L/min are not uncommon during sustained vigorous exercise. Fatigue occurs when energy supply is exceeded by metabolic load. Causes of fatigue include increased ventilation demands, inadequate energy generation by the muscles, and increased work of breathing.

Generally, the body responds to increased ventilatory demand with increased circulation of arterial blood to the muscles (Box 3–17).

Dyspnea is the major complaint when the respiratory muscles become fatigued. Clinical signs include increased respiratory rate, rapid shallow breathing, and an early fall in $Paco_2$.

As muscular fatigue progresses, diaphragm movement reduces, and the accessory muscles have to take over (respiratory alternans) and work even harder. Paradoxical res-

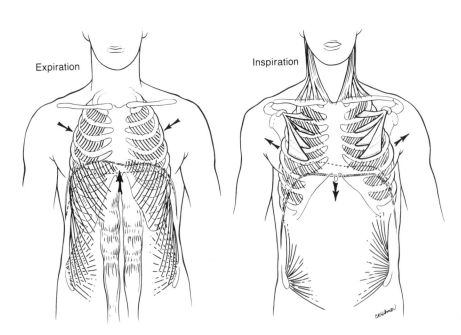

FIGURE 3–37 • Respiratory muscles of inspiration and expiration.

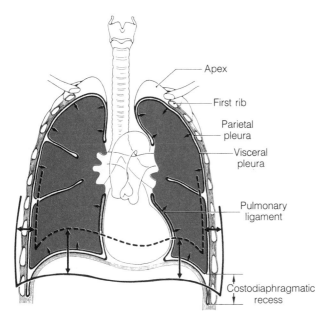

FIGURE 3–38 • Frontal section of the chest showing the location of the chest cage, lungs, mediastinum, and diaphragm. The dotted lines and arrows indicate the descent of the diaphragm during inspiration and the recoil during expiration. (Fishman AP. *Assessment of Pulmonary Function.* New York: McGraw-Hill; 1980. Reproduced with permission of The McGraw-Hill Companies.)

piration occurs when the diaphragm is severely fatigued and the negative pressure created by the accessory muscles pulls up the flaccid diaphragm on inspiration, causing the abdomen to move inward (instead of out) on inspiration.

Finally, there is a decrease in tidal volume, respiratory rate, and minute volume, accompanied by hypoventilation and respiratory acidosis.

Inspiration is an active process, with contraction of the inspiratory muscles, which increases the volume of the chest, decreasing pleural pressure, and with increasing lung volume, which decreases alveolar pressure, drawing air into lungs above functional residual capacity (Fig. 3–39).

During quiet breathing, expiration results from passive recoil of the lungs and thorax. Expiratory muscles cause active decreases in lung volume and include the internal in-

Box • 3–17 PATHOPHYSIOLOGIC PERSPECTIVE

Hyperinflation (found with emphysema and some asthma attacks) flattens the diaphragm, making muscular contraction less effective in pumping air into the lungs. With severe hyperinflation, diaphragmatic contraction may actually pull in the lower ribs, causing an expiratory effect on the thorax. In such cases, the total work of ventilation defaults to the secondary muscles of inspiration.

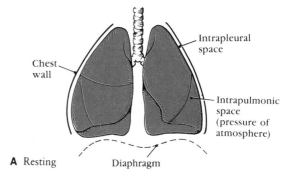

A Resting

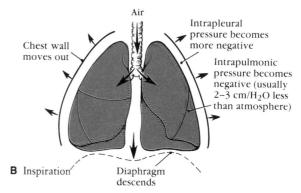

B Inspiration

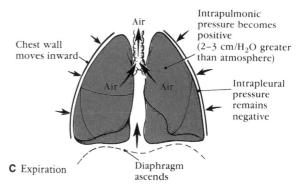

C Expiration

FIGURE 3–39 • Phases of ventilation. (*A*) No movement of air (resting). (*B*) Air moves from the environment to the intrapulmonic space (inspiration). (*C*) Air moves from the intrapulmonic space to the environment (expiration).

tercostals, which pull ribs down from the horizontal to reduce thoracic volume, and the abdominal muscles (rectus abdominis, external and internal obliques, and transversus abdominis), which depress the lower ribs while compressing the abdominal contents to push up the diaphragm from below.

Lung Volumes and Capacities

The air spaces within the lung are classified in terms of four lung volumes that do not overlap. These volumes are then used to define four lung capacities that do overlap.

The tidal volume (V_T) is the normal volume of normal, quiet breathing. For most adults, the V_T is about 500 mL. Inspiratory reserve volume is the additional volume of gas that can be inhaled above the V_T and may be as great as

RESIDUAL VOLUME MEASUREMENT

Because the residual volume always remains in the lungs and cannot be exhaled, indirect means are required to measure the residual volume and any of the capacities that include the residual volume. These methods include body plethysmography, nitrogen washout, helium dilution, and radiographic estimates of volume.

3000 mL. Expiratory reserve volume is the amount of air that can be exhaled below the V_T. These three volumes can be measured directly during inspiration or expiration with a device called a spirometer. The residual volume is the quantity of air that remains in the lung after a maximal expiration, which cannot be exhaled without collapsing the lung (Box 3–18 and Fig. 3–40).

Lung zones are used to describe the relative role of gas in the lungs. The conducting zone is the volume of gas that fills the airways down through the terminal bronchioles. This volume of gas is also known as dead space and is about 150 mL in adults. The respiratory zone, or "live" space, is the volume of gas filling the respiratory bronchioles and acini, available to participate in active gas exchange (respiration). The transitory zone is a mix of dead and live space, which varies based on changes in ventilation, perfusion, position, and disease states.

$$\text{Ventilation} = \text{volume} \times \text{frequency}$$

$$\dot{V}_D = f \times V_D$$

$$\dot{V}_A = f \times V_A = f \times (V_T - V_D)$$

$$\dot{V}_E = \dot{V}_D + \dot{V}_A$$

There are four types of dead space (V_D). Anatomic dead space ($V_{D_{anat}}$) is the gas in the structures of the conducting airways. Alveolar dead space ($V_{D_{alv}}$) is gas in alveoli that are not perfused by the pulmonary circulation and not actively participating in gas exchange. Physiologic dead space ($V_{D_{phys}}$) is the total volume of dead space, including $V_{D_{anat}}$ and $V_{D_{alv}}$. Instrumental dead space ($V_{D_{inst}}$) is the volume of external tubing that is connected to the patient's airway through which two-way gas flow occurs.

Pleura

The pleura are serous membranes lined on their free surfaces with a single layer of mesothelium that covers the lung (visceral pleura) and lines the chest wall, diaphragm, and mediastinum (parietal pleura). The subserous layer of the pleura contains elastic tissue, blood vessels, lymphatics, and nerve fibers. The pleura are airtight and both separate and connect the lungs with the thoracic cavity structures. There is about 15 to 50 mL of pleural fluid between the two pleura, and no air. This fluid lubricates the pleura, allowing them to move with minimal friction, and creates the surface tension between the pleural surfaces that allows the thoracic cage to pull the lung open while the lung pulls in the rib cage. This interface creates an intrapleural pressure that is subatmospheric, usually about 4 cm H_2O. This pressure is greater at the top of the lung and less in the gravity-dependent areas.

The fall in pleural pressure during inspiration helps to suck open the vena cavae and right atria, aiding venous re-

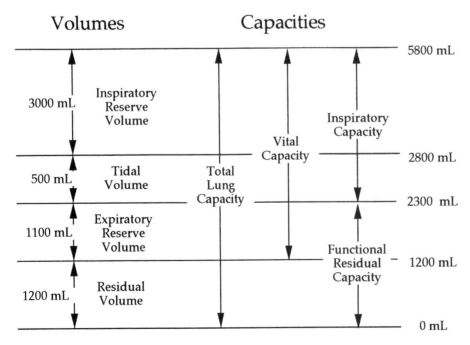

FIGURE 3–40 • Lung volumes and capacities.

turn to the heart. This pressure also helps the lymphatic system drain to the thoracic duct.

The bronchial arteries supply blood to the visceral pleura, whereas venous blood returns through the pulmonary venous system. The internal and intercostal mammary arteries supply the parietal pleura, with return through corresponding veins. The lymphatics of the pleura are integral to the lungs and thoracic cage. The visceral pleura are innervated from the autonomic pulmonary plexus, and the parietal pleura are supplied by the intercostal nerves. The parietal pleura have many pain fibers, which may produce sharp pains on irritation.

Pressure–Volume Relationships

Intrapleural pressure (P_{pl}) is the negative (subatmospheric) pressure created by opposing forces attempting to expand intrapleural space. The lung and chest wall are elastic structures with different equilibrium positions. The lung is constantly trying to become smaller, whereas the chest wall is trying to expand. The surface tension between the two pleurae join the surfaces of the two structures, so that at functional residual capacity, the chest wall expands the lung, and the lung pulls the chest wall in.

Alveolar pressure (P_{alv}) is the pressure in the alveolar space when the airway is patent to the atmosphere (P_{atm}).

When P_{alv} is less than P_{atm}, air flows into the lung. When P_{alv} is more than P_{atm}, air flows out of the lung. The greater the difference in the pressures, the greater the magnitude of airflow, usually expressed in liters per second.

Pulmonic pressure (P_{pul}) is the pressure in the larger central airways between the alveoli and the atmosphere. Changes in P_{pul} are similar but of a lesser magnitude than changes in P_{alv}. Airflow occurs with dynamic changes in P_{pl}. During a normal respiratory cycle, dynamic phases occur at 1 and 3 seconds, whereas there is no flow (static) at 0, 2, and 4 seconds. Airflow occurs only with a P_{atm}–P_{pl} gradient.

Work of Breathing

Three major components of work are elastic, frictional, and inertial work (Fig. 3–41). Elastic work is the work required to overcome the elastic recoil from lung, the displacement of the thoracic cage, and abdominal organ displacement.

Airflow resistance is the greatest single factor in frictional work, with viscous resistance (eg, friction of the lobes) and pleural friction posing secondary issues.

Inertial work is required to overcome changes in acceleration and deceleration of air and in chest wall and lung. These factors are negligible.

$$\text{Work} = \text{force} \times \text{distance pressure} \times \text{volume} \div 2$$

With this formula, no matter how much pressure is applied, if there is no distance, there is no work. In Figure 3–41, the area of the shaded triangle is the elastic work; the area of the lower semicircle is the resistive work during inspiration; and the area of the upper semicircle is the resistive work during expiration. Total work is associated with both elastic work and inspiratory flow-resistive work.

CRITICAL THINKING CHALLENGES
Case Scenario

There is normally no air within the chest outside of the lung. When there is air in the pleural space, the lung tends to collapse to its normal contracted size, and the rib cage tends to expand, creating a pneumothorax. When there is an abnormal volume of fluid in the pleural space, the lung is displaced by fluid, and the pressure–volume relationship may be compromised.

Pneumothorax occurs when gas accumulates in the pleural space. Pleural effusion is fluid in the pleural space. In both cases, the increasing volume of gas or fluid separates the pleura, making the pleural pressure less negative. The result is that the opposing force of the chest wall is not communicated to the lung, and the lung tends to collapse, creating atelectasis.

If the gas in the pleural space accumulates to the point of creating positive pressure, the lung is actively compressed (tension pneumothorax). As pressure builds, the affected lung first collapses and is then pushed toward the unaffected side, shifting the trachea and rotating the mediastinum. This is a life-threatening condition that can be alleviated by creating a path for air to escape the pleural space.

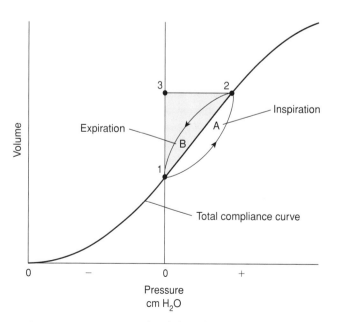

FIGURE 3–41 • Work of breathing. (Kacmarek RM. *Respir Care.* 1988; 33:99–120.)

Elastance is defined as the ability of the lung to resist change in shape and the ability to return to the original shape after having been deformed. A steel bar is more elastic than a balloon. The lung acts as an elastic structure that resists volume change and returns to prechange volumes. The elastic properties in the lung are associated with elastin, collagen, and surface tension forces at the alveoli. The elastance of the lung and chest wall represent the total elastance of the pulmonary system.

Surface tension is created by the contraction of molecules on the surface of gas–liquid interfaces. The greater the attraction between molecules, the smaller the surface area. This surface tension of water creates a skin on which one can float a steel needle. It is this same surface tension that causes bubbles to take the smallest surface area.

Detergents decrease surface tension by reducing the cohesive forces between molecules. Surface tension at the alveolar level effects alveoli size and volume.

Figure 3–42 shows that because the surface area of the alveoli (lung volume) is the smallest, the molecules at the air–blood surface are the closest together, requiring greater pressure to expand the lung. As the surface area increases, the attractive forces between the molecules are reduced, and the larger changes in lung volume require less change in pressure.

Pulmonary surfactant is created by the alveolar type II pneumocytes. These phospholipids float on the alveolar

Box • 3–19 PATHOPHYSIOLOGIC PERSPECTIVE

Lack of surfactant results in alveolar collapse (atelectasis). Prematurity at birth is associated with insufficient surfactant levels in the lung to maintain stable alveoli during the respiratory cycle, resulting in extreme increases in work of breathing. Any condition in which the lung stops producing surfactant or in which the surfactant is denatured or washed out results in unstable alveoli that tend to collapse on exhalation. Application of positive pressure during the expiratory cycle is often used to splint open the alveoli to prevent collapse. The pressure at which the alveoli remain open during expiration is the *lower inflection point.*

epithelium, which exerts a detergent action, reducing cohesive forces, decreasing overall elastance of the lung, reducing opening pressures of the alveoli, and allowing alveoli of differing sizes to be connected, without emptying from the small unit to the larger one (Box 3–19).

Compliance is the reciprocal of elastance ($C = 1/E$), or the ability to change shape in response to applied force. The balloon is more compliant than the steel bar. For the pulmonary system, compliance is a change in volume for a change in pressure. There are three types of pulmonary compliance: chest wall ($C_{\text{chest wall}}$), lung (C_{lung}), and the combination of the chest wall and lung (C_{total}). Figure 3–43 shows the three compliance curves (change in volume versus change in pressure).

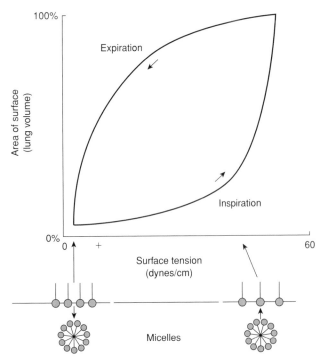

FIGURE 3–42 • Surface tension and the effect on lung volume. (From *Physiology of Respiration* by Michael D. Hlastala and Albert J. Berger. Copyright © 1996 by Oxford University Press, Inc. Used by permission of Oxford University Press, Inc.)

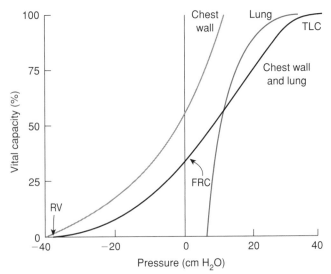

FIGURE 3–43 • Pulmonary compliance, change in volume per change in pressure, for the chest wall, lung, and the combination. (TLC, total lung capacity.) (Murray. *Normal Lung,* 2nd ed. Philadelphia: WB Saunders, 1986.)

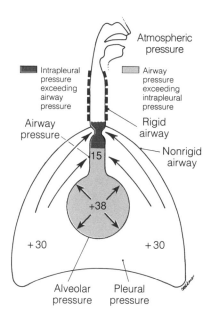

F I G U R E 3 – 4 4 • Mechanisms that limit maximal expiratory flow rate.

Airflow

The cross-sectional area of the airways increases exponentially with each generation, whereas forward airflow velocity decreases.

Flow (mL/s) = velocity [sectional area (cm²) × (mL/cm³)]

Reynold's number (N_R) = (density × mean velocity × diameter) ÷ viscosity

Turbulent flow for air exists when N_R is more than 3000, typically in the first 6 generations of the airway. Laminar flow exists with an N_R that is less than 2000, which is normally found from generations 7 through 17. Diffusive flow with cardiogenic mixing has an N_R of 0 for the peripheral airways from generations 18 through 23.

Airway resistance decreases with each generation of the airway (after the first 5 generations) down to the terminal bronchioles.

Resistance decreases with increases in lung volume. Stretching airways with increased lung volumes increases the radii of the airways, reducing resistance. Half of the resistive work of breathing is generated in the nose. The next greatest source of resistance is in the first 5 generations of the airway.

Dynamic Compression of the Airways

During active forced expiration, $P_{pleural}$ can exceed P_{airway}, creating compression of the airway and decreasing the ra-

dius, normally with no change in airflow (Fig. 3–44). Compression occurs first in the smaller, cartilage-free airways, at the equal pressure point (Box 3–20).

Restrictive and Obstructive Diseases Increase Work of Breathing

Restrictive or low-compliance diseases have increased elastic work with normal-flow resistive work, increasing the total work of breathing.

Obstructive diseases with high airflow resistance have normal elastic work and increased flow-resistive work, resulting in increased total work of breathing.

Box • 3–20 PATHOPHYSIOLOGIC PERSPECTIVE

In diseases with weak or floppy airways, dynamic compression on expiration can collapse the airway, obstructing expiratory flow and trapping gas distal to the collapse. Use of pursed lips or a restricted orifice during expiration can develop positive pressure in the airway, splinting the airway open, and moving the expiratory positive pressure closer to the mouth.

Bibliography

Berne RM, Levy MN. *Principles of Physiology,* 2nd ed. St. Louis: Mosby-Year Book; 1996.

Comroe JH. *Physiology of Respiration.* Chicago: Year Book Medical Publishers; 1968.

Fidone SJ, Gonzalez C. The respiratory system: Control of breathing. In: *Handbook of Physiology.* Baltimore: American Physiological Society; 1986.

Grondins FS, Yamashiro SM. *Respiratory Function of the Lung and Its Control.* CITY: Macmillan; 1978.

Hlastala MP, Berger AJ. *Physiology of Respiration.* London: Oxford University Press; 1996.

Hollinshead WH, Rosse C. *Textbook of Anatomy,* 4th ed. Philadelphia: Harper & Row; 1985.

Junqueira LC, Carneiro J, Kelley RO. *Basic Histology,* 8th ed. CITY: Appleton & Lange; 1995.

Levitzky MG. *Pulmonary Physiology.* New York: McGraw-Hill; 1982.

Mount Castle VA. *Medical Physiology,* 12th ed. St. Louis: CV Mosby; 1968.

Porth CM. *Pathophysiology: Concepts of Altered Health States.* Philadelphia: JB Lippincott; 1994.

Rhoades RA, Tanner GA. *Medical Physiology.* Boston: Little, Brown; 1995.

Selkurt EE. *Physiology,* 5th ed. Boston: Little, Brown; 1984.

Slonim NB, Hamilton LH. *Respiratory Physiology,* 5th ed. St. Louis: CV Mosby; 1987.

Staub NC. *Basic Respiratory Physiology.* CITY: Churchill Livingstone; 1991.

West JB. *Pulmonary Pathophysiology: The Essentials,* 3rd ed. Baltimore: Williams & Wilkins; 1987.

West JB. *Pulmonary Pathophysiology: The Essentials,* 5th ed. Baltimore: Williams & Wilkins; 1995.

Diagnostic Procedures at the Bedside

Gerald E. Hunt

Key Terms

acidemia
alkalemia
alveolar plateau
capacity
capnography
capnometry
curare cleft
dysfunctional hemoglobin
expiratory reserve volume
fractional saturation
functional residual capacity
functional saturation
hypoxemia
inspiratory capacity
inspiratory reserve volume
metabolic acidosis
metabolic alkalosis
residual volume
respiratory acidosis
respiratory alkalosis
tidal volume
total lung capacity
vital capacity

Objectives

- Describe the basic operational characteristics of the measurement devices that may be used to obtain bedside measurements of pulmonary function.
- Recall the lung volumes, capacities, and flow measurements that are commonly measured by bedside spirometry.
- Describe the technique for performing forced spirometry.
- Describe the criterion for response to a bronchodilator as recommended by the American Thoracic Society.
- Describe the procedure for performing radial artery puncture for arterial blood gas sampling.
- Evaluate acid–base and oxygenation status.
- Describe the basic operational principles of pulse oximetry.
- Recall the indications and contraindications for pulse oximetry.
- Describe the basic principles of capnography.
- Recall the clinical indications for capnography.
- Evaluate capnographic waveform morphology.

A variety of bedside diagnostic procedures are available to assist the practitioner in the assessment of a patient's cardiopulmonary status and to aid in the evaluation of the effect of therapeutic interventions. Techniques that are commonly performed at the adult patient's bedside include the following:

- Bedside pulmonary function testing
- Blood gas analysis and interpretation
- Pulse oximetry
- Capnometry, capnography, and end-tidal carbon dioxide measurement

BEDSIDE PULMONARY FUNCTION TESTING

Pulmonary function studies commonly performed at the bedside include the measurement of spontaneous parameters of ventilation, such as respiratory rate, tidal volume, minute volume, and maximal inspiratory pressure. In addition, with appropriate instrumentation, spirometry, lung volume measurement, and flow–volume loops may be obtained at the bedside. Spirometry frequently includes the measurement of slow vital capacity (SVC), forced vital capacity (FVC), forced expiratory volume in 1 second (FEV_1), and a forced expiratory flow measurement, such as the forced expiratory flow from 200 mL to 1200 mL of the FVC ($FEF_{200-1200}$) or the forced expiratory flow between 25% and 75% of the FVC ($FEF_{25\%-75\%}$). The data obtained from these measurements, when compared with a patient's predicted normal values, enable the practitioner to identify characteristic patterns of pulmonary dysfunction. In addition, the practitioner may use the results of bedside pulmonary function values, such as the peak expiratory flow rate (PEFR), and the FEV_1 to evaluate the efficacy of current therapy and to provide objective evidence for modifications of the therapeutic regimen.

MEASUREMENT TECHNOLOGY

Volume Displacement Spirometers

Water-Sealed Spirometer

Figure 4–1 illustrates a Stead-Wells water-sealed spirometer. A lightweight plastic cylinder is positioned in a well between a larger outer cylinder that is open at the top and a smaller inner cylinder that has one or two holes in the top. The well between the outer and inner cylinders is filled with water. The water serves as an airtight, low-friction seal for the plastic cylinder. The plastic cylinder, frequently referred to as the *bell*, moves up and down in proportion to gas that the patient exhales and inhales into the spirometer. A pen connected to the bell allows a tracing of the bell's movement to be recorded on a kymograph. In many systems, the bell is attached to a linear potentiometer

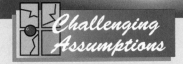

CRITICAL THINKING CHALLENGES

Challenging Assumptions

How Deep Are You Breathing?

Many clinicians mistakenly assume that they can rely on their senses and experience to evaluate a patient's tidal volume or vital capacity without the aid of mechanical devices. It is the rare clinician who can estimate volumes within 50% of the actual volume (if you doubt it, try estimating and measuring volumes in patients who are breathing spontaneously). Two examples of situations in which estimating without measurement can cause problems are evaluating patients (1) with an endotracheal tube and (2) during lung expansion therapy, such as intermittent positive-pressure breathing (IPPB). Estimating volumes without a spirometer can result in a patient being extubated when the volumes are too low to support extubation, requiring reintubation and added patient discomfort and risk. The primary goal of IPPB therapy is to increase volumes during therapy; guessing volumes often results in actually delivering smaller volumes than the patient was taking spontaneously. Guessing is not acceptable when measurements are available. If you do not have the appropriate devices to evaluate your patient, you are placing the patient, yourself, and your institution at risk. You cannot do the job if you do not have the tools.

that provides an analog signal to a recording device or for analog-to-digital signal conversion. Water-seal spirometers can be used to measure spirometric values and, when appropriately equipped, are able measure lung volumes by the helium dilution method.

The use of water-sealed spirometers at the bedside may be limited by the size and weight of the device. Problems that can occur when using a water-sealed spirometer include leaks in the tubing and bell, inadequate water level in the device, and improper positioning of the bell before the start of a test. When a leak is present in the spirometer system, gas is lost because of the effect of gravity on the bell. If the bell is positioned too high or too low at the start of the test, it may be forced out of place during exhalation or completely depleted, with resultant movement of water into the spirometer tubing during inspiration.

Bellows-Type Spirometer

Figure 4–2 illustrates a vertically expanding bellows-type spirometer. The device consists of a collapsible bellows,

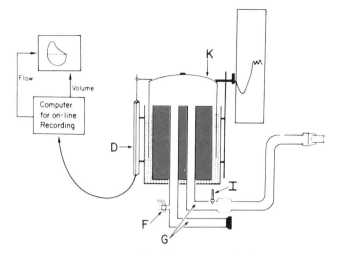

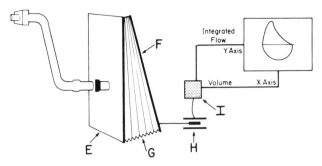

FIGURE 4–1 • Stead-Wells water-sealed volume displacement spirometer. The Stead-Wells spirometers use a lightweight plastic bell (K) and a water seal to contain the exhaled air. A pen is attached directly to the spirometer bell and produces a volume–time tracing upside down from that produced by the chain-compensated spirometer. A stopcock is available for adding special gases (F), and a thermometer (I) is placed in an inlet for ambient temperature recording. A linear potentiometer(D) is attached to the spirometer bell and produces a voltage output proportional to volume as the bell moves up and down. This voltage output may be used by a computer for automatic processing of test results. The computer can integrate the volume signal to obtain flow, and these outputs may be sent to an X–Y recorder for display. G indicates the spirometer's tube, one of which is stoppered.

FIGURE 4–3 • Typical bellows or Wedge spirometer. This spirometer uses an accordian-type folding bellows (G) to attach a lightweight movable bellows plate (F) to a fixed front plate (E). As gas enters the spirometer, the bellows unfolds, and the bellows plate moves outward. A rod attached to the bellows plate is attached to a linear potentiometer (H), which provides an output voltage to the spirometer electronics (I) that is proportional to volume. This spirometer also contains differentiating circuitry that provides for direct recording for computer processing.

Figure 4–3 illustrates a horizontally expanding bellows-type spirometer. The horizontally expanding configuration permits the bellows to be placed in the midposition to allow for measurement of both expiratory and inspiratory volumes as well as flow rates. Like the vertically expanding bellows, the moving end of the horizontally expanding bellows is attached to a recording device.

Problems that may develop with bellows-type spirometers are leaks in the bellows, sticking of the bellows due to aging of the bellows material, and accumulation of moisture and dirt within the folds of the bellows.

Rolling-Seal Spirometer

Figure 4–4 illustrates a dry rolling-seal spirometer. A lightweight piston, supported by a rod, is mounted within a cylinder and sealed by silicone plastic material that rolls on itself as the piston moves within the cylinder. As the pa-

constructed of flexible plastic material, that expands as the patient exhales into it. The vertically expanding configuration is most commonly used to measure FVC, FEV_1, and expiratory flow rates. Attached to the expanding end of the bellows is a recording pen that inscribes on a timed, moving graph, recording the bellows movement. The bellows may also be attached to a linear or rotating potentiometer that provides an analog signal to a recording device or for analog-to-digital signal conversion.

FIGURE 4–2 • Cross-sectional diagram of a vertically expanding bellows-type spirometer. (Ruppel GL. *Manual of Pulmonary Function Testing.* 5th ed. St. Louis: Mosby–Year Book; 1991.)

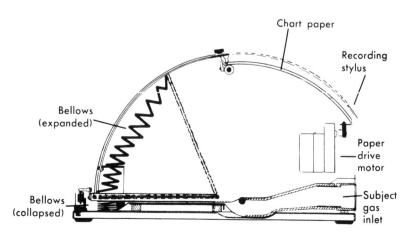

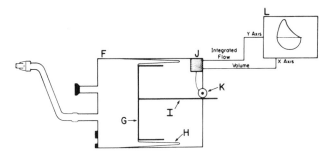

F I G U R E 4 – 4 • Typical rolling-seal spirometer. This spirometer (F) uses a lightweight aluminum piston (G) attached to the inside of a cylinder by a soft, flexible seal (H). As the patient forcefully exhales, the seal rolls between the piston and the sides of the cylinder. A rod (I) attached to the piston causes the voltage on a rotational potentiometer to change, producing a voltage output proportional to the volume change in the spirometer. The volume signal is also differentiated electronically (J) and made available as a flow signal. Thus, both a flow and a volume signal are available as outputs from this spirometer. One or both of these signals may be displayed on an X-Y recorder (L) or input into a computer for automatic processing. These spirometers also have a built-in electronic calibration signal for external display devices, as well as electronics that adjust the spirometer output signal from ambient temperature and pressure, saturated (ATPS) to body temperature and pressure, saturated (BTPS).

tient exhales into the spirometer, the piston is proportionately displaced within the cylinder, and the rod attached to the end of the piston moves forward. The rod can be directly attached to a mechanical recording device or, more commonly, it is attached to a linear or rotating potentiometer that provides an analog signal to a recording device or for analog-to-digital signal conversion. The most common problems encountered with the dry rolling-seal spirometer

CRITICAL THINKING CHALLENGES

Shifting Care Plans

Technology Options in Spirometry

Direct measurement
  Volume displacement
    Water seal
    Wedge bellows
    Rolling seal
Indirect measurement
  Flow versus time
    Rotometer
  Pressure change
  Temperature change
    Heated element anemometer
  Vortex shedding

result from sticking of the rolling-seal or leaks in the seal material.

Respirometers

Measurement of volume by a respirometer (rotameter or turbine flow sensor) is accomplished by the rotation of a thin, lightweight vane as gas molecules flow through the body of the instrument. The rotation of the vane is transmitted, by a gearing mechanism, to a display on the face of the instrument. Figure 4–5 illustrates a Wright respirometer. This device is appropriate for measuring an unforced vital capacity (or SVC) and parameters of resting ventilation, such as the tidal volume (V_T) and exhaled minute volume ($\dot{V}_E$).

Because of inertia of the vane and gearing mechanism of the Wight respirometer, gas flows of less than 3 L/min can cause errors in measurement. At flow rates greater than 300 L/min, distortion of the vane and damage to the gearing mechanism can occur. This upper flow rate limitation generally limits the use of this device to unforced measurements. The practitioner should be familiar with the resolution limits of the device used to prevent erroneous measurement and potential damage to the equipment.

Figure 4–6 illustrates a turbine flow sensor. A rotating turbine blade is positioned between a light source and a photodetector cell. As the speed of the gas flow increases, the number of revolutions of the turbine blade increases. An electronic circuit counts the number of interruptions in the photoelectric beam, per unit of time, and converts the information into flow.

Differential Pressure Pneumotachometer

Figure 4–7 illustrates a Fleisch differential pressure pneumotachometer. Gas flow through this device is proportional to the magnitude of a pressure drop across a fixed resistance. As flow increases, in either direction, the difference in pressure across the fixed resistance increases. This change in pressure is sensed by a pressure transducer, and a signal is sent to a device that can record flow and integrate volume. The resistance offered by the fixed element is small enough that it is not sensed by the patient, yet is of sufficient magnitude to provide a measurable pressure drop. In the Fleisch pneumotachometer, the resistive element consists of a bundle of capillary tubes. Other types of resistive element may be composed of mesh screens (Silverman pneumotachometer) or a wrapped corrugated element.

To achieve an accurate measurement, gas flow through the resistive element of a differential pressure pneumotachometer must be laminar. The pneumotachometer housing may be tapered at each end in an attempt to reduce turbulent flow. Frequently, the resistive element is heated to 37°C to prevent condensation within the element. Moisture on the element changes the resistance of the element and creates measurement error. In some measurement systems

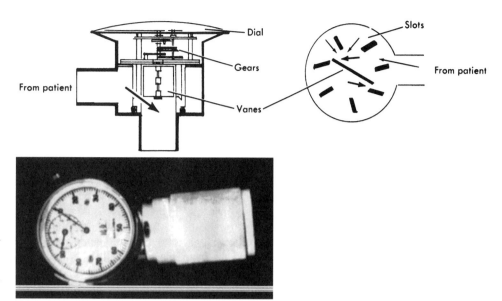

FIGURE 4–5 • Wright respirometer. (McPherson SP. *Respiratory Care Equipment.* 5th ed. St. Louis: Mosby–Year Book; 1995.)

that employ a differential pressure pneumotachometer, a length of large-bore tubing is placed between the patient and the pneumotachometer to trap moisture and other debris in the tubing before they reach the device. Changes in the density or viscosity of the gas can affect measurement accuracy.

Heated Element Anemometer

Figure 4–8 illustrates a heated element anemometer. Also known as a *hot wire anemometer* or *temperature drop pneumotachometer,* measurement is based on the cooling effect of gas flow on a heated element. The element is commonly composed of a platinum wire or a small thermistor bead. The mass of the heated element is small to detect low gas flow rates and to reduce the resistive effect that the element may offer to gas flow through the instrument. Cooling of the heated element is proportional to the magnitude of gas flow past the element. As the element cools, the amount of electrical current supplied to the element, to maintain the element at a constant temperature, is in-

creased. Increases and decreases in the electrical current required to maintain the element at a constant temperature are directly proportional to gas flow. The element temperature is usually heated to a value significantly above 37°C to eliminate any effect that condensation may have on the accuracy of measurement.

Like the differential pressure pneumotachometer, the accuracy of a heated element anemometer may be affected by turbulent gas flow. To reduce the effect of nonlaminar flow through the instrument, the housing may be tapered at each end, or a length of tubing may be placed between the patient and the anemometer. Changes in gas density and viscosity can also alter measurement accuracy.

Ultrasonic Flow Sensor

Figure 4–9 illustrates an ultrasonic flow sensor. Also known as a *vortex device,* gas flow is measured by the vortex shedding principle. As gas flowing through a tube

FIGURE 4–6 • Turbine flow sensor. (Sullivan WJ, Peters GM, Enright PL. Pneumotachographs: Theory and clinical application. *Respir Care.* 1984;29:736–749.)

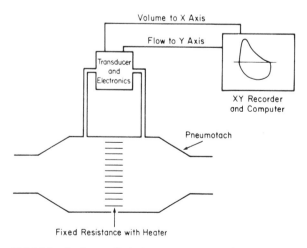

FIGURE 4–7 • Fleisch-type pneumotachometer.

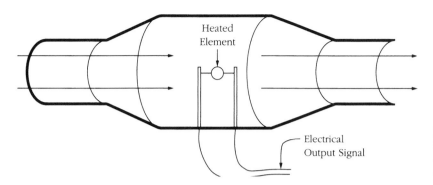

FIGURE 4–8 • Basic design of a thermal anemometer. (Madama VC. *Pulmonary Function Testing and Cardiopulmonary Stress Testing.* Albany, NY: Delmar; 1993.)

meets an obstruction, such as a baffle or strut, vortices are formed. Located downstream from the obstruction created by the baffle or strut is an ultrasonic crystal that emits high-frequency sound waves. Directly across the tube from the emitting crystal is a receiving crystal that detects pulses in the high-frequency sound waves that are created by the vortices. The number of vortices that are created is proportional to gas flow.

Accuracy of the ultrasonic flow transducer is not significantly affected by the humidity content, temperature, or composition of the gas being measured. The design and measurement characteristics of the transducer make it inconsistent in the measurement of low flow rates. The accumulation of condensation on the baffle or strut or on the ultrasonic crystals can produce measurement error. Ultrasonic flow transducer crystals are frequently heated to prevent condensation.

Peak Expiratory Flowmeters

The PEFR can be measured in a number of ways. The measurement can be obtained from a forced spirogram or a flow–volume loop. In addition, the PEFR can be measured by use of a dedicated peak flowmeter. The use of dedicated peak flowmeters has increased dramatically since the publication of the National Institutes of Health (NIH) Asthma Guidelines in 1991.[1] The measurement of PEFR is a cornerstone in the NIH asthma guidelines for both the inpatient and outpatient management of asthma. The PEFR provides an objective indication of deterioration in pulmonary function and information that helps to regrade the efficacy of therapeutic interventions. As such, the availability of dedicated, single-patient peak flowmeters has increased significantly. The two basic types of dedicated peak expiratory flowmeters that are available are the Wright types and single-patient disposable instruments.

Wright Peak Flowmeter

Figure 4–10 illustrates the Wright peak flowmeter. This instrument measures the PEFR using a vane-type mechanism. As the patient exhales through the mouthpiece, a rotating vane is pushed forward by the patient's exhaled gas. As the vane moves forward, a progressively larger leak is created around the vane, and at some point, the leak is of such a magnitude that the bulk of the patient's exhaled gas is vented from the instrument. At this point, the vane fails to move any further, and the PEFR is indicated on the instrument's scale.

The Wright peak flowmeter is a delicate, nondisposable instrument that is intended for use with multiple patients. Appropriate infection control and disinfectant procedures should be performed to prevent cross-contamination by this instrument. Instructing the patient not to inspire through the instrument and use of a low-resistance, disposable mouthpiece that incorporates a one-way valve reduce the possibility of cross-contamination.

Single-Patient Peak Flowmeter

Figure 4–11 illustrates an example of one of the many available single-patient disposable peak flowmeters. Most of these instruments use a movable disk or plate that is propelled forward by the patient's exhaled gas. Measurement is obtained as the disk or plate moves an indicator device along the instrument's scale. The indicator remains at the point of highest flow, and the disk or plate is returned to the starting position by a spring. Before each measurement, the indicator device must be returned to the minimum scale position. The performance of a peak flow maneuver is relatively simple; however, as described later in this chapter, it is effort dependent.

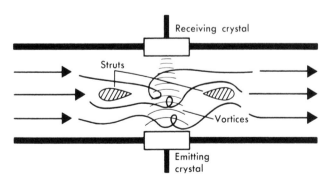

FIGURE 4–9 • Ultrasonic flow sensor. (Ruppel GL. *Manual of Pulmonary Function Testing.* 5th ed. St. Louis: Mosby–Year Book; 1991.)

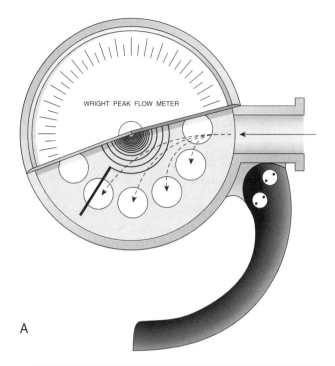

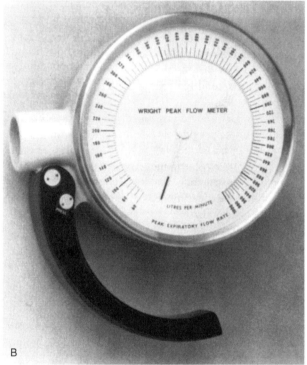

FIGURE 4-10 • (*A*) Schematic of the Wright peak flowmeter. (*B*) Professional model Wright peak flowmeter. (*B* from Madama VC. *Pulmonary Function Testing and Cardiopulmonary Stress Testing.* Albany, NY: Delmar; 1993.)

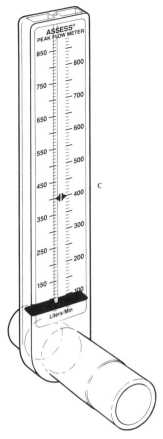

FIGURE 4-11 • Portable single-patient peak flowmeter. (Courtesy of Health Scan Products Inc., Cedar Grove, NJ.)

imal inspiratory pressure. Indices of ventilatory efficiency, derived from the measurement of spontaneous breathing parameters, such as the rapid shallow-breathing index of Yang and Tobin,[2] can provide additional information on which to base therapeutic interventions and make decisions regarding the need for continuation or implementation of mechanical ventilatory support.

The manifestation and progression of pulmonary disease exhibit characteristic changes in the size and relation of lung volumes, timed expiratory volumes, and expiratory flow rates during a forced expiratory maneuver. Spirometry and the flow–volume loop can provide information regarding the extent of existing pulmonary disease, the risk of pulmonary complication after thoracic or upper abdominal surgery, and the efficacy (or inefficacy) of a particular therapeutic intervention or regimen.

Spontaneous Breathing Parameters

Respiratory Rate

Spontaneous respiratory rate is an essential yet frequently undervalued component of any evaluation of pulmonary function. The respiratory rate can serve as a sensitive indicator of the cardiopulmonary system's attempt to compen-

MEASUREMENT AND INTERPRETATION OF BEDSIDE PULMONARY FUNCTION TESTS

Adequacy of ventilatory effort can be assessed, in part, by measurement of such spontaneous breathing parameters as respiratory rate, tidal volume, minute ventilation, and max-

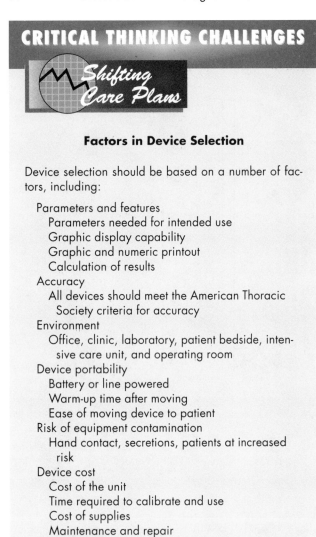

CRITICAL THINKING CHALLENGES

Shifting Care Plans

Factors in Device Selection

Device selection should be based on a number of factors, including:

Parameters and features
    Parameters needed for intended use
    Graphic display capability
    Graphic and numeric printout
    Calculation of results
Accuracy
    All devices should meet the American Thoracic
        Society criteria for accuracy
Environment
    Office, clinic, laboratory, patient bedside, intensive care unit, and operating room
Device portability
    Battery or line powered
    Warm-up time after moving
    Ease of moving device to patient
Risk of equipment contamination
    Hand contact, secretions, patients at increased
        risk
Device cost
    Cost of the unit
    Time required to calibrate and use
    Cost of supplies
    Maintenance and repair
Ease of use
    Computer versus manual computation
    Minimal maintenance
    Calibration requirements

---

sate for alterations in pulmonary function. As an example, the titration of the pressure support level applied to the spontaneous breaths of a patient being supported by mechanical ventilation is frequently based on maintaining a spontaneous respiratory rate of less than 30 breaths/min in adults. In addition, most weaning and extubation protocols use spontaneous respiratory rate as an important part of their evaluation. Weaning attempts that result in maintenance of blood gas parameters yet result in an excessive respiratory rate are likely to fail in the long run as the patient fatigues as a result of the increased workload. Too low a respiratory rate may indicate that significant muscle fatigue already exists or that respiratory drive has been altered by some form of central nervous system depression (eg, medication, head injury, neuromuscular disease).

In addition to the absolute rate of breathing (breaths/min), the pattern (rhythm) of breathing is requisite information. The pattern of breathing can provide potential information regarding the pathophysiology of cardiopul-

monary dysfunction as well as metabolic derangement (eg, Kussmaul's breathing in diabetic ketoacidosis) and neurologic disease (eg, Biot's breathing associated with increased intracranial pressure).

Tidal Volume and Minute Ventilation

Measurement of tidal volume and minute ventilation can be accomplished in several different ways. In the patient without an artificial airway, a mouthpiece or full-face mask may be interfaced with a respirometer or one of a number of electronic spirometers that make provision for recording tidal volume and minute volume. When using a mouthpiece, nose clips should also be used. Some instruments allow for the direct connection of the device to an artificial airway, such as an endotracheal tube or a tracheostomy tube. Many mechanical ventilators allow for the display or recording of spontaneous tidal volume and minute ventilation when placed in the continuous positive airway pressure mode. Caution should be exercised when using the display capabilities of a mechanical ventilator for obtaining spontaneous breathing parameters because the work of breathing imposed by the ventilator may be excessive, and inaccurate measurement may result.

In situations in which the patient requires supplemental oxygen to maintain clinically acceptable arterial oxygen saturation (SaO_2) or partial pressure of arterial oxygen (PaO_2), an alternate source of oxygen must be provided during any measurement. Failure to provide adequate supplemental oxygen may give rise to erroneously high values owing to stimulation of the peripheral chemoreceptors by hypoxemia. In some instances, a one-way valve system may be necessary to prevent the measurement of both inspiration and expiration with instruments that measure bidirectional flow. By permitting the measurement of exhaled gas only, a one-way valve system also reduces the potential for cross-contamination. As with any piece of equipment, the practitioner is encouraged to become familiar with the product literature, operational characteristics, and local institutional procedures for the specific instrument being used.

When measuring spontaneous respiratory rate and minute ventilation, an average value for tidal volume can be obtained by dividing the minute volume by the respiratory rate. Minimum and maximum values for tidal volume can also be measured. The information obtained can be used, in conjunction with other parameters, to evaluate the efficacy of spontaneous ventilation. Table 4–1 provides an example of conventional adult extubation parameters, including spontaneous respiratory rate, tidal volume, and minute ventilation.

Maximum Inspiratory Pressure

The measurement of maximum inspiratory pressure (MIP) provides an indication of the adequacy of a patient's inspiratory muscle strength. The measurement is made using a manometer attached to a mouthpiece or mouth seal, a full-

Table • 4–1   PHYSIOLOGIC PARAMETERS THAT SUGGEST WEANING IS POSSIBLE

Tests of Mechanical Ability

Maximal inspiratory pressure	>-20 cm H_2O
Vital capacity	>15 mL/kg
FEV_1	>10 mL/kg
Resting $\dot{V}E$	<10 L/min
Compliance on ventilator	>30 mL/cm H_2O
Maximum voluntary ventilation	Twice spontaneous $\dot{V}E$
Spontaneous VT	>5 mL/kg
Spontaneous respiratory rate	<30 breaths/min and >6 breaths/min
Rate: VT ratio	<100

Tests of Gas Exchange

PaO_2 on $\leq40\%$ O_2	≥60 mmHg
PaO_2/FIO_2	>200
$PaO_2/PA\bar{O}_2$	>0.20
$Qs/\dot{Q}T$	<0.15
VD/VT	<0.60

face mask, or a manometer that is interfaced with an artificial airway. Nose clips are necessary when a mouth piece or mouth seal are used. A one-way valve system can be used to allow exhalation and to provide immediate airway occlusion on inspiration. The one-way valve system is necessary when performing an MIP measurement in an uncooperative or obtunded patient. Figure 4–12 is an example of such a one-way valve system. When making a measurement using a mouthpiece or mouth seal, a small, controlled leak should be incorporated between the patient and the device to reduce the impact of the cheek muscles on the MIP value obtained.

The patient is instructed to exhale to residual lung volume. When exhalation is complete, the airway is occluded, and the patient is instructed to provide a maximal inspiratory effort. Once measurement is started, it should continue

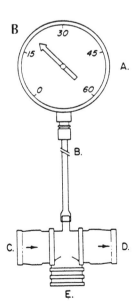

FIGURE 4–12 • One-way valve system for maximum inspiratory pressure measurement. (Kacmarek RM, *Respir Care.* 1989;34:868.)

for 15 to 20 seconds.[3,4] Hemodynamically labile patients should be monitored during the procedure for signs of instability, and the measurement should be halted if significant decompensation occurs. The most negative value observed during the procedure should be recorded.

A healthy male adult can generate an MIP of greater than -100 cm H_2O. A decline in MIP is noted with advancing age. MIP declines in situations of respiratory muscle fatigue, chronic lung hyperinflation, kyphoscoliosis and other severe chest wall deformities, and neuromuscular disease and as a result of certain medications. Clinically, the MIP is used to assess the progress of weaning, readiness for extubation, and progression of neuromuscular disease (eg, Guillain-Barré syndrome). An MIP of -20 cm H_2O or less is considered an indication for ventilatory support.[5]

Bedside Spirometry

Lung Volume Measurement

The total lung volume is divided into several volumes and capacities. There are four lung volumes: residual volume (RV), expiratory reserve volume (ERV), tidal volume (VT), and inspiratory reserve volume (IRV). Lung **capacity** is defined as the sum of any two or more adjacent lung volumes. There are four lung capacities: total lung capacity (TLC), vital capacity (VC), inspiratory capacity (IC), and functional residual capacity (FRC).

Tidal volume is the amount of gas that is inhaled and exhaled with each breath during normal resting breathing. VT is about 8% to 10% of TLC.

Inspiratory reserve volume is the maximum amount of gas that can be inhaled above a normal tidal volume inhalation. IRV is about 50% of TLC.

Expiratory reserve volume is the maximum amount of gas that can be exhaled after a normal tidal volume exhalation. ERV is about 20% of TLC.

Residual volume is the amount of gas remaining in the lungs after a maximal exhalation. This volume cannot be directly measured by simple spirometry. The determination of RV must be done indirectly, as follows: FRC must be determined by the open-circuit or closed-circuit helium dilution method or by measurement of thoracic gas volume, at end expiration, with a body plethysmograph. The value for ERV, as determined by spirometry, is subtracted from the value obtained for FRC, yielding a value for RV (RV = FRC − ERV). RV is about 20% of TLC.

Functional residual capacity is the sum of the RV and ERV. It is from this lung level that normal tidal ventilation occurs. FRC is about 40% of TLC.

Vital capacity is the sum of IRV, VT, and ERV. When this capacity is exhaled forcefully, it is termed the FVC. When the VC is exhaled slowly, it is referred to as the SVC. VC is about 80% of TLC.

Inspiratory capacity is the maximum amount of gas that can be inhaled from resting VT. IC is the sum of VT and IRV. IC is about 60% of TLC.

Total lung capacity is the amount of gas in the lungs after a maximal inspiration. TLC can be viewed as the sum of all four lung volumes (TLC = RV + ERV + VT + IRV) or as the sum of IC and FRC.

Although it is not possible to measure RV, and thus FRC, at the bedside with spirometry, it is important to have an appreciation for how the lung volumes and capacities vary with specific pulmonary disease states. A normal spirogram is depicted in Figure 4–13. Note the relations of the various lung volumes and capacities. Note that the spirogram does not measure RV.

When an RV measurement has been obtained through helium dilution or body plethysmography, a ratio of the relation between the RV and TLC can be helpful in the evaluation of lung volumes. This residual volume/total lung capacity ratio (RV/TLC%) is usually between 20% and 35% in healthy young adults. The RV/TLC% is calculated as follows:

$$\frac{RV}{TLC} \times 100$$

An RV/TLC% greater than 35% indicates an increase in RV or a decrease in TLC resulting from loss of VC.

A spirogram that is representative of a restrictive lung volume pattern is illustrated in Figure 4–14. Note that the values for TLC, VC, FRC, and RV are all decreased. If pure restrictive lung disease is present, a normal relation exists in the RV/TLC%. Box 4–1 lists potential causes of a restrictive lung volume pattern.

The spirogram in Figure 4–15 represents the lung volume pattern associated with hyperinflation. Hyperinflation is most frequently the result of an obstructive airway disease, such as asthma, emphysema, or chronic bronchitis.

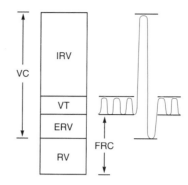

FIGURE 4–14 • Spirogram of a restrictive disorder.

The RV is significantly elevated, and this results in an increase in FRC. In hyperinflation, the VC remains relatively normal, and the TLC is significantly increased. The RV/TLC% is increased.

Figure 4–16 is the spirogram associated with air trapping. Air trapping, like hyperinflation, is associated with obstructive lung disease. The RV and FRC are elevated; however, the VC is decreased, and the TLC is relatively normal. The RV/TLC% is increased in this situation.

An example of a mixed restrictive and obstructive pattern is illustrated in Figure 4–17. In this example, the TLC and VC are decreased, and the RV and FRC are relatively increased. The RV/TLC% is increased. An example of the pathophysiology of a mixed disorder is smoking-induced

---

Box • 4–1 POTENTIAL CAUSES OF A RESTRICTIVE LUNG VOLUME PATTERN

Intrapulmonic
  Interstitial fibrosis
  Pneumonia
  Pulmonary edema
  Vascular congestion
  Sarcoidosis
  Pneumoconiosis
Extrapulmonic
  Thoracic
    Kyphoscoliosis
    Rheumatoid spondylitis
    Pleural effusion
  Abdominal
    Obesity
    Peritonitis
    Ascites
  Neuromuscular
    Myasthenia gravis
    Guillain-Barré syndrome
    Poliomyelitis

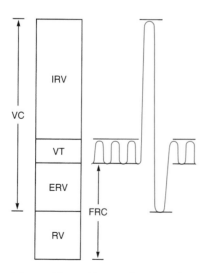

FIGURE 4–13 • Normal lung volumes and capacities in relation to a spirogram.

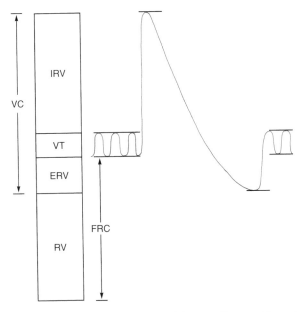

FIGURE 4–15 • Spirogram of hyperinflation. Note the prolonged expiratory time that is associated with the obstructive component of the lung disease.

chronic obstructive pulmonary disease that is coexistent with a disorder such as severe obesity, severe kyphoscoliosis, tracheal stenosis, or a pneumoconiosis (eg, coalminer's lung). Unfortunately, the assessment of mixed disorders is not always straightforward. Within a particular disorder, some volumes are normal, some increased, and some decreased. The use of timed expiratory volume and flow rate studies is helpful in the diagnosis and assessment of mixed disorders.

Table 4–2 provides a basic interpretation scheme for classifying obstructive, restrictive, and mixed disorders, based on a comparison of lung volume measurement to predicted normal values.

In addition to assessing VT, VC, IRV, and ERV, spirometry allows for the measurement of timed expiratory vol-

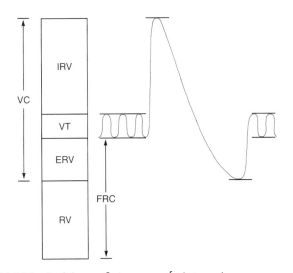

FIGURE 4–16 • Spirogram of air trapping.

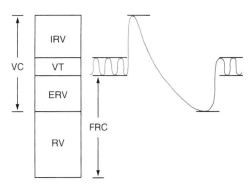

FIGURE 4–17 • Spirogram of mixed restrictive and obstructive disorder.

umes and expiratory flow rates. At the bedside, the most commonly measured timed expiratory volume is the FEV_1. The most frequently measured expiratory flow rates are the PEFR and the $FEF_{25\%–75\%}$.

Forced Expiratory Volume in 1 Second

The FEV_1 is the volume of gas that can be exhaled in 1 second from the start of an FVC maneuver. Other time intervals may be measured, such as 0.5 second, 2 seconds, and 3 seconds; however, the FEV_1 is the most frequently assessed timed measurement obtained at the bedside. The FEV_1 is reduced in airway obstruction caused by bronchospasm, edema, inflammation, or secretion accumulation. In conditions that result in a loss of lung elasticity and radial tethering of the small airways, such as emphysema, the FEV_1 is decreased. When compared with the FVC, the FEV_1 obtained from a patient with significant airway obstruction is less than 65% of the FVC. The comparison of FEV_1 to FVC is the FEV_1/FVC ratio, also known as the $FEV_{1\%}$, and is computed as follows:

$$FEV_{1\%} = \frac{FEV_1}{FVC} \times 100$$

A healthy young person with normal lung function is able to exhale about 75% to 85% of FVC in 1 second.

Restrictive lung processes, such as pulmonary fibrosis, obesity, neuromuscular disease, and thoracic cage deformities, also reduce the FEV_1. In contrast to obstructive lung pathology, FVC is reduced. The resultant $FEV_{1\%}$ is frequently normal or increased.

Peak Expiratory Flow Rate

The PEFR is the maximum flow achieved during an FVC maneuver. The PEFR is primarily a measure of the function of the large airways. Patients with early small airways obstruction may generate significantly high early flow rates during the FVC maneuver and demonstrate normal values for PEFR. With severe small airways obstruction,

Table • 4–2   LUNG VOLUME CHANGES ASSOCIATED WITH VARIOUS PULMONARY DISORDERS

Volume	Hyperinflation	Air Trapping	Restrictive	Mixed
VC	Normal	Decreased	Decreased	Decreased
TLC	Increased	Normal	Decreased	Normal or decreased
FRC	Increased	Increased	Decreased	Normal or decreased
RV	Increased	Increased	Decreased	Normal or decreased
RV/TLC%	Increased	Increased	Normal	Normal or decreased

the PEFR declines. The PEFR occurs early in the FVC and, as such, is effort dependent. If the patient fails to provide maximum effort, the values obtained are decreased and are likely to be variable over repeated testing. The PEFR may be measured independently of an FVC maneuver with a dedicated instrument, such as the Wright peak flowmeter, or with the use of a single-patient portable peak flowmeter. When a peak flowmeter is used, the patient needs only to exhale with maximal force and does not need to perform a complete FVC maneuver. This can be advantageous when evaluating a person who is short of breath. Values are reported in liters per second or per minute. A healthy young adult can generate a PEFR that exceeds 600 L/min.

Monitoring of PEFR has become an important component of the National Asthma Education and Prevention Program.[6] Many brands of single-patient portable peak flowmeters are available for home and institutional use. PEFR is divided into three zones. The green zone represents a PEFR that is 80% to 100% of the individual personal best. The green zone indicates good control of a patient's asthma. The yellow zone represents a PEFR that is 50% to 80% of the individual personal best. The yellow zone indicates that caution is necessary. Based on a predetermined personal asthma action plan, the patient may increase the dosage of bronchodilator medications or institute steroid therapy. The red zone represents a PEFR that is less than 50% of the individual personal best. The red zone indicates a medical alert. The asthma action plan directs the patient to take immediate action and contact the physician or go to a hospital emergency room.

Measurement of PEFR, using the single-patient portable peak flowmeter, is frequently assessed at the bedside in the hospital emergency room and during hospital admission for exacerbations of asthma. PEFR measurement provides easily obtained objective information about the efficacy of current therapy. The general procedure for performing PEFR measurement is detailed in Box 4–2.

Forced Expiratory Flow Between 25% and 75% of the Forced Vital Capacity

The $FEF_{25\%-75\%}$ is a measure of the average expiratory flow rate during the middle half of an FVC maneuver. The $FEF_{25\%-75\%}$ is thought to be relatively effort independent. As such, it may reflect the status of the small to medium air-

ways. A decrease in the $FEF_{25\%-75\%}$ may signify early small airways obstruction. This measurement has been highly variable from test to test in the same patient. In addition, the $FEF_{25\%-75\%}$ is highly dependent on the FVC. A healthy young adult can generate a $FEF_{25\%-75\%}$ of 4 to 5 L/s.

Spirometric Technique

With the proliferation of hand-held, computerized spirometric equipment, the measurement of spirometric parameters at the bedside has become convenient and greatly simplified. The software programs supplied with most portable spirometers incorporate algorithms that determine whether acceptability and reproducibility criteria have been met, automatically display the results of the largest

---

Box • 4–2   PEAK EXPIRATORY FLOW RATE MEASUREMENT PROCEDURE

Explain the procedure to the subject. PEFR is an effort-dependent procedure, and the patient should be encouraged to produce maximal effort. The practitioner should demonstrate the procedure for the subject.

Zero the peak flowmeter.

Have the patient stand up straight. The sitting position may be substituted for those patients in severe distress who are unable to stand.

Nose clips are *not* required.

Inhale completely.

Quickly place the peak flowmeter into the mouth and make a seal around the mouthpiece with the lips. Make sure that the mouthpiece is past the patient's teeth and not occluded by the tongue.

As soon as a seal is formed around the mouthpiece, the patient should exhale with maximal force. It is not necessary for the patient to exhale completely.

The measurement should be repeated two more times for a total of three measurements.

Results should be compared with the patient's personal best or predicted PEFR.

FVC and FEV_1 at body temperature and pressure, saturated (BTPS), and store multiple records for later download and printing. This miniaturization and computerization have not, however, reduced the need for a competent and methodical practitioner. As discussed later, the spirometric procedure can be technique dependent. Appropriate patient preparation and procedure performance are crucial to the validity of the results obtained.

Patient Preparation

Forced spirometry is an effort-dependent procedure. Results and subsequent interpretation of the test may be compromised if the patient performs the procedure with less than maximal effort or cooperation. Careful description by the practitioner of the purpose of the test, the spirometric procedure, and the importance of maximum effort enhances the acceptability of the data obtained. The practitioner should provide instructions in a simple and understandable fashion. In addition to verbal instructions, the practitioner should demonstrate the procedure for the patient. Correct placement of the mouthpiece and appropriate posture should be practiced by the patient before testing. Any tight-fitting or restrictive clothing should be loosened or removed. A brief patient assessment that includes smoking history, recent illness, current medications, vital signs, height and weight measurements, and race should be obtained.

When performing spirometry to assess the response to a bronchodilator, it is common practice to withhold currently administered bronchodilator medications that may confound the assessment of an acute bronchodilator response. Table 4–3 lists common bronchodilators that may mask a bronchodilator response and the recommended time for withholding these medications before spirometric evaluation.

Performing the Procedure

The measurement of FVC may be accomplished by either the open-circuit or closed-circuit method. The method used is determined by the type and recording capabilities of the spirometer. The vertically expanding bellows-type spirometer is an example of the open-circuit method. The patient inhales maximally away from the spirometer mouthpiece and then places the mouthpiece into the mouth and exhales forcefully and completely. Some patients have difficulty coordinating a breath hold at TLC and the rapid transfer of the mouthpiece into the mouth. Prolonged breath holding at TLC (more than 4 to 6 seconds) should be avoided because this has been shown to reduce the PEFR and FEV_1 in normal patients.

The water-sealed spirometer, an example of the closed-circuit method, allows the patient to tidal breathe while attached to the spirometer. No more than five tidal breaths are recommended because CO_2 may accumulate in the reservoir, unless a CO_2 absorbing material is present. CO_2 accumulation is not an issue when a bidirectional flow transducer, such as a differential pressure pneumotachometer, is used for measurement. After the initial tidal breathing, the patient inhales maximally and exhales forcefully and completely while attached to the spirometer. This method is generally easier for the patient to perform and allows for the additional measurement of inspiratory flow and volume. With this method, the patient has the opportunity to form a tight seal around the mouthpiece before performing the forced portion of the procedure. The general procedure for performing an FVC maneuver is detailed in Box 4–3.

The greatest FVC and FEV_1 should be reported even if they are obtained from different acceptable curves. Other measurements, such as the $FEF_{25\%-75\%}$ and the PEFR, should be obtained from the single best test. The best test is the acceptable curve that has the largest sum of FVC and FEV_1. All values should be reported at BTPS. Patient effort and cooperation should be documented.

Figure 4–19 compares a normal FVC curve with those obtained in obstructive and restrictive disorders. The resultant values for FVC and FEV_1 are compared with the values predicted for the patient based on sex, age, height, and race. Figure 4–20 illustrates a flow diagram for the interpretation of spirometry results using the FVC and FEV_1.

Assessing Bronchodilator Response

Prebronchodilator and postbronchodilator spirometry studies can be performed at the bedside to determine the benefit of bronchodilator administration. As noted previously, currently administered bronchodilator medications should be withheld for an appropriate period of time before the spirometric evaluation (see Table 4–3). Prebronchodilator spirometry is performed in accordance with the procedure detailed previously. After the initial measurements, an aerosolized bronchodilator is administered by small-volume nebulizer or metered dose inhaler with a spacer device. Delivery of the bronchodilator should be observed by the practitioner for correct administration technique. After the medication delivery, it is important to

Table • 4–3 **RECOMMENDED TIMES FOR WITHHOLDING BRONCHODILATOR MEDICATION WHEN ASSESSING BRONCHODILATOR RESPONSE**[7]

Drug	Withholding Time (h)
Salmeterol	12
Ipratropium	6
Terbutaline	4–8
Albuterol	4–6
Metaproterenol	4
Isoetharine	3

Box • 4–3 FORCED VITAL CAPACITY PROCEDURE

Ensure that the spirometer has been appropriately decontaminated since last use.

Ensure appropriate calibration procedures, as recommended by the equipment manufacturer and American Thoracic Society standards, have been performed and are within acceptable limits.

The patient may sit or stand to perform the procedure. Sitting may provide support to unstable patients. When sitting, the subject should place the feet flat on the ground and not cross the legs. When standing, a stable chair (ie, one without rollers) should be placed behind the subject in the event that he or she experiences dizziness or syncope. The patient's position should be noted on the test results.

Nose clips are recommended for use.

Review the procedure with the patient:

Appropriate posture. The patient's chin should be slightly elevated and the neck slightly extended. During the forced exhalation maneuver, the patient should attempt to maintain the appropriate chin and neck position and not be allowed to touch the chin to the chest. The patient should avoid excessive flexion at the waist.

Placement of the mouthpiece. The patient should practice the placement of the mouthpiece. This is especially important with the open-circuit method because the patient must quickly place the mouthpiece into the mouth and form a tight seal with his or her lips. As noted previously, the patient should not remain at TLC for more than 4 to 6 seconds. An airtight seal must be created by the lips around the mouthpiece. The tongue should not obstruct the mouthpiece opening. Patients using a cardboard mouthpiece should be instructed not to bite down on the mouthpiece, or the cardboard tube may collapse, creating an obstruction to flow. Occasionally, a patient's dentures may preclude the formation of an adequate seal round the mouthpiece, which may necessitate their removal during testing.

Open-circuit method. The patient is instructed to inspire maximally with the mouthpiece away from the mouth, and then quickly place the mouthpiece into the mouth and exhale forcefully and completely. Placing the mouthpiece next to the cheek, away from the mouth, may reduce the time that the patient must remain at TLC. In addition, excessive movement of flow-sensing devices, such as a differential pressure pneumotachometer, may be sensed as gas flow.

Closed-circuit method. The mouthpiece is placed into the mouth and the subject tidal breathes for 3 to 5 breaths. The patient is then instructed to inspire maximally and then exhale forcefully and completely.

Coaching. The subject should be advised that the practitioner will be coaching him or her in obtaining a maximal performance. Coaching should be firm and vigorous. Examples of appropriate coaching phrases are "blow all your air out," "keep blowing, keep blowing," "get it all out," and "keep going, keep going."

Perform the maneuver:

Have the subject assume the appropriate position
Place nose clips.

Have the subject inspire maximally and exhale forcefully and completely.

Ensure that mouthpiece placement is in accordance with the method (open-circuit or closed-circuit) being used.

The maneuver should be performed a minimum of three times. Based on the following acceptability criteria, the maneuver may be repeated up to eight times depending on patient tolerance. The spirograms should be inspected for acceptability and reproducibility based on the following American Thoracic Society criteria.[8] Although most computerized spirometers are programmed to alert the practitioner to a test that does not meet one or more of the following criteria, it is important to have an appreciation for what constitutes an acceptable spirogram.

A good test start is observed (Fig. 4-18).

An extrapolated volume of 5% of the FVC or 150 mL is observed, whichever is greater.

Manual calculation of the extrapolated volume requires a volume–time tracing and is beyond the scope of this text. Most modern spirometric equipment relies on computer measurement of this parameter. The reader is referred to one of the excellent comprehensive pulmonary function texts for an in-depth discussion of the back-extrapolation technique.[9,10]

No hesitation or false start is observed.

A rapid start to rise time is observed.

No cough, especially during the first second of the maneuver.

No early termination of exhalation.

A minimum exhalation time of 6 seconds, unless there is an obvious volume plateau of reasonable duration, or the subject cannot or should not continue to exhale.

The two largest FVCs from acceptable maneuvers should not vary by more than 0.200 L.

The two largest FEV_1 from acceptable maneuvers should not vary by more than 0.200 L.

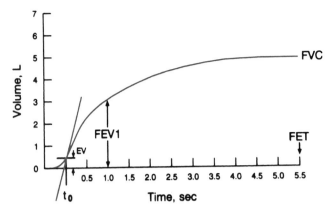

FIGURE 4-18 • Traditional volume–time spirogram. The forced vital capacity (FVC) maneuver starts at the lower left corner at full inhalation. The FVC is the total exhaled volume at the end of the maneuver's plateau (FVC + 5.0 L in this example). The start of the maneuver is determined by "back extrapolation": a tangent is drawn through the steepest portion of the maneuver, intersecting the baseline at the time zero (t_o). The FEV_1 occurs 1 second after time zero (FEV_1 = 3.0 L here). The extrapolated volume (EV = 0.5 L here) and the forced expiratory time (FET = 5.5 seconds here) are measured as quality-control checks. (© Mayo Foundation.)

wait at least 15 minutes before repeating the spirometric measurement.

The recommended criteria for response to a bronchodilator in adults for FVC and FEV_1 is a 12% improvement from baseline *and* an absolute change of 0.200 L.[8] Percentage change in FVC or FEV_1 is calculated as follows:

$$\text{Percentage change} = \frac{\text{Postdrug} - \text{predrug}}{\text{Predrug}} \times 100$$

Example: Prebronchodilator FEV_1 = 2.35 L
Postbronchodilator FEV_1 = 2.83 L

$$\frac{2.83\ \text{L} - 2.35\ \text{L}}{2.35\ \text{L}} \times 100 = 20\% \text{ change}$$

Figure 4–21 is an example of prebronchodilator and postbronchodilator FVC curves. Figure 4–22 is an example of a prebronchodilator and postbronchodilator spirometry report.

Flow–Volume Loops

Figure 4–23 illustrates a normal flow–volume loop. Flow is indicated on the vertical axis and volume on the horizontal axis. The inspiratory loop is shown below the horizontal axis, and the expiratory loop is shown above the horizontal axis. Values for PEFR and peak inspiratory flow rate can be read directly from the graph. Instantaneous flows, such as the forced expiratory flow at 50% of FVC ($FEF_{50\%}$), may also be read directly from the graph. The flow–volume loop provides a simple visual evaluation of pulmonary disease states.

As can be noted in Figure 4–24, the flow–volume loop manifests a characteristic shape in certain pulmonary diseases. In restrictive lung disease, the primary change in the loop is a decrease in volume. In obstructive lung disease, the expiratory portion of the loop becomes concave as small airways collapse from dynamic compression during the FVC maneuver. In addition, note that the PEFR and peak inspiratory flow rate are significantly decreased. Figure 4–25 illustrates a prebronchodilator and postbronchodilator study using expiratory flow–volume curves.

INVASIVE MONITORING OF GAS EXCHANGE

Blood Gas Analysis

Blood gas analysis allows the practitioner to evaluate the body's acid–base balance and the effectiveness of the lungs' ability to oxygenate the blood and ventilate excess

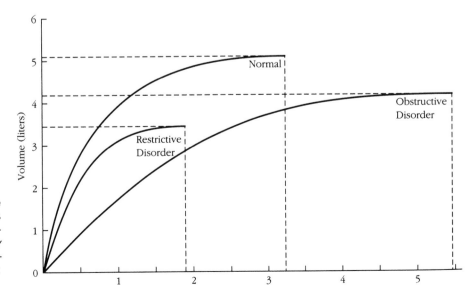

FIGURE 4-19 • Volume–time tracing demonstrating the effects of restrictive and obstructive disorders. (Madama VC. *Pulmonary Function Testing and Cardiopulmonary Stress Testing.* Albany, NY: Delmar; 1993.)

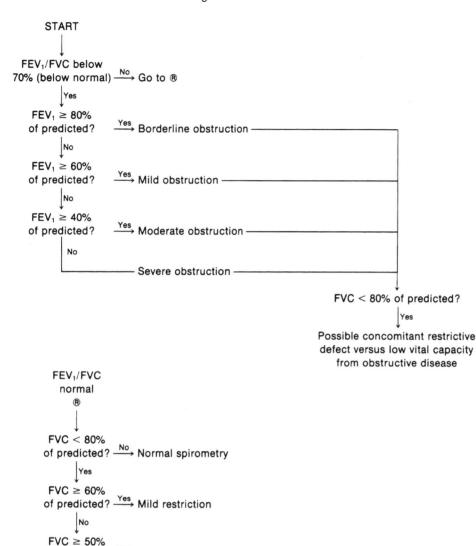

FIGURE 4–20 • Spirometry interpretation. Always start by using the FEV_1/FVC ratio to determine if obstruction exists. Grade the degree of obstruction using the percentage of predicted FEV_1. If the FEV_1/FVC ratio and the FVC are above the lower limit of normal range, spirometry is normal. (© Mayo Foundation.)

CRITICAL THINKING CHALLENGES

Go Figure

Assessing Response to Bronchodilators

A patient with severe disease has an FVC of 1.2 L and an FEV_1 of 600 mL. Twenty minutes after albuterol was administered, the postbronchodilator FVC was 1.3 L with an FEV_1 of 750 mL. What is the percentage improvement in FEV_1? What percentage change is required to be considered significant? Why might this patient's response *not* be considered significant according to the American Thoracic Society?

carbon dioxide from the body. Arterial blood is sampled most frequently because it contains oxygen and carbon dioxide levels that are a reflection of lung function. Mixed venous blood may be sampled from the pulmonary artery by a Swan-Ganz catheter. Mixed venous oxygenation parameters ($P\overline{v}O_2$ and $S\overline{v}O_2$) are used to calculate the mixed venous oxygen content ($C\overline{v}O_2$). $C\overline{v}O_2$ can be used, in conjunction with arterial oxygenation values, in the determination of the arterial–mixed venous content difference $[C(a-v)\ O_2]$ and the calculation of intrapulmonary shunt ($\dot{Q}s/\dot{Q}T$). Sampling of peripheral venous blood may provide useful information about pH or serum lactate level. The use of peripheral venous blood to assess oxygenation is not generally helpful.

Routine arterial blood gas analysis directly measures blood pH, partial pressure of carbon dioxide ($PaCO_2$), and partial pressure of oxygen (PaO_2). In addition, various oxy-

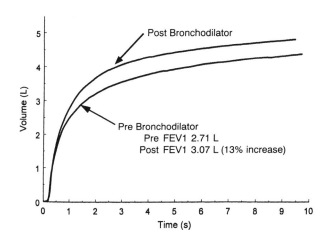

FIGURE 4–21 • Prebronchodilator and postbronchodilator FVC curves. Note that the postbronchodilator FEV_1 meets the American Thoracic Society criterion for a bronchodilator response (13% improvement and an increase of 0.360 L). (National Asthma Education and Prevention Program. *Expert Panel Report II: Guidelines for the Diagnosis and Management of Asthma.* Bethesda, MD: National Institute of Health, 1997.)

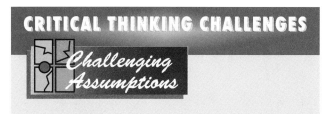

Waiting for Bronchodilator Response

Postbronchodilator spirometry should be performed at least 15 minutes after the bronchodilator is administered. Although 15 minutes may be long enough for fast-acting β-agonists such as albuterol (which has 85% of effect within the first 10 minutes), it may be too short with other formulation. Ipratropium bromide (Atrovent) is an anticholinergic that requires up to 45 minutes to take full effect. To determine response to salmeterol, a long-acting agent that lasts 12 hours, full effect may take 1.5 hours. So the amount of time you wait before performing postbronchodilator spirometry should be based on the onset and time to peak effect of the specific bronchodilator administered.

genation and acid–base parameters can be calculated from the directly measured values. Accurate determination of some calculated parameters require additional data provided by the practitioner or input from a hemoximeter (CO-oximeter). Table 4–4 lists directly measured arterial blood gas parameters and gives examples of commonly calculated arterial parameters.

The calculated value for HCO_3^- is derived from the Henderson-Hasselbalch equation:

$$pH = pK + \log\left(\frac{HCO_3^-}{PaCO_2 \times 0.03}\right),$$

where pK = 6.1 dissociation constant, and
0.03 = solubility coefficient for CO_2
(converts mmHg to mEq/L)

When the direct measurement of oxyhemoglobin saturation is not available, the conventional blood gas analyzer uses a complex formula based on the oxyhemoglobin dissociation curve to estimate oxyhemoglobin saturation. Under certain conditions, such as the presence of a significant level of carboxyhemoglobin, the arterial oxyhemoglobin saturation calculated by the blood gas analyzer overesti-

		Pre Bronchodilator					Post Bronchodilator		
Study: bronch ID:			Test Date: 8/7/96	Time: 9:38 am	Study: bronch ID:			Test Date: 8/7/96	Time: 11:42 am
Age: 59	Height: 175 cm		Sex: M	System: 7 20 17	Age: 59	Height: 175 cm		Sex: M	System: 7 20 17
Trial	FVC	FEV_1	$FEV_1/FVC\%$		Trial	FVC	FEV_1	$FEV_1/FVC\%$	
1	4.34	2.68	61.8%		1	4.68	3.00	64.0%	
2	4.40	2.59	58.9%		2	4.73	2.94	62.2%	
3	4.44	2.62	58.9%		3	4.59	2.95	64.3%	
4	4.56	2.69	58.9%		4	4.76	3.07	64.5%	
5	4.55	2.71	59.6%		5	4.78	3.04	63.5%	
Best Values	4.56	2.71	59.4%		Best Values	4.78	3.07	64.3%	
Predicted Values-1	4.23	3.40	80.5%		Reference Values	4.56	2.71		
LLN-2	3.10	2.62	69.9%		Difference (L)	0.22	0.36		
Percent Predicted	107.8%	79.7%	73.8%		Difference (%)	4.8%	13.4%		

Interpretations: Pre-shift

FEV/FVC results are below the normal range. The reduced rate at which air is exhaled indicates obstruction to airflow.
1 – Predicted values from Knudson et al., *Am Rev Respir Dis* 1983.
2 – LLN is the Lower Limit of the Normal range (95th percentile).

Interpretations: Bronchodilator Response

Significant increase in FEV_1 with bronchodilator (≥12% increase after bronchodilator indicates a significant change).

FIGURE 4–22 • Report of spirometry findings before and after bronchodilator administration. (National Asthma Education and Prevention Program. *Expert Panel Report II: Guidelines for the Diagnosis and Management of Asthma.* Bethesda, MD: National Institute of Health, 1997.)

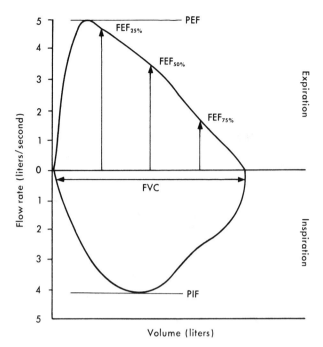

FIGURE 4-23 • The forced vital capacity on a flow–volume graph. (Scanlon CL, et al. *Egan's Fundamentals of Respiratory Care.* 6th ed. St. Louis: Mosby–Year Book; 1995.)

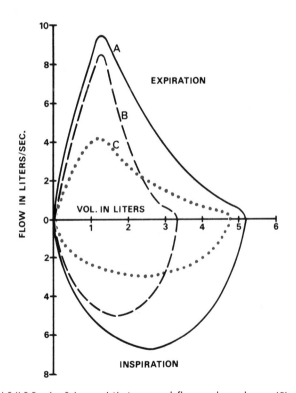

FIGURE 4-24 • (*A*) A normal flow–volume loop. (*B*) A flow–volume loop in restrictive lung disease. (*C*) A flow–volume loop in an obstructive lung disease. Flow–volume loops afford a rapid visual evaluation of the overall disease state. (Kacmarek RM, et al. *The Essentials of Respiratory Care.* 3rd ed. St. Louis: Mosby–Year Book; 1990.)

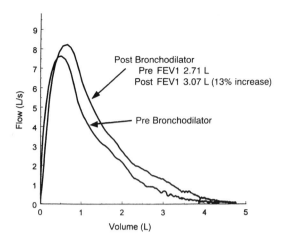

FIGURE 4-25 • Prebronchodilator and postbronchodilator response demonstrated using expiratory flow–volume curves. (National Asthma Education and Prevention Program. *Expert Panel Report II: Guidelines for the Diagnosis and Management of Asthma.* Bethesda, MD: National Institute of Health, 1997.)

mates the actual saturation. The value obtained for CaO_2 would also be overestimated in this situation.

Hemoximetry provides direct spectrophotometric measurement of total hemoglobin (tHb), oxyhemoglobin saturation (O_2Hb), carboxyhemoglobin saturation (COHb), and methemoglobin saturation (metHb). Under most conditions, hemoximetry provides a reliable estimation of oxyhemoglobin saturation and allows accurate calculation of oxygen content.

Table 4–5 lists normal arterial and mixed venous blood gas measurements.

Indications for arterial blood gas sampling and analysis include the need to (1) evaluate the adequacy of a patient's ventilatory ($PaCO_2$), acid–base (pH and $PaCO_2$), or oxygenation (PaO_2 and O_2Hb) and O_2-carrying capacities; (2)

Table • 4–4   MEASURED AND COMMONLY CALCULATED ARTERIAL BLOOD GAS PARAMETERS

Parameter	Description
Directly Measured	
pH	H^+ concentration in the blood
$PaCO_2$	Partial pressure of CO_2 in the arterial blood (mmHg)
PaO_2	Partial pressure of O_2 in the arterial blood (mmHg)
Calculated	
HCO_3^-	Plasma bicarbonate concentration (mEq/L)
BE	Base excess (mEq/L)
SaO_2	Percentage arterial oxyhemoglobin saturation (%)
CaO_2	Arterial oxygen content (mL O_2/dL)
PAO_2	Partial pressure of alveolar O_2
$PAO_2 - PaO_2$	Alveolar-arterial O_2 partial pressure difference

Table • 4–5 NORMAL ARTERIAL AND VENOUS BLOOD GAS VALUES

Arterial	Mixed Venous
pH 7.35–7.45	7.34–7.36
PCO_2 35–45 mmHg	44–46 mmHg
HCO_3^- 22–26 mEq/L	24–30 mEq/L
PO_2 80–100 mmHg	38–42 mmHg
SO_2 >95%	70%
P_B = 760 mmHg	
FiO_2 = 0.21	

assess the response to therapeutic interventions, such as oxygen therapy and mechanical ventilation; and (3) monitor the severity and progression of disease.[11]

Arterial Sampling Technique

The radial artery is the most frequently sampled vessel for obtaining arterial blood, for the following reasons: (1) the artery is relatively superficial and easy to stabilize after the puncture; (2) properly performed, puncture of the radial artery is relatively pain free; and (3) collateral circulation to the hand by the ulnar artery is usually good and easy to evaluate.

About 3% to 5% of the population does not have adequate collateral circulation to the hand because of an incomplete palmer arch. Before radial artery puncture, the degree of collateral circulation to the hand should be assessed by performing a modified Allen test (Box 4–4). This test can be performed on infants and patients who are unable to cooperate. An assistant forms the patient's hand into a fist and squeezes the hand while the examiner proceeds with the test.

Other arteries that may be sampled in adults include the brachial, femoral, and dorsalis pedis arteries. If the radial arteries are inappropriate or unavailable for sampling, the brachial arteries are generally considered to be the sampling sites of second choice. There are important considerations to keep in mind when sampling the brachial artery: (1) the artery is less superficial than the radial artery, (2) the course of the median nerve closely parallels the artery, and (3) inadvertent venous sampling is possible because of the close proximity of large veins.

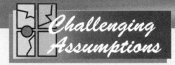 **CRITICAL THINKING CHALLENGES**

Challenging Assumptions

Acid–Base Interpretation Made Easy

Interpretation of arterial blood gas values can be confusing for practitioners as well as physicians. Here is a simple but effective strategy based on the fact that whatever the acid–base status of the body (pH), it is caused by either the respiratory ($PaCO_2$ is the respiratory acid) or the metabolic (HCO_3^- and base excess [BE] are the prime metabolic buffers) components. If a component is acid or alkaline and agrees with the body, it is causative. If a component disagrees, it is compensating for the abnormality. If a component is normal, it is a neutral factor.

Look at the total body pH and determine whether it is acid, normal, or alkaline.

Is the respiratory component ($PaCO_2$) acid, normal, or alkaline? Does it agree or disagree with the body pH?

Is the metabolic (HCO_3^- and BE) acid normal or alkaline? Does it agree or disagree with the body?

When either (or both) of the components agree with the body, it is a cause of the body's condition.

When either the respiratory or metabolic components disagree with the body, it is a compensatory mechanism.

Compensation is complete when the body pH is within normal range (7.35 to 7.45). Compensation is partial when the pH remains out of range (but is closer than if there was no compensation).

For example:

- When the body pH is acid (<7.35) and the $PaCO_2$ is acid (>45 mmHg), the respiratory component *agrees* with the body. This would be respiratory acidosis.

- When the body pH is acid (<7.35) and the $PaCO_2$ (<35 mmHg) is alkaline, the respiratory component disagrees with the body. This would be respiratory compensation.

- When the body pH is alkaline (>7.45) and the HCO_3^- is alkaline (>26 mEq/L or the BE is >+4 mEq/L), the metabolic component *agrees* with the body. This would be metabolic alkalosis. (Note that when the BE is negative there is less buffer), it is acid, positive (more buffer) is alkaline, and 0 ±2 is normal.

- When the body pH is alkaline (>7.45) and the HCO_3^- is acid (<22 mEq/L with BE <−4 mEq/L), the metabolic component *disagrees* with the body. This would be metabolic compensation.

- If both components agree with the body, they are both causative. That would be a mixed acidosis or alkalosis.

- If both components disagree with the body, *something is wrong*. Remember, at least one of the components has to agree with the body to be causing the body pH to be acidic or alkaline.

Box • 4–4 MODIFIED ALLEN TEST PROCEDURE
1. Have the patient form a tightly closed fist.
2. Apply pressure to both the radial and ulnar arteries to occlude blood flow.
3. Elevate the patient's hand (with the fist still clenched) above the level of the heart.
4. Lower the patient's hand below the level of the heart, and instruct the patient to open the fist slowly to reveal the blanched hand.
5. The pressure occluding the ulnar artery is removed while pressure is maintained to occlude the radial artery.
6. Flushing of the palm and fingers within 10 to 15 seconds indicates that adequate blood flow to the hand can be supplied by the ulnar artery in the event of radial artery occlusion or reduction of flow secondary to clotting, spasm of the vessel, or hematoma formation around the artery.

The femoral arteries are generally reserved for sampling during emergency situations or when radial or brachial sampling is not possible. As with sampling of the brachial artery, there are significant considerations when sampling the femoral artery: (1) there is virtually no collateral circulation available to the lower leg if the artery should become occluded, (2) the courses of the femoral vein and femoral nerve closely parallel that of the artery, and (3) after puncture, large amounts of blood may seep from the artery and go unnoticed because of its deep emplacement.

Arterial blood may also be obtained from an indwelling arterial catheter. The radial artery is the most common site for such a catheter, but using the brachial and femoral arteries is not uncommon. Mixed venous blood may be obtained from the distal lumen of a Swan-Ganz pulmonary catheter. As an example, mixed venous blood gas analysis is necessary to compute the difference between arterial and mixed venous oxygen content [$C(a-v)O_2$] and in calculating the percent intrapulmonary shunt ($\dot{Q}s/\dot{Q}T$).

Before performing arterial puncture, the practitioner should verify that the fraction of inspired oxygen (FiO_2) or oxygen liter flow is correct for those patients receiving supplemental oxygen. In addition, the practitioner should ascertain whether the patient is currently receiving anticoagulant or thrombolytic therapy.

Radial Artery Sampling

The procedure for radial artery sampling is given in Box 4–5.

Basic Interpretation of Blood Gas Measurements

pH

The pH is a measure of the hydrogen ion concentration ([H^+]) in the plasma. As the [H^+] increases, the pH decreases, and conversely, as the [H^+] decreases, the pH increases. This inverse relation between pH and [H^+] is based on the following definition of pH:

$$pH = \log\left(\frac{1}{[H^+]}\right), or$$

$$pH = -\log[H^+]$$

Because pH is a logarithmic function, large changes in [H^+] result in small changes in the numeric value of pH. As an example, a decrease in pH of 0.3 units represents a doubling of the [H^+].

The normal pH value of arterial blood pH is 7.35 to 7.45. A pH value below 7.35 is classified as **acidemia.** A pH value above 7.45 is classified as **alkalemia**. A significant decrease in pH can depress organ function, decrease myocardial contractility, promote the development of ventricular dysrhythmias, and depress the central nervous system. A significant increase in pH can also depress organ function and promote cardiac arrhythmias. In addition, an increased pH produces central nervous system and neuromuscular overexcitability.

PaCO₂

The normal value of arterial $PaCO_2$ is 35 to 45 mmHg. A $PaCO_2$ value above 45 mmHg is classified as **respiratory acidosis.** A $PaCO_2$ value below 35 mmHg is classified as **respiratory alkalosis.**

This relation of $PaCO_2$ to pH is based on the CO_2 hydrolysis reaction, as follows:

$$H_2O + CO_2 \rightleftharpoons H_2CO_3 \rightleftharpoons HCO_3^- + H^+$$

When CO_2 combines with water, carbonic acid is formed. The carbonic acid rapidly dissociates into bicarbonate and hydrogen ions. The equilibrium of this reaction can be shifted to the right or the left depending on the relative concentration of CO_2. In the healthy person, significant changes in $PaCO_2$ level can be accomplished within minutes. This ability to modify $PaCO_2$ level quickly can be an important compensatory mechanism when metabolic acidosis or alkalosis occurs.

When CO_2 is retained (hypercapnia), it is usually the result of alveolar hypoventilation. As ventilation falls in the face of constant CO_2 production, or when ventilation is unable to keep up with increased CO_2 production, an increase in the $PaCO_2$ is the result. As the level of CO_2 increases, the equilibrium of the CO_2 hydrolysis reaction is shifted to the right. The result is an increase in [H^+] and a resultant decrease in pH. Box 4–6 lists common causes of respiratory acidosis.

Box • 4–5 RADIAL ARTERY SAMPLING PROCEDURE

1. Assemble the appropriate equipment for the arterial blood gas kit:

    70% isopropyl alcohol prep pads

    3- to 5- mL preheparinized syringe

    20- to 25-gauge needle

    2×2 gauze pads

    Container with ice slush (cup, plastic bag, or disposable emesis basin)

    Rubber syringe cap

    Blood gas data form and label

    Gloves

2. Properly identify the patient (always check the name band).

3. Explain the procedure to the patient.

4. The patient should be seated or lying down in the event that syncope occurs.

5. Wash hands, and put on gloves.

6. Perform the modified Allen test, and document adequate collateral blood flow.

7. Prepare the syringe and select the appropriate needle:

    Most ABG kits contain vented, preheparinized syringes that require the syringe barrel to be withdrawn only to the desired sample volume. When glass, nonheparinized syringes are used, a small amount of heparin (1000 units/mL) is aspirated into the syringe and distributed by pulling the plunger in and out several times. The heparin is then expelled from the syringe. The heparin that remains in the dead space of the syringe, and the needle is adequate to anticoagulate samples (4 mL). Ideally, blood samples should be 2 to 4 mL when liquid heparin is used.

    20- and 21-gauge needles are recommended for adult and adolescent puncture procedures. 22- to 25-gauge needles may be used without affecting accuracy, but some gentle aspiration may be required with smaller-gauge needles, especially if the patient is hypotensive.

8. Position the patient's wrist in mild extension (about 30 degrees). A rolled towel placed under the wrist helps to maintain the proper position.

9. Palpate the radial artery with the tips of the index and middle fingers.

10. After identification of an adequate pulse, cleanse the puncture site with alcohol. Use a circular motion, starting from the center of the site and working outward about one-half inch around the intended site. Do not use an up-and-down or side-to-side motion.

11. Repalpate the artery with one hand, and hold the syringe with the other. The syringe should be held in the same manner as holding a pencil. The needle should be at an angle of about 45 degrees with the bevel upward (Fig. 4-26).

12. Advance the needle through the skin into the artery. As the needle enters the artery, a flash of blood appears in the hub of the needle, and blood begins to pulsate into the syringe. Occasionally, the needle passes completely through the artery. In this instance, a flash of blood is seen in the needle hub, but blood fails to enter the syringe. In an attempt to remedy this situation, the needle should be withdrawn slowly until blood is observed flowing into the syringe. Allow the pulsatile flow to fill the syringe to the desired volume.

13. Once the syringe is filled, the needle should be withdrawn, and immediate pressure should be applied to the puncture site with a sterile 2×2 gauze. Firm pressure should be applied for a minimum of 5 minutes. Patients receiving anticoagulant or thrombolytic therapy and those with disorders of coagulation require that pressure be applied for a minimum of 10 to 15 minutes or longer, until bleeding has stopped. It is prudent to reexamine the puncture site 2 to 5 minutes after the release of pressure. If blood is observed oozing from the site, pressure should be reapplied until the leakage has subsided.

14. The needle should be removed from the syringe and capped with a rubber syringe cap. It is inadvisable to attempt to stick the needle into a rubber stopper, cork, or plastic block or to recap the needle because these practices are dangerous owing to the potential for practitioner needlestick injury. Air that may be present in the syringe should be expelled gently to reduce any air–blood interface. Gently roll or tilt the syringe from side to side to distribute and mix the anticoagulant with the blood. Do not shake the sample violently because this may create foam out of any small air bubbles that may still be present.

15. Sample cooling is generally not required if analysis is to be undertaken within 10 to 15 minutes. If the analysis is to be delayed beyond 15 minutes, the sample should be placed into an ice-water slush. Iced samples should be analyzed within 1 hour. In situations in which the patient's white blood cell count is significantly elevated, such as the leukocytosis associated with leukemia, the sample should be iced immediately and analyzed as soon after puncture as possible.

16. Label the sample, and transport it to the appropriate location for analysis.

Box • 4–6 COMMON CAUSES OF RESPIRATORY ACIDOSIS

Chronic obstructive pulmonary disease
Severe $\dot{V}/\dot{Q}$ mismatch
Neuromuscular disorders
  Guillain-Barré syndrome
  Myasthenia gravis
  Poliomyelitis
Neurologic disorders
Drug overdose
  Narcotics
  Barbiturates

Box • 4–7 COMMON CAUSES OF RESPIRATORY ALKALOSIS

Restrictive lung disorders
  Pulmonary fibrosis
  Pneumonia
  Congestive heart failure
Neurologic disorders
  Anxiety
  Fear
Hypoxemia

A decrease in CO_2 (hypocapnia) is usually the result of alveolar hyperventilation. If ventilation remains constant as metabolic production of CO_2 falls or ventilation outpaces CO_2 production, a decrease in $PaCO_2$ results. As the level of CO_2 decreases, the equilibrium of the CO_2 hydrolysis reaction is shifted to the left. The result is a decrease in $[H^+]$ and a resultant increase in pH. Box 4–7 lists common causes of respiratory alkalosis.

HCO_3^-

The level of plasma bicarbonate ion is generally a reflection of the metabolic constituent of acid–base balance. The normal value for arterial HCO_3^- is 22 to 26 mEq/L.

Values less than 22 mEq/L are classified as a **metabolic acidosis,** and values greater than 26 mEq/L are classified

as **metabolic alkalosis**. The renal system is the primary mechanism that regulates HCO_3^- level.

The relation among pH, $PaCO_2$, and HCO_3^- is demonstrated by the Henderson-Hasselbalch equation:

$$pH = 6.1 + \log \left(\frac{HCO_3^-}{PaCO_2 \times 0.03} \right),$$

where $PaCO_2 \times 0.03$ equals dissolved CO_2 in mEq/L.

If normal values are substituted for HCO_3^- and $PaCO_2$, the following equation applies:

$$pH = 6.1 + \log \left(\frac{24 \text{ mEq/L}}{1.2 \text{ mEq/L}} \right) = 7.40$$

In this equation, the ratio of HCO_3^- to dissolved CO_2 is 20:1. To maintain the pH at the normal value of 7.40, this 20:1 ratio must be maintained. In the case of a metabolic acidosis, such as lactic acidosis that results from anaerobic metabolism, the HCO_3^- level falls as the bicarbonate ions buffer the increase in hydrogen ions. This fall in HCO_3^- alters the ratio of HCO_3^- to dissolved CO_2, and the pH falls. The following equation is an example of this:

$$pH = 6.1 + \log \left(\frac{18 \text{ mEq/L}}{1.2 \text{ mEq/L}} \right) = 7.28$$

In a person with a normal respiratory drive and adequate respiratory muscle strength, it is unlikely that the $PaCO_2$ would remain normal. To compensate for the fall in pH, the body increases the alveolar minute ventilation in an attempt to lower the $PaCO_2$ and alter the ratio of HCO_3^- to dissolved CO_2 toward the normal ratio of 20:1. If the person in the example above were to hyperventilate, decreasing the $PaCO_2$ to 32 mmHg, then the dissolved CO_2 would be 0.96 mEq/L (32 mmHg $\times$ 0.03 = 0.96 mEq/L dissolved CO_2), and the plasma pH would be within the normal range.

$$pH = 6.1 + \log \left(\frac{18 \text{ mEq/L}}{0.96 \text{ mEq/L}} \right) = 7.37$$

Box 4–8 lists common causes of metabolic acidosis.
Metabolic alkalosis is caused by the excessive loss of fixed acid from the body, or an accumulation of HCO_3^-

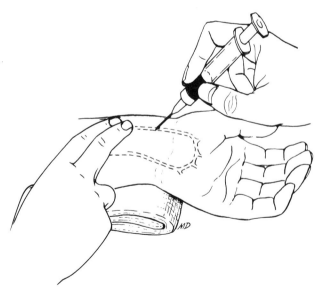

FIGURE 4–26 • Radial puncture. The wrist is extended to about 30 degrees with the palm upward. The puncture is made at a 45-degree angle opposite the blood flow with the bevel facing upward. (Malley WJ. *Clinical Blood Gases: Applications and Noninvasive Alternatives.* Philadelphia: WB Saunders. 1990.)

Box • 4–8	COMMON CAUSES OF METABOLIC ACIDOSIS

Ketoacidosis
Lactic acidosis
Toxic ingestion
   Acetylsalicylic acid
   Methanol
Renal tubular necrosis

ions. As an example, the excessive loss of HCl by prolonged gastric suctioning results in an increase in blood base. For instance, if the HCO_3^- is 29 mEq/L and the $PaCO_2$ is normal at 40 mmHg, an increase in pH is the result:

$$pH = 6.1 + \log\left(\frac{30 \text{ mEq/L}}{1.2 \text{ mEq/L}}\right) = 7.50$$

To return the pH to within the normal range, the body decreases the alveolar minute ventilation in an attempt to increase the $PaCO_2$ and alter the ratio of HCO_3^- to dissolved CO_2 toward the normal value of 20:1. If the person in the previous example were to hypoventilate, increasing the $PaCO_2$ to 46 mmHg, the dissolved CO_2 would be 1.38 mEq/L (46 mmHg $\times$ 0.03 = 1.38 mEq/L dissolved CO_2), and the plasma pH would be within the normal range.

$$pH = 6.1 + \log\left(\frac{30 \text{ mEq/L}}{1.38 \text{ mEq/L}}\right) = 7.44$$

Box 4–9 lists common causes of metabolic alkalosis.

As previously noted, changes in HCO_3^- are mediated by the renal system. As such, the ability to respond to rapid changes in pH is limited. Compensatory changes in the HCO_3^- level in response to chronic changes in $PaCO_2$ generally requires 12 to 24 hours to occur.

If a patient were to retain CO_2 acutely, such as occurs with the hypoventilation associated with a drug overdose ($PaCO_2$ = 55 mmHg), the plasma pH would be decreased because the ratio of HCO_3^- to dissolved CO_2 is 14.5:1.

$$pH = 6.1 + \log\left(\frac{25 \text{ mEq/L}}{1.65 \text{ mEq/L}}\right) = 7.26$$

Box • 4–9	COMMON CAUSES OF METABOLIC ALKALOSIS

Loss of gastric fluid
   Vomiting
   Gastric drainage
Hypokalemia

The HCO_3^- increases or decreases slightly as a result of acute changes in $Paco_2$. This change in HCO_3^- is mediated by the CO_2 hydrolysis reaction:

$$H_2O + CO_2 \rightleftharpoons H_2CO_3 \rightleftharpoons HCO_3^- + H^+$$

As the CO_2 increases, the equilibrium of the reaction is shifted to the right, and a rapid, yet small, increase in HCO_3^- occurs. Conversely, as the CO_2 decreases, the equilibrium of the reaction is shifted to the left, and a small decrease in HCO_3^- occurs. In general, for every 5 mmHg acute decrease in $PaCO_2$, the HCO_3^- decreases by 1 mEq/L; and for every 10 mmHg acute increase in $PaCO_2$, the HCO_3^- increases by 1 mEq/L.

In the patient with chronic CO_2 retention, such as that seen in the end-stage ventilatory failure of chronic obstructive pulmonary disease, the renal system retains HCO_3^- to maintain the pH within the normal range. As an example, if the $PaCO_2$ is chronically 55 mmHg and the HCO_3^- is 31 mEq/L, the pH is in within the normal range because the ratio of HCO_3^- to dissolved CO_2 is 18.8:1.

$$pH = 6.1 + \log\left(\frac{31 \text{ mEq/L}}{1.65 \text{ mEq/L}}\right) = 7.37$$

The body does not generally overcompensate to maintain the pH within the normal range. As an example, if a chronic respiratory acidosis with a $PaCO_2$ of 50 mmHg were to exist, renal compensation would occur, and HCO_3^- would increase just enough to return the pH to a level of 7.35 to 7.36. In this instance, the pH compensation is about half of what the pH would be if the respiratory acidosis were acute and no compensation had taken place.

As a rule, maximum compensation for chronic respiratory and metabolic acidosis is about half of the acute uncompensated value for the pH. Compensation for metabolic alkalosis is slightly less than half, and compensation for respiratory alkalosis is slightly greater than half of the acute uncompensated value for the pH.

PaO_2

At a barometric pressure of 760 mmHg and an FIO_2 of 0.21, the normal adult value for PaO_2 is 80 to 100 mmHg. A PaO_2 value less than 80 mmHg is considered **hypoxemia**. With advancing age, the ability of the lungs to oxygenate the blood declines progressively. For each year beyond the age of 60 years, 1 mmHg is subtracted from the lower limit of the normal PaO_2. For example, a 70-year-old person would not be considered hypoxemic until the PaO_2 was less than 71 mmHg.

Hypoxemia can be further categorized as mild, moderate, or severe. In an adult (60 years old) breathing room air, the limits of hypoxemia are listed below[12]:

Mild hypoxemia: PaO_2 < 80 mmHg
Moderate hypoxemia: PaO_2 < 60 mmHg
Severe hypoxemia: PaO_2 < 40 mmHg

CRITICAL THINKING CHALLENGES

Go Figure

Interpret the following arterial blood gas values:

Body: pH	Respiratory: $PaCO_2$	Metabolic: HCO_3^-	Interpretation: Base Excess
7.20	60	24	0
7.51	29	23	0
7.05	12	5	−30
7.25	90	38	+8
7.58	45	40	+15
7.36	33	18	−5
7.41	27	16	−6

For each year after 60 years of age, 1 mmHg is subtracted from the limits for mild and moderate hypoxemia. A PaO_2 of less than 40 mmHg indicates severe hypoxemia regardless of age.

Clinically significant hypoxemia is considered to exist when the PaO_2 is less than 60 mmHg. This is based on the relation of arterial oxyhemoglobin saturation (SaO_2) to PaO_2. At a PaO_2 of 60 mmHg, the SaO_2 is about 90%. Normally, there is no clinically significant advantage to increasing the SaO_2 to the normal value of more than 95% because this will not significantly increase the arterial oxygen content. This is a particularly important consideration

Box • 4–10 CLINICAL INTERPRETIVE STRATEGY

1. Classify the pH
     Normal: 7.35 to 7.45
     Acidemia: <7.35
     Alkalemia: >7.45
2. Classify the $PaCO_2$
     Normal: 35–45 mmHg
     Respiratory acidosis: >45 mmHg
     Respiratory alkalosis: <35 mmHg
3. Classify the HCO_3^-
     Normal: 22–26 mEq/L
     Metabolic acidosis: <22 mEq/L
     Metabolic alkalosis: >26 mEq/L
4. If the pH is normal, are the $PaCO_2$ and HCO_3^- values within the normal range? If yes, normal acid–base balance likely exists.
5. If the pH is out of range, is it because of respiratory, metabolic, or combined disorder? Has partial pH compensation occurred?
6. If the pH is normal and the $PaCO_2$ or HCO_3^- are out of range, pH compensation has occurred. Determine the primary disorder.
     pH 7.35–7.40: Primary disorder is likely an acidosis ($PaCO_2$ >45 mmHg or HCO_3^- <22 mEq/L)
     pH 7.40–7.45: Primary disorder is likely an alkalosis ($PaCO_2$ <35 mmHg or HCO_3^- >26 mEq/L).
7. Classify the PaO_2
     Does hypoxemia exist?
     If receiving supplemental oxygen, is the hypoxemia corrected? Excessively corrected?

Box • 4–11 ACID–BASE CLASSIFICATIONS

pH <7.35, $PaCO_2$ >45 mmHg, HCO_3^- 22–26 mEq/L = Uncompensated respiratory acidosis

pH >7.45, $PaCO_2$ <35 mmHg, HCO_3^- 22–26 mEq/L = Uncompensated respiratory alkalosis

pH <7.35, $PaCO_2$ >45 mmHg, HCO_3^- >26 mEq/L = Partially compensated respiratory acidosis

pH >7.45, $PaCO_2$ <35 mmHg, HCO_3^- <22 mEq/L = Partially compensated respiratory alkalosis

pH 7.35–7.40, $PaCO_2$ >45 mmHg, HCO_3^- >26 mEq/L = Compensated respiratory acidosis

pH 7.40–7.45, $PaCO_2$ <35 mmHg, HCO_3^- <22 mEq/L = Compensated respiratory alkalosis

pH <7.35, $PaCO_2$ 35–45 mmHg, HCO_3^- <22 mEq/L = Uncompensated metabolic acidosis

pH >7.45, $PaCO_2$ 35–45 mmHg, HCO_3^- >26 mEq/L = Uncompensated metabolic alkalosis

pH <7.35, $PaCO_2$ <35 mmHg, HCO_3^- <22 mEq/L = Partially compensated metabolic acidosis

pH >7.45, $PaCO_2$ >45 mmHg, HCO_3^- >26 mEq/L = Partially compensated metabolic alkalosis

pH 7.35–7.40, $PaCO_2$ <35 mmHg, HCO_3^- <22 mEq/L = Compensated metabolic acidosis

pH 7.40–7.45, $PaCO_2$ >45 mmHg, HCO_3^- >26 mEq/L = Compensated metabolic alkalosis

pH <7.35, $PaCO_2$ >45 mmHg, HCO_3^- <22 mEq/L = Combined acidosis

pH >7.45, $PaCO_2$ <35 mmHg, HCO_3^- >26 mEq/L = Combined alkalosis

when potentially toxic levels of oxygen are required to maintain an adequate PaO_2. Under these circumstances, the use of the lowest FiO_2 that will produce a PaO_2 of 60 to 65 mmHg may be warranted.

When supplemental oxygen is administered, the classification of hypoxemia is modified[12]:

Uncorrected hypoxemia: $PaO_2 < 60$ mmHg
Corrected hypoxemia: $PaO_2 > 60$ mmHg; <100 mmHg
Excessively corrected hypoxemia: $PaO_2 > 100$ mmHg; $<$ minimally acceptable level

This classification reflects the fact that the patient would be hypoxemic if he or she was breathing room air. As an example, if a patient had a PaO_2 of 72 mmHg and an FiO_2 of 0.30, it can be assumed that hypoxemia would occur on room air. This is based on knowledge of the minimally acceptable PaO_2 for a particular FiO_2. In the normal lung, an increase in FiO_2 of 0.10 increases the partial pressure of alveolar oxygen (PAO_2) by about 50 mmHg. In the previous example, the minimally acceptable PaO_2 at an FiO_2 of 0.30 would be about 150 mmHg. This can be computed easily for any FiO_2 by multiplying the FiO_2 by 500 (or oxygen percentage by 5). Box 4–10 lists a basic clinical interpretive strategy. Box 4–11 lists the pH, $PaCO_2$, and HCO_3^- para-

meters for basic acid–base classification. Figure 4–27 illustrates a flow-chart approach to acid–base interpretation.

NONINVASIVE MONITORING OF GAS EXCHANGE

Pulse oximetry and capnography are noninvasive monitoring techniques that can provide the practitioner with moment-to-moment, real-time information regarding the oxygenation and ventilation status of patients in a variety of clinical situations. Proper use and the appropriate interpretation of noninvasively obtained gas exchange data require that the practitioner be well versed in the operational principles involved in the measurement technique. In concert with a firm grasp of the physiology of gas exchange, the practitioner can make clinically relevant decisions regarding the validity and utility of noninvasively obtained data.

Pulse Oximetry

Operational Principles

Pulse oximetry provides continuous, noninvasive information regarding of the amount of arterial oxygen that is com-

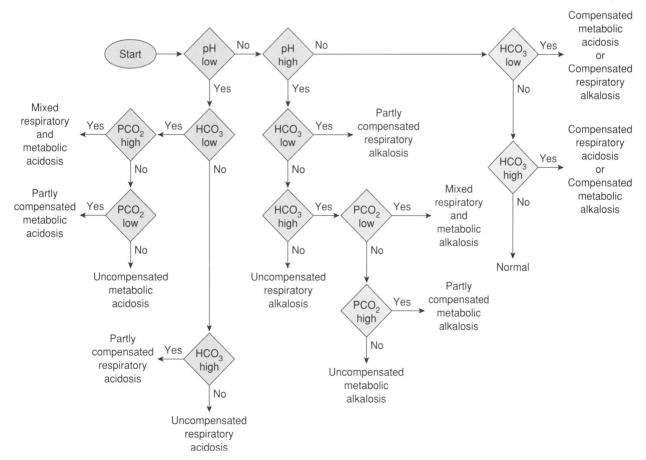

FIGURE 4–27 • Acid–base interpretation flow chart. (Chatburn RL, Lough MD. *Handbook of Respiratory Care.* 2nd. ed. St. Louis: Mosby–Year Book; 1990.)

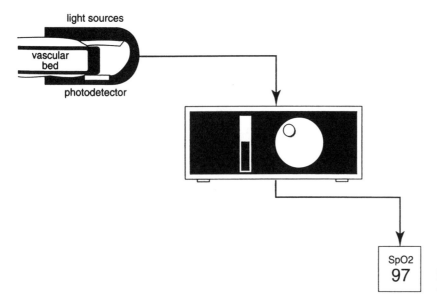

light sources

vascular
bed

photodetector

SpO2
97   FIGURE 4–28 • Pulse oximetry application.

bined with hemoglobin (SpO$_2$). Measurement is accomplished by placing two light-emitting diodes, one that emits light in the red wavelength (about 660 nm) and one that emits light in the infrared wavelength (about 920 nm), on one side of a pulsatile vascular bed. A photodetector is placed on the opposite side of the vascular bed and measures the intensity of the transmitted light through the optical pathway (Fig. 4–28).

The principles of optical plethysmography and spectrophotometry are used in pulse oximetry to determine the SpO$_2$ values. Optical plethysmography measures the changes in light absorption caused by the change in volume of a pulsatile vascular bed, to differentiate arterial from venous blood. Components of the optical pathway, such as venous blood, bone, tissue, and skin, are normally nonpulsatile. This nonpulsatile absorbance is used as a baseline by the pulse oximeter. During systole, the vascular bed dilates, the blood volume increases, and the light absorption increases. The pulse oximeter's microprocessor assumes that only pulsatile absorbance is arterial blood (Fig. 4–29).

The amplitude of the plethysmographic pulse is indicated in a number of different ways by the various manufacturers

of pulse oximeters. Some monitors use an auditory signal that changes in intensity or pitch with changes in pulse amplitude. Other monitors display a lighted, vertical bar that increases or decreases in height in proportion to the pulse amplitude. Many monitors graphically display the arterial pulse waveform as a confirmation of arterial pulsation. The assessment of adequate arterial pulse amplitude is important in obtaining valid measurement of SpO$_2$.

Spectrophotometry uses various wavelengths of light to determine the absorption of different substances. Oxygenated hemoglobin (O$_2$Hb) and deoxygenated hemoglobin (Hb) possess different light-absorption characteristics. Red light is readily absorbed when passed through deoxygenated hemoglobin; little red light is absorbed when passed through oxygenated hemoglobin. Infrared light passed through oxygenated hemoglobin is absorbed; little infrared light is absorbed when passed through deoxygenated hemoglobin. The pulse oximeter calculates the SpO$_2$ by comparing the amount of infrared light absorbed with the amount of red light absorbed.

Oxygen saturation measured by two-wavelength pulse oximeters is termed **functional saturation**. Functional sat-

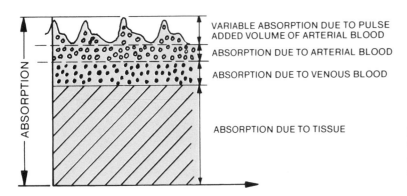

VARIABLE ABSORPTION DUE TO PULSE
ADDED VOLUME OF ARTERIAL BLOOD

ABSORPTION DUE TO ARTERIAL BLOOD

ABSORPTION DUE TO VENOUS BLOOD

ABSORPTION DUE TO TISSUE

FIGURE 4–29 • When light is passed through tissue, some of that light is absorbed by each constituent of the tissue, but the only variable light absorption is due to arterial blood. (Courtesy of Ohmeda Inc., Madison, WI.)

uration is the ratio of oxyhemoglobin to the total hemoglobin (sum of deoxyhemoglobin and oxyhemoglobin) available for binding with oxygen.

$$\text{Functional saturation} = \frac{O_2Hb}{Hb + O_2Hb}$$

When compared with measurement by a CO-oximeter, a multiple-wavelength oximeter, the pulse oximeter fails to detect certain species of dysfunctional (non–oxygen-binding) hemoglobin. The multiple-wavelength CO-oximeter measures **fractional saturation**, which is the ratio of oxyhemoglobin to the total number of hemoglobin molecules present. In this case, total hemoglobin represents the sum of oxyhemoglobin, deoxyhemoglobin, and dysfunctional hemoglobins. The two most commonly measured dysfunctional hemoglobins are carboxyhemoglobin (COHb) and methemoglobin (metHb).

$$\text{Fractional saturation} = \frac{O_2Hb}{Hb + COHb + metHb + O_2Hb}$$

In the presence of a significant amount of dysfunctional hemoglobin, such as may be seen in the patient with smoke inhalation, the functional saturation, as obtained by pulse oximetry, may be significantly different from the fractional saturation that would be obtained by CO-oximetry. Recognizing this difference would be of clinical importance in that the saturation obtained by pulse oximetry could significantly overestimate the true oxyhemoglobin saturation.

Clinical Indications

The American Association for Respiratory Care Clinical Practice Guideline on the use of pulse oximetry provides three general indications for performing pulse oximetry[13]:

- The need to monitor the adequacy of arterial oxyhemoglobin saturation
- The need to quantitate the response of arterial oxyhemoglobin saturation to therapeutic intervention or a diagnostic procedure
- The need to comply with mandated regulations or recommendations of authoritative groups

Pulse oximetry provides a continuous, real-time trend of the patient's oxyhemoglobin saturation. When the information obtained from pulse oximetry is coupled with other clinical information, such as direct patient assessment, hemoglobin concentration, and information from other noninvasive monitors of gas exchange (capnography or transcutaneous gas monitoring), decisions can be made regarding oxygen supplementation requirements and the need to obtain more definitive information by arterial blood gas analysis.

Pulse oximetry is also used for oxygenation monitoring during surgery and surgical recovery, in emergency medicine, for prescribing oxygen for hospitalized patients, during sleep studies and exercise testing, for prescribing and evaluating long-term home oxygen therapy, and in monitoring infants and children.

Application Technique

Various configurations of pulse oximetry probes are available (Fig. 4–30). Single-patient probes are available for use in adults, children, and infants. These probes are usually placed on the finger of an adult or child. The great toe, foot, or palm is usually used for probe placement in infants. When the probe is applied, it should be placed snugly around the digit, yet not so tight as to affect circulation. When using any oximetry probe for continuous monitoring, the probe site should be inspected frequently to detect any alterations in circulation or skin integrity. The probe site should be changed if any abnormalities are noted. The probe's light-emitting diodes should be placed directly across the vascular bed from the photodetector. Care should be taken to avoid misalignment because this may result in erroneous readings.

In situations resulting in poor peripheral perfusion, such as hypotension, the administration of vasoactive drugs, or hypothermia, specially designed monitoring probes are available that may allow for adequate pulse detection. An adult nasal sensor is available that samples a vascular bed supplied by a branch of the carotid artery. During low peripheral perfusion states, it may be possible to obtain an adequate signal with the nasal sensor to permit accurate SpO_2 measurement.

In addition to the single-patient probes, a number of nondisposable, reusable probes are available. These probes are variously held in place by spring-loaded clips, special tape configurations, Velcro fasteners, or tape. As with the single-patient probes, care must be taken to align the light-emitting diodes directly across the vascular bed from the photodetector.

Regardless of the type of probe used, the manufacturer's directions for use should be followed closely. Specifically, the patient weight guidelines for the particular probe should be followed. In addition, probes from one manufacturer should not be used with another manufacturer's monitor unless the equipment's operational manual specifically permits the practice.

Measurements of SpO_2 may be made continuously or may be obtained by spot-checking. Continuous measurement of SpO_2 is of particular value in monitoring the oxygenation status of critically ill respiratory patients who are being mechanically ventilated. When a pulse oximeter is being used for continuous monitoring, it is necessary to set appropriate saturation alarm limits.

The proper performance of the pulse oximetry spot-check deserves additional discussion. When obtaining SpO_2 spot-check readings, the practitioner should perform the measurement in duplicate. The difference between the two measurements should not differ more than $\pm2\%$. In

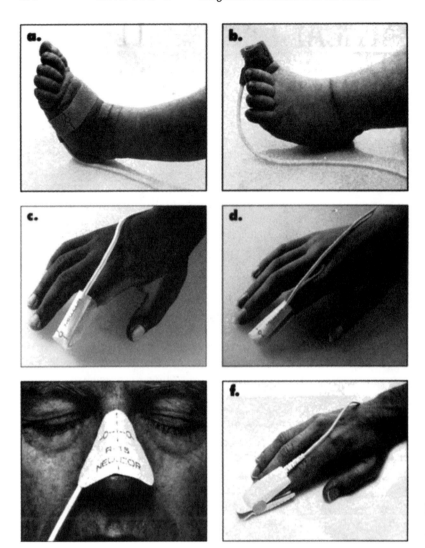

FIGURE 4-30 • Pulse oximetry probes. (Courtesy of Nellcor Puritan Bennett, Pleasanton, CA.)

CRITICAL THINKING CHALLENGES

Case Scenario

Pulse Oximetry

You are called to the emergency department to evaluate a patient. The patient appears to be short of breath and hypotensive with cold and clammy skin. The pulse oximetry shows an SpO_2 of 94% and a pulse of 84 beats/min. What can you do at the bedside to determine if the oximeter is working properly for this patient?

Answer: Check the pulse rate. If the palpated pulse rate is within 5 beats/min of the oximeter readout, there is usually adequate perfusion to measure oxygen saturation.

addition, a manually obtained pulse or an electrocardigram pulse should agree within ±5 beats/min with the oximeter pulse reading. Failure to obtain an adequate correlation may cast doubt on the accuracy of the SpO_2 measurement and indicate the need to change the sampling site or obtain arterial blood for blood gas analysis.

Interpretation

An examination of the oxygen content equation quickly reveals that hemoglobin is the primary transport mechanism for delivering oxygen to the tissues.

$$\text{Oxygen content} = (Hb \times 1.36 \times SO_2) + (PO_2 \times 0.003)$$

Hb = hemoglobin (g/dL blood)

1.34 = mL of O_2 carried by 1 g/dL blood of fully saturated hemoglobin

SO_2 = oxygen saturation of hemoglobin

PO_2 = partial pressure of O_2 in plasma

0.003 = mL O_2/dL blood carried as dissolved O_2 per mmHg PO_2

When normal values for arterial blood are entered into this equation, it becomes apparent that most oxygen is bound to hemoglobin and little is transported as oxygen dissolved in plasma.

$$\text{Arterial oxygen content (CaO}_2) = (15 \text{ g/dL} \times 1.34 \times 0.97)$$
$$+ (100 \text{ mmHg} \times 0.003)$$

In this example, the CaO_2 is 19.8 mL O_2/dL blood or 19.8 vol%. Of this amount, only 0.30 mL O_2/dL blood is carried as dissolved oxygen in the plasma (1.5% of the total oxygen carried).

Hemoglobin oxygen saturation is a function of the partial pressure of oxygen in the blood. This relation can be seen in the oxyhemoglobin dissociation curve (Fig. 4–31). As PO_2 increases, the oxyhemoglobin saturation increases in a relatively linear fashion until the saturation reaches about 85% to 90%. Above this point, large changes in PO_2 produce relatively small changes in oxyhemoglobin saturation. This insensitivity to elevated PO_2 makes pulse oximetry inappropriate when monitoring for hyperoxemia is the goal. The normal adult value for arterial oxygen saturation (SaO_2) is more than 95%. In clinical practice, an SaO_2 of 90% is generally acceptable.

Limitations

Motion artifact is a frequent cause of erratic measurement and spurious alarm conditions. Frequent movement of the extremity being sampled, shivering, seizure activity, and transport situations may be associated with motion artifact. Identification of motion artifact may be made by observing an erratic pulse rate on the oximeter or by comparing the pulse rate displayed with that obtained manually or by an electrocardiographic monitor. Some models of pulse oximeters display an arterial waveform obtained from the plethysmographic measurement of the vascular bed being sampled. Inspection of this waveform may also aid in the detection of motion artifact. Reduction of motion artifact may be accomplished by: (1) ensuring that the sensor is placed correctly, (2) using an adhesive sensor in situations in which motion is likely, (3) stabilizing the sensor by immobilizing the sensor site, or (4) moving the sensor to a less active site.

Low perfusion states caused by poor peripheral blood flow may not provide the oximeter with an adequate arterial pulse signal. As a result, the oximeter may display readings that are intermittent or absent. Reduction in pulse signal may also render the oximeter more susceptible to the effects of motion artifact. Common situations that result in decreased peripheral perfusion include hypotension, hypovolemia, hypothermia, and the administration of vasoconstrictor agents. Blood flow to the fingers or toes may be improved by placing warm towels over the extremity. The use of a central sensor, such as a nasal or reflectance sensor, or sampling the earlobe may provide an adequate pulse signal during low perfusion states.

Dysfunctional hemoglobins may result in an inaccurately measured SpO_2. The two most commonly encountered dysfunctional hemoglobin species are COHb and metHb. The presence of significant amounts of COHb results in falsely high SpO_2 readings. In clinical situations in which COHb is suspected, such as carbon monoxide poisoning as a result of smoke inhalation, SaO_2 should be evaluated by fractional measurement with a multiple-wavelength CO-oximeter. Clinically, the formation of significant levels of metHb is most commonly associated with the administration of dapsone or primaquine. The direction of the SpO_2 change due to metHb is difficult to predict. Depending on the patient's actual oxygen saturation and the concentration of metHb present, the SpO_2 may be either falsely high or falsely low. As was noted for the presence of COHb, measurement of the SaO_2 in situations in which metHb is suspected should be performed by CO-oximetry.

Ambient light sources, such as direct sunlight, fluorescent lights, infrared heat lamps, and phototherapy lamps, may interfere with the accuracy of pulse oximetry readings. Ambient light interference is characterized by a lack of correlation between the displayed oximeter pulse and the patient's actual pulse rate. Carefully covering or wrapping the sensor site with gauze or a towel can eliminate ambient light interference.

Nail polish colors that absorb the red light transmitted by the pulse oximeter can significantly lower oximetry readings. Blue, black, green, and brown are the colors associated with inaccurate oximetry measurement. Polish in these colors should be removed or an alternate probe site selected.

Dark skin pigmentation may affect the accuracy of pulse oximetry measurements. Technical difficulties with mea-

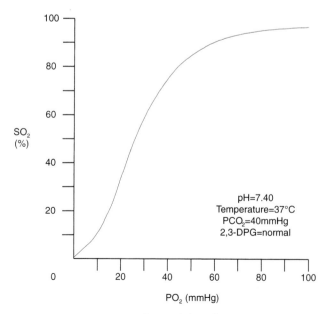

FIGURE 4–31 • Oxyhemoglobin dissociation curve.

surement have occurred when sampling is performed on patients with darkly pigmented skin.[14]

Capnometry and Capnography

Operational Principles

Capnometry is the measurement and numerical display of airway carbon dioxide concentration or partial pressure during the ventilatory cycle. Capnometry is limited to the assessment of alveolar ventilation (peak CO_2 concentration) and detection of rebreathing (inspired minimal CO_2 concentration). Capnometry is limited in its clinical utility because of the inability of the practitioner to confirm the validity of the measured CO_2 concentration.

Capnography is the graphic display of airway CO_2 concentration or partial pressure measurement as a function of time. The resulting waveform is called a *capnogram.* The evaluation of the configuration of the capnogram may be useful in the assessment of the adequacy of alveolar ventilation, integrity of the airway, cardiopulmonary function, and ventilator function. The capnogram provides a measure of the end-tidal partial pressure of CO_2 ($PetCO_2$), which is frequently a reliable estimate of the arterial partial pressure of CO_2 ($PaCO_2$).

Analysis of CO_2 concentration is commonly performed by two methods: infrared absorption spectrophotometry and mass spectrometry. Most capnographic equipment used in respiratory care measures CO_2 concentration by infrared absorption spectrophotometry. In an infrared absorption system, a beam of infrared light passes through the gas to be sampled. CO_2 molecules that are present in the light path absorb some of the infrared light. To determine the concentration of CO_2 in the sample, a comparison is made between the amount of infrared energy absorbed as the light passes through the sample and the amount of light absorbed by a CO_2-free reference cell.

Mass spectrometry can be used to measure multiple gas concentrations, including inspired and expired carbon dioxide, oxygen, nitrogen, and anesthetic gases. The use of mass spectrometry is generally limited to the operating room, pulmonary function laboratory, and special research situations because of the high cost of the equipment.

Clinical Indications

Box 4–12 lists the numerous indications for the measurement and graphic display of exhaled CO_2.[15]

Application Technique

Two techniques of sampling are used with infrared absorption systems: sidestream and mainstream. The sidestream (diverting or aspirating) capnogram withdraws gas from the patient's airway, using a sampling adapter and fine-bore tubing, to the capnogram (Fig. 4–32). An infrared

---

---

light source and photodetector are located in a measurement chamber within the capnogram. Because the gas sample must be transported to a remote measurement site, a delay in measurement occurs. The major factor that determines the response time of sidestream capnograms is the flow rate at which the sample gas is aspirated from the airway. Most capnograms use a sampling flow rate of between 50 to 150 mL/min. Sample gas transport through the fine-bore tubing may be reduced or occluded by condensed water vapor or accumulated airway secretions. Gas sampling flow rates that are too slow may result in artifacts in the capnographic waveform.

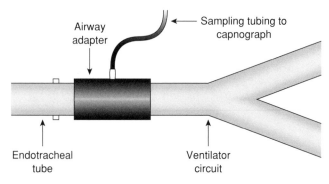

FIGURE 4–32 • Sidestream capnographic sampling technique.

The mainstream (nondiverting or in-line) capnogram uses a sample measurement chamber that is placed in-line with the patient's airway (Fig. 4–33). The measurement chamber houses an infrared light source and a photodetector and is attached to the patient's airway by a windowed airway adapter. The delay in response time of the mainstream capnogram is negligible. Mainstream sample chambers can be bulky, impose additional weight on the airway, and add significant mechanical dead space by the airway adapter. Mainstream sample chambers are delicate and may be easily damaged if dropped or handled roughly. Recently developed mainstream sensors now available are more durable, are more lightweight, and have less dead space.

Interpretation

Under the circumstance of a normal ventilation–perfusion ($\dot{V}/\dot{Q}$) relation, the venous blood entering the pulmonary circulation has a partial pressure of CO_2 ($PvCO_2$) of 46 mmHg. CO_2 rapidly moves across the alveolar-capillary membrane to the alveolus. By the time the blood leaves the alveolar lung unit, the PCO_2 in the end-capillary blood and that in the alveolus ($PACO_2$) are in equilibrium. The $PACO_2$ approximates the partial pressure of CO_2 in the arterial blood ($PaCO_2$) when the $\dot{V}/\dot{Q}$ relation is normal. The $P_{et}CO_2$ approximates the average value of $PACO_2$ of all functional lung units. Based on the relation of $PaCO_2$ to $PACO_2$ and the relation of $PACO_2$ to $P_{et}CO_2$, the $P_{et}CO_2$

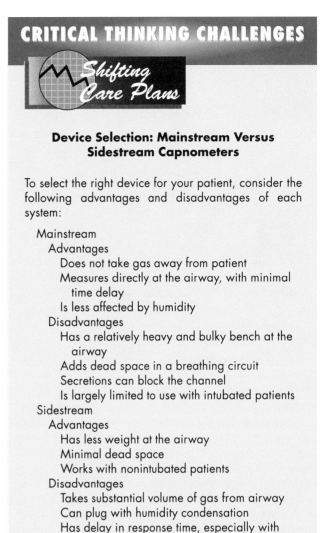

closely approximates the $PaCO_2$. The difference between the $PaCO_2$ and the $P_{et}CO_2$ is the arterial to end-tidal difference ($P[a-et]CO_2$). The value for the $P(a-et)CO_2$ is normally 5 mmHg or less.[16]

The difference between the $PaCO_2$ and the $P_{et}CO_2$ may be affected significantly by changes in $\dot{V}/\dot{Q}$ matching. The primary $\dot{V}/\dot{Q}$ disturbance causing changes in the $P(a-et)CO_2$ is dead-space ventilation. Dead space exists when lung units are ventilated but not perfused (high $\dot{V}/\dot{Q}$). The lung units that lack perfusion, yet continue to be ventilated, have CO_2 concentrations similar to that of atmospheric air (Fig. 4–34). The resultant dilution of the end-tidal gas causes $P_{et}CO_2$ values to be lower and the $P(a-et)CO_2$ difference to widen. Clinical situations that may result in dead-space ventilation are listed in Box 4–13.

Shunt perfusion occurs when lung units have absent or decreased ventilation compared with perfusion (low $\dot{V}/\dot{Q}$). In situations of low $\dot{V}/\dot{Q}$, ventilation is increased in normally perfused lung units to maintain a relatively normal $PaCO_2$ (Fig. 4–35). A small increase in the $P(a-et)CO_2$

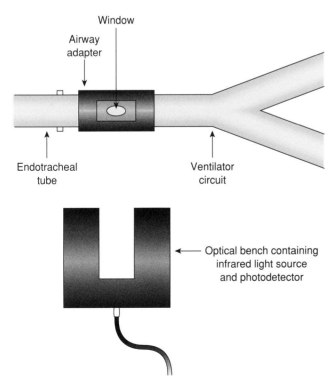

Window
Airway adapter
Endotracheal tube
Ventilator circuit
Optical bench containing infrared light source and photodetector

FIGURE 4–33 • Mainstream capnographic sampling technique.

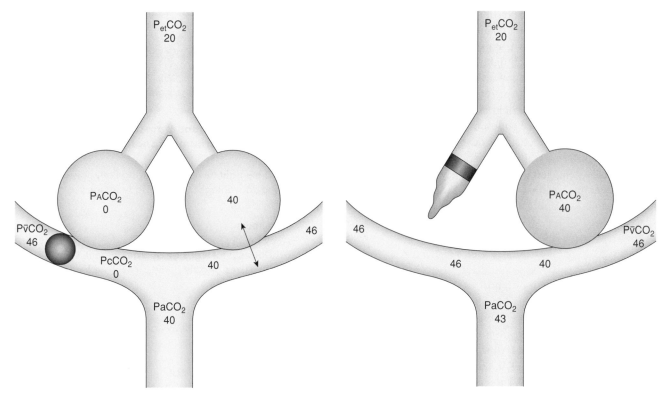

FIGURE 4-34 • Dead-space ventilation effect on P(a − et) CO$_2$ difference.

FIGURE 4-35 • Shunt perfusion effect on P(a − et) CO$_2$ difference.

gradient may occur with shunt perfusion because of the admixture of mixed venous blood to arterial blood. In general, the increase in the P(a−et)CO$_2$ difference is relatively small compared with the effect that shunt perfusion has on arterial oxygen saturation. Infants and children with large intracardiac shunts may exhibit a large P(a−et)CO$_2$ that is in proportion with the degree of mixing.

A normal capnogram is illustrated in Figure 4–36. On the ordinate, concentration is expressed as partial pressure of CO$_2$ in millimeters of mercury. On the abscissa, time is expressed in seconds. As the patient begins to exhale (see segment A-B in Fig. 36), the initial sample contains CO$_2$-free gas from tracheal dead space that has not been involved in gas exchange. As exhalation continues, CO$_2$ concentration begins to rise as gas from alveoli with rapid

time constants begin to empty (see segment B-C in Fig. 4–36). As alveolar gas begins to dominate the exhaled gas volume, the change in CO$_2$ concentration decreases significantly. This slowly changing CO$_2$ concentration produces the **alveolar plateau** (see segment C-D in Fig. 4–36). The P$_{et}$CO$_2$ is measured at the point of highest CO$_2$ concentration (see point D in Fig. 4–36). This value for P$_{et}$CO$_2$ represents the ventilation weighted average of CO$_2$ concentration for all ventilated lung units. If significant maldistribution of ventilation is not present, the value of P$_{et}$CO$_2$ is taken as the best approximation of PACO$_2$ and thus an estimate of PaCO$_2$. When inspiration occurs, the CO$_2$ concentration declines rapidly as CO$_2$-free gas is entrained into the airway (see segment D-E in Fig. 4–36). The essentials of a normal capnogram are listed in Box 4–14.

Box • 4–13	CLINICAL SITUATIONS THAT RESULT IN DEAD-SPACE VENTILATION

Pulmonary embolism
Hypotension
Hemorrhage
Pulmonary hypoperfusion
Cardiac arrest

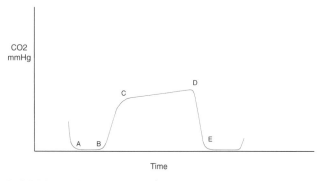

FIGURE 4–36 • Normal capnogram.

Box • 4–14 ESSENTIALS OF A NORMAL CAPNOGRAM

A zero baseline
A rapid, sharp uprise
An alveolar plateau
A rapid, sharp downstroke

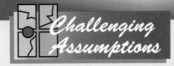

CRITICAL THINKING CHALLENGES

Challenging Assumptions

Role of Capnography in Chronic Obstructive Pulmonary Disease

Although capnometry can provide a good indication of changes in $PaCO_2$ through measurement of $P_{et}CO_2$ in select patients, the value of such measurements in patients with COPD has been called into question. The problem appears to be that the air trapping and uneven emptying of the lungs combine to provide erratic and sometimes erroneous trending of $P_{et}CO_2$. In fact, a good end-tidal measurement may not be attainable in patients with severe disease, in whom air trapping occurs. Consequently, capnometry with an end-tidal alarm may not provide reliable monitoring of patients with severe COPD during mechanical ventilation. Although the waveform may indicate trapping, the changes in values may not be directly related to changes in alveolar ventilation or CO_2 production.

Examination of the capnographic waveform morphology is important in validating the reliability of the $P_{et}CO_2$ measurement and diagnostically in conditions of altered cardiopulmonary function, changes in airway integrity, and ventilatory equipment malfunction. Initially, the $P(a-et)CO_2$ should be established by simultaneous capnographic and arterial blood gas measurement. If the $P(a-et)CO_2$ gradient is acceptable (usually less than 6 mmHg), the value for $P_{et}CO_2$ may be used as a reasonable estimation of $PaCO_2$. After $P(a-et)CO_2$ correlation, if a significant increase or decrease in $P_{et}CO_2$ occurs, the capnographic waveform should be examined to determine that the measurement is valid. In situations of hypoventilation or hyperventilation, the capnographic waveform appears normal in morphology. The ascending limb of the waveform retains its steepness, and the alveolar plateau is nearly horizontal. The value for $P_{et}CO_2$ is elevated in hypoventilation and decreased in hyperventilation (Fig. 4–37). Conditions that increase the production of CO_2, such as sepsis, fever, seizures, and increased metabolic rate, exhibit a normal capnographic waveform with an elevated $P_{et}CO_2$. A transient increase in $P_{et}CO_2$ may be the result of bicarbonate administration or the release of a limb tourniquet. Conversely, clinical conditions that cause reduced CO_2 production, such as hypothermia, exhibit a normal capnographic waveform with a decreased $P_{et}CO_2$.

Alterations in cardiopulmonary function widen the $P(a-et)CO_2$ difference. The $P_{et}CO_2$ is significantly lower than the $PaCO_2$. Situations that result in dead-space ventilation (high $\dot{V}/\dot{Q}$), such as pulmonary embolism, hemorrhage, cardiac arrest, pulmonary hypoperfusion, and hypotension, exhibit a normal capnographic waveform. As the dead-

space fraction increases, the $P(a-et)CO_2$ difference increases, and the $P_{et}CO_2$ decreases.

Integrity of the airway and the distribution of ventilation may be assessed by analysis of the capnographic waveform morphology. In situations of airflow obstruction, such as bronchospasm, the capnographic waveform is characterized by an increased slope or absence of the alveolar plateau (Fig. 4–38). The $P_{et}CO_2$ may be elevated in severe obstruction; however, if significant air trapping occurs, the $P_{et}CO_2$ may be significantly less than the $PaCO_2$. Without concomitant inspection of the capnographic waveform, the decrease in airflow and gas trapping may go unrecognized if only the $P_{et}CO_2$ is noted. Observing changes in the slope of the alveolar plateau, before and after the administration of an aerosolized bronchodilator, may allow for evaluation of the efficacy of the therapy. When significant maldistri-

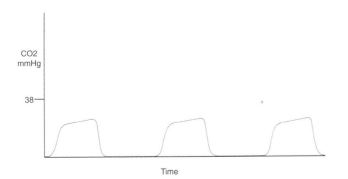

FIGURE 4–37 • Hyperventilation.

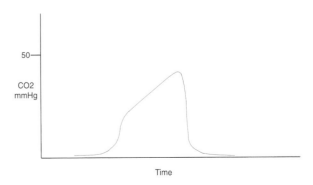

FIGURE 4–38 • Airflow obstruction.

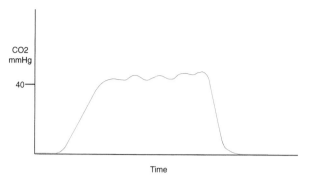

FIGURE 4–39 • Uneven alveolar emptying due to maldistribution of ventilation.

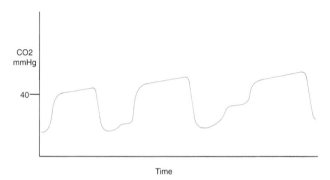

FIGURE 4–40 • Rebreathing of exhaled carbon dioxide.

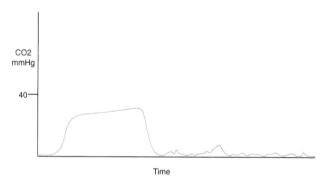

FIGURE 4–41 • Sudden loss of capnographic waveform.

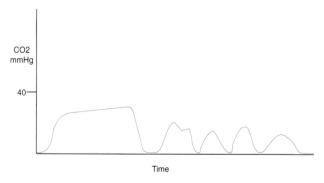

FIGURE 4–42 • Partial airway obstruction or leak in the airway system.

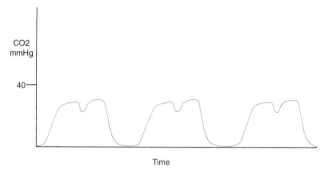

FIGURE 4–43 • Curare cleft.

bution of ventilation occurs, the ascending limb of the capnographic waveform may lose its steepness, and the alveolar plateau may appear to waver because of the uneven emptying of various alveolar time constants (Fig. 4–39).

Elevation of the capnographic waveform baseline is indicative of rebreathing of previously exhaled gas. As the baseline CO_2 concentration increases, so does the $P_{et}CO_2$ (Fig. 4–40). Causes of rebreathing include the addition of excessive mechanical dead space, a malfunctioning expiratory valve, or inadequate gas flow through a T-piece system.

Sudden loss of the capnographic waveform and a near-zero or zero $P_{et}CO_2$ may indicate a complete airway disconnection from a mechanical ventilator, complete ventilator malfunction, or a totally obstructed or kinked endotracheal tube (Fig. 4–41).

Sudden loss of the capnographic waveform and a decrease in the $P_{et}CO_2$ to a low but nonzero value may indicate an endotracheal tube in the hypopharynx, a partial airway obstruction, a partial ventilator circuit disconnect, or a leak in the airway system (Fig. 4–42).

The appearance of a downward cleft (**curare cleft**) in the alveolar plateau of the capnographic waveform may be observed in patients recovering from neuromuscular blockade (Fig. 4–43). This cleft may also be observed in the nonparalyzed patient when the patient is breathing out of synchrony with a mechanical ventilator or when the ventilator assist sensitivity is set too high.

References

1. National Asthma Education and Prevention Program. *Expert Panel Report: Guidelines for the Diagnosis and Management of Asthma.* Bethesda, MD: National Institutes of Health; 1991.
2. Yang KL, Tobin MJ. A prospective study of indexes predicting the outcome of trials of weaning from mechanical ventilation. *N Engl J Med.* 1991;324:1445.
3. Kacmarek RM, Cycyk-Chapman MC, Young-Palazzo PJ, Romagnoli DM. Determination of maximal inspiratory pressure: A clinical study and literature review. *Respir Care.* 1989;34:868–878.
4. Hess D. Measurement of maximal inspiratory pressure: A call for standardization. *Respir Care.* 1989;34:857–859. Editorial.
5. Madama VC. *Pulmonary Function Testing and Cardiopulmonary Stress Testing.* Albany, NY: Delmar Publishers; 1993.

6. National Asthma Education and Prevention Program. *Expert Panel Report II: Guidelines for the Diagnosis and Management of Asthma.* Bethesda, MD: National Institutes of Health; 1997.

7. American Association for Respiratory Care. Clinical practice guideline: Spirometry, 1996 update. *Respir Care.* 1996;41:629–636.

8. American Thoracic Society. Standardization of spirometry: 1994 update. *Am J Resp Crit Care Med.* 1995;152:1107–1136.

9. Wagner J. *Pulmonary Function Testing: A Practical Approach.* 2nd ed. Baltimore: Williams & Wilkins; 1992.

10. Ruppel GL. *Manual of Pulmonary Function Testing.* 7th ed. St. Louis: CV Mosby; 1998.

11. American Association for Respiratory Care. Clinical practice guideline: Sampling for arterial blood gas analysis. *Respir Care.* 1992;37:913–917.

12. Shapiro BA, Peruzzi WT, Templin R. *Clinical Application of Blood Gases.* 5th ed. St. Louis: CV Mosby; 1994.

13. American Association for Respiratory Care. Clinical practice guideline: Pulse oximetry. *Respir Care.* 1991;36:1406–1409.

14. Jubran A, Tobin MJ. Reliability of pulse oximetry in titrating supplemental oxygen therapy in ventilator-dependent patients. *Chest.* 1990;97:1420–1425.

15. American Association for Respiratory Care. Clinical practice guideline: Capnography/capnometry during mechanical ventilation. *Respir Care.* 1995;40:1321–1324.

16. Hess D. Capnometry and capnography: Technical aspects, physiologic aspects and clinical application. *Respir Care.* 1990;35:557–573.

Bibliography

Adams A, McArthur C, eds. Pulmonary function testing: Trends and techniques. *Respir Care Clin North Am.* 1997;3.

American Association for Respiratory Care. Clinical Practice Guideline: In-vitro pH and blood gas analysis and hemoximetry. *Respir Care.* 1993;38:505–510.

Gravenstein JS, Paulus DA, Hayes TJ. *Capnography in Clinical Practice.* Boston: Butterworth Scientific; 1989.

Hicks GH, ed. Applied noninvasive respiratory monitoring. *Probl Respir Care.* 1989;2.

Kacmarek RM, Hess D, Stoller JK. *Monitoring in Respiratory Care.* St. Louis: CV Mosby; 1993.

Malley WJ. Clinical blood gases: Application and noninvasive alternatives. St. Louis: CV Mosby; 1990.

Peruzzi WT, Shapiro BA, eds. Blood gas measurements. *Respir Care Clin North Am.* 1995;1.

Welch JP, DeCesare R, Hess D. Pulse oximetry: Instrumentation and clinical application. *Respir Care.* 1990;35:584–601.

Wilkins RL, Krider SJ, Sheldon RL. *Clinical Assessment in Respiratory Care.* 3rd ed. St. Louis: CV Mosby; 1995.

Respiratory Pathophysiology

James B. Fink • Patrick Fahey

Key Terms

airway hyperresponsiveness
blue bloater
bronchiectasis
cor pulmonale
obstructive sleep apnea
pendelluft motion
pink puffer
pleural effusion
pneumothorax

Objectives

- Describe the differences between acute and chronic diseases of the chest.

- Differentiate characteristics of obstructive and restrictive diseases.

- Provide a differential diagnosis of common diseases.

- Use laboratory and assessment criteria to identify acute airway infection, chronic obstructive pulmonary disease, asthma, chronic bronchitis, emphysema, bronchiolitis, cystic fibrosis, interstitial lung disease, neuromuscular disease, infectious lung disease, tuberculosis, acute respiratory failure, and adult respiratory distress syndrome.

- Associate common approaches to treatment for patients with these diseases.

- Differentiate among therapies that support the patient, provide relief, and actually treat the underlying problem.

This chapter covers the common problems that affect most patients identified with respiratory disease. Diseases are defined in terms of their underlying pathology, causes, and effects on lung and body function. This information is intended to provide the foundation for differential diagnosis through assessment and diagnostic testing. Also discussed are the major issues in medical management, in broad terms, with more specific focus on respiratory care interventions and their relative value in supporting the patient, relieving symptoms, and controlling or treating the underlying disease.

ACUTE RESPIRATORY INFECTION

Most acute respiratory infections are viral. Although some viruses are associated with regular clinical patterns, the symptoms can vary considerably depending on age of the patient, severity of infection, and preexisting disease.

Types

The common cold is a viral infection that presents with stuffy, runny nose (rhinorrhea), conjunctivitis, and sore throat.

Acute pharyngitis, the common sore throat, is often accompanied by fever and some degree of malaise, with inflammation of the throat, soft palate, and tonsils. Tonsilar lymph nodes may be enlarged. Sore throat is often caused by a virus or hemolytic streptococcal infection. Bacterial sore throat may benefit from antibiotic therapy.

Acute tracheobronchitis is an inflammation of the upper airway in which the major symptom is cough, often with a barking sound due to inflammation of the larynx. Hoarseness and inspiratory stridor may result, depending on the degree of laryngeal obstruction. In young children, the inflammation and edema of the structures in the larynx can produce a life-threatening acute obstruction called epiglottitis, which is usually bacterial (*Haemophilus influenzae*) and of sudden onset. Examination of the pharynx reveals a red, swollen epiglottis. Severe obstruction may require bypassing the upper airway by tracheostomy. These patients should be observed closely.

Acute bronchiolitis is a lower airway inflammation that usually occurs in infants less than 6 months old. It is preceded by upper respiratory symptoms, followed by cough, wheezing, and grunting respiratory distress. Although exhaustion may require ventilatory support, bronchopneumonia is relatively rare.

Pneumonia is an inflammation of the lung parenchyma. Fever, tachypnea, and cough with pleural pain may be associated with clinical and radiologic signs of consolidation or infiltrates. Pneumonias are discussed in greater detail later in the chapter.

Influenza refers to an acute illness in which symptoms of malaise, myalgia, and nausea overshadow the initial respiratory tract symptoms. Patients may be "flat on their backs" for 3 to 5 days, requiring up to several weeks to recover fully.

Treatment

For viral infections, the medical course is typically to try to alleviate symptoms and wait for the infection to run its course, whereas bacterial infections may be treated with antibiotics. With moderate obstruction from mucosal swelling, the use of cold aerosols may reduce swelling. Antiinflammatory drugs may also help to reduce swelling. The use of α-adrenergic receptor drugs has been advocated to reduce swelling through localized vasoconstriction in the mucosa. Such therapy may be short lived and result in a rebound effect as the drug "wears off," resulting in even greater edema. Some airway spasm may respond to bronchodilators, especially if the patient has a preexisting disease with a component of reversible bronchospasm. Palliative measures include decongestants, gargles, and washes to soothe inflamed throat tissue.

OBSTRUCTIVE PULMONARY DISEASE

As the name implies, obstructive pulmonary diseases are diseases of the lung that obstruct or reduce the flow of air in or out of the lungs (Box 5–1). Airway obstruction, or narrowing of the bronchial lumen, is caused by one of three mechanisms:

Extramural: The bronchus is compressed by external pressure (eg, enlarged lymph node or space-occupying lesion, compressing neighboring airways; Fig. 5–1).
Mural: The airway is narrowed by inflammation or lesions within the bronchial walls (eg, bronchogenic carcinoma, chronic bronchitis, or asthma).
Intraluminal: The bronchus is obstructed by foreign objects or thick secretions within the airway.

Complete obstruction cuts off airflow in both directions, leading to shunt of dependent areas and atelectasis. The more central the airway, the more acute and critical the effect. Complete obstruction of the trachea is not compatible with life, whereas obstruction of a bronchiole presents less

---

Box • 5–1   OBSTRUCTION

Obstruction may be acute or chronic due to the following factors:

- Reduced lung elasticity or lung recoil
- Airway closure
- Inflammation of the airway
- Fixed airway obstruction (such as a tumor)
- Variable airway obstruction (secretions)
- Smooth muscle contraction

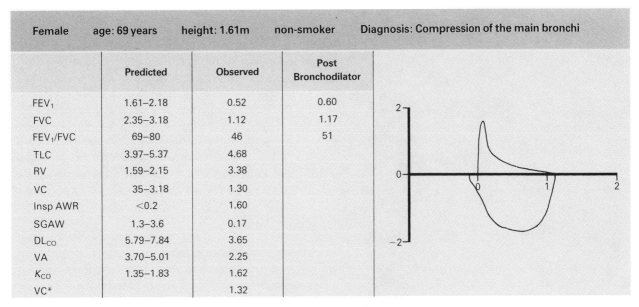

	Predicted	Observed	Post Bronchodilator
FEV₁	1.61–2.18	0.52	0.60
FVC	2.35–3.18	1.12	1.17
FEV₁/FVC	69–80	46	51
TLC	3.97–5.37	4.68	
RV	1.59–2.15	3.38	
VC	35–3.18	1.30	
Insp AWR	<0.2	1.60	
SGAW	1.3–3.6	0.17	
DL_CO	5.79–7.84	3.65	
VA	3.70–5.01	2.25	
K_CO	1.35–1.83	1.62	
VC*		1.32	

Female   age: 69 years   height: 1.61m   non-smoker   Diagnosis: Compression of the main bronchi

FIGURE 5–1 • Compression of the main bronchi.(*Color Atlas of Respiratory Diseases.* St. Louis: Gower, F2.13.)

severe problems because of the smaller volume of dependent lung affected.

Partial obstruction of an airway impairs gas flow and movement of secretions. This increases the work of breathing on both inspiration and expiration. In addition, the normal airway expands on inspiration and compresses on expiration. With partial airway obstruction, an airway may open enough to let air in on inspiration but compressed enough to trap gas on expiration. This can lead to gas trapping and overdistention of lung tissue distal to the obstruction.

Upper Airway

Obstructive Sleep Apnea

Obstructive sleep apnea is estimated to affect 3% to 4% of the population and is more prevalent in adults older than 40 years (Fig. 5–2). Apnea is defined as periods without airflow of more than 10 seconds. This is considered clinically significant with five or more episodes per hour during sleep.

The forms of sleep-related breathing disorders are as follows (Fig. 5–3):

Central apnea: Lack of respiratory effort
Upper airway obstructive apnea: Absent airflow despite respiratory muscle movement
Mixed apnea: Combination of lack of muscle movement followed by unsuccessful respiratory efforts

Obstructive sleep apnea is commonly associated with obese men but can occur in many other patients as well. The obstruction correlates to a loss of muscle tone in the pharynx during deep sleep, resulting in structures such as the tongue blocking the airway. Therapeutic options in-

clude application of continuous positive-pressure ventilation, medications, use of prosthetic devices to keep tissue from occluding the airway, surgical interventions (such as tracheostomy), and weight reduction.

Inhalation of Foreign Objects

Localized acute airway obstruction is most commonly the result of aspiration of a foreign body. This occurs fre-

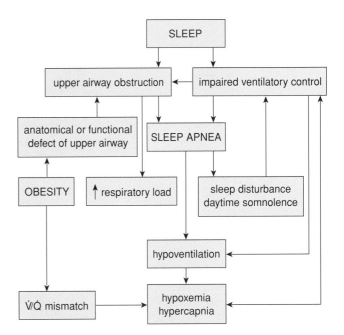

FIGURE 5–2 • Schematic demonstration of pathogenesis of sleep apnea syndrome. (Farzan S. *A Concise Handbook of Respiratory Disease.* 3rd ed. Reston, VA: Reston Publishers; 1992.)

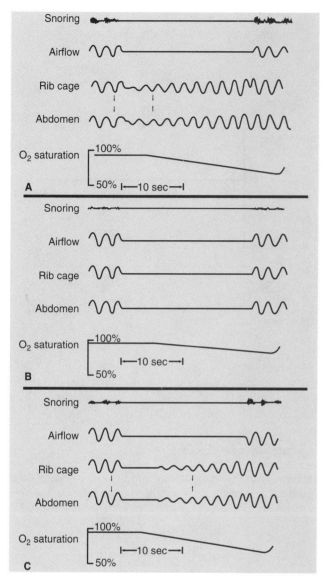

FIGURE 5–3 • Types of sleep apnea. (*A*) Obstructive apnea is characterized by loud intermittent snoring, complete cessation of airflow, paradoxical movement of the chest and abdomen, and moderate to severe oxygen desaturation. (*B*) In central apnea, snoring and simultaneous cessation of airflow and respiratory effort are absent. Usually, only mild to moderate oxygen desaturation is present. (*C*) In mixed apnea, an initial central apnea is followed by an obstructive apnea that usually produces moderate to severe oxygen desaturation.

quently with small children (less than 4 years of age) and inebriated or obtunded adults. Ranging from toys to food, the first line of defense against inhaled objects is the cough. Because of the angle of the airways, 70% of aspirated objects go down the right mainstem bronchus, 25% enter the left bronchus, and 5% stay in the trachea.

Immediately apparent symptoms of acute airway obstruction include coughing, choking, gagging, temporary aphonia, and wheezing. Laryngospasm is a natural defense mechanisms, which typically lasts for several seconds.

Hoarseness or a brassy cough may indicate objects lodged in the larynx.

In cases of total acute obstruction of the airway, use the Heimlich maneuver to dislodge the occluding object. This consists of a rapid compression of the thoracic contents (through compression of the abdomen or thorax) to pressurize air in the lungs to expel the obstruction. A lodged object that cannot be expelled through cough may be removed with postural drainage, blind aspiration of the airway (suctioning), or direct visualization using bronchoscopy. Failure to clear the airway may require use of an emergency tracheostomy.

Lower Airway

Asthma, chronic bronchitis, and emphysema are the three major diseases broadly referred to as chronic obstructive pulmonary disease (COPD). These diseases are often described in a patient population that overlaps, with some patients being affected by one, two, or all three diseases (Fig. 5–4). Bronchiectasis and cystic fibrosis are also COPDs.

Asthma

Asthma is a chronic inflammatory disorder of the airway that is characterized by increased responsiveness of the airways to various stimuli, resulting in narrowing airways and airflow obstruction secondary to mucosal edema, constricted smooth muscles, and thick secretions that can plug small airways (Box 5–2 and Fig. 5–5).

Airways are infiltrated with eosinophils and mononuclear cells, and there is vasodilation and evidence of mi-

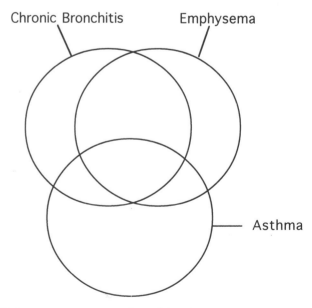

FIGURE 5–4 • Overlay of the clinical manifestations of chronic bronchitis, emphysema, and asthma in chronic obstructive pulmonary disease.

Box • 5–2 ASTHMA

The working definition of asthma from National Heart Lung Blood Institute (1995) is as follows: Asthma is a chronic inflammatory disorder of the airways in which many cells and cellular elements play a role, in particular mast cells, eosinophils, T lymphocytes, macrophages, neutrophils, and epithelial cells. In susceptible individuals, this inflammation causes recurrent episodes of wheezing, breathlessness, chest tightness, and coughing, particularly at night or in the early morning. These episodes are usually associated with widespread but variable airflow obstruction that is often reversible either spontaneously or with treatment. The inflammation also causes an associated increase in the existing bronchial hyperresponsiveness to a variety of stimuli (NHBLI, 1995). Moreover, recent evidence indicates that subbasement membrane fibrosis may occur in some patients with asthma and that changes contribute to persistent abnormalities in lung function (Roche, 1991).

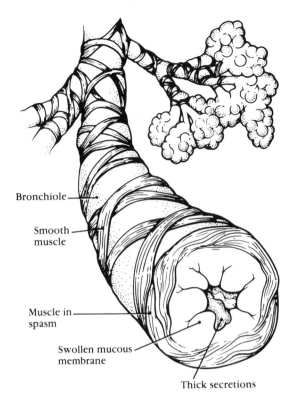

Bronchiole

Smooth muscle

Muscle in spasm

Swollen mucous membrane

Thick secretions

FIGURE 5–5 • Key factors in asthma include: inflammation and swelling of the mucosa, smooth muscle hyperactivity, and thick secretion.

crovascular and epithelial disruption. The airway smooth muscle is often hypertrophied, which is characterized by new vessel formation, increased numbers of epithelial goblet cells, and deposition of interstitial collagens beneath the epithelium. These changes may not be completely reversible (Box 5–3).

Airway hyperresponsiveness is the tendency for airways to narrow too easily and too much. Exposure to allergens, environmental irritants, cold air, exercise, or viral infection leads to clinical symptoms of wheezing and dyspnea. The level of airway responsiveness often correlates with the clinical severity of asthma; causative factors are shown in Figure 5–6.

Inflammation is an early and persistent component of asthma. Therapy to suppress the inflammation should be long-term and consistent. Symptoms of asthma range from simple cough to severe wheezing with dyspnea. Severity of symptoms can range from occasional cough to life-threatening exacerbations, which may require extensive emergency department and critical care unit intervention, up to and including intubation and mechanical ventilation.

Asthma is a chronic disease that has been estimated to affect more than 5% (15 million overall, 4.8 million children) of the population in the United States; however, in specific populations, such as schoolchildren in urban Chicago, estimates exceed 17% of the population. Asthma accounts for 5000 deaths annually, 470,000 hospitalizations, and 100 million days of restricted activity. The incidence and morbidity of asthma appears to be on the rise worldwide.

Asthma can manifest at any age. Although about half of the cases develop in childhood, another third are adult on-

set, at or before the age of 40 years. About 10% of asthma cases develop after the age of 65 years. Increasing evidence supports the statement that once you have asthma, you have it for life. Many children with asthma appear to have fewer symptoms in their teens and are thought to have outgrown their asthma, only to have recurring symptoms in their adult years.

Asthma is an inflammatory disease, with cellular infiltration and edema, characterized by airway hyperreactivity and smooth muscle contraction. This has been a critical revelation in the treatment and control of the disease. As recently as the 1980s, the primary treatment of moderate asthma was the use of bronchodilators to relieve the bron-

Box • 5–3 IMMUNOHISTOPATHOLOGIC FEATURES OF ASTHMA

Mast cell activation
Inflammatory cell infiltration
   Neutrophils
   Eosinophils
   Lymphocytes
Edema
Denudation of airway epithelium
Collagen deposition beneath the basement membrane

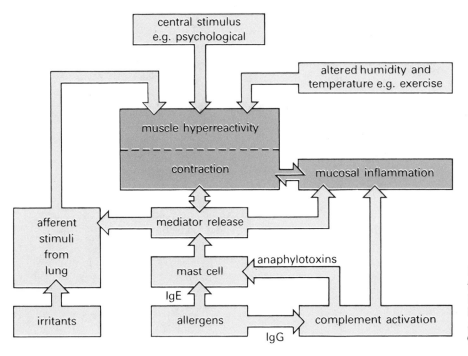

FIGURE 5–6 • Factors and interaction leading to muscle hyperreactivity in asthma. IgE, immunoglobulin E; IgG, immunoglobulin G. (*Color Atlas of Respiratory Diseases.* St. Louis: Gower, F15.4.)

chospastic component of the disease, without addressing the underlying inflammatory component.

The goals of asthma therapy are listed in Box 5–4.

CONTROL OF TRIGGERS

Asthma symptoms and exacerbations have been shown to increase with exposure to allergens and irritants. Finding the allergens or irritants that "trigger" a patient's asthma can be essential to help control it. Inhalant allergens are associated with animals, dust mites, cockroaches, fungi, molds, and pollens. Other irritants include tobacco smoke and common environmental pollutants. The workplace can provide exposure to chemicals or irritants that trigger asthma. Food allergies (sulfite-containing foods and oth-

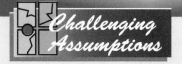

CRITICAL THINKING CHALLENGES
Challenging Assumptions

Many patients with chronic bronchitis and emphysema also have reversible bronchospastic disease that appears in many respects to be like asthma, responding to many of the same medications. This relationship has been described as three rings (representing populations of patients with chronic bronchitis, asthma, and emphysema) that overlap, representing a large number of patients who have elements of two or more chronic obstructive pulmonary diseases. Some definitions of asthma would exclude bronchospastic components of chronic bronchitis. Practitioners responsible for treating patients with obstructive lung disease should follow a simple rule of thumb: if it looks like asthma, feels like asthma, and responds like asthma, treat it like asthma.

Box • 5–4   ASTHMA THERAPY: GOALS AND MANAGEMENT STRATEGIES

GOALS

- Prevent chronic symptoms.
- Maintain near-normal pulmonary function.
- Maintain normal activity and exercise levels.
- Prevent recurrent exacerbation, and minimize need for emergency room visits.
- Provide effective medical care with no adverse effects.
- Meet patient and family's expectations of good asthma care.

MANAGEMENT STRATEGIES

- Identify factors that trigger asthma and minimize exposure when possible.
- Control the underlying inflammation of the airways.
- Relieve the symptoms with bronchodilator therapy.

CRITICAL THINKING CHALLENGES

Shifting Care Plans

Animal Control

Many patients with asthma are allergic to their pets. Advising the patient to remove the family pet from the home is often unacceptable to the patient or family. The next best bet is to keep the animals out of the patient's bedroom, creating a safe zone that is relatively free of the animal's allergens. Most people spend 8 hours a day sleeping, so keeping the bedroom allergen free (as much as possible) is a good step. Keep the bedroom door closed, and consider using filters in air ducts to catch danders from central air or heating.

ers) can also trigger asthma, and exposure to identified foods should be avoided. Cold air and exercise are also potent triggers of asthma symptoms in some patients.

Substantially reducing exposure to these triggers can reduce inflammation of the airways, symptoms, and the need for medical intervention.

As opposed to pets, most patients would love to get rid of their dust mites. Unfortunately, they are microscopic critters found in mattresses, upholstery, pillows, carpets, and bedding. If patients are sensitive to mites, several actions can be taken, including the following:

- Keep house humidity at less than 50%.
- Encase mattress in an allergen-impermeable cover (this can also be done with the pillows).
- Wash pillows, sheets, and blankets weekly in hot water (more than 54.4°C [130°F]). An alternative for pillows is to place them in a hot dryer for 1 hour each week. It is also helpful to minimize the use of upholstered furniture, carpets, and rugs in the asthmatic patient's bedroom.

MEDICATION

In most patients, asthma can be controlled with consistent application of appropriate medications. We have the technology to reduce mortality and morbidity significantly with proper medical management.

The strategy of medication (discussed in more detail in Chapter 8) is based on disease severity, representing a stepwise approach to managing asthma in adults and children older than 5 years of age.

Let us review these steps, starting with mild intermittent asthma, step 1, in which the patient may need only a short-acting bronchodilator twice a week to provide symptomatic relief. With increasing severity, in step 2, we add medications for long-term control in the form of antiinflammatory drugs (inhaled corticosteroids at low doses, cromolyn, or nedocromil) and possibly leukotriene inhibitors. In step 3, we may increase the dosage of inhaled antiinflammatory drugs and add long-acting bronchodilators, such as salmeterol or sustained-release theophylline, to allow patients to sleep through the night. With severe persistent asthma, we add corticosteroid tablets.

Use this system two ways: (1) step up until the patient gets the asthma under control, and (2) step down after the patient's symptoms are under control, reviewing the treatment plan at 1- to 6-month intervals to determine whether gradual reduction in treatment may be possible.

EDUCATION

Patients need to be taught the facts about asthma. They need to understand what causes the disease and how to identify signs of onset as well as what triggers their asthma and how to avoid those triggers. The need to understand what each prescribed medication is and to know how to administer each medication safely is essential. Written medication plans, treatment action plan, and use of symptom diaries with peak flow monitoring have all been shown to

CRITICAL THINKING CHALLENGES

Challenging Assumptions

Asthma is 10% medication and 90% education. Asthma is relatively straightforward to diagnose, and we have a full tool chest of medications that, with strict patient adherence to the medication plan, reduce the severity of asthma from severe persistent to moderate and from moderate to mild. The problem is twofold: (1) most people tend to stop taking their medication when they start to feel good, and (2) most patients do not know how to take their medication properly. Both of these problems are addressed with patient education, so after the diagnosis is made and the medications prescribed, the real work begins. Patient education has to extend beyond how to use a peak flowmeter or metered dose inhaler to a thorough understanding of what medications are being prescribed and why they are important. Written medication and action plans, when they are understood and followed, serve to reduce emergency visits and hospital stays. Patient instruction may require as much as 40 minutes for the initial session and 20 minutes or more with every follow-up visit. The big problem is that few health care providers are willing (or able) to provide the resources required for this level of education.

Box • 5–5   WHAT YOU SHOULD TELL YOUR PATIENTS ABOUT ASTHMA

Asthma is a chronic inflammatory disease of the airways.

Asthma is not contagious.

Asthma can be controlled with good management.

Good management of asthma can reduce your symptoms from severe to moderate and from moderate to mild.

You may prevent asthma attacks and control asthma symptoms by:

Identifying and reducing exposure to triggers

Using medications that relieve asthma symptoms, as needed.

Using medications that control asthma by eliminating or reducing the occurrence of symptoms by reducing inflammation of the airway. (These medications must be taken regularly, even when the patient is feeling good.)

Having regular communication and follow-up with your health care provider to adjust your treatment plan to meet your needs, even when your asthma is well controlled.

Box • 5–6   WHAT HEALTH CARE PROFESSIONALS SHOULD PROVIDE TO HELP PATIENTS CONTROL THEIR ASTHMA

A written explanation of each medication prescribed, with dose, frequency, desired action, and potential side effects as well as what the patient should do if they occur.

A written medication plan that explains the following:

• Dose and frequency for each medication when the patient feels good
• What the patient should do when he or she feels bad
• When the patient should seek help
• How to get help

A demonstration of the proper use and cleaning of aerosol delivery devices and accessories (holding chambers or spacers), including the following:

• Metered dose inhalers and accessory devices
• Nebulizers and compressors
• Dry powder inhalers, as prescribed

Demonstrate the proper use of peak flowmeters and a symptom diary, and explain how to use them to determine the patient's personal best and when the patient needs to adjust his or her medications.

Explain what asthma triggers are, how to identify what triggers the patient's asthma, and how to avoid those triggers.

This information should be provided by the physician, nurse, office or clinic staff, or other health care professional or asthma support group referred to the patient for asthma education.

---

help patients care for themselves better and meet their treatment goals (Box 5–5).

The national guidelines also recommend that specific information, instruction, and written information should be provided to every patient (or family care provider for a patient) with asthma (Box 5–6).

Patients or their families should be able to determine whether the goals for asthma management are being met. The Chicago Asthma Consortium, a nonprofit collaboration of more than 130 organizations, developed a self-evaluation to help patients determine whether they were getting what they need to meet realistic expectations and to help guide patients in getting what they need from their health care providers or to find providers who will help them meet those needs (Box 5–7).

Chronic Bronchitis

Chronic bronchitis is a clinically diagnosed disease of patients afflicted with cough and sputum production on most days for 3 or more months per year for 2 successive years.

In its early stages, patients may be free of symptoms except for cough after viral upper respiratory tract infections. The cough may persist for increasing lengths of time, and the infection may be associated with wheezing. Chronic sputum production is often associated with colonization by *H. influenzae* and *Streptococcus pneumoniae.*

As the disease progresses, there is a chronic reduction in the FEV_1, with at least partial reversibility after administration of bronchodilators. At this stage, chronic bronchitis is difficult to distinguish from bronchiectasis.

In the severe stages, constant wheezing, sputum production, and dyspnea are associated with episodes of respiratory failure. These patients are described as **blue bloaters**, in that they are often obese and cyanotic, with chronic hypoventilation and hypoxia-induced polycythemia.

The major causative factor for chronic bronchitis is cigarette smoking, followed by environmental pollution, genetic make-up, and chronic occupational exposure to high concentrations of irritating gases. Structural and immunologic predisposition to recurrent bronchial infection and genetic make-up appear to be factors for some patients.

An early change found in the airways with chronic bronchitis is an increase in size and number of the goblet cells and cells in the mucosal glands. The mucous gland/wall thickness ratio (Reid index, see Chapter 3) increases from 0.26 to more than 0.60. Hypertrophy and hyperplasia of secretory cells are associated with epithelial squamous metaplasia. Goblet cells appear in the terminal bronchioles (where they are not usually found). There is a net increase in sputum produced. Chronic inflammation causes an increase in bronchial wall thickness, reducing the diameter of the airway, especially in airways less than 2 mm in diameter. This is the basis of reduced airflow and, in some patients, of low ventilation–perfusion ($\dot{V}/\dot{Q}$) mismatching.

Pulmonary function changes are shown in Figure 5–7 and include frequency dependence of compliance, increased closing volumes, and diminished maximal expiratory flow rates at low lung volumes. During symptomatic periods, FEV_1 and $FEF_{25\%–75\%}$ may be reduced, and partial reversibility is seen with bronchodilator therapy.

In early or mild chronic bronchitis, the chest radiograph is normal, with increased lung marking and peribronchial thickening as the disease progresses.

Increased sputum production is associated with hypertrophied mucous glands that increase in number in response to the chronic irritation of the airway.

Secretions within the airway lumen increase airflow restriction and $\dot{V}/\dot{Q}$ mismatching. Hypoxemia in these patients is associated with right ventricular hypertrophy, cor pulmonale, and polycythemia. To avoid chronic bronchitis, the patient should not smoke cigarettes and should avoid environmental exposure to tobacco smoke.

A treatment plan for chronic bronchitis should include the following:

- No smoking
- Inhaled steroids
- Bronchodilators
- Theophylline
- Antibiotics to treat infections
- Oxygen to treat hypoxemia
- Bronchial hygiene to assist in removing secretions

Emphysema

Emphysema is a chronic disease that involves distention and destruction of the alveolar walls (Fig. 5–8). Reduced elastic recoil results in airways no longer being pulled open by surrounding airways, with a tendency for the airways to collapse during exhalation, presenting a large amount of intrinsic hyperinflation (Fig. 5–9). Alveoli that are distended also tend to obliterate their associated pulmonary capillary bed. The $\dot{V}/\dot{Q}$ may be matched well in these units, so that hypoxemia does not typically occur.

A genetic predisposition is found in a small percentage of patients with α_1-antitrypsin deficiency (more recently called antiprotease inhibitor deficiency). This deficiency is found in 0.06% of the population and is responsible for between 1% and 10% of all cases of emphysema.

Emphysema is a pathologic entity, and its diagnosis is made by a combination of clinical signs, symptoms, chest radiographic findings, and abnormal pulmonary function. In the early stages of the disease, mild dyspnea on exertion is the primary symptom. With more advanced disease, the patient may be described in terms of the **pink puffer**: underweight and barrel chested. Supraclavicular fossae are hollowed, and accessory muscles are hypertrophied. The patient remains pink, even while in acute distress, and the chest is hyperresonant on percussion. Chest radiographs reveal hyperinflation, pulmonary oligemia, and bullae; increased anteroposterior diameter; flattening of the diaphragm; elongation of the mediastinum; and increased width of the retrosternal space.

Centrilobular, panlobular, and paraseptal classifications are made on the basis of gross and microscopic observations, with no differentiation in clinical presentation (Fig. 5–10). Therapeutic approaches are the same for all except the panlobular type, which is associated with a deficiency of protease inhibitors.

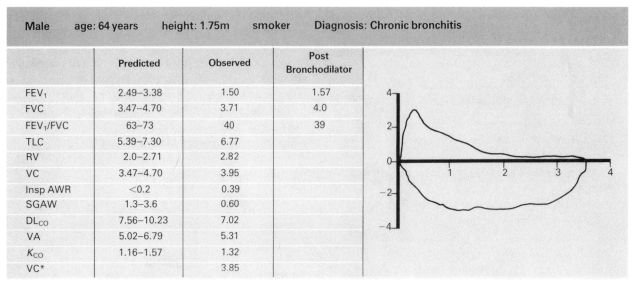

	Predicted	Observed	Post Bronchodilator
FEV$_1$	2.49–3.38	1.50	1.57
FVC	3.47–4.70	3.71	4.0
FEV$_1$/FVC	63–73	40	39
TLC	5.39–7.30	6.77	
RV	2.0–2.71	2.82	
VC	3.47–4.70	3.95	
Insp AWR	<0.2	0.39	
SGAW	1.3–3.6	0.60	
DL$_{CO}$	7.56–10.23	7.02	
VA	5.02–6.79	5.31	
K_{CO}	1.16–1.57	1.32	
VC*		3.85	

Table header: Male   age: 64 years   height: 1.75m   smoker   Diagnosis: Chronic bronchitis

FIGURE 5–7 • Flow volume loop and characteristic changes associated with chronic bronchitis. (*Color Atlas of Respiratory Diseases.* St. Louis: Gower, F2.3.)

The primary defect underlying emphysema is derangement of lung elastin by neutral proteases such as elastase (Fig. 5–11). Elastase is produced by polymorphonuclear leukocytes and alveolar macrophages in response to lung inflammation. Chronic or recurrent infections, environmental irritants, cigarette smoking, and occasionally α_1-antitrypsin deficiency result in degrading of elastin in the distal airways and alveoli. With the loss of basic elastin structure, septal walls are lost, and blood vessel density is reduced.

With emphysema, the loss of elastin reduces elastic recoil and subsequently gas exchange at the respiratory bronchioles, alveolar ducts, and alveolar septa, resulting in increased volume of air trapped, reduced pulmonary vasculature, and reduced total surface area for gas exchange.

Pulmonary function tests show an increased total lung capacity and residual volume at the expense of decreased vital capacity with a reduction in expiratory flow rates (Fig. 5–12). Unless there is an element of asthma, flow obstruction does not reverse with bronchodilator administration. Single breath–diffusing capacity for carbon monoxide reflects a reduction in gas exchange surface area proportional to the loss of alveolar capillary area.

Because the underlying mechanism is structural, there is no therapy to reverse emphysema. Treatment is oriented toward reducing irritation and making the patient comfortable. In that most patients have a combination of bronchitis and emphysema, treatment with bronchodilators is common. Focus should be on the use of ipratropium bromide (Atrovent), β-adrenergic receptor agonists, and theophylline. The use of inhaled steroids is commonly prescribed, with increasing evidence supporting their use. Other therapeutic options include breathing retraining, building inspiratory muscle endurance, and using pursed-lip breathing or fixed orifice resistors to stabilize the airway and reduce gas trapping. Oxygen may also be administered to relieve hypoxemia.

Bronchiectasis

Bronchiectasis is permanent dilation of one or more bronchi due to destruction of the bronchial wall secondary to chronic infection (Fig. 5–13). Sputum production is

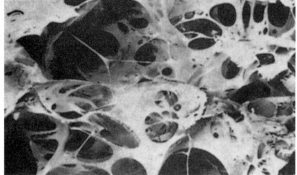

FIGURE 5–8 • Scanning electron micrographs of normal (*top*) and emphysematous (*bottom*) lung tissue.

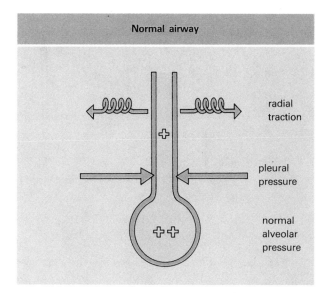
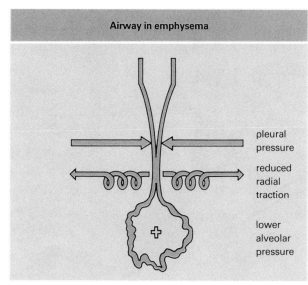

FIGURE 5-9 • Comparison of airway calibers between normal airways and airways in emphysema. Airway caliber depends on intraluminal pressure, radial traction (elastic tissue surrounding the airway pulling it open), and pleural pressure. With emphysema, airways tend to collapse on exhalation because of reduction in radial traction due to loss of neighboring alveoli and reduction in intraluminal pressure due to lower elastic recoil of the affected airway. In addition, pleural pressures actually increase secondary to hyperinflation. (*Color Atlas of Respiratory Diseases.* St. Louis: Gower, F9.25; F9.26.)

markedly increased, with secretions that are often foul smelling and purulent.

Bronchiectasis often presents with a chronic cough and production of large quantities of purulent sputum; exacerbations of symptoms is common with fever and malaise. Bacterial pneumonia, without antibiotic treatment, can lead to permanent damage of the airway, with dilation of the airway and pooling of secretions. These pooled secretions became the perfect growth medium for bacteria and

the site for chronic infection, leading to further destruction of the airway.

The sputum is characteristic, with purulent, mucoid, and formed elements that settle out into as many as five layers when left to stand.

Bronchography can reveal changes in bronchial anatomy consistent with bronchiectasis but is not necessary to make the diagnosis. Cough, sputum production, and recurrent pulmonary infections are primary diagnostic criteria.

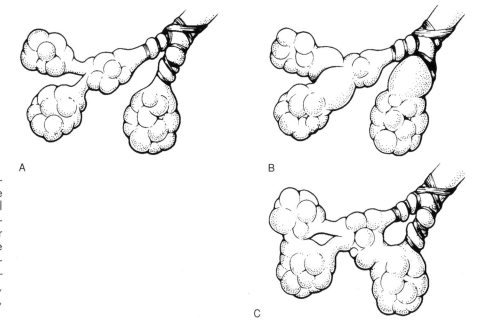

FIGURE 5-10 • Emphysema has several characteristic alterations of the structure of the airway. (*A*) A normal airway. (*B*) Dilation of the respiratory bronchioles with centrilobar emphysema. (*C*) Destruction of the alveolar walls with panlobular emphysema. (From Cotran et al. *Robbins' Pathologic Basis of Disease,* 4th ed. Philadelphia: WB Saunders, 1989: 769.)

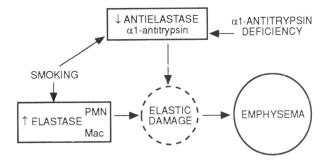

FIGURE 5–11 • Protease–antiprotease mechanisms of emphysema. Smoking inhibits antielastase and favors the recruitment of leukocytes and release of elastase. PMN, polymorphonuclear leukocyte; Mac, alveolar macrophage. (Cotran RS, Kumar V, Robbins SL. *Robbins' Pathologic Basis of Disease.* 4th ed. Philadelphia: WB Saunders; 1989:769.)

In the antibiotic era, most diffuse bronchiectasis is found in relatively young patients who are not cigarette smokers, with no episodic bronchospasm.

Several rare syndromes are associated with bronchiectasis. Kartagener's syndrome (sinusitis, bronchiectasis, and situs inversus) appears to be affected by ciliary immotility.

Cylindrical, varicose, and saccular bronchiectases have been differentiated through bronchograms. Cylindrical appears to be the earlier stage with the greater chance of reversibility.

Therapy is directed at controlling cough, sputum production, and infection. A treatment plan typically includes the following:

- Antibiotic therapy to control and clear infections
- Secretion clearance techniques to minimize buildup of secretions in the affected airways, including directed cough, active cycle of breathing, positive expiratory pressure, and postural drainage

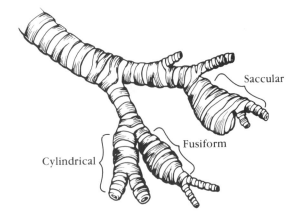

FIGURE 5–13 • Three classic types of bronchiectasis.

- Bronchodilator therapy, only in the presence of reversible airway obstruction

Surgery may be indicated in patients with advanced bronchiectasis that is localized in a lobe secondary to recurrent infections.

Cystic Fibrosis

Cystic fibrosis (CF) is a chronic obstructive pulmonary disease associated with dysfunction of the pancreas and liver; it is genetically transmitted (autosomal recessive). CF is the most common lethal genetic disease among white children, affecting one in 2000 white infants. Between 10,000 and 20,000 cases have been identified. In the 1950s, typical life expectancy was 4 years after diagnosis; today, many CF patients live well into their third decade. Earlier diagnosis and more aggressive and effective treatment have been credited with the dramatic increase in longevity.

Male	age: 72 years	height: 1.83m	ex-smoker	Diagnosis: Emphysema
	Predicted	**Observed**	**Post Bronchodilator**	
FEV$_1$	2.53–3.42	0.61	0.60	
FVC	3.68–4.98	2.21	2.31	
FEV$_1$/FVC	60–70	28	26	
TLC	5.92–8.02	11.22		
RV	2.30–3.12	8.22		
VC	3.68–4.98	3.00		
Insp AWR	<0.2	0.32		
SGAW	1.3–3.6	0.35		
DL$_{CO}$	7.85–10.62	2.87		
VA	5.51–7.46	4.89		
K_{CO}	1.07–1.45	0.59		
VC*		2.75		

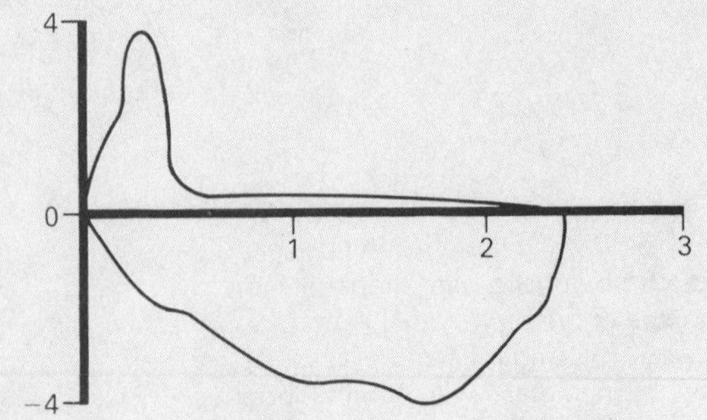

FIGURE 5–12 • Flow volume loop and characteristic changes associated with emphysema. (*Color Atlas of Respiratory Diseases.* St. Louis: Gower, F2.3.)

CF affects all organ systems with exocrine function, including the small intestine, biliary tract, pancreas, uterine cervix, paranasal sinuses, and mucus-secreting glands in both the digestive and respiratory tracts. It also affects the male genital tract, with a high incidence of sterility. Primarily an exocrine disease, CF affects digestion and nutritional status; secondary effects on the lungs include secretion and retention of thick secretions in the airways.

Decreased water content or increased electrolyte content of secretion, disturbed autonomic secretory control, or production of abnormal mucous glycoproteins have been speculated to account for the large amount of thick secretions with abnormal viscoelastic characteristics. The stasis and retention of secretions is also affected by ciliary dyskinesia. Mucous plugging of airways leads to inflammation followed by colonization of bacteria and subsequent obliteration of the small airways. Retained secretions are associated with colonization of *Escherichia coli* and *Pseudomonas aeruginosa,* producing purulent secretions and predisposing the patient to development of bronchiectasis. Bronchiectasis and peribronchial fibrosis are the products of chronic infection.

CF is diagnosed by a "sweat test," documenting high sodium concentrations in sweat. Some patients may demonstrate increased closing volume, decreased maximal expiratory flow rates, and increased alveolar–arterial O_2 gradient, consistent with small airway obstruction.

Inflammation of the airway, increased smooth muscle tone, reduced elastic recoil, and obstruction from impacted secretions combine to make CF an obstructive disease. The progression of the lung disease with CF is shown in Figure 5–14.

CF often presents with recurrent pulmonary infections at an early age, with a chronic cough, nonproductive at first, but eventually with increased sputum, particularly at night.

Impaired nutrition from gastrointestinal dysfunction contributes to lower weights, short stature, and delayed maturation. With progression of the disease, complications include hemoptysis, atelectasis, recurrent pneumonia, mucous impaction of the bronchi, pneumothorax, and cor pulmonale.

Respiratory treatment is oriented toward bronchial hygiene, mobilization, and hydration of secretions. Nebulized bronchodilators, antibiotics, and mucolytics (eg, DNAse) may be administered to improve airflow and ciliary transport, reduce infection, and reduce viscosity of secretions.

RESTRICTIVE PULMONARY DISEASE

Restrictive pulmonary diseases restrict lung expansion, resulting in reduced lung volumes. Expiratory flows may be limited secondary to the reduced lung volumes rather than an obstructive process in the airways. Table 5–1 summarizes restrictive lung diseases.

Stiffening of Lung Tissue: Interstitial Lung Diseases

Pulmonary Fibrosis (Cryptogenic Fibrosing Alveolitis)

Pulmonary fibrosis is a condition of unknown cause characterized by an inflammatory exudate of the alveolar wall with a tendency to develop fibrosis.

Three broad causative categories are (1) fibrogenic dusts, such as silica and asbestos; (2) granulomas, caused by hypersensitivity pneumonitis, sarcoidosis, and berylliosis; and (3) chronic exudates, ranging from chronic left ventricular failure, chronic renal failure, and certain drugs, which may result in alveolar wall fibrosis (Fig. 5–15). A

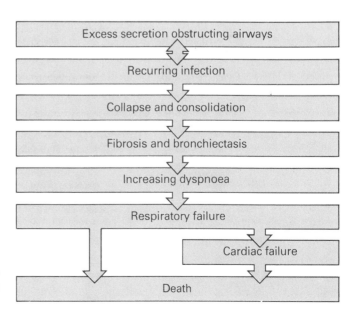

FIGURE 5–14 • Progress of lung disease in cystic fibrosis. (*Color Atlas of Respiratory Diseases.* St. Louis: Gower, F11.18.)

Table • 5–1   RESTRICTIVE DISEASES

Category	Examples	Pathogenesis	Assessment of Findings
Respiratory center depression	Narcotic and barbiturate dependence	Direct depression of respiratory center	Respiratory rate: <12/min; associated signs of hypoventilation
	Central nervous system lesions, head trauma	Injury to or impingement on respiratory centers	Hyper- or hypoventilation; cerebral edema and its signs
Neuromuscular	Guillain-Barré syndrome	Acute toxic polyneuritis; intercostal paralysis leads to diaphragmatic breathing; vagal and SNS paralysis lead to reduced ability of bronchioles to constrict, dilate, react to irritants	Reduced negative inspiratory pressure, VT, VC, compliance, breath sounds; hypoxemia, hypercapnia
	Duchenne muscular dystrophy	Genetic; thoracoscoliosis; paralysis of intercostals, abdominal muscles, diaphragm, accessory muscles	Pulmonary symptoms appear late; reduced IC, ERV, VC, VT, FRC, compliance PO_2; elevated PCO_2; abnormal respiratory patterns
Restriction of thoracic excursion			
Thoracic deformity	Kyphoscoliosis, pectus excavatum	Deformity of chest compresses lung tissue and limits thoracic excursion	Reduced breath sounds in affected areas, probably with rales; reduced compliance, TLC, VC, ERV; signs of hypoventilation, hypoxemia, increased work of breathing
Traumatic chest wall instability	Flail chest	Fracture of a group of ribs leads to unstable chest wall; reduced intrathoracic pressure on inspiration pulls area in and causes pressure on parenchyma; this increases work of breathing and hypoventilation	Obvious flail, unequal chest excursion, bruising, skin injuries, localized pain on inspiration, dyspnea, reduced breath sounds with rales and rhonchi; reduced compliance, ERV, TLC, VC, PO_2
Obesity	Obesity hypoventilation syndrome (pickwickian syndrome)	Excess abdominal adipose tissue impinges on thoracic space and diaphragmatic excursion; reduced respiratory drive; increased weight of chest restricts thoracic excursion	Somnolence, twitching, periodic respirations, polycythemia, right ventricular hypertrophy or failure; reduced compliance, ERV, TLC, VC, PO_2; elevated PCO_2; distant breath sounds
Pleural disorders	Pleural effusion	Accumulation of fluid in pleural space secondary to altered hydrostatic or oncotic forces	Unequal chest expansion; dullness and reduced breath sounds in affected area; may be constant chest discomfort; dyspnea if amount of fluid large; if over 250 mL, shows on radiographs; if large, bulging of intercostal space
	Pneumothorax	Accumulation of air in pleural space with proportional lung collapse	Hyperresonance; reduced breath sounds; tracheal deviation away from pneumothorax; tachycardia; unequal chest expansion; breath sounds reduced or absent; shows on radiographs
Disorders of lung parenchyma	Pulmonary fibrosis	Many possible causes: occupational sarcoid, etc.	Reduced compliance, hypoxemia, hypercapnia, and their consequences
	Tuberculosis	Bacterial invasion leads to scarring, reduced compliance, and reduced lung function	Visible on films; positive skin test, sputum; malaise, weight loss, fatigue, evening fever with night sweats, cough, hemoptysis
	Atelectasis	Obstruction of bronchioles, shrunken airless alveoli; reduced compliance; right-to-left shunting	Dyspnea, tachycardia, cough, fever, decreased chest wall expansion, hypoxemia, radiologic evidence
	Adult respiratory distress syndrome (ARDS)	Widespread atelectasis; loss of surfactant; interstitial edema, formation of hyaline membrane	Dyspnea, tachypnea, grunting, labored respirations, hypoxemia, occasional hypercapnia, cyanosis; radiographs show bilateral patchy infiltrates
	Pulmonary edema	Increased pulmonary capillary pressure leads to interstitial and alveolar edema	Hypoxemia, tachypnea; signs of congestive heart failure, radiologic butterfly infiltrates, rales
	Aspiration pneumonia	Chemical irritant from aspirant leads to bronchoconstriction, necrosis, and fibrosis of airways	Hypoxemia, signs of ARDS, wheezing, tachypnea, tachycardia
	Pneumoconiosis	Inhalation of pollutants, results in scarring, fibrosis, and secondary emphysema	Slow developing pulmonary signs of dyspnea, hypoxemia, hypercapnia, cor pulmonale
	Bacterial pneumonia	Virulent bacteria, especially pneumococcal; inflammatory exudate with congestion and edema; poor ventilation in consolidated areas	Rapidly developing fever, chest pain, cough, blood-streaked or rusty-colored sputum; responds well to antibiotic treatment
	Viral pneumonia	Rapid onset of inflammation of alveoli and terminal and respiratory bronchioles; secondary bacterial infection common	Respiratory distress with or without fever; much more severe in children with fever, dehydration, and respiratory failure, especially in those under 2 years of age

SNS, sympathetic nervous system; IC, inspiratory capacity; ERV, expiratory reserve volume; FRC, functional residual capacity; TLC, total lung capacity.

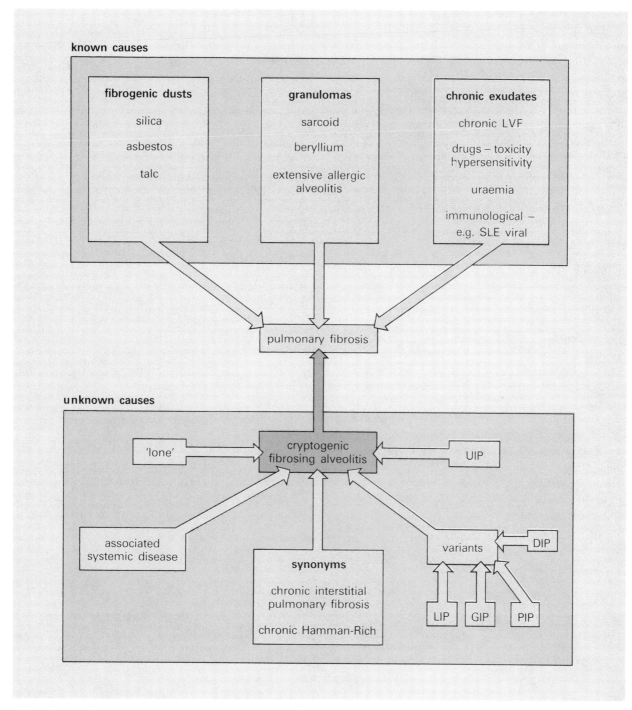

FIGURE 5–15 • Common causes of pulmonary fibrosis. LVF, left ventricular failure; SLE, systemic lupus erythematosus; UIP, usual interstitial pneumonia; DIP, desquamative interstitial pneumonia; GIP, giant cell interstitial pneumonia; LIP, lymphocytic interstitial pneumonia; PIP, plasma cell interstitial pneumonia. (*Color Atlas of Respiratory Diseases.* St. Louis: Gower, F21.1.)

number of connective tissue disorders (eg, systemic lupus erythematosus, rheumatoid arthritis, and sclerosis) can induce a fibrosing alveolitis that is histologically indistinguishable from cryptogenic fibrosing alveolitis. For our purposes, the effects on the lungs are similar. Commonly, the alveolar walls show fibrosis and inflammatory infiltration, with progressive destruction of lung tissue as large areas of fibrosis replace individual alveoli, with large air spaces creating a honeycomb appearance on radiograph. Collagen infiltrates the pulmonary epithelium, endothelium, and interstitium.

Pulmonary fibrosis affects patients of any age; twice as many men are affected as women, and the typical patient is in his or her mid-50s and presents with progressive dyspnea and, subsequently, a dry cough. Examination reveals fine Velcro-like basal crepitations (crackles, in 90% of patients) and finger clubbing (70% of patients). Pulmonary function tests reveal a restrictive pattern; the FEV_1/FVC ratio is often higher than 90% (Fig. 5–16).

Corticosteroids and immunosuppressant drugs provide some symptomatic relief, but only 20% of patients show physiologic improvement after this treatment. Fibrosis has a serious prognosis; 60% of patients die from respiratory failure or terminal infection within 5 years of diagnosis.

Thoracic Expansion Restriction

Abnormalities that affect movement of the thorax include obesity and various forms of thoracic cage deformity.

OBESITY

Obese patients have a reduced expiratory reserve volume because of the pressure of tissue on the thorax and abdomen. This combines with decreased thoracic compliance, respiratory muscle inefficiency, and increased oxygen requirements to result in a sequence of events (Fig. 5–17) leading to obesity-related hypoventilation syndrome. With tidal ventilation close to residual volume, there is a tendency toward reduced ventilation at the bases, with increased atelectasis and subsequent hypoxemia. These problems are greater in the supine, as opposed to the upright, position. Obese patients are also at high risk of developing obstructive sleep apnea.

KYPHOSIS AND SCOLIOSIS

Kyphosis and scoliosis are conditions associated with a curving of the spine. The greater the angle of the spine between the upper and lower limbs, the greater the severity of the disease, reducing the total lung capacity, primarily because of changes in chest wall compliance (Fig. 5–18). Mild scoliosis (angle less than 35 degrees) is relatively common, affecting 0.1% of the population. In 0.01% of the population, moderate scoliosis (more than 75 degrees) is associated with respiratory problems. Severe (more than 120 degrees) scoliosis is associated with cardiopulmonary failure. The greater the angle, the greater the severity of the disease. An angle of 100 degrees is associated with a 40% decrease in total lung capacity, vital capacity, and functional residual capacity. Residual volume stays close to normal. Hypoxemia is usually minimal but may be worse during rapid-eye-movement sleep. Increases in $Paco_2$ levels in patients with severe deformity are associated with tidal volume decreases. As tidal volume decreases, anatomic dead space volume remains stable, increasing the total dead space (Vd/Vt). Treatment for associated respiratory failure includes nighttime ventilation, which has been associated with improved clinical symptoms as well as longevity.

ANKYLOSING SPONDYLITIS

Ankylosing spondylitis, rheumatoid inflammation of the vertebrae, results in decreased chest wall compliance. Unlike other forms of chest wall deformities, functional residual capacity is elevated by as much as 1 L as the rib cage stiffens at a level that is closer to the normal resting level

Male	age: 49 years	height: 1.75m	non-smoker	Diagnosis: Fibrosing alveolitis

	Predicted	Observed	Post Bronchodilator	
FEV₁ (l)	2.89–3.91	1.0	1.0	
FVC (l)	3.75–5.08	1.21	1.14	
FEV₁/FVC (%)	68–79	83	88	
TLC (l)	5.39–7.30	2.06		
RV (l)	1.79–2.42	0.96		
VC (l)	3.75–5.08	1.10		
Insp AWR (kPa/l/s)	<0.2	0		
SGAW (kPa/s)	1.3–3.6	>3.6		
DL_CO (mmol.min/kPa)	8.42–11.39	1.73		
VA (l)	5.02–6.79	1.74		
K_CO (mmol.min/kPa/l)	1.33–1.80	0.99		
VC* (l)		1.10		

FIGURE 5–16 • Flow volume loop and characteristic changes associated with fibrosing alveolitis. (*Color Atlas of Respiratory Diseases.* St. Louis: Gower, F21.9.)

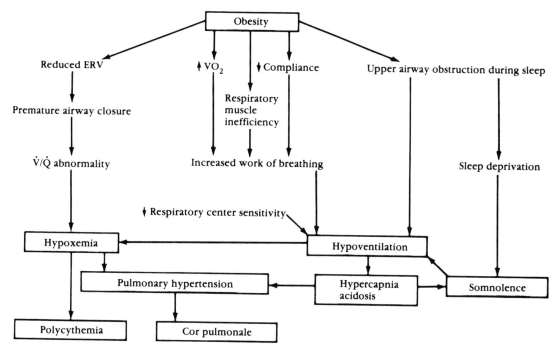

FIGURE 5-17 • Obesity-related hypoventilation syndrome. ERV, expiratory reserve volume. (Farzan S. *A Concise Handbook of Respiratory Disease*. Reston, VA: Reston Publishers; 1978.)

of the ribs. These patients rarely develop respiratory failure without other superimposed pulmonary disease.

RESPIRATORY MUSCLE DISORDERS

Neuromuscular Disease

Patients with respiratory muscle weakness present with a restrictive pattern of pulmonary function testing and with decreased vital capacity (40% to 70% of predicted), total lung capacity, and functional residual capacity. Pulmonary compliance is thought to decrease because of microatelectasis associated with reduced lung volumes, whereas chest wall compliance is decreased as a result of stiffening of rib cage ligaments and tendons, ankylosis of costosternal and thoracovertebral joints, or even spasticity of the intercostal muscles. Pulmonary gas exchange is usually well maintained until respiratory muscle strength falls to 30% of the

Female	age: 20 years	span: 1.60m	non-smoker	Diagnosis: Scoliosis

	Predicted	Observed	Post Bronchodilator
FEV$_1$	2.83–3.83	1.30	1.27
FVC	3.05–4.13	1.37	1.45
FEV$_1$/FVC	80–93	95	88
TLC	4.24–5.73	2.37	
RV	1.18–1.60	1.06	
VC	3.05–4.13	1.31	
Insp AWR	<0.2	0	
SGAW	1.3–3.6	>3.6	
DL$_{CO}$	7.98–10.80	4.48	
VA	3.95–5.34	1.65	
K$_{CO}$	1.64–2.22	2.72	
VC*		0.95	

FIGURE 5-18 • Flow volume loop and characteristic changes associated with scoliosis. (*Color Atlas of Respiratory Diseases*. St. Louis: Gower, F2.7.)

predicted value, and Pa_{CO_2} levels rise. With respiratory muscle weakness, rapid shallow breathing with infrequent sighs is common.

Myasthenia Gravis

Myasthenia gravis is an autoimmune disease in which antibodies to the acetylcholine receptor impair neuromuscular function, leading to progressive muscular weakness that decreases with rest. There is progressive decrease in the muscle action potential with repetitive stimulation of the motor nerve. Respiratory muscle weakness becomes significant in 60% of cases. A myasthenic crisis, or acute exacerbation of the disease, may occur as a result of infection, drugs, or even pregnancy.

Treatment includes oral anticholinesterase inhibitors, such as neostigmine. During crisis, weakness may result in respiratory failure, requiring support with mechanical ventilation.

Guillain-Barré Syndrome

Guillain-Barré syndrome is an acute inflammatory polyneuritis that results in progressive symmetric weakness; it accounts for more than half of patients with neuromuscular disease admitted to the intensive care unit.

Progression of the disease for 2 to 4 weeks may lead to reduction of vital capacity requiring ventilatory support (25% of patients). With proper support, there is only a 2% mortality rate, and less than 15% of patients have any residual disability.

Tetanus

Tetanus is caused by an exotoxin of *Clostridium tetani,* an organism commonly found in soil and feces. The organism enters the body in wounds that contain foreign bodies, manure, or soil and replicates, producing toxins that spread through the blood to the nervous system, with an incubation period of 2 to 21 days. The toxin binds to the presynaptic terminal, interfering with the release of inhibitory transmitter substances. This results in increased muscle tone, loss of coordination, and simultaneous contraction of both agonist and antagonist muscle groups.

Moderate to severe tetanus may present with dysphagia and intense seizures, with many patients requiring intubation and mechanical ventilation. In patients on ventilatory support, autonomic nervous system problems are the leading cause of mortality and include fluctuating hypertension, tachycardia, sweating, hyperexia, and arrhythmias. Even with optimal intensive care unit support, these patients have a 20% mortality rate.

Muscular Dystrophies

Muscular dystrophies are a group of genetically determined, painless degenerative myopathies characterized by weakness and atrophy of the muscles without involvement of the nervous system. Respiratory involvement is greatest with limb-girdle, myotonic, and Duchenne dystrophy, predisposing to increased CO_2 levels, with up to 75% of patients dying from respiratory failure.

Amyotrophic lateral sclerosis (ALS), a disease involving the anterior horn cell, leads to progressive respiratory muscle weakness. ALS patients have a restrictive ventilation pattern, rapid shallow breathing, and decreasing muscle strength with a decreasing ventilatory response to CO_2. Respiratory failure is the primary cause of death from amyotrophic lateral sclerosis.

Mechanical ventilation is used to support these patients, sometimes for many years.

ELECTROLYTE DISTURBANCES

When electrolytes are out of balance, the function of nerves and muscles and their communication may be affected. Water is 60% of body weight and is either intracellular fluid (ICF; 66%) or extracellular fluid (ECF; 34%). Only 8.4% of body water (about 25% of ECF) is in the plasma. Sodium and chloride are found in the ECF space, whereas blood, blood proteins, and colloids are restricted to the intravascular space.

Types of Electrolyte Disturbances

Sodium

Sodium and its major anions chlorine and bicarbonate (HCO_3) are more than 90% of the solute of the ECF. Sodium has a normal serum level of 136 to 145 mEq/L, whereas intracellular levels are much lower (10 mEq/L) because of an active sodium pump. Changes in sodium concentration change the osmolarity of both the ECF and ICF compartments as well as ECF volume. Hyponatremia (sodium concentration less than 135 mEq/L) with a low serum osmolarity can progress to neurologic manifestations owing to brain swelling that occurs with sodium concentrations lower than than 120 mEq/L. Symptoms include lethargy and weakness that can rapidly progress to seizures, coma, and death. Treatment of hyponatremia includes replacement normal or hypertonic saline using the formula:

$$\text{Na required} = (140 - \text{patient's Na}) -$$
$$(0.6 \times \text{body weight in kilograms})$$

Usually, half the calculated dose is given over 8 to 12 hours, so that serum levels do not increase more than 2 mEq/h.

Hypernatremia (sodium concentration higher than 150 mEq/L) usually occurs in patients who are unable to respond to thirst. The symptoms occur because of cellular dehydration of the central nervous system, resulting in somnolence, confusion, respiratory paralysis, and death.

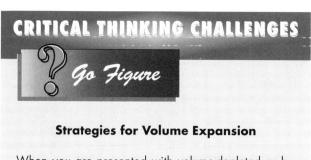

Strategies for Volume Expansion

When you are presented with volume-depleted or hypotensive patients, several common strategies are available to increase their blood volume.

- Dextrose, given intravenously, distributes throughout all the fluid in the body. If you administer 1 L of dextrose, how many milliliters will end up in the intravascular space?
- Saline and Ringer's solution are crystalloids that stay in the extracellular fluid. If 1 L of Ringer's solution is given intravenously, how much (in milliliters) will remain in the intravascular space?
- Colloids stay in the intravascular space when administered. If you administer 1 L of colloids, how much (in milliliters) will remain in the intravascular space? Based on your calculations, which solution would you give the volume-depleted, hypotensive patient?

Potassium

Potassium is the primary cation in the ICF, with 3500 mEq in the body, and less than 1% in the intravascular space (serum potassium concentration normally is 3.5 − 5.0 mEq/L). The ratio of ICF to ECF potassium is determined by insulin, aldosterone, epinephrine, cell membrane integrity, and pH. Potassium is excreted by the kidneys (90%) and the intestine (10%). Hypokalemia, a decrease of serum potassium of 1 to 2 mEq/L, may be due to decreased intake, renal losses (diuretic therapy, renal disease, or antibiotics), gastrointestinal losses (vomiting, diarrhea) and skin losses (sweat and burns). Internal alterations of potassium balance can occur with respiratory or metabolic alkalemia, β-adrenergic receptor agonists, vitamin B_{12} therapy, acute leukemia, and delirium tremens. Clinical features of hypokalemia include impaired neuromuscular function (weakness, paralysis, respiratory insufficiency, intestinal dilation and ileus, and myoglobinuria), cardiovascular disturbances (arrhythmias and conduction defects), and nephropathy (impaired urinary concentrating ability). Hyperkalemia can also cause weakness, flaccid paralysis, paresthesias, alteration in mental status, life-threatening arrhythmias, and cardiac-conducting defects.

Calcium

Calcium is stored primarily in bone (99%), where it is released into the circulation to normal serum levels of 9 to 10.5 mg/dL). In the serum, 45% is active (ionized), and 40% is bound to protein or complexing ions, such as citrate (5% to 15%). Serum levels are maintained through parathyroid hormone and vitamin D. Common causes of hypocalcemia include hypoparathyroidism, magnesium depletion, malabsorption syndrome, decreased vitamin D intake or activation, and acute pancreatitis. Neuromuscular features include tetany, paresthesias, muscle cramps, and seizures. Hypercalcemia can be caused by hyperparathyroidism, malignancies, sarcoidosis, tuberculosis, histoplasmosis, hyperthyroidism, renal disorders, immobilization, and acquired immunodeficiency syndrome. Symptoms include lethargy, muscle weakness, hyporeflexia, confusion, coma, hypertension, bradycardia, arrhythmias, and potentiation of digitalis toxicity.

Phosphate

Phosphate (PO_4) is the major intracellular anion that plays a role in intracellular respiration and metabolism, with the high-energy compounds adenosine phosphatase and adenosine triphosphatase; derangements can affect virtually every organ of the body. The body contains about 800 g of phosphate, with 85% in the bone; normal serum levels are 3 to 4.5 mg/dL. Hypophosphatemia can be due to decreased intake (starving, antacids, vomiting, malabsorption), increased urinary losses, respiratory alkalosis, sepsis, diabetic ketoacidosis, and alcoholism. Symptoms include weakness, hyporeflexia, paresthesias, seizures, respiratory failure, congestive heart failure, decreased 2,3-diphosphoglycerate, and hepatic dysfunction.

Symptoms of hyperphosphatemia are similar to those seen with hypocalcemia.

Magnesium

Magnesium is found mostly in intracellular bone and muscle, with total body stores of 200 mEq. Serum levels of 1.3 to 2.1 mEq/L are a poor estimation of total body levels. Hypomagnesemia is often associated with alcoholism, decreased intake, renal losses, and endocrine problems and presents with altered mental status, tetany, hyperactive reflexes, tremor, ataxia, and seizures. Hypermagnesemia is usually due to a combination of renal insufficiency, iatrogenic factors (antacids, enemas, laxatives), and increased tissue breakdown, with severe diabetic ketoacidosis, burn, or tissue trauma. Symptoms are most commonly seen with renal insufficiency and include nausea, vomiting, progressive neurologic abnormalities, respiratory depression, hypotension, and cardiac arrhythmias.

Treatment

Treatment of electrolyte disturbances is directed at underlying causes and at providing appropriate levels of supplements.

SPINAL CORD INJURY

Spinal cord injury results from extreme flexion or extension coupled with rotation. Complete cord transection is rare, and the primary lesion is usually a small vessel injury producing a contusion that results in ischemic or hypoxic necrosis of the cord minutes to hours after the initial insult. The most common causes of spinal cord injury are vehicular accidents, falls, and sports-related activities. In the United States, there are about 10,000 survivors of spinal cord injury each year. Rapid evacuation, transportation and treatment are key to limiting damage after injury.

Patients with lesions of the middle cervical cord (C3 to C5) suffer paralysis of the diaphragm and depend on their neck muscles for spontaneous ventilation. In these patients, there is considerable inward (paradoxical) motion of the lower rib cage and abdomen on inspiration, and changing from erect to supine position causes respiratory distress secondary to a 50% reduction in vital capacity.

Lower cervical (C6 to C8) and upper thoracic (T1 to T6) cord lesions leave the diaphragm and neck muscles intact but cut off control of the intercostal and abdominal muscles. This allows diaphragmatic breathing but severely hampers the ability to perform forced expiratory maneuvers, such as those required to cough and clear the airway of secretions. Unlike those with high cord lesions, these patients have reduced dyspnea with changes from the upright to supine position as their vital capacity increases by 16%. This is most likely caused by the weight of the abdominal contents pressing the diaphragm toward the lung during exhalation. Pulmonary function with low cord lesions (below C5) has been shown to improve over time, from 30% of predicted value immediately after injury to 60% 5 months after injury.

Unilateral diaphragmatic paralysis presents as an elevated hemidiaphragm, with lung volumes reduced by about 20%. Unilateral diaphragmatic paralysis may be caused by trauma, malignancy, pneumonia, herpes zoster virus, or other, unknown (idiopathic) causes. Diagnosis is made either by fluoroscopy, looking for the affected side to rise paradoxically during a sniff maneuver, or by a delayed phrenic nerve conduction time.

The degree of respiratory impairment depends on the level of the lesion. High cervical lesions (C1 to C2) paralyze the diaphragm, abdominal muscles, scalenes, and intercostals. This leaves only the trapezius and sternomastoid muscles (innervated by the 11th cranial nerve) to support ventilation. Mechanical ventilation is often required initially, but patients may ultimately be trained to breathe with these neck muscles while awake for periods of hours. These patients may also be ventilated with a diaphragmatic pacemaker. Lesions of the middle cervical cord (C3 to C5) cause paralysis of the diaphragm that cannot respond to pacing.

PLEURAL DISEASE

The integrity of the pleura and of the chest wall are essential to maintaining the integrity of the thoracic pump. Instability of the chest wall, such as occurs with multiple rib fractures, can reduce the ability of the pump to bring air into the lung on the affected side (Fig. 5–19). Similarly, air or fluid in the pleural space can reduce the efficiency of the pump.

Closed Pneumothorax

Pneumothorax, or air in the pleural space, may come from a bronchopleural fistula or an opening in the thoracic wall (penetrating wound). An open pneumothorax has an open communication of air from the pleural space to the atmosphere (Fig. 5–20). The lung collapses, and the chest wall enlarges. The mediastinum may shift to the unaffected side, where the pressure is lower, especially during inspiration. This **pendelluft motion** may allow rebreathing of air

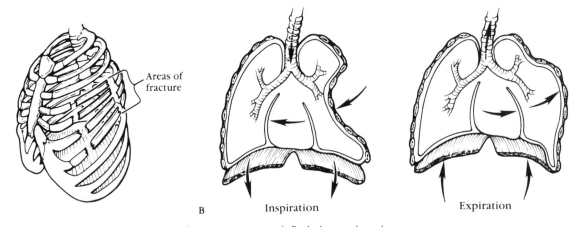

A   B   Inspiration   Expiration

FIGURE 5–19 • Paradoxical breathing can occur with flail chest, when three or more ribs are broken in two or more places. Similarly, pneumothorax on one side can cause pendelluft breathing with air moving from the collapsed lung to the good lung.

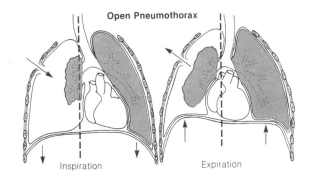

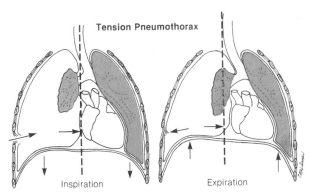

FIGURE 5–20 • Open or communicating pneumothorax (*top*) and tension pneumothorax (*bottom*). In an open pneumothorax, air enters the chest during inspiration and exits during expiration. There may be slight inflation of the affected lung due to a decrease in pressure as air moves out of the chest. In tension pneumothorax, air can enter but not leave the chest. As the pressure in the chest increases, the heart and great vessels are compressed, and the mediastinal structures are shifted toward the opposite side of the chest. The trachea is pushed from its normal midline position toward the opposite side of the chest, and the unaffected lung is compressed.

from the good lung to the affected lung and back with each respiratory cycle, placing the patient at risk.

A closed pneumothorax implies that the air in the pleural cavity is not in communication with the atmosphere. A closed pneumothorax may pose a serious threat to the patient, with air continuously entering the pleural space and with no way for the air to escape. Tension can develop, compressing the lung tissue and pressing the mediastinum toward the unaffected lung. As the mediastinum is pushed over, it rotates, causing two problems: (1) cardiac tamponade from the pressure, reducing venous return to the heart; and (2) in severe cases, tearing of the aorta secondary to the rotation of the mediastinum.

Manifestations depend on the volume of air space. With spontaneous pneumothorax, pleuritic pain may be the initial sign, with increased respiratory and heart rates. Asymmetry of the chest may be apparent, with a lag of chest movement on the affected side on inspiration. Percussion is hyperresonant, with decreased breath sounds over the affected area. Diagnosis of pneumothorax is confirmed by chest radiograph. With tension, the position of the trachea

reflects mediastinal shift, away from the pressure and toward the unaffected lung.

Treatment varies with the cause and extent of the lung collapse. Primary treatment of a closed pneumothorax is to make it an open pneumothorax by venting it to the outside, usually with some form of seal that allows air to escape but not to enter the pleural space. Small pneumothoraces (less than 30%) can reabsorb over a period of days. Tension pneumothorax requires immediate action with insertion of a large-bore needle or chest tube and attachment of a closed drainage system.

Pleural Effusion

Pleural effusion is the accumulation of fluid in the pleural space (Fig. 5–21). When the serous fluid (transudate from the pleural capillaries) in the pleural space exceeds the reabsorption rate of the venules and lymphatics in the pleura, the accumulating fluid forms a pleural effusion. Secretions and reabsorption are affected by hydrostatic pressure, oncotic pressure, capillary permeability, and effectiveness of lymphatics for drainage.

Thin clear transudate may be formed with increased venous pressures secondary to cardiac decompensation or hypoproteinemia (due to low osmotic pressure). Transudate is thin and clear, with less than 3% protein; specific gravity is less than 1.015; and only a few lymphocytes and few pathogens are cultured. Transudate tends to accumulate when the normal hydrostatic pressure is increased in the pulmonary capillary bed (with left heart failure) or when the oncotic pressure is reduced (eg, hypoproteinemia, cirrhosis, or nephrosis).

Pleural exudate is more viscous and less translucent and may clot on standing, with more than 3% protein and a specific gravity of more than 1.015. It tends to accumulate as a

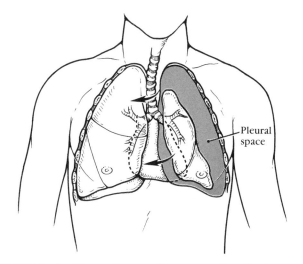

FIGURE 5–21 • Pleural effusion can allow fluid to accumulate in the pleural space and, in some cases, to compress the lung and shift and rotate the mediastinum, much like tension pneumothorax.

result of capillary wall damage by inflammation or infection (eg, pneumonia or tuberculosis) or interference with lymphatic drainage (eg, neoplasm).

The following is a list of types of pleural effusion:

Chylothorax: Collection of chyle (milky-white, opalescent fluid consisting largely of emulsified fats) caused by lymphoma or obstruction of the thoracic duct

Empyema: Pus or purulent pleural fluid that requires drainage and treatment with antibiotics

Hemorrhagic effusions: Frank blood in the pleural space or hemothorax, associated with trauma or pulmonary infarction; may also be associated with neoplasm

Malignant effusions: Pleural metastasis of adenocarcinomas generating from the lung, breast, ovary, and stomach; also primary pleural malignancy mesothelioma. In both cases, survival after diagnosis averages less than 4 months. Effective therapy is not available.

Parapneumonic effusions: Found in about half of all pneumonias; exudative; usually resolved with pneumonia

Pneumothorax: Small effusion in about one fourth of cases of pneumothorax; exudate from irritation as a result of exposure to air

Thoracentesis, or aspiration of fluid from the pleural space, is both diagnostic and therapeutic. Treatment should be directed at the cause of the disorder, with thoracentesis used in large effusions to permit reexpansion of the lung. If the effusion is secondary to a malignancy, a sclerosing agent (that basically "fries" the secretory glands) is injected in the pleural space to reduce fluid reduction as a palliative measure.

PULMONARY VASCULAR DISEASE

Congestive Heart Failure

Left heart failure is common after myocardial infarction affecting the left ventricle and after mitral valve stenosis. Failure of the left heart results in higher pressures building up in the pulmonary vascular bed. Increased pulmonary vascular pressures increase the work load on the right side of the heart, which may also become hypertrophied, causing increased systemic venous pressures. Right-sided heart failure manifests as increased venous pressure, backing up in the capillaries and pushing fluid into the interstitial space. This creates pedal edema in dependent areas and is also seen with distention of the great veins.

Pulmonary hypertension, whether secondary to disease or hypoxemia, increases hydrostatic pressure in the pulmonary capillaries and can increase pressures in the right ventricle, which can hypertrophy or fail over time.

When the left heart fails, pressure builds up in the pulmonary vasculature, causing fluid to lead in the extravascular space, precipitating pulmonary edema, with symptoms described previously (Fig. 5–22).

Cor pulmonale is heart failure secondary to increased pulmonary resistance, increasing end-diastolic pressures and resulting in right ventricular enlargement and hypertrophy. Increased pulmonary resistance is typically due to hypoxic pulmonary vasoconstriction from severe, end-stage obstructive or restrictive lung disease.

Treatment

Treatment is directed at reducing alveolar hypoxia with administration of oxygen. Diuretics may be used to reduce fluid load and edema.

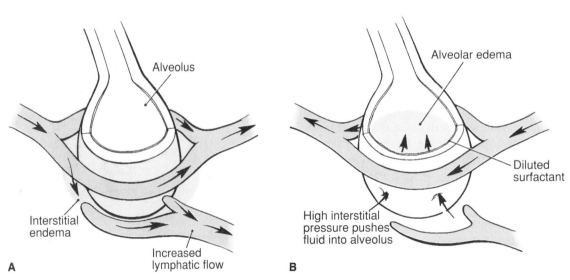

A

B

FIGURE 5–22 • Illustrations of stages of pulmonary edema, both interstitial (*A*) and alveolar (*B*).

Pulmonary Embolus

A pulmonary embolus is caused by any obstructing material (eg, blood clot, air bubble, fat, tumor cells) that becomes lodged in the pulmonary vascular system, obstructing blood flow to the dependent lung beyond. Any foreign or dislodged material in the systemic circulation is filtered by the pulmonary vasculature.

The pulmonary circulation serves the function of filtering the systemic circulation to remove debris and foreign matter in the blood, protecting major organs from embolization. The smaller the emboli, the smaller the blood vessel in which it lodges, and the less disruption in pulmonary blood flow. Large objects can reduce blood flow to large areas of the lung. Large thrombi that lodge in the bifurcation of the pulmonary artery (saddle thrombi) can occlude blood flow to both lungs.

Pulmonary emboli can block blood flow through the pulmonary vessel, and if the blockage persists, pulmonary infarction and tissue necrosis can ensue in tissue not supplied by bronchial circulation. Blood clots or thrombi, often from deep veins in the lower part of the body, break loose and are carried by the venous blood to the right side of the heart and into the pulmonary artery. With long bone fracture, fat emboli are formed that can also lodge in the lung. In response to pulmonary embolism, humoral agents, such as serotonin and prostaglandin, are released into the blood, causing bronchial constriction (reducing ventilation to the area of reduced perfusion).

Predisposing factors for pulmonary embolism are listed in Box 5–8.

Dyspnea and chest pain are common symptoms of pulmonary embolism. Hemoptysis may occur with pulmonary tissue infarction. Hypoxemia may result from $\dot{V}/\dot{Q}$ mismatching secondary to humoral-induced bronchospastic changes in airway pressure. Normal ventilation or hyperventilation secondary to dyspnea, and increased respiratory rate despite increased VD/VT are also symptoms.

Box • 5–8 FACTORS THAT PREDISPOSE TO PULMONARY EMBOLISM

Venous stasis
Varicose veins
Thrombophlebitis
Long periods of immobilization (bedrest, long car or airplane rides)
Long bone fractures
Postoperative period after hip or abdominal surgery
Multiple myeloma
Polycythemia
Neoplasms

Pulmonary emboli can be diagnosed by radionuclide ventilation–perfusion scans, which compare areas of normal ventilation with areas of decreased perfusion. Ventilation is shown by having the patient breath xenon-133 and scanning the lung. Perfusion is shown by injecting radiolabeled particles (technetium) injected into the venous blood. Areas of reduced perfusion show less radiation.

In patients with COPD or other causes of poor ventilation–perfusion relationships, pulmonary arteriography may be required. This involves running a catheter into the pulmonary artery and injecting radiopaque die while chest radiographs are taken.

When the source is thought to be thrombus, preventive measures, such as anticoagulant therapy (heparin or warfarin sodium), are used both short- and long-term. When emboli cause severe hemodynamic compromise, thrombolytic agents, such as streptokinase and urokinase, are used to dissolve the clots. The surgical alternative of embolectomy is considered only as a last resort for severe acute obstruction.

Ventilatory Regulation Defects

Problems in ventilatory regulation may be due to problems in the ventilatory control center or the central or peripheral chemoreceptors but are often associated with some other form of pulmonary disease (vascular, obstructive, or restrictive). These disorders should be suspected when there are abnormal responses to hypoxia or hypercapnia. Frequency and chronicity of ventilatory disorders can be estimated by the presence of metabolic compensation for respiratory acidosis. In general, problems with ventilatory regulation can be confirmed by breathing low O_2 or high CO_2 mixtures in the laboratory and looking for an abnormal response.

Ventilatory regulation disorders, both hypoventilation and hyperventilation, may be central (neurologic problems in the brain-stem control centers caused by vascular insufficiency, infection, trauma or tumors) or chemically induced (respiratory depressants and stimulants).

INFECTIOUS LUNG DISEASE

Pneumonia

Pneumonia is an infectious process that results when a pathogen overwhelms the host defenses of the respiratory system and involves the lung parenchyma. An infectious process restricted to the large airways is considered tracheobronchitis (discussed earlier). Before the era of antibiotics, pneumonia was associated with a mortality rate of more than 80%; this rate decreased to less than 15% with the discovery of penicillin. Pneumonias are often classified as *community acquired* (patient presents with an infection), *hospital acquired* (60% of critically ill patients develop pneumonia after being admitted to the hospital, and more than 40% of those die), *immunocompromised hosts* (subject to infection from a wider range of pathogens, many of which do not infect others), and *aspiration* (caused by aspiration of acidic gastric contents).

The lungs are often considered to be pathogen free below the larynx because of the efficiency of the normal defense mechanisms. In any disease state or condition in which the defenses are compromised, such as chronic bronchitis, bronchiectasis, and CF, the airway becomes colonized with bacteria, resulting in acute and chronic infections. Bacteria can also reach the lungs through the circulation and with aspiration of gastric contents or oral secretions. Aerosols from coughing and contaminated respiratory care devices, can transport pathogens deep into the lungs. If these pathogens are not swept clear or effectively taken "out of commission" by the macrophages, infection and inflammation can result.

A number of infectious agents are associated with pneumonia. Viral and bacterial agents are most common, however, mycobacterial (tuberculosis), fungal, parasitic, and protozoan (*Pneumocystis carinii*) infections can also occur, especially in sick and immunocompromised patients. Immunocompromised hosts are most susceptible to infections and are most likely to experience mortality or morbidity.

Viral infection of the airways is the most common cause of pneumonia in children; in adults, it accounts for less than 10% of hospital admissions for pneumonia, and influenza is the most common agent. Influenza-related pneumonia is of greatest risk to the elderly; patients with chronic lung, heart, or kidney disease; and women in the last trimester of pregnancy. Cytomegalovirus has been identified as a major problem in small children with chronic lung disease and in immunocompromised patients (eg, those with acquired immunodeficiency syndrome and transplanted lungs), in whom the mortality rate can reach 50%. Influenza-related pneumonia typically occurs 1 to 2 days after onset of influenza symptoms, with a dry cough, dyspnea, generalized discomfort, and an interstitial pattern on chest radiograph. Viral serology is seldom of clinical value.

Pneumococcal pneumonia is the most common bacterial type, with streptococci found in the noses of more than 25% of healthy adults. These bacteria most commonly affect patients with chronic lung disease, diabetes, and renal failure. Clinical signs include fever, chills, cough, respiratory distress, pulmonary consolidation, and confusion. Chest radiographs may reveal lobar consolidation or patchy bronchopneumonic processes (Fig. 5–23). Sterile pleural effusions are found in 25% of patients, empyema is found in less than 2%, and abscesses are rare. Leukocytosis (15,000 to 30,000 cells/mm³) with neutrophilia is common.

Staphylococcus aureus accounts for less than 5% of community-acquired and 11% of hospital-acquired pneumonias,

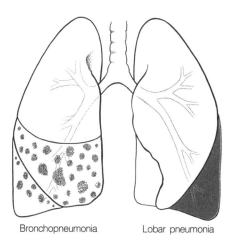

Bronchopneumonia   Lobar pneumonia

FIGURE 5–23 • Distribution of lung involvement in lobar and bronchopneumonia patterns.

with a higher incidence for bacterial pneumonias that follow a viral infection. Staphylococcal pneumonia has a presentation similar to that of pneumococcal pneumonia with the addition of necrosis and abscess of parenchymal tissue (more than 25% of cases) and more frequent empyema (10%).

Gram-negative bacilli are often infectious agents of great consequence in patients with debilitating chronic diseases and in hospitalized patients. *P. aeruginosa* is common in CF and COPD, *E. coli* is associated with urinary tract and intestinal bacteremias, and *Klebsiella pneumoniae* is associated with alcoholism. These pathogens are relatively common in the upper airways, making sputum analysis less than reliable. Diagnosis usually relies on specimens with organisms from the blood, pleural fluid, or lung tissue (bronchial alveolar lavage or bronchoscopy). These pneumonias have a high incidence of pleural reactions.

Legionella are gram-negative bacilli that are often found in water; outbreaks of infection are associated with air-conditioner condensers, water supplies, and even hospital faucets and shower heads. Increased risk is associated with chronic diseases, compromised immunity, and malignancy. After an incubation period of 2 to 10 days, patients present with dry cough, respiratory distress, fever, malaise, weakness, confusion, and gastrointestinal disturbance. There is often multiorgan involvement, with failure to respond to antibiotics other than erythromycin.

Mycoplasma pneumoniae is a common problem in young adults but is more commonly diagnosed from extrapulmonary symptoms, such as myalgias, skin lesions, myringitis, hemolytic anemia, and neurologic complications ranging from meningitis to encephalitis. Pulmonary findings look like viral pneumonia and are only reported by 10% of the infected patients.

Pneumocystis carinii is caused by a protozoan parasite that forms a 5-µm cyst containing sporozoites. Severe infection is secondary to reactivation of latent infection due to immunosuppression. Patients present with dyspnea, dry cough, and diffuse patchy infiltrates. *P. carinii* is a causative agent in about one third of immunocompromised patients with patchy infiltrates. Diagnosis is definitive with bronchoalveolar lavage or transbronchial biopsy. Treatment with aerosolized pentamidine is effective in bringing about recovery and providing prophylaxis in more than 75% of patients.

Fungi are not commonly associated with pneumonias, but the lungs are often affected by systemic fungal infections. *Histoplasma capsulatum, Coccidioides immitis*, and *Blastomyces dermatitidis* occur in normal hosts, whereas *Aspergillus* and *Candida* species are more common in immunocompromised hosts.

Medical management of pneumonia is based on identification of the causative agent, a determination of drug sensitivities, and implementation of appropriate antibiotic, antiviral, or antifungal therapy. Respiratory care, unless antibiotic agents are administered by aerosol, is limited to supportive and palliative interventions. Lung expansion and bronchial hygiene may be appropriate, as may treatment of reversible bronchospasm exacerbated by the acute infection of the airway. Systemic hydration is essential, whereas administration of bland aerosols is seldom appropriate, unless there is a bypassed upper airway. In severe infections, respiratory failure may ensue, requiring mechanical ventilation.

Tuberculosis

Once thought to be on the verge of eradication in the United States, tuberculosis is on the rise worldwide. Tuberculosis is an infectious disease caused by *Mycobacterium tuberculosis*, which are slender, rod-shaped, acid-fast bacteria that protect themselves with a waxy outer capsule that permits the organisms to remain alive even in old calcified lesions. Tuberculosis can infect any organ but is most commonly associated with the lungs (Fig. 5–24). *M. tuberculosis* is an airborne infection that is spread by small aerosol particles (droplet nuclei) commonly less than 3 µm in diameter. These small particles can be produced with coughing, talking, singing, or sneezing and can remain suspended in the air for hours.

After inhalation, the droplet nuclei enter the lungs and implant in a respiratory bronchiole; the bacillus is soon engulfed by macrophages. A granulomatous lesion forms and, over a 3-week period, forms a cheese-like necrosis. This is often coincidental with converting to a positive skin test. The tubercle bacilli may drain through the lymph system to the tracheobronchial lymph nodes. The hypersensitivity response limits replication of the bacillus. The small quantity of bacilli inhaled often results in encapsulation and containment of the primary lesion, which becomes calcified and can then be seen on radiograph.

The lung lesion may progress to invasion of a bronchus, forming an air-filled cavity that is 10 to 15 cm in diameter, permitting spread of the disease and allowing the bacteria to enter the sputum.

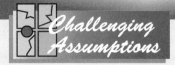

Patients with pneumonia often develop cough, complain of difficulty clearing secretions, and may have evidence of consolidation or infiltrates on chest radiograph. Some clinicians have propagated the practice of ordering chest physical therapy (postural drainage and percussion) for these patients. As discussed in Chapter 13, there is no evidence to support postural drainage and percussion therapy in pneumonia patients unless there is underlying chronic pulmonary disease with daily production of more than 30 mL/d. Pneumonia patients with scant secretions, with or without chronic obstructive pulmonary disease, have not been shown to benefit from this therapy. There remains, however, a strong rationale for frequent turning, aggressive mobilization, good hydration, instructional deep breathing, and coughing.

Primary tuberculosis may be asymptomatic and detected by a positive Mantoux skin test or by the calcified lesions seen on chest radiograph. Patients may present with low-grade fevers, night sweats, easy fatigue, weight loss, and anorexia. A cough may develop, which starts out dry and later becomes productive of purulent and sometimes bloody sputum. Dyspnea and orthopnea develop with progression of the disease.

Diagnosis is made by chest radiographs, skin tests, and sputum inductions. Drug sensitivity studies may be done when drug-resistant strains are suspected. The Mantoux skin test involves intradermal infection of a purified pro-

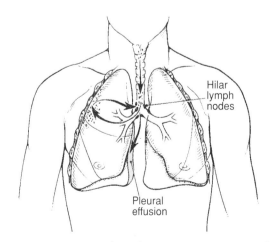

FIGURE 5–24 • Tuberculosis organisms are usually deposited in the lung periphery, either in the lower part of the upper lobe or in the upper part of the lower lobe. Arrows indicate entrance, deposition, spread to hilar lymph nodes, and pleural effusion.

tein derivative of tuberculin. A positive reaction is a discrete area of skin inflammation or skin elevation of greater than 10 mm. In immunosuppressed patients, a skin reaction of 5 mm or greater can be indicative. Patients with tuberculosis may have 15- to 20-mm skin reactions.

Primary treatment is drug therapy with isoniazid (INH), rifampin, ethambutol, streptomycin, and pyrazinamide. INH is the most widely used drug. Multiple drugs are recommended in treating resistant strains, and active tuberculosis requires multiple drugs. Failure to take the drugs over the months of treatment can result in the development of resistant strains. Uncomplicated tuberculosis is generally treated for 6 to 9 months.

Respiratory care for patients with tuberculosis is largely diagnostic, with induced sputum using hypertonic saline, and involves educational intervention. Teaching patients to contain their germs is important. Tissues are to tuberculosis as condoms are to sexually transmitted diseases. Aspects of limiting exposure and practitioner safety are addressed in Chapter 9.

CARCINOMA OF THE LUNG

Four types of pulmonary neoplasms account for 95% of all lung cancers: squamous cell, adenocarcinoma, large cell, and oat cell. As many as 75% of patients have metastasis at the time of diagnosis, with cancer spreading to the pleura, mediastinum, lymph nodes, liver, bone, and brain. These carcinomas have one thing in common: they are all progressive, unrelenting, and often fatal. Most patients do not have symptoms for a long time, then present with cough and bloody sputum, often with enlarged lymph nodes; they may also have chest pain, dyspnea, and hoarseness. Radiologic evidence on routine chest radiographs may be the first sign. Once the tumor is advanced enough to see on chest radiographs, it usually has invaded other areas. Sputum cytology and bronchoscopy confirm the diagnosis.

Management may range from surgery to chemotherapy and radiation therapy. Respiratory care is largely palliative in these patients.

SMOKE INHALATION

Each year in the United States, smoke inhalation is the cause of more than 6000 deaths and plays a factor in a significant number of the 2 million burn injuries treated. The primary cause of smoke inhalation injury is the toxic byproducts (organic acids, aldehydes, and gases) from incomplete combustion that chemically injure the mucosa, causing edema and bronchoconstriction. Carbon monoxide is the most common immediate cause of death in fire victims, with 200 times greater affinity for hemoglobin than oxygen, limiting the oxygen-carrying capacity and shifting the oxygen dissociation curve to the left (Table 5–2). A problem associated with burning plastics is the release of cyanide, which blocks cellular metabolism of oxygen. At

Table • 5–2 CARBON MONOXIDE LEVELS: CLINICAL FEATURES AND TREATMENT

COHb%	Clinical Features	Treatment
0–10	None	None
10–20	Headache	High flow, High F_IO_2 oxygen, 1 hour
20–30	Severe headache, nausea, vomiting	High-flow oxygen, high F_IO_2, 1 hour
40–50	Visual disturbance, altered mental state	Hyperbaric oxygen if available, 2 atmosphere, F_IO_2 1.0, for 30 minutes
>50	Coma, convulsions, respiratory and cardiovascular depression Central nervous system damage	
>70	Almost always fatal	

temperatures of 350° to 500°C, dry air causes injury primarily to the upper airway. The respiratory tract is so efficient in conditioning inhaled gas that it cools the gas sufficiently so that the gas does not cause burns by the time it reaches the trachea. On the other hand, steam has considerably more thermal capacity, overwhelming the heat exchange capacity of the upper airway and resulting in injury to the tracheobronchial tree and lung parenchyma.

Inhalation injury should be suspected in patients with facial burns, singed nasal hair, stridor, hoarseness, wheezing, or black flecks of carbon or charred material in their sputum. Eight to 24 hours after burn injury, tracheobronchitis presents in the large and medium airways with mucosal edema, hemorrhage, sloughing of tissue, pseudomembranes, and bronchiolitis.

Treatment includes administration of oxygen for carbon monoxide poisoning, protecting the airway, aggressive bronchial hygiene, and possibly ventilatory support.

INHALED IRRITANTS

A wide variety of gases and chemicals are toxic to the airway. The site of damage depends in large part on whether the irritants are water soluble (Fig. 5–25). Water-soluble irritants (eg, ammonia, sulfur dioxide, and low concentrations of chlorine) have an immediate effect on the upper respiratory tract and bronchi, where they contact a respiratory tract that is largely bathed in aqueous secretions (mucus), creating mucosal edema and irritation (warning the subject that there is irritant gas so he or she can flee the area). Insoluble irritants (eg, phosgene, oxides of nitrogen, and cadmium oxide) are not dissolved in the moist upper airway and end up reaching the lung parenchyma without warning, so that exposure may be prolonged, resulting in damage of the alveoli and development of pulmonary edema.

Treatment consists of getting the subject away from the irritant, medical management of mucosal and alveolar

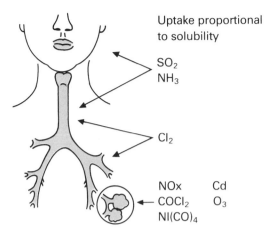

Uptake proportional
to solubility

SO_2
NH_3

Cl_2

NOx   Cd
$COCl_2$ O_3
$NI(CO)_4$

FIGURE 5–25 • Site of damage from respiratory irritants. Sulfur dioxide and ammonia in the upper airway; chlorine in the main branch; and nitric oxide, ozone and other irritants in the lung parenchyma. (*Color Atlas of Respiratory Diseases*. St. Louis: Gower, F18.2.)

edema, palliative efforts to soothe the airway with cool aerosols, and bronchodilators, if bronchospasm is evident and shown to be reversible.

DROWNING

The initial response to drowning appears to be closing the epiglottis (10% of victims die from asphyxia, with no water in lungs). Others aspirate fluid, develop pulmonary edema, intrapulmonary shunt, and possibly profound hypoxemia, identical to that seen in adult respiratory distress syndrome. Aspiration of fresh water can cause transient hypervolemia as water passes from the lungs to the intravascular space. In salt water, fluid crosses from the blood into the lungs, creating pulmonary edema and hypovolemia. Serum electrolytes and hematocrit rarely present major clinical problems. Neurologic impairment depends on the duration of immersion and the temperature of the water. In very cold water (less than 20°C), victims have recovered from as much as 40 minutes of submersion, perhaps because of the diving reflex (bradycardia when the face is immersed in cold water).

Resumption of ventilation after immersion is key. Keep the patient's airway open, oxygenate liberally until an arterial blood gas level is measured, and ventilate as necessary.

ACUTE RESPIRATORY FAILURE

Respiratory failure is characterized by an inability to eliminate CO_2 (type I) or an inability to oxygenate (type 2). Ventilatory failure is associated with a $PaCO_2$ of 50 mmHg and a pH 7.25. Chronic respiratory failure allows time for metabolic compensation, presenting with high $PaCO_2$ and normal pH. Acute respiratory failure is not compensated and is often superimposed on chronic respiratory failure. As CO_2 levels increase, O_2 levels fall, adding hypoxemia

to the equation. Acute respiratory failure, if not treated in a timely manner, can result in death. Figure 5–26 shows two types of respiratory failure in patients with chronic airflow obstruction. Clinical signs of respiratory failure are presented in Figure 5–27.

Hypercapnia occurs when alveolar ventilation decreases (due to decreased minute volume or increased dead space) or when CO_2 production increases (fever, exercise, or increased metabolism.) Normally, when VCO_2 increases, ventilation increases to compensate and maintain normal CO_2 levels. When the need to increase ventilation exceeds a patient's capacity to "blow off" the CO_2, ventilatory failure ensues.

Failure to oxygenate occurs when a patient is unable to maintain a PaO_2 of 50 mmHg on ambient air. Increasing $PaCO_2$ from 40 to 60 mmHg results in a decrease in PAO_2 from 90 to 70 mmHg, and an alveolar arterial gradient of 20 mmHg would bring the PaO_2 to 50 mmHg, representing failure to oxygenate.

Acute respiratory failure is treated by increasing minute ventilation, decreasing VD, or reducing CO_2 production.

Minute volume can be improved by reducing lung obstruction (bronchodilators, mucolytics, secretions removal), reducing restriction (lung expansion), or improving ventilatory control. In extreme cases, mechanical ventilation (noninvasive or with intubation) may be required. VD can be reduced by increasing tidal volume.

Reduction of CO_2 production is achieved by reducing fever, treating infection, administering antipyretic drugs (aspirin), and decreasing muscle activity (agitation or shivering).

ACUTE RESPIRATORY DISTRESS SYNDROME

Acute respiratory distress syndrome (ARDS) has been described as diffuse pulmonary infiltrates that occur after acute lung injury, including blunt chest trauma, septic shock, hypoperfusion, aspiration of gastric contents, fat embolism after long bone fractures or surgery, severe pneumonias of any cause, smoke inhalation, or radiation or chemical exposure. Prolonged exposure to high concentrations of oxygen (more than 60% O_2 for more than 24 hours) produces events that are difficult to differentiate from ARDS.

In patients with ARDS, there is generally a change in alveolar capillary membrane permeability secondary to inflammatory response of the type I cells. The flooding of fluid across the alveolar–capillary membrane washes out surfactant as it alters the ability of type II cells to produce surfactant. Without surfactant, there is a tendency of alveoli to collapse (diffuse atelectasis), reducing lung volume and compliance. This increases shunting, producing refractory hypoxemia (Fig. 5–27).

Diagnostic criteria for ARDS include generalized infiltrates on chest radiograph (Fig. 5–28), total thoracic compliance less than 50 mL/cm H_2O, and refractory hy-

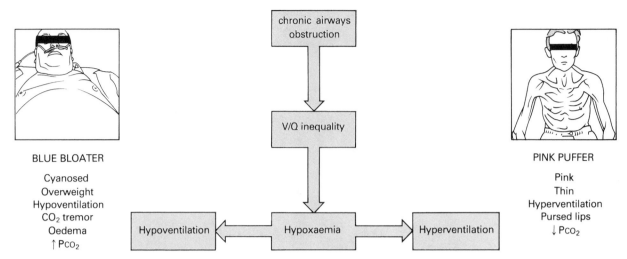

BLUE BLOATER

Cyanosed
Overweight
Hypoventilation
CO_2 tremor
Oedema
↑PCO_2

chronic airways
obstruction

V/Q inequality

Hypoventilation ← Hypoxaemia → Hyperventilation

PINK PUFFER

Pink
Thin
Hyperventilation
Pursed lips
↓PCO_2

FIGURE 5–26 • The clinical extremes of respiratory failure in chronic airflow obstruction with the blue bloater and the pink puffer. (*Color Atlas of Respiratory Disease.* St. Louis: Gower, F10.8.)

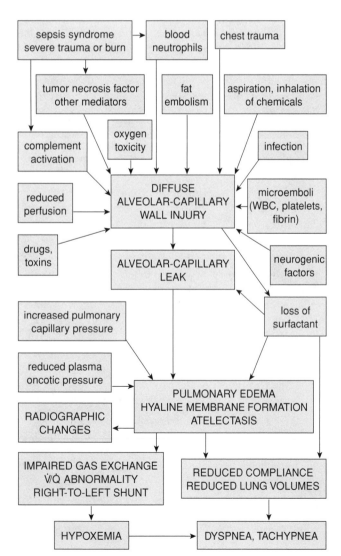

FIGURE 5–27 • Pathogenesis and pathophysiology of adult respiratory distress syndrome. (Farzan S. *A Concise Handbook of Respiratory Disease.* 3rd ed. Reston, VA: Reston Publishers; 1992.)

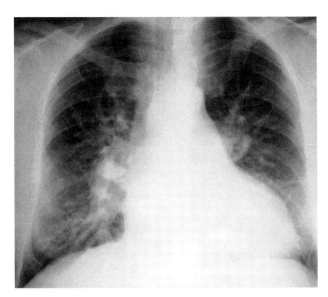

FIGURE 5-28 • Radiograph from a patient with acute respiratory distress syndrome. (*Color Atlas of Respiratory Diseases*. St. Louis: Gower, F10.10)

poxemia, with a PaO_2/PAO_2 ratio of less than 0.33. Pulmonary artery wedge pressure is normal.

Sepsis is a common cause of ARDS and a major risk factor (50% of patients with ARDS). The sepsis syndrome consists of clinical and laboratory findings indicative of a systemic response to sepsis, temperature higher than 39°C or lower than 35°C, white blood cell count of less than 12,000 or less than 3000 cells/mm³, positive blood culture, and documented source of infection. This is accompanied by unexplained hypotension (systolic arterial pressure of less than 90 mmHg for more than 2 hours), systemic vascular resistance of less than 800 dyne/s/cm⁵, or unexplained metabolic acidosis, with base deficit of more than 5 mEq/L.

Treatment is aimed at expanding the lung with positive airway pressure (continuous positive airway pressure or positive end-expiratory pressure) to a level at which the alveoli do not collapse during exhalation. This application of pressure increases lung volumes, reduces shunt, and increases lung compliance, reducing hypoxemia and work of breathing. Although ARDS is often diffuse through the lungs, it is not homogeneous; that is, not all alveoli are equally affected. Consequently, the pressure required to expand surfactant-depleted alveoli may cause more normal alveoli to be overdistended. The lower inflection point is that pressure at which the compliance of the lung improves with the application of positive airway pressure. This is discussed in greater detail under mechanical ventilation. Oxygen is required but should be administered with care to minimize the risk of oxygen toxicity. The administration of intravenous fluid is an important part of initial resuscitation, but an increase in microvascular permeability can increase lung edema, even with a low wedge pressure.

Bibliography

Bates B. *A Guide to Physical Examination and History Taking.* 6th ed. Philadelphia: JB Lippincott; 1995.

Brewis RAL. *Lecture Notes on Respiratory Disease.* Oxford, UK: Blackwell Scientific; 1980.

Burton GC, Hodgkin JE, Ward JJ. *Respiratory Care: A Guide to Clinical Practice.* 4th ed. Philadelphia: JB Lippincott; 1996.

Des Jardins T. *Clinical Manifestations of Respiratory Disease.* Chicago: Year Book Medical Publishers; 1984.

George RB, Light RW, Matthay MA, Matthay RA. *Chest Medicine.* Baltimore: Williams & Wilkins; 1995.

Porth CM. *Pathophysiology: Concept of Altered Health States.* 4th ed. Philadelphia: JB Lippincott; 1994.

Tobin MJ. *Essentials of Critical Care Medicine.* New York: Churchill Livingstone; 1989.

Turner-Warwic, M, Hudson ME, Corrin B, Kerr IH. *Clinical Atlas Respiratory Diseases.* London: Gower Medical Publishing; 1989.

Wanner A, Sackner MA. *Pulmonary Diseases: Mechanisms of Altered Structure and Function.* Boston: Little, Brown; 1983.

West JB. *Pulmonary Pathophysiology: The Essentials.* 5th ed. Baltimore: Williams & Wilkins; 1995.

Assessing Signs and Symptoms of Respiratory Dysfunction

Joyce Anderson • James B. Fink

6

Key Terms

cyanosis
dyspnea
fremitus
hemothorax
infiltrate
pallor
palpation
peak flow
percussion
pleural effusion
pneumothorax
tachypnea

Objectives

- Identify sequential steps in the decision-making pathway necessary to the effective management of respiratory dysfunction.

- Identify components of an assessment.

- Identify the clinical evaluation components necessary to completing an assessment.

- Identify the diagnostic investigations necessary to completing an assessment.

- Identify normal and abnormal findings in completing a respiratory assessment.

- Identify the respiratory diagnosis.

- State the treatment plan based on assessment findings.

- Evaluate the effectiveness of treatment based on assessment findings.

MANAGING RESPIRATORY DYSFUNCTION

The emerging roles of the respiratory care practitioner (RCP) include the roles of assessor, evaluator, educator, and consultant. Essential to fulfilling these roles is the ability to assess and diagnose skillfully the signs and symptoms of respiratory dysfunction and to assess body system contributions to respiratory dysfunction. This chapter focuses on steps in a systematic approach to managing signs and symptoms of respiratory dysfunction, with a primary focus on assessment and diagnostic skills for a beginning RCP.

The sequence of the chapter is as follows: sequential steps in a decision-making pathway, components of an assessment, clinical evaluation components necessary to completing an assessment, diagnostic investigations necessary to completing an assessment, documentation of assessment findings, identification of a respiratory diagnosis, statement of a management plan based on assessment findings, and evaluation of the effectiveness of therapy based on assessment findings.

SEQUENTIAL STEPS IN A DECISION-MAKING PATHWAY

Developing a systematic approach to decision making is a key strategy in effective management of respiratory dysfunction. The RCP who has incorporated a regular systematic approach in managing respiratory dysfunction has taken the first essential step in delivering quality care to patients.

The essence of patient management of respiratory dysfunction is to identify problems, define solutions, implement solutions, and evaluate the effectiveness of implemented solutions. Figure 6–1 is an outline of an approach to the management of abnormalities in respiratory function.

COMPONENTS OF AN ASSESSMENT

The underlying goals of a respiratory assessment are to identify abnormalities in respiratory function, to identify systemic and metabolic factors that affect respiratory function adversely, and to identify deficits in knowledge by the patient that impact on self-care and respiratory function.

---

1. Immediately recognize and make a decision regarding the severity of the patient's condition.
   ↓
2. Perform a clinical evaluation of the patient's respiratory function.
   ↓
3. Perform or seek diagnostic evaluations of respiratory function.
   ↓
4. Formulate a respiratory diagnosis.
   ↓
5. Decide and implement management strategies based on respiratory diagnosis.
   ↓
6. Evaluate efficacy of management strategies based on identified, desired outcomes.

FIGURE 6–1 • Outline of an effective strategy for identifying and managing abnormalities in respiratory function.

Box • 6–1   PATIENT DIAGNOSTIC INTERVIEW

Demographics
  Age
  Occupation
Past medical history
  Smoking history
  History of respiratory or cardiac disease
  History of systemic disease
  Medications
  Home oxygen
Allergies
History of present illness
  Symptoms
    Description
    Onset
    Duration
    Severity
    Aggravating factors
    Intermittent or continuous
  When respiratory difficulties started
  Medications and therapy taken to relieve symptoms
  Whether the patient adhered to plan and, if not, why
  Whether the treatment worked
  Assess cough
    Frequency
    Strength
    Effectiveness
      Quantity of sputum
      Color
      Consistency
      Odor
  Assess dyspnea—subjective scale
  Apparent work of breathing
  Whether respiratory symptoms limit activities
  Patient's goals for treatment
  Mental status
    Confused
    Lethargic
    Irritable
    Obtunded

CRITICAL THINKING CHALLENGES

Case Scenario

Mr. B. is a 50-year-old who presents to the emergency room complaining of difficulty breathing. The RCP is called to assess Mr. B. and suggest a plan of treatment to the emergency room physician. List questions and information that you need to complete your assessment.
- Past medical history
- History of present illness
- Physical examination
- Diagnostic evaluations

On questioning Mr. B., you find out that he has smoked two packs of cigarettes per day for 11 years. He had asthma when he was a child but has not had an attack since he was 17 years old. He has not previously been on any medications. His respiratory rate is 28 breaths/min, his pulse oximeter reading is 89%. His CBC shows a hemoglobin level of 12.8, hematocrit of 39, and white blood cell count of 22,000. His breath sounds are clear. His chest radiograph shows an infiltrate in his right middle lobe. His temperature is 101.8°F.

What is your respiratory diagnosis? What would you suggest as treatment for Mr. B.? How would you follow up on your suggested treatment for Mr. B.?

Table • 6–1 DYSPNEA INDEX

Degree of patient perceived difficulty breathing (perceived dyspnea).

Grade	Description	
	Difficulty	Exertion
0	No difficulty	Very, very light
1	Mild	Fairly light
2	Moderate	Somewhat hard
3	Severe	Hard
4	Very severe	Very, very hard

The most effective strategy in identifying abnormalities in respiratory function is to be thoroughly familiar with what is considered normal respiratory function.

Primary components of a respiratory assessment include identifying any past medical history that impacts on respiratory function and any history of present illness relating to respiratory function, performing a physical examination of the patient, and making diagnostic evaluations of respiratory function.

Information on the past medical history can be obtained by reading the patient's medical record and by asking the patient questions related to the past medical history. Information on the history of present illness can be obtained from the patient's medical record and by asking the patient.

The physical examination of the patient includes the use of four techniques: inspection, auscultation, percussion, and palpation. The beginning RCP needs to develop skills in the use of inspection and auscultation.

Diagnostic investigations include laboratory and other procedures that can provide information and assist in formulating a respiratory diagnosis (Box 6–1).

CRITICAL THINKING CHALLENGES

Case Scenario

Tom J. is a 16-year-old in the pediatric ward who has been admitted with a diagnosis of status asthmaticus. You are called to assess him for treatment. What assessment parameters will you assess and document?

Assessment Parameters

Your assessment findings of Tom J. are as follows: Dyspnea index 3 out of 4. He is alert. His respiratory rate is 20 breaths/min. His heart rate is 112 beats/min. His pulse oximeter reading is 88%. His peak flow reading is 180. You auscultate expiratory wheezing over the right posterior lobes. What is your respiratory diagnosis? What treatment plan would you recommend for Tom J.? How would you follow up on Tom. J.?

Two hours later, you are called stat to assess Tom J. His respiratory rate is 30 breaths/min. Breath sounds show wheezing bilaterally. His peak flow reading is 180. His pulse oximeter reading is 97% on a nasal cannula at 2 L/min. His dyspnea index is 2 out of 4. What is your respiratory diagnosis? What would you suggest as treatment?

CRITICAL THINKING CHALLENGES

Case Scenario

Mrs. A. is a 66-year-old with a history of chronic obstructive lung disease. She has been admitted to 6 north and the doctor has ordered albuterol administered by metered dose inhaler at 4 puffs q.i.d. You are here to start her treatments. Your assessment findings are as follows: respiratory rate 18 breaths/min, breath sounds diminished throughout, and arterial blood gas values of PO_2, 69; PCO_2, 58; pH, 7.39; HCO_3, 29. Her best personal peak flow is 240; her peak flow today is 180. She has stated that she took her "green" top medicine (meaning her Atrovent) at home and that it did not help her at all. What are your respiratory diagnoses? What is your plan of care?

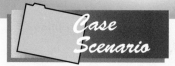

CRITICAL THINKING CHALLENGES
Case Scenario

Mr. J. is a 28-year-old asthmatic patient. He calls you while on duty at 1 AM. He states that he has taken three albuterol treatments in the last 2 hours. His peak flow is 220 after his last treatment. His best personal peak flow is 650. What would you suggest that he do? Why?

CRITICAL THINKING CHALLENGES
Go Figure

Cyanosis occurs when there is 5 g% or more of desaturated hemoglobin. A patient with polycythemia may become cyanotic with relatively moderate hypoxia (blue bloater), whereas a patient who is anemic may actually die of hypoxia while still in the pink (pink puffer). If the patient has a hemoglobin concentration of 10 g, at what saturation will the patient become cyanotic?

Past Medical History

In assessing the patient's past medical history, the RCP should determine smoking history, history of cardiac or respiratory disease, and history of any systemic disease that might affect respiratory function (eg, ascites or renal disease). Note whether the patient is on home oxygen as well as the patient's activities of daily living. Ask if the pa-

tient is on any medicines at home and, if so, what they are, how often medicines are being used, and the last time any respiratory medicines were taken. Note allergies to any medications.

History of Present Illness

In the history of present illness, the RCP should pay attention to the following parameters: severity of symptoms,

(text continues on page 150)

Box • 6–2 PHYSICAL ASSESSMENT

Vital signs
  Body temperature
  Pulse rate
  Blood pressure
  Respiratory rate
Inspection
  Breathing pattern
  Chest (shape and condition)
  Use of respiratory muscles
    Inspiration/exhalation ratio
    Use of accessory muscles
    Flaring
    Retractions
  Skin color
  Clubbing
  Edema
Palpation
  Symmetry of chest expansion
  Position of the trachea
  Fremitus
Percussion
  Density of lung tissue
    Resonant
    Dull
    Hyperresonant
  Diaphragmatic excursion
Auscultation
  Normal breath sounds
  Adventitious sounds

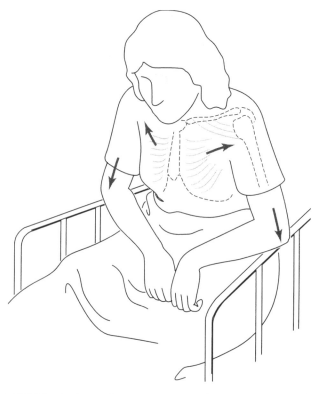

FIGURE 6–2 • Patient position and posture may provide clues to use of accessory muscles. Note position—leaning forward on elbows, fixing arms to allow optimal movement of chest wall with use of pectoralis major muscles.

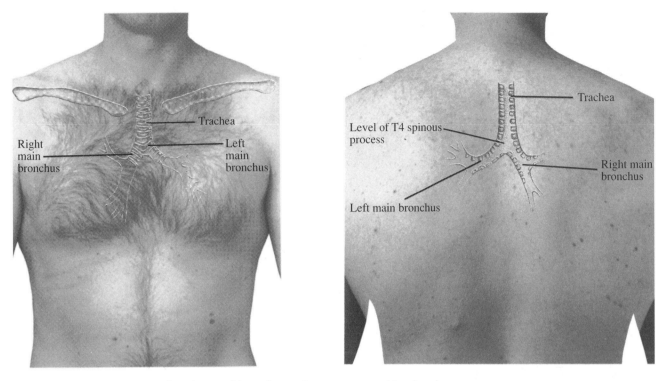

FIGURE 6–3 • Position of trachea and bronchi in relation to external landmarks.

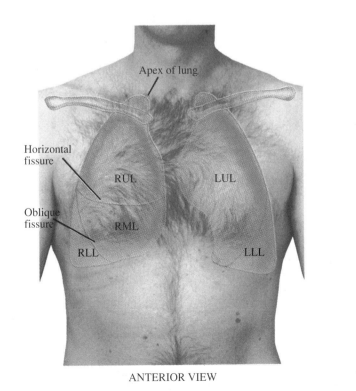

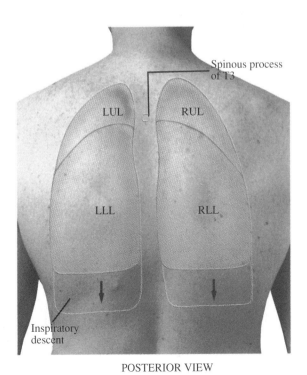

ANTERIOR VIEW   POSTERIOR VIEW

FIGURE 6–4 • Position of lungs in relation to internal and external landmarks.

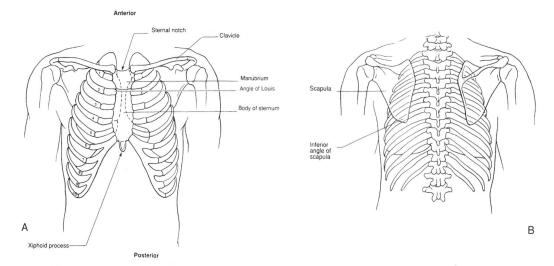

FIGURE 6-5 • Structures of the bony thorax in relation to key landmarks.

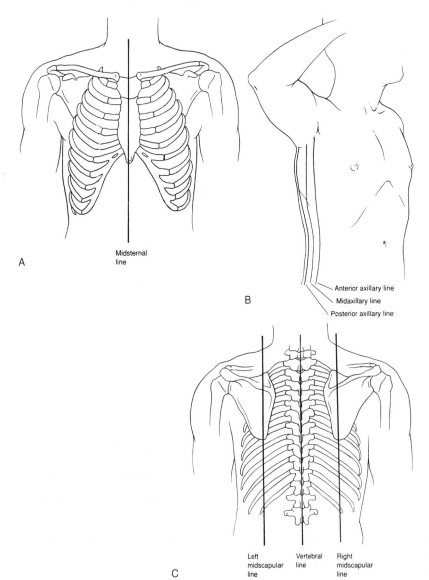

FIGURE 6-6 • Vertical lines with key landmarks used to describe position on chest wall.

Inspiration Expiration

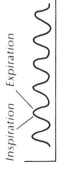

Normal

The respiratory rate is about 14–20 per min in normal adults and up to 44 per min in infants.

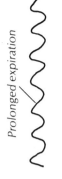

Slow Breathing *(Bradypnea)*

Slow breathing may be secondary to such causes as diabetic coma, drug-induced respiratory depression, and increased intracranial pressure.

(illustration: Rapid Shallow Breathing waveform)

Rapid Shallow Breathing
(Tachypnea)

Rapid shallow breathing has a number of causes, including restrictive lung disease, pleuritic chest pain, and an elevated diaphragm.

(illustration: Rapid Deep Breathing waveform)

Rapid Deep Breathing
(Hyperpnea, Hyperventilation)

Rapid deep breathing has several causes, including exercise, anxiety, and metabolic acidosis. In the comatose patient, consider infarction, hypoxia, or hypoglycemia affecting the midbrain or pons. *Kussmaul's breathing* is deep breathing due to metabolic acidosis. It may be fast, normal in rate, or slow.

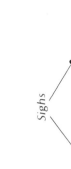

Hyperpnea   *Apnea*

Cheyne–Stokes Breathing

Periods of deep breathing alternate with periods of apnea (no breathing). Children and aging people normally may show this pattern in sleep. Other causes include heart failure, uremia, drug-induced respiratory depression, and brain damage (typically on both sides of the cerebral hemispheres or diencephalon).

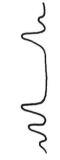

Sighs

Sighing Respiration

Breathing punctuated by frequent sighs should alert you to the possibility of hyperventilation syndrome—a common cause of dyspnea and dizziness.

Occasional sighs are normal.

Prolonged expiration

(illustration: Obstructive Breathing waveform)

Obstructive Breathing

In obstructive lung disease, expiration is prolonged because narrowed airways increase the resistance to air flow. Causes include asthma, chronic bronchitis, and COPD.

(illustration: Ataxic Breathing waveform)

Ataxic Breathing *(Biot's Breathing)*

Ataxic breathing is characterized by unpredictable irregularity. Breaths may be shallow or deep, and stop for short periods. Causes include respiratory depression and brain damage, typically at the medullary level.

FIGURE 6–7 • When observing respiratory patterns, think in terms of rate, depth, and regularity of the patient's breathing. Describe what you see in these terms. Traditional terms, such as *tachypnea*, are given so that you will understand them, but simple descriptions are recommended for use.

what aggravates the symptoms, what alleviates the breathing problem, changes in respiratory status from previous level, cough, sputum, hemoptysis, fever, dyspnea, presence of confusion, and any medicines that the patient is taking.

Cigarette smoking has an adverse effect on respiratory function. Knowing the smoking history is an important part of the information needed to assess respiratory function.

In the history of present illness, the severity, onset, and precipitating and aggravating factors of the symptoms provide clues to establishing a respiratory diagnosis and formulating treatment goals, outcomes, and implementation strategies. Note when the patient's respiratory difficulty started, medicines taken to relieve the problem, whether the medicines helped, whether the patient ever had an attack this severe, and what precipitated the attack.

Difficulty breathing at intermittent intervals results from events that may be related to bronchoconstriction, whereas persistent difficulty breathing is more often related to chronic respiratory disease. Nocturnal shortness of breath may be related to asthma and congestive heart failure. Difficulty related to activity can have a number of causes but may be indicative of exercise-induced asthma.

Changes in respiratory status from a previous level may indicate the progression of disease to a more severe state or may indicate an acute exacerbation brought on by infection, change in environment, or other precipitating factors.

Coughing is an important defense mechanism and is not found commonly in healthy people. The primary method of clearing the airway is through use of the mucociliary mechanism of the epithelial lining of the airway. Coughing serves two purposes: to clear secretions from the airway and to prevent foreign material from entering the airway. When the coughing mechanism is ineffective, abnormalities in gas exchange, atelectasis, and pneumonia may be the end result.

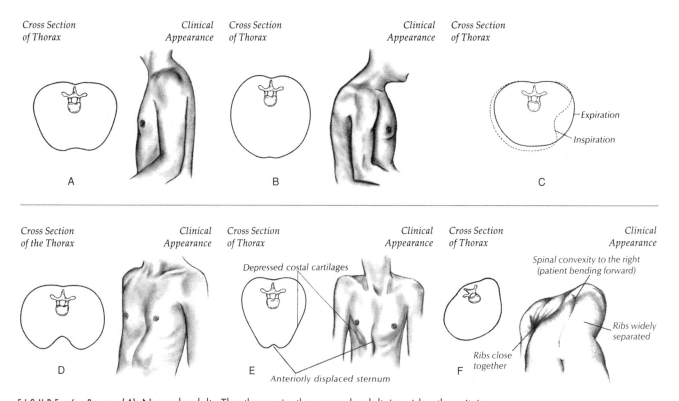

FIGURE 6–8 • (*A*) Normal adult. The thorax in the normal adult is wider than it is deep, that is, its lateral diameter is larger than its anteroposterior diameter. (*B*) Barrel chest. A barrel chest has an increased anteroposterior diameter. This shape is normal during infancy and often accompanies normal aging and chronic obstructive pulmonary disease. (*C*) Traumatic flail chest. If multiple ribs are fractured, paradoxical movements of the thorax may be seen. As descent of the diaphragm decreases intrathoracic pressure on inspiration, the injured area caves inward; on expiration, it moves outward. (*D*) Funnel chest (pectus excavatum). A funnel chest is characterized by a depression in the lower portion of the sternum. Compression of the heart and great vessels may cause murmurs. (*E*) Pigeon chest (pectus carinatum). In a pigeon chest, the sternum is displaced anteriorly, increasing the anteroposterior diameter. The costal cartilages adjacent to the protruding sternum are depressed. (*F*) Thoracic kyphoscoliosis. In thoracic kyphoscoliosis, abnormal spinal curvatures and vertebral rotation deform the chest. Distortion of the underlying lungs may make interpretation of lung findings difficult.

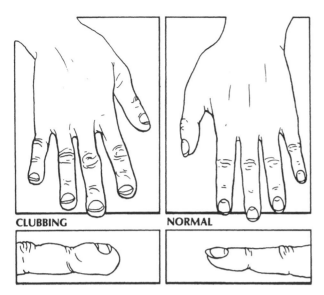

FIGURE 6–9 • Digital clubbing.

In the history of present illness, the RCP seeks information on the frequency of the cough, productivity of secretion and amount, consistency and color of the secretions, and acuteness of the cough. Infection of the respiratory tract might yield secretions that are green, gray, or yellow. This is abnormal and needs to be investigated further. Normal secretions should be clear and thin. Amounts of expectorant greater than 30 mL/d are probably indicative of bronchiectasis. Chronic bronchitis is probably the diagnosis if the patient is expectorating on a daily basis.

Fever may be indicative of a respiratory or systemic infection. Sputum cultures have an essential role in identifying the source and pathogenicity of a possible respiratory infection.

The presence of **dyspnea**, or shortness of breath, may result from abnormalities in respiratory function as a primary source, but other sources contributing to dyspnea must also be investigated. Cardiac disorders may manifest as **tachyp-nea** (rapid respiratory rate) and **cyanosis** (bluish discoloration of the skin). Metabolic disturbances, such as metabolic acidosis, may manifest as changes in respiratory rate and rhythm. Ascites and abdominal distention may manifest as tachypnea and shallow breathing. The presence of dyspnea dictates an overall systemic appraisal to determine its cause. The use of a dyspnea index (Table 6–1) helps to determine the degree of dyspnea present in the patient. It also provides a reference point to determine improvement or deterioration of respiratory status.

Confusion and mental status changes in a patient are often the first clues of respiratory dysfunction. Information relating to mental status changes can be assessed by asking questions related to time, place, and person.

Medicines that a patient is taking may impact on respiratory function. Information on the name of the medicine, frequency of use, last time used, effects of use, and adverse effects (if any) is needed to assess efficacy of medicine; appropriate use of inhaled bronchodilators, anticholinergics, and steroids; and compliance with medication regimens.

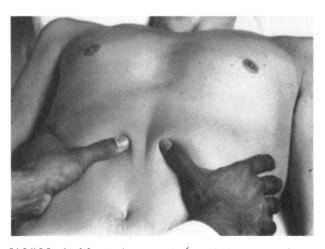

FIGURE 6–10 • Assessment of respiratory expansion.

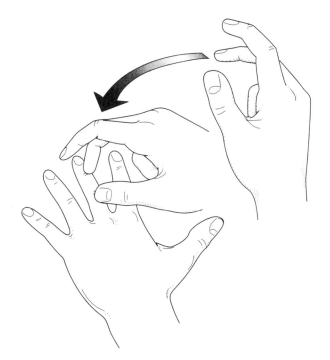

FIGURE 6-11 • Technique for chest percussion.

Physical Examination

Physical examination of the patient by the beginning RCP makes use primarily of the skills of inspection and auscultation (Box 6–2).

The physical examination performed by the RCP should include assessment of the following: general overall status of the patient, vital signs, the respiratory system, the car-

diovascular system, and any body system that might affect respiratory function adversely.

In the general overall assessment, evaluate the patient's appearance, mental status, respiratory rate and rhythm, and work of breathing.

Appearance: Inspect the patient for dyspnea, degree of apprehension, and skin color. Severe apprehension, dyspnea, and abnormal skin coloring (especially cyanosis) may indicate life-threatening difficulties.

Mental status: One of the first indications of respiratory dysfunction is an altered mental status. Confusion, irritability, and lethargy are deviations from normal and if observed in the patient may indicate abnormalities in respiratory function.

Respiratory rate and rhythm: Deviations from normal rates and rhythms indicate the presence of respiratory dysfunction. Rates above 25 breaths/min may indicate primary respiratory dysfunction (eg, pneumonia), metabolic disturbances (eg, ketoacidosis), or systemic disturbances (eg, shock or sepsis). Rates less than 10 breaths/min are indicative of central nervous system or metabolic disturbance.

Work of breathing: Note the use of neck muscles, intercostal muscles, and abdominal muscles during inspiration. Use of these muscles indicates an increased work of breathing. Posture of the patient combined with use of accessory muscles may be a key to hyperinflation (Fig. 6–2).

Note whether a fever is present. Fever may indicate that a respiratory or systemic infection is present. In the presence of fever, the body uses and needs additional oxygen.

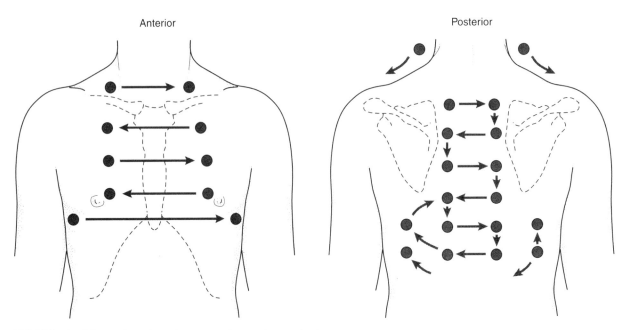

FIGURE 6-12 • Locations for percussion and auscultation.

Normally Air-Filled Lung

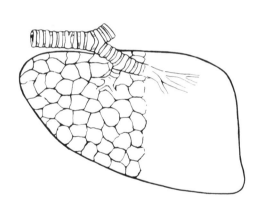

Airless Lung, as in Lobar Pneumonia

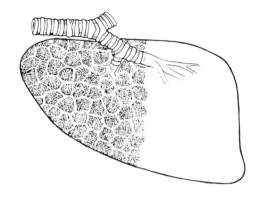

Breath Sounds

Predominantly vesicular

Bronchial or bronchovesicular over the involved area

Transmitted Voice Sounds

Spoken words muffled and indistinct

Spoken words louder, clearer (bronchophony)

Spoken "ee" heard as "ee"

Spoken "ee" heard as "ay" (egophony)

Whispered words faint and indistinct, if heard at all

Whispered words louder, clearer (whispered pectoriloquy)

Tactile Fremitus

Normal

Increased

FIGURE 6–13 ● Breath sounds in air-filled and airless lungs. The origins of breath sounds are still unclear. According to leading theories, turbulent airflow in the central airways produces the tracheal and bronchial breath sounds. As these sounds pass through the lungs to the periphery, lung tissue filters out their higher-pitched components, and only the soft and lower-pitched components reach the chest wall. There, they are heard as vesicular breath sounds. Normally, tracheal and bronchial sounds may be heard near their anatomic origins; vesicular breath sounds predominate elsewhere. When lung tissue loses air, it transmits high-pitched sounds much better. If the tracheobronchial tree is open, bronchial breath sounds may replace the normal vesicular sounds in areas that overlie airless lung. This change may be caused by lobar pneumonia, in which the alveoli fill with fluid, red blood cells, and white blood cells—a process called *consolidation*. Other causes include pulmonary edema or hemorrhage. The appearance of bronchial breath sounds usually correlates with an increase in tactile fremitus and transmitted voice sounds.

Table • 6–2   CHARACTERISTICS OF BREATH SOUNDS

	Duration of Sounds	Intensity of Expiratory Sound	Pitch of Expiratory Sound	Locations Where Heard Normally
Vesicular*	Inspiratory sounds last longer than expiratory ones	Soft	Relatively low	Over most of both lungs
Broncho-vesicular	Inspiratory and expiratory sounds are about equal	Intermediate	Intermediate	Often in the 1st and 2nd interspaces anteriorly and between the scapulae
Bronchial	Expiratory sounds last longer than inspiratory ones	Loud	Relatively high	Over the manubrium, if heard at all
Tracheal	Inspiratory and expiratory sounds are about equal	Very loud	Relatively high	Over the trachea in the neck

*The thickness of the bars indicates intensity; the steeper their incline, the higher the pitch.

Inspection

To identify abnormal findings in the physical examination, the RCP must be familiar with normal findings.

The physical examination starts with inspection of the chest. During inspection of the chest, it is important for the practitioner to be able to visualize the structures of the thorax in context of the anatomic landmarks (Figs. 6–3 and 6–4). It is also of value to be able describe any abnormal findings in terms of those landmarks shown in Figures 6–5 and 6–6. With the patient in a sitting position (if possible), note the rate, depth, regularity, and effort of breathing (Fig. 6–7). Normal breathing is quiet and even.

Note the anteroposterior diameter of the chest in proportion to its lateral diameter, normally a ratio of 1:2. Note the shape of the chest (Fig. 6–8). Each side in the normal chest is symmetric to the other side. Asymmetry may be indicative of kyphoscoliosis (abnormal curvature the spine). The "barrel chest" is often seen in patients with pulmonary emphysema. Observe the ribs and intercostal spaces between the ribs to see if there is abnormal retraction of the spaces between the ribs during inspiration (seen in asthma, emphysema, or tracheal obstruction) or abnormal bulging of the intercostal spaces during expiration (seen in asthma, emphysema, or pleural effusion).

Inspect the membranes of the mouth and the nail beds for cyanosis or **pallor** (paleness of the skin). Both are abnormal conditions and may indicate decreased oxygenation or decreased hemoglobin available to transport oxygen.

Inspect the feet and ankles for peripheral edema (swelling), which may indicate systemic disorders that can manifest as respiratory dysfunction. Inspect the fingers for clubbing (a decrease or loss of the 15-degree angle that the nail makes with the cuticle), which may indicate a primary respiratory dysfunction or a systemic disorder with respiratory manifestations (Fig. 6–9).

Inspect the abdomen for distention or large size, which can interfere with the ability of the lungs to descend and inflate, resulting in respiratory dysfunction.

Palpation

In **palpation,** the practitioner uses his or her hands to touch the patient to assess thoracic expansion, position of key structures, and tactile fremitus.

The assessment of thoracic expansion involves placing the hands on both sides of the chest, with thumbs toward the midline, below the ribs (anterior; Fig. 6–10) or below the scapula (posterior), and asking the patient to take a deep breath. The practitioner looks for normal symmetry of chest expansion and notes variances.

The position of the trachea is normally in the midline but may be pushed or pulled from midline because of a variety of problems. Tension pneumothorax and effusions may push the trachea from midline, whereas atelectasis or open pneumothorax may pull the trachea to the affected lung. The trachea may also be pushed aside by space-occupying lesions.

(text continues on page 158)

Table • 6–3   ADVENTITIOUS LUNG SOUNDS

	Duration	Intensity	Pitch
Discontinuous†			
Fine crackles (. . . . .)	Very brief	Soft 5–10 ms	High
Coarse crackles (• • • • •)	Not as brief 20–30 ms	Somewhat louder	Lower
Continuous‡			
Wheezes (⋀⋀⋀⋀⋀⋀⋀)	Longer than >250 ms	Louder crackles	Relatively high
Rhonchi (⋁⋁⋁⋁)	Longer than >250 ms	Louder crackles	Relatively low

*The thickness of the bars indicates intensity; the steeper their incline, the higher the pitch.

†Discontinuous sounds (crackles) are intermittent, nonmusical, and brief, like dots in time.

‡Continuous sounds are like dashes in time but do not necessarily persist throughout the respiratory cycle. Unlike crackles, they are musical.

Crackles

Crackles have two leading explanations. (1) They result from a series of tiny explosions when small airways, deflated during expiration, pop open during inspiration. This mechanism probably explains the late inspiratory crackles of interstitial lung disease and early congestive heart failure. (2) Crackles result as air bubbles flow through secretions or lightly closed airways during respiration. This mechanism probably explains at least some coarse crackles.

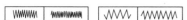

Inspiration   Expiration

Late inspiratory crackles may begin in the first half of inspiration phase but must continue into late inspiration. They are usually fine, fairly profuse, and repeat themselves from breath to breath. These crackles appear first at the bases of the lungs, spread upward as the condition worsens, and shift to dependent regions with changes in posture. Causes include interstitial lung disease (such as fibrosis) and early congestive heart failure.

Early inspiratory crackles appear soon after the start of inspiration and do not continue into late inspiration. They are often but not always coarse and are relatively few in number. Expiratory crackles are sometimes associated. Causes include chronic bronchitis and asthma.

Midinspiratory and expiratory crackles are heard in bronchiectasis but are not specific for this diagnosis. Wheezes and rhonchi may be associated.

Wheezes and Rhonchi

Wheezes occur when air flows rapidly through bronchi that are narrowed nearly to the point of closure. They are often audible at the mouth as well as through the chest wall. Causes of wheezes that are generalized throughout the chest include asthma, chronic bronchitis, COPD, and congestive heart failure (cardiac asthma). In asthma, wheezes may be heard only in expiration or in both phases of the respiratory cycle. Rhonchi suggest secretions in the larger airways. In chronic bronchitis, wheezes and rhonchi often clear with coughing.

Occasionally in severe obstructive pulmonary disease, the condition worsens to the point that the patient is no longer able to force enough air through the narrowed bronchi to produce wheezing. The resulting silent chest should raise concern and not be mistaken for improvement.

A persistent localized wheeze suggests a partial obstruction of a bronchus, as by a tumor or foreign body. It may be inspiratory, expiratory, or both.

Stridor

A wheeze that is entirely or predominantly inspiratory is called stridor. It is often louder in the neck than over the chest wall. It indicates a partial obstruction of the larynx or trachea, and demands immediate attention.

Pleural Rub

Inflamed and roughened pleural surfaces grate against each other as they are momentarily and repeatedly delayed by increased friction. These movements produce creaking sounds known as a pleural rub (or pleural friction rub).

Pleural rubs resemble crackles acoustically, although they are produced by different pathologic processes. The sounds may be heard as discrete, but sometimes are so numerous that they merge into an apparently continuous sound. A rub is usually confined to a relatively small area of the chest wall, and typically is heard in both phases of respiration. When inflamed pleural surfaces are separated by fluid, the rub often disappears.

Mediastinal Crunch
(Hamman's Sign)

A mediastinal crunch is a series of precordial crackles synchronous with the heart beat, not with respiration. Best heard in the left lateral position, it is due to mediastinal emphysema (pneumomediastinum)—often a medical emergency.

FIGURE 6–14 • Adventitious (added) lung sounds.

Table • 6–4   PHYSICAL SIGNS IN SELECTED CHEST DISORDERS

The teal boxes in this table suggest a framework for clinical assessment. Start with the three boxes under Percussion Note: resonant, dull, and hyperresonant. Then move from each of these to other boxes that emphasize some of the key differences among various conditions. The changes described vary with the extent and severity of the disorder. Abnormalities deep in the chest, moreover, usually produce fewer signs than do superficial ones, and may cause no signs at all. Use the table for the direction of typical changes, not for absolute distinctions.

Condition	Trachea	Percussion Note	Breath Sounds	Tactile Fremitus and Transmitted Voice Sounds	Adventitious Sounds
Normal The tracheobronchial tree and alveoli are clear; the pleurae are thin and close together; the mobility of the chest wall is unimpaired.	Midline	Resonant	Vesicular, except perhaps bronchovesicular and bronchial sounds over the large bronchi and trachea, respectively	Normal	None, except perhaps a few transient inspiratory crackles at the bases of the lungs
Chronic Bronchitis The bronchi are chronically inflamed, and a productive cough is present. Airway obstruction may develop.	Midline	Resonant	Normal	Normal	None; or scattered coarse crackles in early inspiration and perhaps expiration; or wheezes or rhonchi
Left-Sided Heart Failure *(Early)* Increased pressure in the pulmonary veins causes congestion and interstitial edema (around the alveoli). The bronchial mucosa may become edematous.	Midline	Resonant	Normal	Normal	Late inspiratory crackles in the dependent portions of the lungs; possibly wheezes
Consolidation The alveoli fill with fluid or blood cells, as in pneumonia, pulmonary edema, or pulmonary hemorrhage.	Midline	Dull over the airless area	Bronchial over the involved area	Increased over the involved area, with bronchophony, egophony, and whispered pectoriloquy	Late inspiratory crackles over the involved area

Condition and Process	Trachea and Mediastinum	Percussion Note	Breath Sounds		Adventitious Sounds
Atelectasis *(Lobar Obstruction)* — When a plug in a mainstem bronchus (as from mucus or a foreign object) obstructs air flow, the affected lung tissue collapses into an airless state.	May be shifted toward the involved side	Dull over the airless area	Usually absent when the bronchial plug persists. Exceptions include right upper lobe atelectasis, where adjacent tracheal sounds may be transmitted.	Usually absent when the bronchial plug persists. In exceptions, eg, right upper lobe atelectasis, may be increased	None
Pleural Effusion — When fluid accumulates in the pleural space, it separates the air-filled lung from the chest wall and blocks the transmission of sound.	Toward the opposite side in a large effusion	Dull to flat over the fluid	Decreased to absent, but bronchial breath sounds may be heard near the top of a large effusion.	Decreased to absent, but may be increased toward the top of a large effusion	None, except a possible pleural rub
Pneumothorax — When air leaks into the pleural space, usually unilaterally, the lung recoils from the chest wall. Pleural air blocks the transmission of sound.	Toward the opposite side if much air	Hyperresonant or tympanitic over the pleural air	Decreased to absent over the pleural air	Decreased to absent over the pleural air	None, except a possible pleural rub
Emphysema — This is a slowly progressive disorder in which the distal air spaces are enlarged and the lungs become hyperinflated. Chronic bronchitis is often associated.	Midline	Diffusely hyperresonant	Decreased to absent	Decreased	None, or the crackles, wheezes, and rhonchi of associated chronic bronchitis
Asthma — Widespread narrowing of the tracheobronchial tree diminishes airflow to a fluctuating degree. During attacks, airflow decreases further, and the lungs hyperinflate.	Midline	Normal to diffusely hyperresonant	Often obscured by wheezes	Decreased	Wheezes, possibly crackles

Fremitus is the palpable vibration from the patient's vocal cords that travels through the tracheobronchial tree and lung parenchyma. Fremitus is increased with consolidated or fluid-filled lung and decreased with obstructed airways, hyperinflation, fibrosis, pneumothorax, or a thick chest wall.

Percussion

Percussion, as the name implies, consists of striking the chest wall to produce audible sounds in the underlying tissue. The sound varies based on the density of the tissues, down to about 5 cm below the surface. The goal is to use one finger to strike the joint of another placed against a surface, creating an audible vibration. Press the distal joint of the hyperextended middle finger of one hand firmly on the chest wall. With your other hand, use the middle finger to strike a quick, sharp, but relaxed motion on the joint of the finger placed on the chest (see Fig. 6–10). Percussion is performed on the chest wall, over soft (not bony) tissue, in a pattern that allows the practitioner to compare both sides of the chest at both levels (Fig. 6–11).

Air-filled normal lung tissue produces a nice resonant percussion note. When tissue is filled with fluid or solid material (eg, with pleural effusion, fibrosis, consolidation, atelectasis), the percussion note becomes dull, as when you percuss your thigh. Hyperinflated lungs produce a hyperresonant note. When an air-filled space is hyperinflated (as with a tension pneumothorax), it makes a tympanic note (like a tight drum head), which you can hear by percussing your cheek filled with air under pressure.

Percussion can be used to determine diaphragmatic excursion (Fig. 6–12). Determine the level of the diaphragm during quiet breathing (above the diaphragm is normally resonant, below is dull). Direct the patient to take a deep breath and hold it while you determine the new level of the diaphragm, normally 5 or 6 cm lower than with normal breathing. Paralysis of a hemidiaphragm (Fig. 6–13) is detectable by normal movement on one side, with minimal movement of the paralyzed side. A high diaphragm may indicate pleural effusion or atelectasis. A low diaphragm with reduced movement may be indicative of hyperinflation.

Auscultation

Skill in the use of a stethoscope is necessary to listen to breath sounds. A stethoscope with comfortable-fitting ear pieces, thick-walled double tubes about 10 to 12 inches in length, a diaphragm (for hearing most sounds), and a bell (for hearing low-pitched sounds and for use in children) provides an effective tool for auscultating breath sounds.

After warming the diaphragm of the stethoscope in the palms of the hands, gently lay it on the area of the chest to be auscultated (Tables 6–2 and 6–3). Auscultate both

---

Box • 6–3 DIAGNOSTIC INVESTIGATIONS

Assessment of hypoxia
  Pulse oximetry
Arterial blood gases
Clinical laboratory analyses
  CBC
  Blood chemistry
  Electrolytes
Chest radiograph
  Imaging reports
Pulmonary function
  Peak flow, forced vital capacity, FEV_1
    Before and after bronchodilator
    Presence of obstruction or restriction
  Negative inspiratory force
  Tidal volume
Sputum examination
  Gram stain
  Cytology
  Histology
Electrocardiogram
Hemodynamics

Table • 6–5 PHYSIOLOGIC EFFECTS OF HYPOXEMIA

PaO_2 (mmHg)	Function	Abnormality	Sign or Symptom
<60	Heart rate	↑	Tachycardia
	Respiratory rate	↑	Tachypnea
	Na^+ and H_2O excretion	↓	Edema
<55	Cardiac output	↑	Bounding pulses
	Arrhythmias	↑	Tachyarrhythmias Bradyarrhythmias
	Mentation	↓	Somnolence Confusion Pinpoint pupils
	RBC mass	↑	Plethora Erythrocythemia Thromboemboli
	PA pressure	↑	Jugular venous distention Edema RV S_4 Hepatomegaly Abnormal ECG*
<30	Cardiac output	↓	Cyanosis Pulse pressure Shock
	Metabolism	↓	Lactic acidosis

*ECG findings of cor pulmonale (RAE, RVE, rightward shift in ventricular or atrial vectors).

ECG, electrocardiogram; RBC, red blood cell; PA, pulmonary artery; RV, right ventricular.

Box • 6-4	SIGNS AND SYMPTOMS OF HYPERCAPNIA

$PaCO_2$ >50 mmHg
Headache
Depressed tendon reflexes
Confusion and drowsiness
Disorientation
Coma
Tachycardia
Bounding pulses
Tremor
Diaphoresis
Increase in blood pressure
Flushed skin, warm periphery
Small pupils, enlarged retinal veins

the anterior and posterior chest in a systematic fashion, comparing one side with the other. Ask the patient to breathe deeply through the mouth. Listen to the breath sounds.

Normal breath sounds are vesicular, bronchial, bronchovesicular, or tracheal, all heard in different locations of the lung. Vesicular breath sounds are soft, low-pitched sounds heard over most of the chest. Bronchial breath sounds are loud, high-pitched sounds heard normally over the large airways (see Fig. 6–13). Bronchovesicular breath sounds are intermediate between bronchial and vesicular sounds and are heard normally either anteriorly near the first and second intercostal spaces or posteriorly between the scapulae. Tracheal breath sounds are loud, high-pitched sounds heard over the trachea. Abnormal (or adventitious) breath sounds are primarily of two types—continuous (wheezes) or discontinuous (crackles)—and may be heard in any area of the lung (Fig. 6–14). Continuous breath sounds are generated when air passes through narrowed airways. Discontinuous breath sounds are heard when air passes through secretions in the airway.

The observation of physical signs provides effective clues to a variety of chest disorders (Table 6–4). Further diagnostic testing can provide additional vital information.

Diagnostic Investigations

Diagnostic investigations (Box 6–3) are used to complete the overall picture of the assessment and to identify any abnormalities that would indicate respiratory dysfunction. These investigations include laboratory data (arterial blood gases, complete blood count, electrolytes), chest radiographs, pulmonary function tests, cultures and Gram stains of sputum, and additional studies as indicated.

Although the practitioner should be aware of and look for signs and symptoms of hypoxemia (Table 6–5) and hypercapnia (Box 6–4), arterial blood gases provide a more comprehensive perspective of both oxygenation and acid–base balance. Abnormalities in arterial blood gases (Table 6–6) give an indication of the severity of respiratory dysfunction. Decreased oxygen values and increased carbon dioxide values indicate impairment of respiratory function.

Decreases in the complete blood count (CBC) hemoglobin and hematocrit indicate a decreased ability of the body to carry oxygen to the tissues.

Increases in the white blood cell count of the CBC may indicate infection or an inflammatory process in the body. During an infectious process, with an increase in body temperature, the body uses and needs additional oxygen. This usually manifests as an increase in respiratory rate and heart rate.

Abnormalities in electrolytes (sodium, potassium, chloride) alter muscle function and can cause abnormalities in respiratory and cardiac muscle function.

Chest radiographs provide a wide range of information on respiratory function. They are used to confirm infiltrates in the lungs, normal or abnormal lung expansion and diaphragm excursion, **pleural effusions** (abnormal amounts of fluid in the pleural spaces), and **pneumothorax** or **hemothorax** (free air or blood, respectively, in the pleural spaces).

(text continues on page 162)

Table • 6-6 COMPARATIVE VALUES FOR COMPENSATED AND UNCOMPENSATED RESPIRATORY ACIDOSIS

Arterial Blood Gas Components	Normal Values	Compensated Respiratory Acidosis (An Example)	Uncompensated Respiratory Acidosis (An Example)
pH	7.35–7.45	7.35	7.22
PCO_2	35–45 mmHg	54 mmHg	74 mmHg
PO_2	80–100 mmHg	62 mmHg	40 mmHg
O_2 saturation	95%–100%	83%	69%
HCO_3^-	22–26 mEq/L	32 mEq/L	28 mEq/L
H_2CO_3	1.05–1.35 mEq/L	1.8 mEq/L	2.9 mEq/L

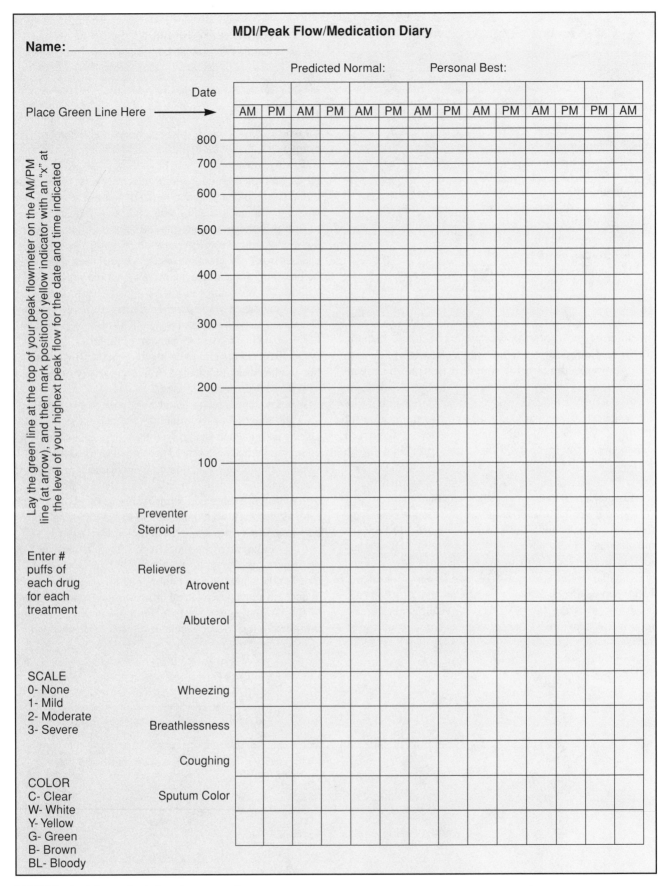

FIGURE 6–15 • Peak flow/symptom diary.

How To Use Your Peak Flow Meter

1. Stand up if possible, or sit upright with **good posture.**
2. Before using the peak flow meter, make sure **the yellow indicator** has been reset. The indicator should be within the diamond outline near the mouthpiece.
3. To **reset** the indicator, hold the meter at the end opposite the mouthpiece. Swing your arm to shake the indicator down toward the mouthpiece. Do this as if you were shaking down a thermometer.
4. Take a **deep breath.**
5. Put the **mouthpiece** between your lips. Seal your lips around the mouthpiece. **Do not stick your tongue into the mouthpiece.**
6. **Blow out** as hard and as fast as you can.
7. **Repeat** steps 4 through 6 two more times. **Do not reset the meter after each maneuver.**
8. The yellow indicator will mark the **highest peak flow** of your three efforts. Note the number at the middle of the yellow indicator. Enter this number on your Peak Flow/Medication Diary.
9. When you have **finished** using the peak flow meter, put it back in its original package or in a baggy. This will protect your peak flow meter from dust and dirt.

(**Note:** These instructions are specific to use of a Truzone peak flow meter.)

How To Use Your MDI - Peak Flow - Medication Diary

The MDI-Peak Flow-Medication Diary is designed to provide a "snapshot" of how you are doing. It also shows how much medication you are taking two times each day. It is not designed for you to record all medication taken throughout the day. Only record what you take when you wake up in the morning and at bedtime.

1. The peak flow diary sheet covers a period of 7 days. Write your name on the line provided. Starting with today's date, write the dates for the next 7 days across the top of the sheet.
2. Under each date is a graph for charting your peak flow for AM and PM (once in the morning upon waking and once in the evening at bedtime) before taking your medications. Begin entering results in your diary in the left most column, filling in subsequent days to the right.
3. A simple method for recording your peak flow is to place the green plastic ring at the end of the flow meter at the level of the DATE line on the diary, aligning the scale on the peak flow meter with the scale on the paper and enter an "x" in the column for today's date and time, next to the middle of the yellow indicator.
3a. An alternative is to read the number on the scale next to the middle of the yellow indicator and enter it in today's column, marking an x at the corresponding number on the scale.
4. Below the peak flow section of the diary, indicate the number of puffs of each medication taken immediately after you measured your peak flow.
5. Next, record how much wheezing, breathlessness and coughing you feel after the treatment, by entering a number between 0 (no symptoms) and 3 (severe symptoms).
6. Finally, take a deep breath and cough. Mark down the color of your sputum, such as clear, white, yellow, green, brown or bloody.
7. Remember to fill out this form every day and bring it with you to your next clinic visit, or any time that you need to go to the Emergency Department or hospital for your breathing.

FIGURE 6–15 • Continued.

Pulmonary function tests provide information on the functional status of the lungs. For the beginning RCP, useful information is provided by looking at the **peak flow**, forced vital capacity, negative inspiratory force, tidal volume, and forced expiratory volume in 1 second (FEV$_1$). Note whether any airway disease has been identified as obstructive (abnormalities in the flow of air into and out of the lungs) or restrictive (abnormalities in lung volumes).

Peak flows are a useful bedside assessment of pulmonary function. The peak flow provides information on how fast the patient is able to move air out of the lungs. Although nomograms are useful in determining what a patient's peak flow should be, in patients with established airway disease, the patient's own best peak flow (under the most optimal circumstances) should be the reference peak flow to determine deviations up and down.

A patient education monitoring system is commonly used to assist the RCP and the patient in monitoring peak flows to detect changes in respiratory status (Fig. 6–15). The system makes use of the stoplight, red-yellow-green system. If a patient's peak flows are in the green zone (80% to 100%

of personal best effort), the patient is advised to continue with his or her regular routine. A yellow zone (50% to 80% of best peak flow effort) indicates caution, and the patient is advised to consult the primary caregiver for advice. Peak flows in the red zone (below 50% of best personal effort) signal a medical alert. Emergency medical attention should be sought by consulting with the primary caregiver.

Pulmonary function tests done before and after bronchodilator therapy provide information on whether the bronchodilator is able to reverse airway obstruction. Peak flow maneuvers also assist in determining this information.

Cultures and Gram stains of the sputum are performed to determine if an infectious process exists in the lungs and to identify the causative organism if present. If an infection is present, the patient will probably be given antibiotics to treat the infection.

Other studies might be indicated to rule out suspected abnormalities of respiratory function and are ordered as the situation indicates.

Once the clinical evaluation has been completed (histories of past and present illness, physical examination, and

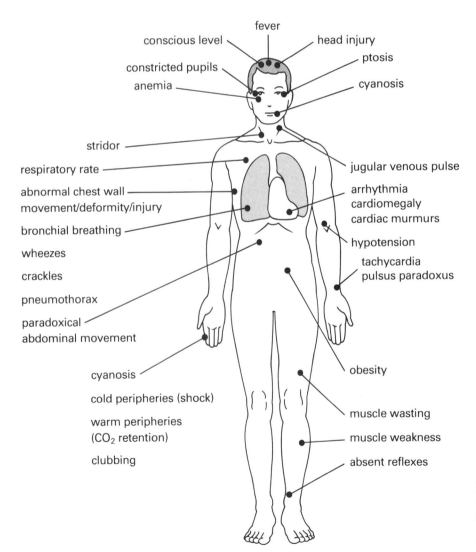

FIGURE 6–16 • Important clinical signs in the assessment of a patient with respiratory failure. (*Color Atlas of Respiratory Diseases.* St. Louis: Gower, F10.12.)

diagnostic evaluations), abnormal data are clustered and analyzed to put together the whole picture of the patient's problem, and a respiratory diagnosis is made (Fig. 6–16). This diagnosis assists in making decisions for appropriate interventions and therapy, the next steps in managing abnormalities in respiratory function.

Last, but not least, assessment of the patient needs to address the patient's ability to understand, learn, and participate in therapeutic interventions and therapy. Box 6–5 identifies the areas necessary to the development and implementation of an effective care plan.

Respiratory Diagnoses

Five categories of respiratory diagnoses cover a wide range of abnormal findings in patients with abnormalities in respiratory function (Box 6–6).

Once a respiratory diagnosis has been made, the other steps in managing respiratory dysfunction (management strategies, implementation, and evaluation) follow in sequence. Table 6–7 provides some common examples of how clinical data and assessment correlate to common treatment plan selection. The treatment plan is initiated in consultation with the physician or primary caregiver based on all assessment findings linked together to make the respiratory diagnosis.

DOCUMENTATION

Once the clinical evaluation, respiratory diagnosis, and treatment plan have been undertaken, essential objective data found during the physical examination, diagnostic evaluation, and implementation of the treatment plan need to be documented in the patient's medical record. Documentation of findings is important for several reasons. It provides information for others involved in the patient's care. Practitioners that will care for the patient after an initial assessment is done are better able to evaluate respiratory status and efficacy of care when previous findings are available to review. Documentation of findings provides a reference point for evaluation of treatment outcomes and alternative therapies if indicated.

After the assessment is documented in the medical record, the practitioner should document the communication of the treatment plan to the patient and the level of comprehension exhibited by the patient. Figure 6–17 is an example of a preprinted patient education and service treatment plan that guides the practitioner through the basic steps associated with teaching a respiratory patient about the medical prescription, tools of administration, use of peak flowmeters, medication and symptom diaries, and treatment plan. Just as documenting assessment findings helps

(text continues on page 167)

Box • 6–5 EVALUATING KNOWLEDGE DEFICIT

Language skills
  Is English the patient's first language?
  What language is the patient most comfortable
    with?
Reading ability
  English
  Primary language
Barriers to learning
  Physical
  Hearing
  Vision
  Speech
  Dexterity
  Emotional
  Cognitive and memory
Patient preference of teaching strategy
  One-to-one
  Pamphlets
  Videos
  Demonstrations
  Groups and classes
Considerations
  Cultural
  Religious
  Financial
Reception to education?
Person responsible for dispensing medications
  Patient
  Spouse or family member
  Other
Patient knowledge of illness
  Diagnosis
  Causative factors
  Care plan
    Medication, dose, frequency, effect, side effects
    Treatments
  Prognosis
  Action plan
Patient expectations of care plan outcome

Box • 6–6 FIVE CATEGORIES OF RESPIRATORY DIAGNOSIS

1. Knowledge deficit
2. Impaired gas exchange
3. Ineffective airway clearance
4. Ineffective breathing pattern
5. High risk for aspiration

Table • 6–7   ASSESSMENTS COMMONLY MADE BY THE RESPIRATORY CARE PRACTITIONER

Objective Clinical Data (Examples)	Assessments (Cause of Objective Clinical Data)	Plan (Common Treatment Selections)
Vital Signs		
↑ breathing, ↑ blood pressure, ↑ pulse	Respiratory distress	Treat underlying cause
Airway		
Wheezing	Bronchospasm	Bronchodilator Tx
Inspiratory stridor	Laryngeal edema	Cool mist
Rhonchi	Secretions in large airways	Bronchial hygiene Tx
Crackles	Secretions in distal airways	Treat underlying cause—eg, CHF
Cough		
Strong cough	Good ability to mobilize secretions	None
Weak cough	Poor ability to mobilize secretions	Bronchial hygiene Tx
Secretions		
Amount: >30 mL/24 h	Excessive bronchial secretions	Bronchial hygiene Tx
White and translucent sputum	Normal sputum	None
Yellow/opaque sputum	Acute airway infection	Treat underlying cause
Green sputum	Old, retained secretions and infections	Bronchial hygiene Tx
Brown sputum	Old blood	Bronchial hygiene Tx
Red sputum	Fresh blood	Bronchial hygiene Tx
Frothy secretions	Pulmonary edema	Treat underlying cause—eg, CHF
Alveoli		
Bronchial breath sounds ⎤	⎡ Atelectasis ⎤	
Dull percussion note ⎥	Infiltrates ⎥	Hyperinflation Tx, oxygen Tx
Opacity on chest radiograph ⎥	Fibrosis ⎦	
Restrictive PFT values ⎦	⎣ Consolidation	No specific, effective respiratory care Tx
Depressed diaphragm on radiograph	Air trapping and hyperinflation	Treat underlying cause
Pleural Space		
Hyperresonant percussion note	Pneumothorax	Evacuate air*
Dull percussion note	Pleural effusion	Evacuate fluid*
Thorax		
Paradoxical movement of the chest wall	Flail chest	Mechanical ventilation*
Barrel chest	Air trapping (hyperinflation)	Treat underlying cause—eg, asthma
Posterior and lateral curvature of spine	Kyphoscoliosis	Bronchial hygiene Tx
Arterial Blood Gases—Ventilatory		
pH ↑, $PaCO_2$ ↓, HCO_3 ↓	Acute alveolar hyperventilation	Treat underlying cause
pH N, $PaCO_2$ ↓, HCO_3 ↓↓	Chronic alveolar hyperventilation	Generally none
pH ↓, $PaCO_2$ ↑, HCO_3 ↑	Acute ventilatory failure	Mechanical ventilation*
pH N, $PaCO_2$ ↑, HCO_3 ↑↑	Chronic ventilatory failure	Low-flow oxygen, bronchial hygiene
Sudden Ventilatory Changes on Chronic Ventilator Failure (CVF)		
pH ↑, $PaCO_2$ ↑, HCO_3 ↑↑, PaO_2 ↓	Acute alveolar hyperventilation on CVF	Treat underlying cause
pH ↓, $PaCO_2$ ↑↑, HCO_3 ↑, PaO_2 ↓	Acute ventilatory failure on CVF	Mechanical ventilation*
Metabolic		
pH ↑, $PaCO_2$ N or ↑, HCO_3 ↑, PaO_2 N	Metabolic alkalosis	Give potassium*—hypokalemia / Give chloride*—hypochloremia
pH ↓, $PaCO_2$ N or ↓, HCO_3 ↓, PaO_2 ↓	Metabolic acidosis	Give oxygen—lactic acidosis
pH ↓, $PaCO_2$ N or ↓, HCO_3 ↓, PaO_2 N	Metabolic acidosis	Give insulin*—ketoacidosis
pH ↓, $PaCO_2$ N or ↓, HCO_3 ↓, PaO_2 N	Metabolic acidosis	Renal therapy*
Indication for Mechanical Ventilation		
pH ↑, $PaCO_2$ ↓, HCO_3 ↓, PaO_2 ↓	Impending ventilatory failure ⎤	
pH ↓, $PaCO_2$ ↑, HCO_3 ↑, PaO_2 ↓	Ventilatory failure ⎥	Mechanical ventilation*
pH ↓, $PaCO_2$ ↑, HCO_3 ↑, PaO_2 ↓	Apnea ⎦	
Oxygenation Status		
PaO_2 <80 mmHg	Mild hypoxemia ⎤	
PaO_2 <60 mmHg	Moderate hypoxemia ⎥	Oxygen Tx and treat underlying cause
PaO_2 <40 mmHg	Severe hypoxemia ⎦	
Oxygen Transport Status		
↓PaO_2, anemia, ↓cardiac output	Inadequate oxygen transport	Oxygen Tx and treat underlying cause

*Physician ordered.
PFT, pulmonary function test; CHF, congestive heart failure.
Des Jardins T, Burton G. *Clinical Manifestations and Assessment of Respiratory Disease Workbook.* St. Louis, CV Mosby, 1996.

VA Department of Veterans Affairs	MEDICAL RECORD	SERVICE TREATMENT PLAN

PATIENT EDUCATION: MDI / HOLDING CHAMBER / PEAK FLOW

RECIPIENT CODES (RC):

P Patient
F Family Member
C Caregiver

LEARNING CODES (LC):

V Verbalizes adequate comprehension of content
D Demonstrates procedures safely
R Requires reinforcement of content/procedures
U Unable to learn*
N/R Not receptive to learning at this time*
U/E Unable to evaluate *
N/A Not applicable
*PN Document additional information on
Progress Notes

SIGNATURE	INITIALS

EDUCATIONAL CONTENT	DATE RC/LC/INIT.	DATE RC/LC/INIT.	DATE RC/LC/INIT.
Understanding of prescription Identify each medication and describe use / purpose Understand frequency and dose for each drug			
Use of Metered Dose Inhaler (MDI) Warm MDI to hand temperature Assemble apparatus Shake canister, hold upright, place inhaler 2 finger distance away from open mouth (aimed into mouth) or place inhaler between lips After normal exhalation, begin to slowly inspire while activating MDI Continue inspiration to fill lungs and hold breath for 10 seconds Wait one minute between puffs			
Use of MDI with holding chamber Warm MDI to hand or body temperature Assemble apparatus Shake canister vigorously and hold canister upright Place holding chamber in mouth or place mask over nose and mouth Breathe through mouth, normally and activate MDI at the beginning of inspiration, take two or three breaths through the holding chamber Wait one minute between puffs			
Signature of patient / family / caregiver **For patient health education this date**			

SIGNATURE / TITLE-PRACTITIONER	Date

Enter in space below - PATIENT IDENTIFICATION - *Treating Facility - Ward No.* Date

OP578 1189b
118 M52

**MEDICAL RECORD
SERVICE TREATMENT
PLAN**

VA Form
Apr 1989 **10-0043a**   027049

* U.S. GPO: 1989-241-638/05852

FIGURE 6–17 • Patient education and service treatment plan.

EDUCATIONAL CONTENT	DATE RC/LC/INIT.	DATE RC/LC/INIT.	DATE RC/LC/INIT.
Use of Peak Flow Meter Shake down indicator Take deep breath, seal mouthpiece between lips Blow out hard and fast Note value on indicator Repeat two more times Write highest value on diary trend sheet Perform twice a day			
MDI / Peak Flow / Medication Diary Record peak flow with accurate numbers Record medication use Record self assessment of wheezing, breathlessness, coughing and sputum color			
Aerosol Medication Treatment Plan Understand indications for each drug Discuss strategy for any changes in dose and current prescription			
Is patient able to reliably self-administer?			
Written Materials Received (circle) a. Post Discharge Self Medication Management Instructions b. How to use your Peak Flow Meter c. How to use your MDI / Peak Flow/Medication Diary d. Drug Information Sheets e. Conquering Asthma f. Guide to Better Breathing g. Specify _____			
Signature of patient / family / caregiver For patient health education this date			

FIGURE 6–17 • Continued.

other members of the team to determine changes in the patient's condition, documentation of patient education is key to letting the team know what has been taught and how the patient responded to the information.

SUMMARY

Steps in the management of abnormalities of respiratory function include identifying the acuteness of the situation; performing a clinical evaluation, including past medical history, history of present illness, and physical examination (with inspection and auscultation); clustering findings to assign a respiratory diagnosis; deciding on management strategies and interventions; and evaluating interventions to determine if treatment goals have been met.

Bibliography

Bates B, Bickley LS, Hoekelman RA. *A Guide to Physical Examination and History Taking*. 6th ed. Philadelphia: JB Lippincott; 1995.

Brewis RAL. *Lecture Notes on Respiratory Disease*. Oxford, UK: Blackwell Scientific; 1980.

Burton GC, Hodgkin JE. Ward JJ. *Respiratory Care: A Guide to Clinical Practice*. 4th ed. Philadelphia: JB Lippincott; 1996.

Des Jardins T. *Clinical Manifestations of Respiratory Disease*. Chicago: Year Book Medical Publishers; 1984.

George RB, Light RW, Matthay MA, Matthay RA. *Chest Medicine*. Baltimore: Williams & Wilkins; 1995.

Kelley, WN, ed. *Textbook of Internal Medicine*. 2nd ed. Philadelphia: JB Lippincott, 1992.

Porth CM. *Pathophysiology: Concept of Altered Health States*. 4th ed. Philadelphia: JB Lippincott; 1994.

Tobin MJ. *Essentials of Critical Care Medicine*. New York: Churchill Livingstone; 1989.

Turner-Warwick M, Hudson ME, Corrin B, Kerr IH. *Clinical Atlas Respiratory Diseases*. London: Gower Medical Publishing; 1989.

West JB. *Pulmonary Pathophysiology: The Essentials*. 5th ed. Baltimore: Williams & Wilkins; 1995.

Physical Properties of Gases and Fluids

Vijay Deshpande • James B. Fink

Key Terms

absolute pressure
absolute zero
combined gas law
compliance
conduction
convection
critical pressure
critical temperature
diffusion
elastance
equivalent weight
gauge pressure
heat of fusion
heat of vaporization
kinetic theory
radiation
Reynold's number
Van der Waals' forces

Objectives

- Contrast solids, liquids, and gases.

- Compare and contrast common system of weights and measures.

- Describe Dalton's law of partial pressures.

- Identify combined gas law, Boyle's law, Charles's law, and Gay-Lussac's law.

- Use Henry's law and Graham's law to describe diffusion and gas solubility.

- Discuss fluid dynamics.

- Contrast laminar and turbulent flow.

- Discuss the role of surface tension.

- Explain Hooke's law, Starling's law, and Poiseuille's law.

- Predict laminar or turbulent flow with Reynold's number.

- Describe the operation of jet mixing.

A knowledge of basic sciences is essential to understanding how the body works in health and disease, as well as the gases and devices used for the diagnosis and treatment of disease. This chapter reviews some of the key concepts in chemistry and physics applied in the practice of respiratory care.

THE ATOM AND THE MOLECULE

The *atom* is the smallest unit of matter for each of the elements, whereas the *molecule* is the smallest stable unit of any compound. Most atoms can combine with other atoms to produce compounds that are different from the individual atoms involved. Atomic and molecular reactions that create various compounds are the basis of chemistry. An atom of oxygen is less stable than a molecule of oxygen (O_2). When two atoms of hydrogen react with one atom of oxygen, the water (H_2O) molecule that results is more stable than the individual atoms composing it.

STATE OF MATTER

Matter exists in three states: solid, liquid, and gas. The state of any matter depends on the strength of intermolecular forces, also known as **Van der Waals' forces**. In solids, these forces are so strong that solids have fixed shapes and volumes. The molecular motion in solids is limited to vibrations around a fixed point (Fig. 7–1*A*). As the cohesive intermolecular forces decrease, the molecules are relatively mobile, as observed in liquids (see Fig. 7–1*B*). In gases, the intermolecular forces are so weak that gas molecules move freely at random (see Fig. 7–1*C*).

CHANGE OF STATE IN MATTER

Application of energy, such as heat energy, facilitates transformation of solids to liquids and to gases, as observed when ice melts to water and, on further heating, the water boils to form steam.

Figure 7–1 indicates molecular forces in solids, liquids, and gases. On application of heat energy, the molecular motion increases as a result of a decrease in intermolecular cohesive forces, and solids are converted into liquids and liquids into gases. The reverse occurs as a result of removing energy by cooling.

GAS PHYSICS
Movement of Gases

Whereas molecules in solids are relatively close together, gas molecules are widely separated and move at high velocities. According to the **kinetic theory**, the movement of gas molecules is random, with the molecules expanding unless they are confined in a container. Gas molecules in a container collide and bounce off one another and the walls of the container. The smaller the size of the container, the greater the number of collisions of gas molecules with each other and with the walls of the container.

Molecular Velocity and Temperature

To physicists, temperature is a measure of average velocity of molecules. Thus, when gas molecules are at a complete standstill, the temperature should be zero. In fact, this hy-

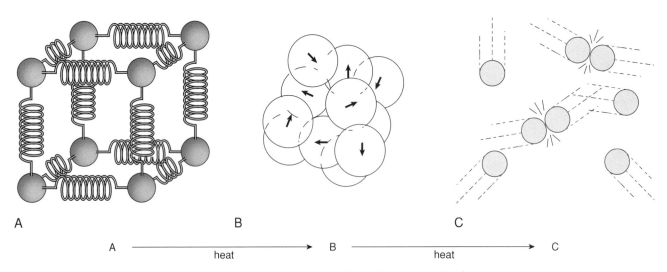

A   B   C

A ——————————→ B ——————————→ C
        heat   heat

FIGURE 7–1 • States of matter. (*A*) Molecules in solids have the highest intermolecular attraction and vibrate only around a fixed point. (*B*) On applying heat energy, the intermolecular cohesive forces are weakened, and the solid is converted into liquid, in which the molecules are relatively free and move over each other. (*C*) Further application of heat energy can reduce the intramolecular forces to a minimum, and the molecules move around in a random motion and collide with each other.

Matter changes its physical state as a result of application of energy such as heat. When ice (solid) is heated, it changes to water (liquid) and on further heating is converted in steam (gas).

Iodine is found in crystalline form at room temperature. On application of heat energy, it sublimes; that is, it is converted from a solid to a gaseous state without going through the normal anticipated transition of solid–liquid–gas. **Explain.**

Answer: The melting point and the boiling point of iodine are the same. This is a characteristic of the element iodine; thus, the solid molecules are transformed directly into the gaseous state. The intramolecular forces in iodine weaken so much on application of heat that the intermediate liquid phase is very unstable, and the molecules are converted into the gaseous state.

Kelvin ($°K = °C + 273$) 0°	−223°	273°	373°
Celsius [$°C = (°F − 32) × 5/9$] −273°	−40°	0°	100°
Fahrenheit −40° ($°F = 9/5 °C + 32$)		32°	212°

FIGURE 7−2 • Reference points used to compare temperature scales.

pothetical temperature is termed **absolute zero** degrees on the Kelvin, or absolute, scale. On applying heat energy to gases, the increase in kinetic energy promotes increased velocity. Conversely, cooling removes energy from the molecules and slows their random motion. Thus, at increased temperatures, molecular velocities are higher than at low temperatures.

Temperature Measurement (Scales)

In practice, molecular velocity is indirectly determined by measuring temperature. Temperature scales are designed to facilitate predicting behavior of molecules at various velocities. For practical purposes, however, two scales of temperature measurement were devised: the Celsius and the Fahrenheit scales. To construct temperature scales, two reference points were essential for calibration. Because water is the most abundant liquid on earth, the freezing point of water to ice and the boiling point of water to steam were selected as the two reference points used to calibrate thermometers (Fig. 7–2).

Temperature scales that are commonly used in medicine are the Celsius (centigrade), Kelvin (absolute), and the Fahrenheit scales. The Celsius scale, the most commonly used scale in medicine, assigns the freezing point of water as 0°C and the boiling point of water as 100°C, with 100 equal intervals between these two points. Normal body temperature is 37°C.

The Kelvin scale is most commonly used to study changes in behavior of gases resulting from changes in gas

velocities (temperature). The Kelvin scale uses the same size degree as the Celsius scale but assigns the zero point at absolute zero (0°K), which is −273°C. Water freezes at 273°K and boils at 373°K. To convert Celsius to Kelvin, simply add 273°.

The Fahrenheit temperature scale is based on the coldest temperature that can be achieved by mixing salt, ice, and water (0°F). The freezing point of water is 32°F, body temperature is 98.6°F, and the boiling point of water is 212°F.

The temperature difference between freezing and boiling water are 180°F and 100°C. Consequently, 1 °C is $^{180}/_{100}$ or $\%$ of 1°F, and 1°F is $\%$ of 1°C. Because the absolute zero points of these scales are different, conversions of scale require the following adjustments:

$$°C = 5/9(°F − 32)$$
$$°F = 9/5(°C + 32)$$
$$°K = °C + 273$$

You are in the emergency department evaluating a child in moderate respiratory distress. You note that her current temperature has been measured at 38.9°C. The child's mother states that she measured her child's temperature at home an hour ago and it was 103.0°F. Has the child's temperature increased, decreased, or remained the same since her mother measured it an hour ago?

Quantification of Heat

The *calorie* (cal) is the quantity of heat required to raise the temperature of 1 g of water 1°C. The "big" calorie, or *kilocalorie,* (kcal) is equivalent to 1000 calories and is used in stating the energy value of foods. The *calorimeter* is an instrument used to measure the heat released when a sample of food or fuel is burned.

The British thermal unit (BTU) is the amount of heat required to raise the temperature of 1 pound of water 1°F.

Latent Heat

The three states of matter differ in terms of molecular motion, with molecules being the most energetic in the gaseous state and less energetic in the solid state. The three states differ in terms of their energy content. Because heat is a manifestation of molecular kinetic energy, we can establish a relationship between states of mater and heat energy.

Heat is absorbed at the freezing point and liberated at the melting point, but the temperature of a substance does not change during the transition. The **heat of fusion** is a form of latent heat, defined as the amount of heat required to melt 1 g of a substance without changing its temperature.

The heat of fusion of ice is 80 cal/g. For each gram of ice that melts, 80 cal are taken from the environment. For each gram of water that freezes, 80 cal of heat are liberated. Latent **heat of vaporization** is the heat required to change a liquid into a vapor or gas. It is defined as the amount of heat needed to vaporize a mass of liquid without changing its temperature. The heat of vaporization for water is 540 cal/g. For each gram of water converted to water vapor, 540 cal are absorbed from the environment. This explains the cooling effect of evaporation.

Heat is transmitted in three ways: by conduction, convection, and radiation. **Conduction** is transmission of heat from molecule to molecule, as in solid metals. **Convection** is transmission of heat through a liquid or gas, in which the gas molecules expand and rise as they are heated, carrying the heat with it as it spreads. **Radiation** requires travel through space as electromagnetic waves at the speed of light and is the mechanism by which the sun heats the earth.

Critical Temperature and Pressure

To convert a gas into liquid and solid, the gas movement has to be decreased. This can be accomplished by cooling the gas molecules, which decreases the velocity of the gas molecules. Each gas has a characteristic temperature at which it can be converted into a liquid by applying pressure. Above this temperature, the gas cannot be liquefied regardless of how much pressure is applied.

Critical temperature is the *highest* temperature above which a gas cannot be liquefied by application of pressure

(Fig. 7–3). **Critical pressure** is the *lowest* pressure necessary at the critical temperature of a substance to maintain it in a liquid state. Table 7–1 lists the boiling points, critical temperatures, and critical pressures of some common liquids.

The commercial manufacture of oxygen is primarily accomplished through a three stage process known as *fractional distillation* of liquid air. Box 7–1 explains this process.

Molecular Collisions and Pressure

When gas molecules collide with each other or with the walls of their container, pressure develops. The greater the number of collisions, the higher the pressure. Factors responsible for increased frequency of collisions of gas molecules include the number of molecules, the velocity of gas molecules, and the size of the container. The greater the number of molecules in a container, the higher the pressure. If gas temperature is increased, the velocity of the molecules increases, the collision of molecules with each other and the walls of the container increases, and pressure increases. If the volume of the container is reduced, the pressure increases. Thus, the factors affecting pressure are the number of molecules, the temperature, and the volume of the container (Fig. 7–4).

Pressure is defined as force per unit surface area (P = F ÷ A). Atmospheric pressure is measured by a barometer, and a manometer measures the pressure of gas mixture. For fluids (liquids or gases), pressure is measured from the column height and the density of a fluid. This concept is the

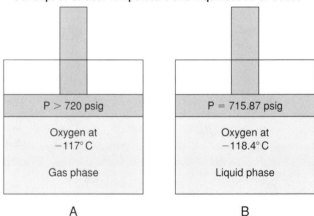

Concept of Critical Temperature and Liquification of Gases

FIGURE 7-3 • The critical temperature for oxygen is −118.4°C. Unless the gas is cooled to or below its critical temperature, the gas will not go into liquid form no matter how much pressure is applied. (A) When oxygen is cooled to −117°C, which is above the critical temperature, and a pressure of over 720 psi is applied, the oxygen molecules remain in a gaseous state. (B) On cooling the gas to its critical temperature, the gas can be liquefied by applying 715.87 psi of pressure.

Table • 7–1   PHYSICAL CHARACTERISTICS OF SOME LIQUIDS

Gas or Liquid	Boiling Point (°C)	Critical Temperature (°C)	Critical Pressure (psig)
Oxygen	−182.96	−118.4	715.87
Nitrogen	−195.80	−147.00	477.50
Helium	−268.90	−267.90	18.50
Carbon dioxide	−78.40	31.00	1057.40
Water	100	374.10	5484.50

Box • 7–1   FRACTIONAL DISTILLATION OF LIQUID AIR

1. PURIFICATION

Using a large compressor, room air is first compressed to 1500 psig. This increase in pressure results in a rise in temperature (according to Gay-Lussac's law) that is dissipated by use of a water-cooled heat exchanger. The air is then further compressed to 2000 psig, passed through an after-cooler, and delivered to a countercurrent heat exchanger at room temperature. By using waste nitrogen as a coolant, the air is cooled to −50°F. This process causes water vapor to freeze and be removed from the system.

2. LIQUEFACTION

In a second heat exchanger, gas is cooled to −40°F by the evaporation of liquid ammonia, eliminating any remaining water vapor. A third heat exchanger cools the air to −265°F, with the pressure remaining at 200 psig. At this point, no liquefaction has taken place because the critical pressure of air is 532 psig. For liquefaction to take place, the air is released into a separator and expanded to 90 psig. Releasing the pressure causes a further reduction in temperature and partial liquefaction.

3. DISTILLATION

In the separator, gas and liquid are pumped through separate streams into the distillation column. The liquid portion enters the top of the distillation column and passes over a series of cylindrical shells that contain metal trays. As the liquid passes down over the trays, vapor from the separator passes through them. The falling liquid becomes richer in oxygen (as nitrogen boils off), and the rising vapor becomes richer in nitrogen. At the bottom of the column, liquid oxygen forms but contains a few impurities. These include the gases argon and krypton. The oxygen is reboiled with precise control of temperature and pressure. These gases evaporate (their boiling points are lower), leaving 99.9% pure oxygen.

Branson R, et al. *Respiratory Therapy Equipment*. Philadelphia: JB Lippincott; 1995 and *Compressed Gas Association: Handbook of Compressed Gases*. 2nd ed. New York: CGA; 1990.

reason that mercury is preferred over water in a barometer. At normal atmospheric pressure, a water barometer rises to a height of over 33 feet, whereas a mercury barometer shows only a 760-mm column (76 cm or 30 inches) because its density is 13.6 times greater than that of water.

Pressure is expressed as gauge pressure or absolute pressure. **Gauge pressure** on a manometer reflects the pressure above or below atmospheric pressure. **Absolute pressure** is the sum of gauge pressure and atmospheric pressure. Conventionally, a pressure of 25 cm H_2O indicates that the pressure will increase a water column to a 25-cm height against atmospheric pressure. Various units of pressure are used and include atmospheres (atm), inches of mercury (in Hg), millimeters of mercury (mmHg), centimeters of water (cm H_2O), kilopascal (kPa), and pounds per square inch (psi). One torr (from Torricelli, the inventor of the mercury barometer) is equivalent to 1 mmHg.

The atmospheric pressure at sea level is relatively stable and provides a baseline pressure that facilitates conversion to other units. One atmosphere, expressed in various units, is equivalent to 760 mmHg, 760 torr, 29.9 in Hg, 1034 cm H_2O, 33.9 feet of fresh H_2O, 14.7 psi, 101.3 kPa, and 1.014×10^6 dynes/cm² (Table 7–2).

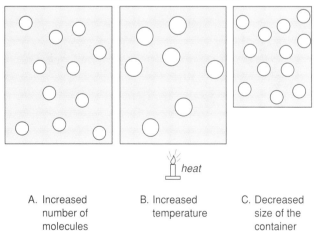

Pressure increases as a result of

heat

A. Increased number of molecules

B. Increased temperature

C. Decreased size of the container

FIGURE 7–4 • Factors responsible for changes in pressure in a container. (*A*) With a higher number of molecules, the molecules collide with each other and with the walls of the container. (*B*) At a higher temperature, the gas velocity increases, which increases the frequency of collisions and thus pressure. (*C*) If the size of the container is decreased, pressure increases.

Table • 7–2   PRESSURE UNITS

1 atmosphere	= 760 mmHg (torr)
	= 1034 cm H_2O
	= 14.7 psi
	= 1.014×10^6 dynes/cm^2
	= 101.3 kPa
1 mmHg	= 1.36 cm H_2O
1 psi	= 51.7 mmHg (torr)
	= 70.34 cm H_2O
1 cm H_2O	= 0.74 mmHg (torr)
1 kPa	= 7.5 mmHg (torr)

Volume

Because gases are invisible and are in constant random motion, quantifying their volumes and weights posed a problem to researchers. Chemists and physicists established a uniform quantitative unit called a *mole*. A mole, or gram molecular weight, corresponds to the molecular weight expressed in grams. One mole of oxygen weighs 32 g, and 1 mole of CO_2 weighs 44 g.

Avogadro's Law

According to Avogadro's law, 1 mole of a gas contains 6.02×10^{23} molecules, and equal volumes of all gases, at the same temperature and pressure, will occupy the same number of moles. Further investigation by Avogadro revealed that 1 mole of a dry gas at STPD (standard temperature and pressure, dry) (0°C and 1 atm pressure, with no water vapor present [dry]) occupies a volume of 22.4 L. Thus, 1 mole of a gas has a mass equal to its molecular weight and the corresponding volume of 22.4 L. The density of any gas can be calculated by dividing its molecular weight by 22.4. Gases with lower molecular weights have

CRITICAL THINKING CHALLENGES

Go Figure

A patient on a mechanical ventilator has a peak airway pressure of 38 cm H_2O. What would that be in mmHg?

A patient is being transferred to your hospital from Germany. The referring physician has called with a pretransport report that includes arterial blood gas measurements for the partial pressures of oxygen (PaO$_2$) and carbon dioxide (PaCO$_2$). The values are reported as follows:

PaO$_2$ 11.5 kPa
PaCO$_2$ 5.2 kPa

What are these values in mmHg?

lower densities. In respiratory care, the density of inspired air can be reduced by employing a helium–oxygen gas mixture (Table 7–3).

Gas Laws

Gas laws predict physical behavior of gases at different temperatures, pressures, volumes, and masses. These laws ignore intermolecular forces and molecular volumes for convenience. Such a condition is represented by ideal gases.

Boyle's Law

At constant temperature, pressure times volume equals constant:

$$P \times V = K$$

At constant temperature and mass, the volume and pressure of a gas are inversely proportional. Thus, an increase in pressure exerted on a volume of gas decreases the volume proportionately. A volume of 800 mL of gas at 1 atmospheric pressure decreases to 400 mL on doubling the pressure, and vice versa.

The most common physiologic application of Boyle's law is observed in normal breathing. Figure 7–5 illustrates the sequence of inspiration and expiration based on Boyle's law. During inspiration, the diaphragm is contracted to increase the intrathoracic volume. Because the temperature is constant at 37°C, according to Boyle's law, the intrathoracic pressure decreases, decreasing the pressure in the lungs and causing gas flow from the atmosphere to the lungs. During expiration, the sequence reverses, and a higher pressure is developed inside the lungs, allowing for exhalation.

Calculation of compressible volumes in the ventilator circuit and measurements of thoracic gas volumes using a body plethysmograph require the use of Boyle's law.

Charles's Law

At constant pressure, volume divided by temperature equals constant:

$$V \div T = K$$

Charles's law describes the relationship between gas volume and temperature. Under the conditions of a constant pressure and mass, gas volume and temperature are directly proportional. In other words, as the temperature is increased, the gas volume increases. The reverse is also true. As gas temperature is decreased, there is a decrease in original volume. This increase or decrease in volume is proportional to $\frac{1}{273}$ of the original volume per degree change in temperature. Thus, theoretically, if the gas is cooled to −273°C or 0°K (absolute zero), the volume decreases to zero. Figure 7–6 demonstrates the effect of increased temperature on gas volume.

Table • 7–3 DENSITIES OF GASES AND GAS MIXTURES

Gas	Molecular Weight	Density (molecular weight ÷ 22.4)
Oxygen	32	1.43 g/L
Nitrogen	28	1.25 g/L
Room air	29	1.29 g/L
Helium	4	0.18 g/L
Helium–oxygen mixture (80% : 20%)*	9.6	0.43 g/L
Helium–oxygen mixture (70% : 30%)	12.4	0.55 g/L

*The 80% helium and 20% oxygen mixture has one third the density of oxygen. This mixture is generally used to treat severely obstructed airways in children with asthma.

The most common example of Charles's law involves collecting expired gas at room temperature. If 1000 mL of air is inspired at room temperature (25°C), the volume of the inspired air expands at body temperature (37°C) to 1040 mL.

Gay-Lussac's Law

At constant volume, pressure divided by temperature equals constant:

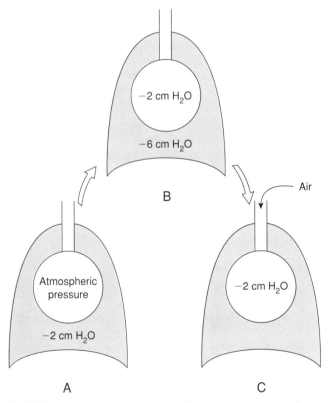

FIGURE 7–5 • Application of Boyle's law in normal mechanics of breathing. (*A*) Normal status of lungs and thorax. (*B*) As the diaphragm descends during inspiration, the intrathoracic volume increases, decreasing the pressure to −6 cm H_2O. (*C*) The negative intrathoracic pressure is transmitted to the lungs, the pressure decreases below atmospheric pressure, and air moves in.

$$P \div T = K$$

According to Gay-Lussac's law, at constant volume and mass, the gas pressure and temperature are in direct proportion. An increase in temperature at constant volume results in increased pressure.

In respiratory care, compressed gas cylinders are commonly used to deliver therapeutic gases. These metal cylinders have a fixed volume. If the temperature of these cylinders is increased, the pressure inside the cylinder increases, presenting the potential danger of explosion. Therefore, most compressed gas cylinder manifold systems are incorporated with a safety feature (frangible disk) that ruptures open at a preset pressure, avoiding explosion (Fig. 7–7).

During transfilling of cylinders, the cylinder receiving gas becomes warm, whereas the cylinder from which the gas is being removed feels cool (Fig. 7–8). This is an example of Gay-Lussac's law. On opening a cylinder valve to deliver gas, the manifold system is cooled because of a decrease in gas pressure to atmospheric pressure. Consequently, the temperature in the system decreases proportionately.

Combined Gas Law

Pressure times volume divided by temperature equals constant:

$$(P \times V) \div T = K$$

By combining the three gas laws given previously, a predictable relationship among pressure, volume, and temperature can be obtained. This is generally known as the **combined gas law**. Knowing that the original conditions of P_1, V_1, and T_1 are equal to the final conditions of P_2, V_2, and T_2, variations in original conditions lead to predictable changes in respective parameters.

$$(P_1 \times V_1) \div T_1 = (P_2 \times V_2) \div T_2$$

Dalton's Law of Partial Pressures

Dalton's law of partial pressures states that the total pressure exerted by a gas mixture is equal to the sum of partial

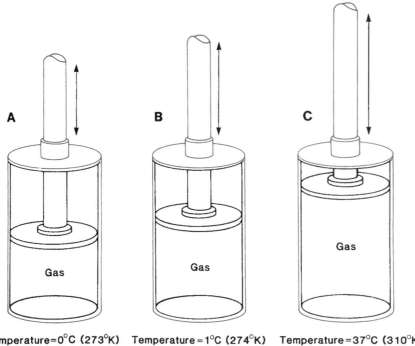

FIGURE 7-6 • Explanation of Charles's law. Constant pressure is applied. The piston is moveable, as indicated by its position at three different volumes. (*A*) Conditions of 0°C and a volume of 273 mL at a set pressure. (*B*) The effect of increasing the temperature by 1°C at the same pressure. (*C*) Increase in volume when the temperature is raised to 37°C. Note that at the constant applied pressure, the volume increases as the temperature is increased.

Temperature=0°C (273°K)   Temperature=1°C (274°K)   Temperature=37°C (310°K)

Volume=273 mL   Volume=274 mL   Volume=310 mL

pressures of each constituent gas. Moreover, the partial pressure exerted by each gas is proportional to the concentration of that gas in the mixture. The most common application of Dalton's law is found in the partial pressures of each constituent gas of the atmosphere.

Figure 7–9 illustrates Dalton's law as it applies to the pulmonary system when breathing room air at sea level and at high altitude.

The atmosphere consists of 20.9% oxygen, 79% nitrogen, and 0.1% trace gases. At sea level, the atmospheric pressure is 760 mmHg. Thus, the partial pressure exerted by oxygen and nitrogen are $760 \times 0.209 = 159$ mmHg and $760 \times 079 = 600$ mmHg, respectively. At high altitudes, the atmospheric pressure decreases, resulting in lower partial pressures of oxygen and nitrogen. Conversely, in hyperbaric conditions, the partial pressure of oxygen is increased.

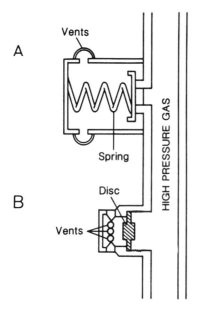

FIGURE 7-7 • Application of Gay-Lussac's law. When the contents (gas) in a cylinder are heated, the gas volume remains the same (fixed), and the pressure rises proportionately. The safety device, the frangible disk, ruptures at specific pressure and releases excess pressure to atmosphere.

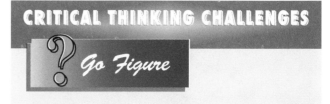

CRITICAL THINKING CHALLENGES

Go Figure

A frangible disk safety system that is incorporated into a cylinder valve is set to rupture at a pressure of 3300 psig. The current temperature is 22°C and the cylinder pressure is 2200 psig. At what temperature (°C) will the pressure in the cylinder equal the rupturing pressure of the frangible disk? Remember, gas law problems require temperature to be expressed in Kelvin (K = °C + 273).

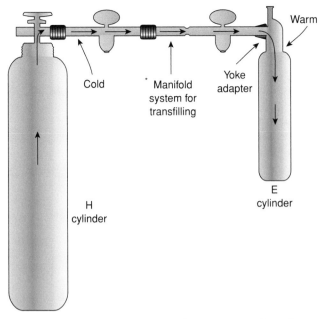

FIGURE 7–8 • Application of Gay-Lussac's law during transfilling of cylinders. As the gas leaves the large cylinder through the manifold system, the pressure drops from cylinder pressure to atmospheric pressure, causing the temperature to drop. The receiving cylinder pressure rises as gas is filled into the cylinder; consequently, the temperature rises. In both cases, the volume of the respective cylinders is constant.

Movement of Gas Molecules

Diffusion

Diffusion is the passive movement of gas molecules from a region of high concentration to a region of low concentration. An increased concentration of gas increases its partial pressure, which increases diffusion.

Fick's Law

Fick's law describes factors influencing diffusion of gases across a tissue membrane. For a gas diffusing across a tissue membrane, the following equation identifies all influencing factors and their relationships to other factors:

$$\text{Volume of gas diffused} \propto (\text{surface area} \times \text{pressure gradient} \times \text{diffusion constant}) \div \text{thickness}$$

As can be seen, the surface area, pressure gradient across the membrane, and thickness of the membrane are important considerations in determining the rate of diffusion. In many pulmonary diseases, the patient becomes hypoxemic owing to a decrease in the total surface area (eg, pulmonary emphysema) or an increase in the thickness of the diffusing membrane (eg, interstitial edema, pulmonary fibrosis). The diffusion constant is dependent on Henry's law of solubility and Graham's law of diffusion.

Figure 7–10 illustrates the effects of changes in surface area and thickness on the diffusion of oxygen.

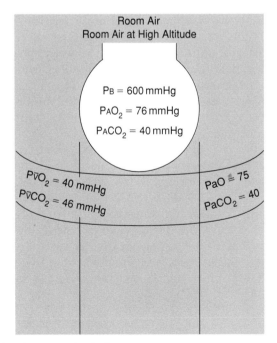

FIGURE 7–9 • Dalton's law of partial pressures as applied to alveolar air. At high altitudes, although the inspired concentration of oxygen is still 21%, the barometric pressure is decreased. As a result, the partial pressure of inspired oxygen is less than normal, leading to inadequate oxygenation of the blood in the pulmonary veins and promoting hypoxemia.

CRITICAL THINKING CHALLENGES

Go Figure

Many patients receiving long-term oxygen therapy use small oxygen gas cylinders. The home care agency periodically replaces empty cylinders with full cylinders. The empty cylinders are filled with oxygen from a large cylinder bank. During transfilling of cylinders, the small cylinder warms up, whereas the large cylinder feels cold. The manifold system becomes very cold. **Explain.**

Henry's Law of Solubility

According to Henry's law, the amount of a gas that dissolves in a liquid is proportional to the partial pressure of the gas and its solubility coefficient. The *solubility coefficient* is the amount of gas that dissolves in 1-mL of a liquid and is inversely proportional to the temperature. The solubility coefficient of oxygen in 1 mL of plasma at 37°C and 760 mmHg pressure is 0.023 mL; for carbon dioxide, 1 mL of plasma can accommodate 0.510 mL of CO_2 in dissolved form.

Graham's Law of Diffusion

Graham's law states that the diffusion of gases through a liquid is inversely proportional to the square root of the molecular weight of the gas. Thus, lighter gas molecules have higher diffusion rates than do heavier gas molecules. When gas diffusion involves liquid medium, both Henry's law and Graham's law are applicable. A classic example of application of these two laws involves diffusion of CO_2 and O_2 across the alveolar-capillary membrane. The oxygen molecules diffuse out of alveoli into pulmonary venous blood; simultaneously, the CO_2 molecules diffuse from the pulmonary venous blood into the alveoli for exhalation. Based on Henry's law and Graham's law, the diffusibility of CO_2 across the alveolar-capillary membrane is $0.510 \div \sqrt{44}$, and that for oxygen is $0.023 \div \sqrt{32}$. It is obvious that CO_2 diffuses 19 times faster than does O_2. Therefore, in pulmonary diseases, an increase in membrane thickness does not affect diffusion of CO_2 as much as it does diffusion of O_2 until the disorder becomes significant.

Elastance and Compliance

Elastance is the ability of a distorted or stretched object to return to its original shape. Elastance is expressed as change in pressure per unit change in volume ($E = \Delta P \div$ ΔV), often in cm H_2O/mL. **Compliance** is the ease with which an object can be distorted and is expressed as a change in volume per unit change in pressure ($C = \Delta V \div$ ΔP), often in mL/cm H_2O. Compliance is the inverse of elastance. $C = 1 \div E$.

The greater the tendency of an object to return to its original shape (high elastance), the more force that is required to distort it (low compliance). The easier it is to distort an object (high compliance), the less tendency the object has to return to its original form (low elastance).

Hooke's law states that an elastic body stretches equal units of length or volume for each unit of weight or force applied to it up to the point that the elastic limit of the system is reached. The *elastic limit* is that point at which each additional unit of weight or force results in smaller changes in length or volume.

Figure 7–11 illustrates the effect of stretching of the elastic fibers in the lung during normal breathing.

In pulmonary physiology, elastance is reflected by the recoiling force of the lungs. Lung compliance is a major factor considered in many pulmonary disorders. A decreased lung compliance is associated with a stiffer lung and requires the generation of greater negative pressure in the intrathoracic space to receive adequate spontaneous tidal volume. This promotes increased work of breathing. Disorders leading to stiff lungs are also associated with increased recoiling force. On the other hand, patients with emphysema have compliant lungs that can be inflated easily, yet these patients experience difficulty in exhaling all the air owing to decreased recoiling force. These patients require longer expiratory time and prefer to exhale with their lips pursed.

Surface Tension

Surface tension is the force that exists at the interface between either a gas and liquid or two liquids. Surface tension results from the intramolecular forces of like molecules being attracted to each other. It causes the molecules of a substance to move away from the interface to occupy the smallest volume possible. Surface tension is commonly expressed in dynes per centimeter.

La Place's law defines the relationship among the surface tension, pressure, and radii of bubbles and spheres: $P = 2ST \div r$.

The pressure inside a sphere or cylinder due to surface tension is greater the smaller the sphere. When two spheres are attached, the smaller sphere tends to empty into the larger sphere until the smaller sphere collapses. This happens with balloons and can happen in the lungs unless a naturally occurring surface active agent, called *pulmonary surfactant,* is present. Pulmonary surfactant coats the alveoli, altering surface tension in such a way as to prevent collapse at small volumes.

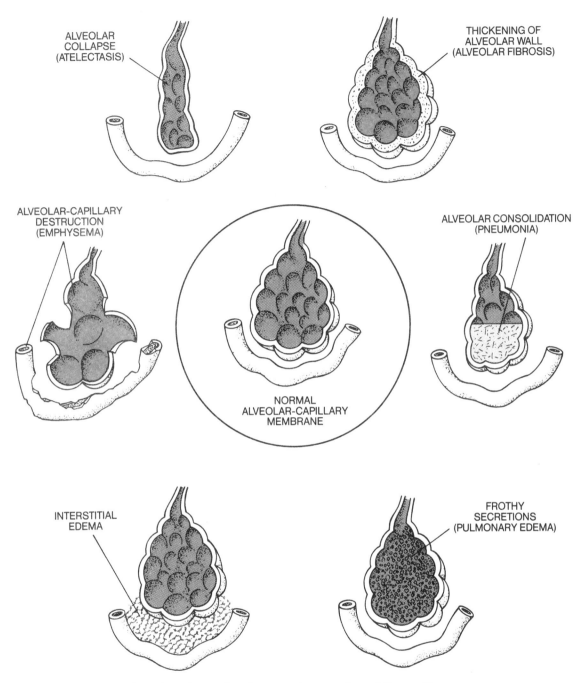

FIGURE 7–10 • Clinical conditions that decrease the rate of gas diffusion. These conditions are known as *diffusion-limited problems.* (DesJardins T. *Cardiopulmonary Anatomy and Physiology.* 3rd ed. Albany: Delmar Publishers; 1997.)

As a structure increases or decreases in volume, it must pass its critical volume, below which the effects of surface tension are so great that the structure collapses. The force required to expand a bubble increases as the volume approaches the critical volume and decreases once the system's volume exceeds the critical volume.

Figure 7–12 illustrates situations in which the surface tensions of different alveoli are the same, with smaller alveoli emptying into larger alveoli as a result of a higher pressure in the smaller alveoli.

Gas Flow Dynamics

When dealing with gases, we generally consider bulk flow that results from a pressure gradient. The higher the pressure gradient, the greater the flow of gas. Velocity and flow

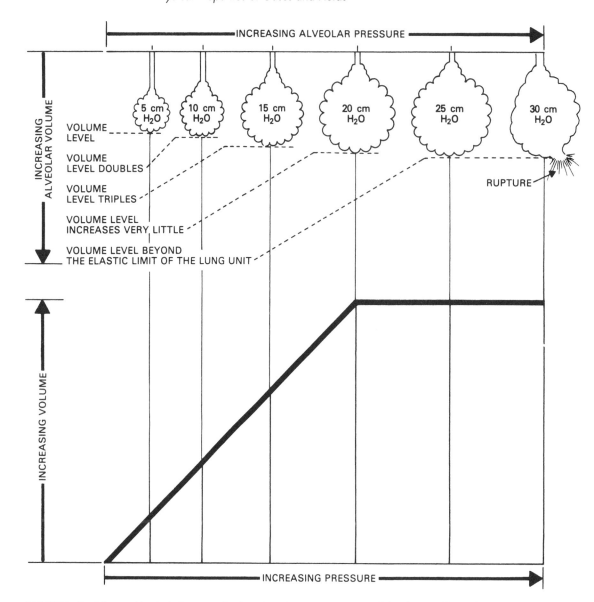

FIGURE 7–11 • Hooke's law applied to the elastic properties of the lungs. Over the normal physiologic range of the lungs, volume changes vary directly with pressure changes. Once the elastic limit is reached, however, little or no volume change occurs in response to pressure changes. (DesJardins T. *Cardiopulmonary Anatomy and Physiology.* 3rd ed. Albany: Delmar Publishers; 1997.)

are different in their units. *Velocity* is a measure of distance covered in a unit of time (velocity equals distance divided by time), whereas *flow* refers to volume moved per unit time (flow equals volume divided by time).

Gas flow = volume ÷ time
     = area × (distance ÷ time)
     = cross-sectional area × (distance ÷ time)
     = cross-sectional area × velocity

Law of Continuity

The product of gas flow and cross-sectional area is the same at all points in a closed system. This continuity may

be observed in inspired air moving into the lungs and in blood flow moving through pulmonary capillaries. During inspiration, the air moves through the trachea with the least cross-sectional area and the highest gas velocity. As the air moves from trachea to mainstem bronchi, segmental bronchi, bronchioles, and finally alveoli, the cross-sectional area increases after each dichotomy, eventually expanding to 70 m² at the alveolar level. All this time, the gas velocity proportionately decreases and finally reaches a minimal level. Similar activity occurs in the pulmonary capillaries. The right ventricle pumps blood through the large pulmonary artery, which gives rise to bifurcations, eventually reaching the level of the pulmonary capillaries. By this time, the cross-sectional area has expanded to a

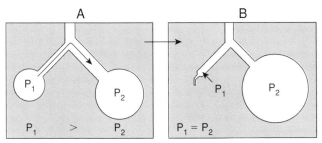

FIGURE 7-12 • Laplace's law. Effect of surface tension in the pulmonary system. If the surface tensions of different-diameter alveoli are the same, smaller alveoli empty into larger alveoli (A) and eventually collapse (B). (Berne RM, Levy MN. *Principles of Physiology.* 1st ed. St. Louis: Mosby; 1990.)

maximum, and the blood flow is at its minimal velocity. The conditions around the alveolar capillary membrane are optimal for gas diffusion between the slow gas velocity in the alveoli and the slowly moving capillary blood (Fig. 7–13).

Laminar Flow

Flow is laminar when it proceeds in a smooth, streamlined manner with few directional changes. This type of flow ex-

ALVEOLAR–CAPILLARY MEMBRANE

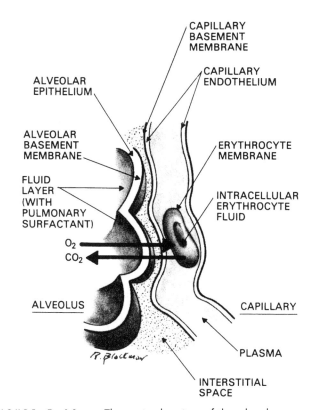

FIGURE 7-13 • The major barriers of the alveolar-capillary membrane through which a gas molecule must diffuse. (DesJardins T. *Cardiopulmonary Anatomy and Physiology.* 3rd ed. Albany: Delmar Publishers; 1997.)

ists in concentric cylindrical layers. As the molecules move along the wall of a rigid tube, the frictional resistance within the wall decreases the forward motion of the molecules closest to the wall. Thus, the layer closest to the wall is almost stationary. The next layer experiences less frictional resistance and thus advances further. The forward velocity of each layer increases from the wall of the tube to the center of the tube. The overall velocity pattern resembles a parabola. The molecules at the center of the tube advance at a greater velocity than those at the sides of the tube (Fig. 7–14).

Laminar flow implies movement of smoothly sliding layers, or lamina, in one direction and parallel to each other. During this type of flow, molecular friction develops between adjacent layers. Slower-moving molecular layers reduce the overall velocity of the faster-moving layers. This phenomenon is called *viscosity.* Laminar flow is observed in tube systems that are rigid, smooth, and unobstructed. The diameter of these tubes is relatively uniform. The pressure gradient required to produce and maintain laminar flow is proportional to the flow and the resistance (Ohm's law). If resistance increases, flow decreases. If the pressure gradient increases, flow increases.

$$\text{Resistance} = \text{pressure gradient} \div \text{flow}$$

Various factors influence flow characteristics and resistance. The relationship of these factors during laminar flow in a rigid cylindrical tube is expressed by Poiseuille's law. Poiseuille's law states that the resistance of flow varies directly with the length of the tube and inversely with the radius of the tube. Radius, however, is quantitatively more important because resistance varies with the fourth power of the radius.

$$\text{Flow} = (\pi \times r^4 \times \Delta P) \div (8 \times n \times l)$$
$$\text{Thus, resistance (R)} = \Delta P \div \text{flow}$$
$$= (8 \times n \times l) \div \pi \times r^4,$$

where r is the radius of the tube, ΔP is the pressure gradient, n is the viscosity, and l is the length of the tubing.

The viscosity of the gas also affects resistance during laminar flow. In clinical practice, however, changes in viscosity are insignificant because the composition of the gas is not changed. Thus, the primary factor that determines airway resistance during laminar flow is the radius of the airways. The radius of the airways remains relatively unchanged unless some form of obstruction, such as increased sputum, tumor, bronchospasm, or foreign body, occurs.

A common clinical example is an asthmatic patient in acute bronchospasm. In this case, the radius of the airway is significantly decreased, increasing the airway resistance. In the case of a spontaneously breathing patient, this increase in resistance increases the work of breathing. During mechanical ventilation, the increase in airway resistance increases the pressure required by the ventilator to deliver the tidal volume.

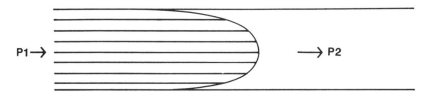

A. Laminar Flow in a smooth rigid tube resulting from a pressure gradient of P1–P2

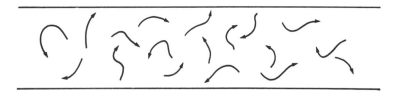

B. Turbulent flow

FIGURE 7–14 • (A) Laminar flow through a rigid tube. Note the advancement of the fluid molecules in a parabolic pattern. (B) In turbulent flow, the molecules move in any direction. The pressure required to maintain laminar flow is lower than that required to maintain turbulent flow of the same magnitude.

In respiratory physiology, the length of the airway is relatively constant. With respiratory equipment applications, it is important to recognize that the length of the conducting tube may not remain constant. If the length of the tube is increased, resistance increases, and flow decreases, unless the pressure gradient is increased. The opposite effect occurs if the length of the tube decreases.

Turbulent Flow

Turbulent flow is characterized by disorderly flowing vortices known as *eddy currents.* The flow moves at a uniform velocity. Molecular movement is more random and rapid. The change from laminar flow to turbulent flow is prompted by an increase in velocity, an increase in gas density, an increase in diameter of the tube, or a decrease in the viscosity of the gas. This relationship is known as **Reynold's number**. A Reynold's number of less than 2000 predicts laminar flow, whereas a number exceeding 2000 predicts turbulent flow.

Reynold's number = (diameter × velocity × density)
÷ viscosity

The driving pressure required to produce turbulent flow varies directly with resistance and the square of flow. Thus, more pressure is required to maintain turbulent flow than to maintain laminar flow. For turbulent flow, resistance is determined by the length of the tube, radius of the tube, and density of the gas.

Turbulent flow is affected by gas density (not viscosity), whereas laminar flow is affected by gas viscosity (but not density). Turbulent flow is sometimes said to be *density dependent*, whereas laminar flow is *density independent*. In the tracheobronchial tree, a laminar flow normally exists in

airways less than 2 mm in diameter. Turbulent flow is observed in the upper respiratory tract and large central airways. Overall tracheobronchial flow is a combination of laminar and turbulent flow.

CRITICAL THINKING CHALLENGES
Case Scenario

In situations in which severe obstruction of the airway exists, such as in acute asthma or the compression of a large airway by a tumor, the likelihood that turbulent flow exists is high. As can be seen by the following equations, the pressure gradient necessary to move a given flow through a tube is much higher when turbulent flow is present. The greater the pressure change necessary, the greater the resulting work of breathing.

Laminar flow: $\Delta P = \dfrac{n\,8\,l\,V}{\pi r^4}$

Turbulent flow: $\Delta P = \dfrac{f\,l\,V^2}{4\pi r^5}$

where n = viscosity, l = length, V = flow, r = radius, and f = friction factor

Looking again at the Reynold's number equation, RN = (diameter × velocity × density) ÷ viscosity, it can be seen that a decrease in the density of the gas may result in a decrease in Reynold's number. A reduction in Reynold's number will reduce the likelihood of turbulent flow and reduce the pressure gradient necessary for gas flow.

In clinical practice, this is done by substituting helium for nitrogen in the inspired air. Helium has a density of 0.18 g/L, and nitrogen has a density of 1.25 g/L.

Acceleration of Flow

An increased pressure gradient enhances gas flow from a higher pressure to a lower pressure. Thus, driving pressure can be increased to accelerate gas flow. Acceleration of gas flow can also be achieved by employing Bernoulli's and Venturi's principles as well as the jet-mixing principle based on viscous shearing forces.

Bernoulli's Principle

Bernoulli's principle states that the sum of the pressure and the kinetic energy has the same value at all points along a streamline. The sum of pressure energy and velocity energy at any given point is the same as that at any other point along the fluid flow in a tube. If a tube is tapered, the fluid velocity is increased, with a resultant decrease in pressure distal to the constriction. As a result of tapering or constriction to gas flow, velocity increases. To conserve the total fluid energy, this acceleration in velocity energy is balanced by a decrease in pressure energy. If the driving pressure is kept constant, the smaller the orifice size of the tubing constriction, the higher the velocity of the fluid and the greater the pressure drop past the orifice (Fig. 7–15).

A physiologic application of Bernoulli's principle is observed in advanced arteriosclerosis. The accumulation of plaque in the inner walls of the coronary artery constricts flow to the heart muscle, whereas the driving pressure is increased, resulting in an increased contraction of the heart. If the delivered velocity is sufficiently high, the lateral wall pressure decreases, collapsing the artery, owing to higher external pressure. The flow is momentarily interrupted, and Bernoulli's effect is eliminated. The blood vessel then reopens owing to arterial pressure. As blood flows through the constricted artery, the internal pressure decreases, and the artery closes again. This periodic closure and opening of the blood vessel is known as *vascular flutter*. In respiratory care devices, gases often flow through a restriction or orifice, resulting in an increase in the velocity of the gas and a corresponding decrease in its pressure.

Venturi's Principle

If flow occurs through constricted tubing, the pressure drop distal to the constriction can be used to entrain a second fluid to mix with the main flow. Venturi's principle states that the pressure drop distal to the constriction can be restored to the driving pressure by funneling immediately distal to the constriction at an angle of divergence of less than 15 degrees. Figure 7–16 depicts the constriction of a Venturi tube. The pressure drop across an obstruction is restored provided the angle of divergence is less than 15 degrees. Furthermore, the flow increases owing to entrainment of the second fluid.

Clinically, Venturi devices are used to increase gas flow. Because a second gas can be entrained using Venturi's prin-

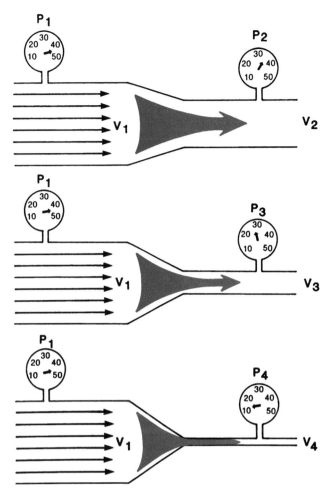

FIGURE 7–15 • As the orifice size of the constriction is decreased, the velocity of the fluid exiting the orifice increases, and a greater pressure drop results: $V_4 > V_3 > V_2 > V_1$ and $P_1 > P_2 > P_3 > P_4$.

ciple, the Venturi tube can be used to deliver a precise oxygen concentration to patients by mixing air with oxygen.

Constant-Pressure Jet Mixing

For many years, the Venturi mask, or air-entrainment mask, has been used to provide high-flow oxygen and air mixtures in a precise and predicable manner. This is a misnomer, however, because the principle of operation for this device is constant-pressure jet mixing. The mixing of air with the driving gas (usually oxygen) occurs at a constant ambient pressure. The entrainment of the ambient air results from viscous interaction between the driving gas flow and the stationary ambient air.

The theory of viscous shearing interaction can be compared with the theory describing laminar flow. A concentric cylindrical forward velocity parabolic pattern develops as a result of frictional resistance offered by the cylindrical wall of the tubing. In this case, the molecules closest to the wall

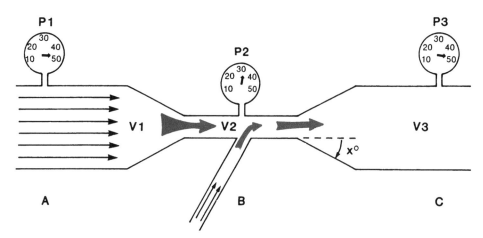

FIGURE 7–16 • Venturi's principle A, B, and C represent three sections of a tube in which section A has a higher cross-sectional area than section B. Gas flow through section A enters section B at a higher velocity, owing to constriction of the tubing. According to Bernoulli's principle, pressure decreases ($P_1 > P_2$). This pressure drop facilitates entrainment of a second fluid into the main flow. The original pressure, P_1, can be restored if the angle of divergence of the tubing (angle X) is less than 15 degrees.

have the slowest forward velocity, and the molecules in the center of the tube have the highest forward velocity. Each layer of molecules is decelerated by the frictional viscous resistance in proportion to the distance of the molecules from the wall. When this principle is applied to two fluids, one moving and the other stationary, the stationary fluid decelerates the moving fluid, whereas the moving fluid attempts to accelerate the stationary fluid. The net result is the development of a viscous shearing layer. Because fluids are

deformed relatively easily, the viscous shearing force promotes movement of layers of the stationary fluid into the path of the moving fluid. As shown in Figure 7–17, layers of ambient air are in a stationary condition outside the jet orifice before initiating any oxygen flow. Velocity refers to the forward, linear movement of the gas molecules per unit time, whereas flow indicates the volume of gas leaving the orifice or nozzle per unit time. On initiating the flow of oxygen, the velocity of the gas increases as it exits the con-

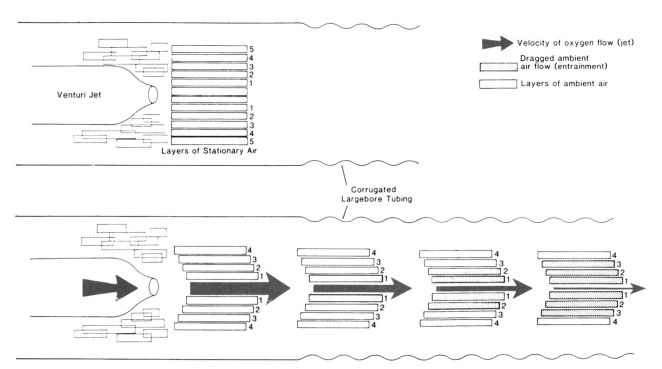

FIGURE 7–17 • Operation of a Venturi mask by jet-mixing principle. Numbers 1, 2, 3, 4, and 5 represent imaginary stationary layers of ambient air at the exit port of the Venturi jet. As the gas flow (oxygen in this case) is initiated, a high-velocity oxygen jet advances through the nozzle, attempting to accelerate adjacent air layers. The stationary layers of air attempt to decelerate the advancing oxygen jet. As the stationary layers of air are deformed, a "staircase" effect develops in the proximity of the main jet flow. Thus, layer 1 advances farther than layer 2 which, in turn, advances farther than layer 3, and so on. Subsequently, these layers are drawn into the main flow of gas produced by the jet, increasing the total flow, and the oxygen flow is diluted by incoming layers of air. The jet mixing is a function of the jet orifice size (jet velocity) and is independent of the jet flow.

stricted port. The high-velocity oxygen flow imparts some of its kinetic energy to the stationary ambient air, distorting adjacent layers of the air. As the forward velocity of oxygen is decelerated by the stationary layers of air, it accelerates the stationary layers, and viscous shearing results in a "staircase" effect on the adjacent layers of the ambient air. This gas dilution is the result of jet mixing due to viscous shearing force and not to the Venturi entrainment based on a pressure-drop phenomenon.

SOLUTIONS

A *solution* is a homogenous mixture of two substances, either two liquids or a liquid and a solid. The *solute* is the substance being dissolved (the solid or the liquid in smallest volume) in the solvent. In most physiologic solutions, water is the solvent. Solutes create an osmotic pressure, increase the boiling point, and reduce the melting point of the solvent. A dilute solution contains only a small amount of solute per volume of solvent. When a solution holds the maximum amount of solute at a given temperature, it becomes *saturated*. When a saturated solution with excess solute is heated to allow the excess solute to dissolve and is then cooled without being agitated, allowing the excess to stay in solution, the solution becomes *supersaturated*. When a supersaturated solution is physically agitated, the excess solute precipitates ("rains out") out of solution to the bottom of the container.

Solutions may be described in several ways, as follows:

- *Volume percent* (vol%) is the number of milliliters of solute per 100 mL of solution.
- *Gram percent* (g%) is the number of grams of solute per 100 mL of solution.
- *Ratio* is the simple ratio between the quantity of solute in grams to the volume of solute in milliliters.
- *Percent weight to volume* (% W/V) is the number of grams of solute per 100 mL of solution.

Equivalent Weights

Equivalent weight is the amount of a substance that will react completely with 1 mole of hydrogen ion (H+) or hydroxyl ion (OH−) or other monovalent substance. For acids, equivalent weights are calculated by diving the molecular weight of the acid by the number of H+ ions replaceable in a chemical reaction.

Equivalent weights are expressed in grams as the gram equivalent weight (GEW) or in milligrams as the milliequivalent weight (mEq). Equivalent weights are used to quantify the volume of acid or base administered to correct acid–base problems.

Osmosis

When two solutions of different concentrations are separated by a semipermeable membrane (a membrane that al-

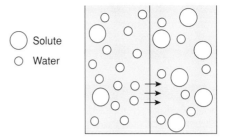

○ Solute
○ Water

FIGURE 7–18 • Osmosis.

lows water molecules to pass, but not solute), water shifts from the area of low concentration to an area of high concentration across the membrane until the concentration is equalized on both sides of the membrane (Fig. 7–18).

Osmotic pressures result from potential pressure differences between water and a solution. The osmotic pressure of a solution is directly related to the quantity of particles dissolved in the solution. To stop osmotic pressure, hydrostatic pressure may be applied. Both hydrostatic and osmotic pressure occur in all body fluids. Hydrostatic pressure is dependent on compartment fluid pressures (arterial, venous, and capillary blood pressures). Osmotic pressure may be caused by a variety of particles, many of which can pass through membranes, with the exception of proteins. Colloid osmotic pressure, or oncotic pressure, is osmotic pressure as a result of proteins.

Starling's Law of Fluid Filtration

Starling's law of fluid filtration describes the forces and factors affecting the movement of fluid across capillaries into the interstitium (Fig. 7–19):

$$\dot{Q} = k \left[(P_{cap} - P_{is}) - \Sigma (\pi_{cap} - \pi_{is}) \right],$$

where $\dot{Q}$ is net fluid movement across the capillary, k is the permeability coefficient of the capillary, P_{cap} is hydrostatic pressure within the capillary, P_{is} is the interstitial hydrostatic pressure, Σ is the coefficient of the membrane's ability to prevent the passage of protein, π_{cap} is the plasma colloid

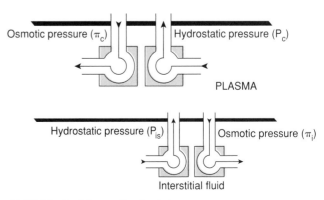

Osmotic pressure (π_c)   Hydrostatic pressure (P_c)

PLASMA

Hydrostatic pressure (P_{is})   Osmotic pressure (π_i)

Interstitial fluid

FIGURE 7–19 • Starling's law.

osmotic pressure within the capillary, and π_{is} is the interstitial colloid osmotic pressure.

Bibliography

Adriani J. *The Chemistry and Physics of Anesthesia.* 2nd ed. Springfield, IL: Charles C Thomas; 1992.

Brooks S. *Integrated Basic Sciences.* 4th ed. St. Louis: CV Mosby; 1979.

Ewen D. *Physics for Career Education.* Englewood Cliffs, NJ: Prentice-Hall; 1974.

Kimball WR. Fluid mechanics. In: Kacmarek RM, Hess D, Stoller JK, eds. *Monitoring in Respiratory Care.* St. Louis: Mosby-Year Book; 1993.

Nave C, Nave B. *Physics for the Health Sciences.* 3rd ed. Philadelphia: WB Saunders; 1985.

Scacci R. Air entrainment masks: Jet mixing is how they work. *Respir Care.* 1979;24:928–933.

Serway RA, Faughn JS. *College Physics.* Philadelphia: WB Saunders; 1985.

Wojciechowski W. *Respiratory Care Sciences - An Integrated Approach.* New York: John Wiley & Sons; 1985.

APPENDIX A

WEIGHTS AND MEASURES

LENGTH

1 micrometer (μm) = 0.000001 meter (m) = 0.001 millimeter (mm) = 0.0001 centimeter (cm)
1 mm = 0.001 m = 0.1 cm = 1,000 μm
1 cm = 0.01 m = 10 mm = 10,000 μm
1 M = 100 cm = 1000 mm = 1,000,000 μm
1 kilometer (km) = 1000 m

WEIGHT

1 microgram (μg) = 0.000001 gram (g) = 0.001 milligram (mg) = 0.0001 centigram (cg)
1 mg = 0.001 g = 0.1 cg = 1,000 μg
1 cg = 0.01 g = 10 mg = 10,000 μg
1 g = 100 cg = 1000 mg = 1,000,000 μg
1 kilogram (kg) = 1000 g = 1,000,000 cg = 1,000,000,000 μg

VOLUME

1 microliter (μL) = 0.000001 liter (L) = 0.001 milliliter (mL) = 0.0001 centiliter (cL)
1 mL = 0.001 L = 0.1 cL = 1000 μL
1 cL = 0.01 L = 10 mL = 10,000 μL
1 L = 100 cL = 1000 mL = 1,000,000 μL
1 kiloliter (kL) = 1000 L = 1,000,000 cL = 1,000,000,000 μL

METRIC–ENGLISH EQUIVALENTS

1 m = 39.37 inches (in)
1 yard = 3 feet (ft) = 36 in = 0.914 m
1 ft = 30.48 centimeters (cm) = 12 in = 0.3048 m
1 cm = 0.3937 in
1 in = 2.54 cm
1 kilometer (km) = 0.62 mile
1 mile = 1.61 km
1 kg = 2.204 pounds (lb)
1 lb = 453.6 g = 0.454 kg
1 ounce (oz) = 28.35 g
1 L = 1.057 liquid quarts (qt)
1 liquid qt = 0.956 L
1 dry qt = 1.01 L

STANDARD DEFINITIONS

	BTPS	ATPS	ATPD	STPS	STPD
Temperature	37°C	Room temp.	Room temp.	0°C	0°C
Pressure	Atmospheric	Atmospheric	Atmospheric	760 mmHg	760 mmHg
Humidity	Saturated	Saturated	Dry	Saturated	Dry

BTPS, body temperature and pressure, saturated; ATPS, ambient temperature and pressure, saturated; ATPD, ambient temperature and pressure, dry; STPS, standard temperature and pressure, saturated; STPD, standard temperature and pressure, dry.

8

Pharmacology Associated With Respiratory Care

Michael Mahlmeister

Key Terms

antimicrobial
bronchodilator
controller
corticosteroid
expectorant
heliox
leukotriene
methylxanthine
mucokinetic agent
parenteral administration
pharmacodynamics
pharmacokinetics
pharmacotherapeutics
polypharmacy
receptor theory
reliever
surfactant
sympathomimetic
systemic administration
therapeutic index

Objectives

- Define terms and principles associated with the study of pharmacology.

- Identify medications commonly administered by aerosol inhalation.

- Describe cardiopulmonary conditions for which aerosol medication administration might be indicated.

- Discuss strategies for optimizing delivery of aerosol medications to achieve expected outcomes.

- Discuss medicolegal considerations associated with drug administration.

- Identify resources available to health care providers to enhance their understanding of cardiopulmonary pharmacology.

This chapter reviews the clinical application of pulmonary pharmacology by respiratory care practitioners (RCPs) and others engaged in the administration of inhaled medications. The safe, effective administration of medications requires an understanding of the general principles of pharmacology. Appendix E provides the reader with general information on drug names, the FDA process, and generic resources for drug information. The reader is encouraged to pursue other resource texts for a more in-depth description of pharmacology principles, which is beyond the scope of this chapter.[1,2] Comprehensive texts are also available on the specific topic of respiratory pharmacology.[3,4] The reader must also integrate the information contained in this chapter with a basic knowledge of chemistry, physics, anatomy, physiology, mathematics, aerosol delivery systems, and clinical respiratory care. Practitioners should also be knowledgeable about published professional resources related to aerosol medication administration, such as the American Association for Respiratory Care (AARC) Aerosol Consensus Statement, AARC Clinical Practice Guidelines, and National Institutes of Health (NIH) Asthma Guidelines.[5–8]

The variety and number of medications administered directly to the lung by aerosol inhalation continues to grow yearly. This chapter discusses **bronchodilators,** which relax airway smooth muscle; **mucokinetic agents,** which facilitate clearance of bronchial secretions; **antimicrobials,** which treat pulmonary infections; and other medications that can be delivered by aerosol inhalation. The scope of this chapter incorporates not only the categorization and properties of cardiopulmonary medications commonly administered by aerosolization but also critical elements related to the clinical application of these medications. Protocols on appropriate administration techniques, titration of medication to clinical response, and issues surrounding the safe administration of aerosol medications are central to the focus of this chapter.

GENERAL CONCEPTS OF PHARMACOLOGY

The human body functions based on an intricate balance of thousands of biochemical interactions taking place simultaneously each second. The movement of our eyes as we read this page and the intellectual processes taking place to comprehend what is read all involve myriad biochemical activities. A *drug* is any substance introduced into the body that alters the biochemical actions of the body. Drugs may be taken for the purpose of treatment, diagnosis, or prevention of illness. *Pharmacology* is the study of how drugs act to change the body's normal biochemical processes. *Respiratory pharmacology* deals with the study of drugs administered via the respiratory system, usually by aerosolization, that have an impact on the pulmonary system. Most drugs delivered to the lungs by inhalation are administered specifically for the management of a pulmonary problem. Ongoing clinical research, however, is establishing the

efficacy and safety of a number of inhaled drug preparations for the treatment of systemic, nonpulmonary conditions. One can anticipate a growing number of nonrespiratory drugs developed for inhalation administration, further enhancing the valuable role of the professional RCP in aerosol medication administration.

The delivery of aerosolized medication to the lung is but one of many routes of drug administration. Pills, tablets, and syrups taken orally, intravenous (IV) or intramuscular (IM) injections (commonly referred to as **parenteral administration**), topical creams, nasal sprays, and skin patches represent some of the other ways to deliver medication to the body. Irrespective of the route of drug administration or of the form that the medication takes, several basic principles of drug actions apply. These are principles of **pharmacokinetics**, **pharmacodynamics**, and **pharmacotherapeutics**.

Pharmacokinetics incorporates four concepts related to drug administration: absorption, distribution, metabolism, and excretion. Various types of drug preparations, coupled with proper patient education, ensure that a particular drug is administered in a manner that optimizes absorption. An excellent illustration of the principle of absorption is seen in nicotine replacement therapy, used as part of a smoking cessation program. Individuals can receive nicotine replacement through the use of transdermal (skin) patches, chewing gum, or nasal sprays. All three preparations are formulated to ensure the same result: effective absorption to achieve a therapeutic, stable dosage of nicotine in the bloodstream. Once absorbed, a drug must achieve distribution to the desired site of action for it to work. Most drugs administered systemically are distributed through the bloodstream. Factors such as the drug's chemistry and dosage and the patient's body weight and cardiac or renal disease can impact on drug distribution.

Metabolism of drugs within the body influences the pharmacologic effects of drugs. The liver serves as the primary site of drug metabolism for drugs taken orally, altering the amount of available active drug or actually producing the drug metabolite that serves as the pharmacologically desired bioactive compound. Multiple factors affect drug metabolism (eg, liver disease, cardiac disease), which in turn affects the volume and potency of the medication ultimately available to exert its desired effect. Inhaled medications delivered directly to the lung bypass the liver's first-pass elimination and are directly available to act on the respiratory system. This in large part explains why a much smaller dose of inhaled β_2-adrenergic receptor bronchodilator is needed to exert its therapeutic effect on the lung than would be needed if the medication were taken orally.

The *elimination* of a drug refers to its clearance from the body or its biotransformation into an inactive state. The kidney is the primary organ for drug elimination, with renal disease playing a significant role in proper drug dosing. The concept of *half-life* (T½) refers to the length of time it normally takes for 50% of a drug to be eliminated from the body. Multiple factors, such as age, gender, diet, and health, contribute to a drug's T½, which can vary from individual to individual or change within the same individual. Knowledge of a drug's T½, coupled with a comprehensive assessment of the patient's history and medical condition, contributes to determining the proper dosage and frequency of medication administration.

A second related concept is that of **therapeutic index** (TI). TI represents a measure of the difference between the therapeutic dose and the toxic (or lethal) dose. Medications with a wide TI possess a large margin of dosing safety. Conversely, drugs with a narrow TI, such as the cardiac drug digitalis, require close attention to dosing strategies and the clinical condition of the patient to ensure safe administration. Fortunately, the types of aerosolized bronchodilators commonly administered possess a relatively large TI.

Pharmacodynamics refers to the principles by which drugs produce their actions on the body. The common theory for how drugs exert their effect is the **receptor theory**. Specific proteins in cell membranes are acted on by the chemical constituents of drugs, producing a cascade of biochemical events that leads to the desired drug action (or to an undesirable side effect). Drugs that elicit the desired receptor stimuli effect are classified as *agonists*; drugs that act on receptors to block the receptor stimuli effect are called *antagonists*. Different drugs within the same category may possess varying *affinity* (binding power) for receptors.

Respiratory medications follow the drug receptor theory. A β_2-adrenergic receptor agonist, such as albuterol, can be administered by inhalation to an asthmatic patient to stimulate β_2-adrenergic bronchial smooth muscle receptors, producing bronchodilation (bronchial smooth muscle relaxation). Conversely, bronchodilation can be produced by administration of an antagonist, or anticholinergic, aerosol bronchodilator, which binds to cholinergic bronchial smooth muscle receptors, suppressing their inherent propensity for airway smooth muscle constriction. Atrovent is an example of an anticholinergic bronchodilator.

Pharmacotherapy refers to the clinical application of drugs. The primary focus of this chapter is on how respiratory pharmacology is applied clinically. A knowledge of respiratory drugs, administration equipment and techniques, and clinical protocols that articulate appropriate outcome-oriented care contributes to a strong pharmacotherapy foundation. The reader is referred to Chapters 10 and 12, both of which contribute information relevant to pharmacotherapy concepts discussed in this chapter.

Drug Prescriptions

A drug prescription represents a medication order written by a physician or other legally authorized provider, such as an advanced practice nurse (ie, nurse practitioner or nurse midwife) or a physician assistant. In in-patient settings such as the hospital or skilled nursing facility, the prescription is written as an order in the patient's medical record, usually on a special physician order sheet created by the institution. Traditionally, orders usually included the following:

- Name of medication (generic name preferred but not mandatory)
- Medication dose (and strength if multiple concentrations are available)
- Route of administration, such as oral, IV, aerosolized
- Frequency of administration, such as t.i.d. (three times/day) or q 1 h (every hour)

The evolution of the respiratory care profession has led to modifications in written orders for aerosolized medications. Certain therapeutic interventions, such as "hand neb" or "MDI," imply medication administration by aerosol inhalation because hand-held nebulizer (HHN) and metered dose inhaler (MDI) therapy represent two types of commonly understood aerosol medication delivery techniques. Consequently, route of administration is usually not part of an order. The order may merely read "hand neb with 0.5 mL albuterol t.i.d.," or "unit dose albuterol t.i.d." Refer to Appendix A for a list of commonly used abbreviations.

What follows is a typical medication order received by an RCP:

0.5 mL albuterol & 3 mL N/S by SVN f/b 4 puffs Azmacort q.i.d.

In this order, 0.5 mL of albuterol indicates the amount of bronchodilator medication to be administered; & 3 mL N/S indicates that 3 mL of normal saline should be used as a diluent; by SVN indicates that the medication should be administered as an aerosol treatment using a small-volume, acorn-type hand nebulizer; f/b 4 puffs Azmacort means followed by 4 puffs of the corticosteroid medication Azmacort from a metered dose inhaler; q.i.d. indicates that this dose should be administered four times per day, during normal waking hours. Refer to Appendix B for an overview of concepts of medication dosages and calculations.

Further evolution in aerosol medication administration orders has been based on the use of patient care protocols. These protocols use a system by which the physician writes a generic order in the patient's medical record for the patient care assessment and treatment protocol or bronchodilator protocol. A preestablished protocol is then implemented by the practitioner, which may authorize the practitioner to evaluate the patient and to determine the type, dose, and frequency of medication and the type of aerosol administration technique. The practitioner would then automatically initiate therapy, assess patient response, and modify the care plan as needed. Some form of written (and perhaps verbal) communication would occur with the physician regarding the care plan. Protocol systems place added responsibility for the medication prescription in the hands of the practitioner, who is at the bedside evaluating the patient, rather than carrying out a standard physician-generated order for a specific treatment.

The use of protocols for medication administration has become widespread, and the legal ramifications of this change in drug prescribing have not been fully defined. At the minimum, practitioners who provide protocol care in institutions must ensure that those protocols are approved at the highest level within the institution (eg, by the executive medical board) and that they delineate the following:

- The role and limitations of the practitioner in selecting and administering medications
- How communication with the physician and documentation in the medical record occurs
- Under what circumstances the protocols will be applied
- Detailed information on how the practitioner applies the protocols
- The education involved in training practitioners to deliver medications competently by following the protocols

Appendix C illustrates two examples of protocol care for bronchodilator therapy: a therapy protocol for implementing metered dose inhaler therapy and a disease management protocol for the emergency department care of a patient with asthma.

PRINCIPLES OF AEROSOL MEDICATION ADMINISTRATION

The administration of a medication directly to the lung by aerosol inhalation offers several advantages over **systemic administration** by injection or oral routes (Box 8–1). Aerosol drug delivery serves as a primary treatment for a number of respiratory conditions. Achieving the desired therapeutic outcomes of aerosolized medication administration requires an understanding of aerosol physics, administration equipment, and techniques of aerosol medication delivery. Multiple variables contribute to the degree of effectiveness of inhaled medications, and failure

Medico-Legal Alert #1

The RCP has medicolegal responsibility for identifying the accuracy and completeness of medication orders and for clarifying orders that fall outside of standard practice. The RCP is responsible for serving as a patient advocate, and as such *must* question medication orders that are incomplete, are inaccurate, stipulate other than standard doses, or are, in the judgment of the RCP, not indicated or have the potential for patient harm. The courts recognize RCPs for their expertise in the area of respiratory pharmacology and aerosol drug administration, and as such hold them responsible for exercising independent judgment regarding all physician orders.

Box • 8–1   ADVANTAGES OF AEROSOL DELIVERY OF MEDICATIONS

Medication is delivered directly to the desired site of action

Effective dose is lower than if administered by oral or injectable route
(Ratio of dose to effect is high)

Fewer systemic side effects when delivered directly to lung

Allows for immediate cessation of drug delivery if side effects do occur

Convenient, simple, inexpensive route of administration

Available route in all patient populations

---

to recognize these factors can decrease the clinical benefits and increase the risks of side effects of therapy.

Figure 8–1 illustrates the respiratory system as it pertains to inhalation of aerosol particles. The particle size determines the site of maximal aerosol drug deposition. The treatment of a pulmonary condition located in the lower

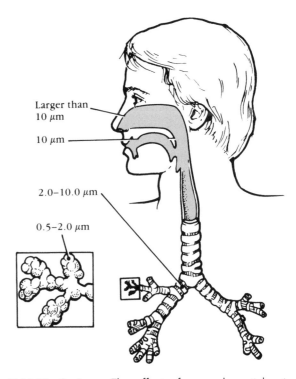

Larger than 10 μm

10 μm

2.0–10.0 μm

0.5–2.0 μm

FIGURE 8–1 • The effect of aerosol particle size on area of preferential deposition within the airways. Particles with a mass median aerodynamic diameter of greater than 10 μm are filtered by the nose, whereas particles larger than 15 μm are filtered with mouth breathing. Particles entering the airway that are between 5 and 10 μm deposit in the trachea and in the first six generations of the bronchi. Particles between 0.5 and 2 μm deposit in the lung parenchyma, and particles smaller than 1 μm commonly are exhaled.

airways requires generating particles in the range of 1 to 5 μm. Conversely, the treatment of postextubation stridor is optimized when particles are in the 5- to 10-μm range, allowing for maximal deposition in the upper airway and larynx. Some of the factors that affect particle size produced during an aerosol treatment include type and volume of medication being aerosolized, the aerosol delivery device used, and the delivery flow rate.

Several devices commonly are employed to administer aerosolized medications. These include small-volume nebulizers (SVNs), atomizers, MDIs (propellant and breath actuated), dry powder inhalers, ultrasonic nebulizers, and positive-pressure devices. Health care providers responsible for the administration of aerosolized medications must have a thorough knowledge of these devices, including operational characteristics of different brands within a category. Studies have shown that different brands of SVNs have significantly different performance characteristics, which could affect pharmacologic efficacy and therapeutic outcomes.[9,10] A comprehensive review of these devices and of general principles of aerosol therapy can be found in Chapter 12.

RESPIRATORY DYSFUNCTION AND AEROSOLIZED MEDICATIONS

A variety of conditions affecting the respiratory system can be safely and effectively treated by aerosol medication administration, as either a primary or secondary line of therapy. Inhaled bronchodilators and steroids represent a first-line therapy for the management of asthma. The NIH Asthma Guidelines, initially published in 1991 and updated in 1997, contain elaborate medication algorithms for managing the full spectrum of asthma severity classifications, incorporating both nebulizer and MDI techniques (see Appendix D). Other conditions in which *airway hyper-reactivity* ("twitchy airways") exist, such as chronic obstructive pulmonary disease (COPD) and cystic fibrosis (CF), often benefit from aerosol bronchodilator therapy. Bronchodilator therapy may also have a role in the treatment of such conditions as acute respiratory distress syndrome (ARDS), respiratory syncytial virus (RSV) pneumonia, and bronchopulmonary dysplasia, in which airway reactivity and reversible bronchospasm may be present.

The pathophysiology associated with CF and chronic bronchitis includes the chronic production of a large volume of pulmonary secretions. Patients with these conditions may benefit from the use of inhaled mucokinetic agents, such as dornase alfa (Pulmozyme) or, rarely, *N*-acetylcysteine (Mucomyst), to help facilitate mobilization of these secretions. The instillation of *N*-acetylcysteine has also been used successfully in patients with artificial airways in place, who have thick, tenacious secretions unresponsive to optimal humidity therapy.

Aerosolized antimicrobials are used to manage a variety of pulmonary infections. Once again, patients with CF, whose lungs are chronically colonized with gram-negative organisms, may benefit from aerosolized antibiotics, such as gentamycin or tobramycin. RSV pneumonia often responds to the aerosol administration of the antiviral drug ribavirin. Patients with acquired immunodeficiency syndrome (AIDS) may receive regular aerosol treatments with pentamidine for prophylaxis against *Pneumocystis carinii* pneumonia. Aerosolized amphotericin B has been used on occasion in patients who are immunocompromised as prophylaxis against nosocomial fungal pneumonia.

Several studies have looked at the role of aerosolized **surfactant** replacement therapy in patients ranging from newborns with respiratory distress syndrome to adults with ARDS. Experimental studies have been conducted looking at the inhalation of recombinant interferon-γ as an agent to alter the body's immune response. Superoxide dismutase, an antioxidant, has been studied for the treatment of certain lung diseases. Aerosolized heparin has been studied for the role it may play in preventing hypoxia-induced pulmonary hypertension. Morphine has been aerosolized in compassionate use cases to manage pain in patients with cancer. As mentioned earlier, coming years will likely produce an ever-growing range of medications available for aerosol administration, enhancing the role of the RCP as a respiratory pharmacology resource. Studies are under way looking at the use of aerosol medication administration to treat nonrespiratory conditions ranging from diabetes to osteoporosis, hepatitis, and multiple sclerosis.

Although a variety of pulmonary conditions have been associated with the common use of aerosol drug therapy, the administration of medications should occur on a case-by-case basis. Each patient should undergo physical assessment to establish clinical need, identify outcome goals, and implement an individualized care plan, rather than automatically ordering drug therapy based on a global disease diagnosis, tradition, or habit. Outcomes management represents a rationale approach to aerosol medication administration, impacting positively on quality, safety, and cost of care. Aerosol drug therapy can best be accomplished within the context of protocol care, whereby the expert assessment by the practitioner is followed by selection of the most appropriate, cost-effective, and safe therapeutic intervention available. In the hands of a trained, competent practitioner, a protocol that affords the clinician the authority to select and adjust drug type, dosage, technique, and frequency may produce the highest level of care. The AARC Clinical Practice Guideline on Aerosol Therapy, the NIH Asthma Guidelines, and the AARC Aerosol Consensus Statement represent resources that health care providers have used to develop scientifically sound aerosol medication administration protocols. Figure 8–2 illustrates a protocol for aerosolized medication administration in patients with asthma, incorporating the elements described previously.

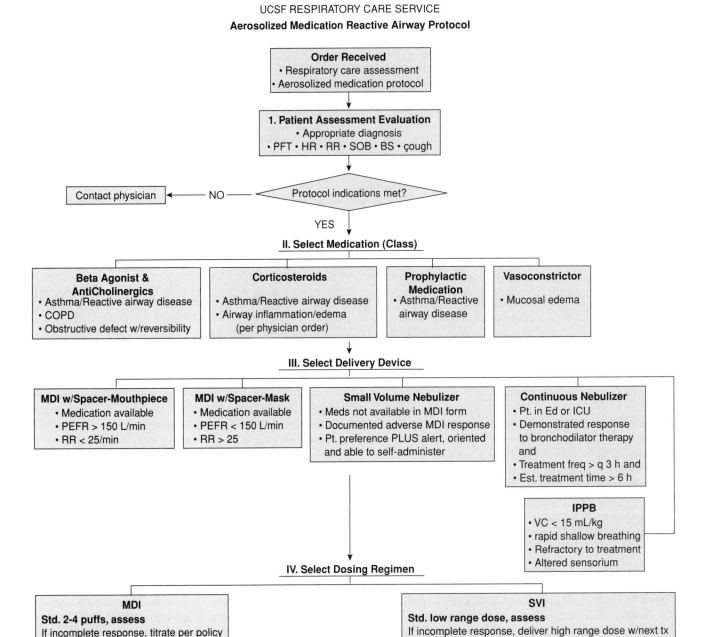

FIGURE 8–2 • Aerosolized Medication and Reactive Airway Protocol. (Courtesy of University of California, San Francisco, Respiratory Care Department.)

MEDICATIONS SPECIFIC TO RESPIRATORY CARE

The Autonomic Nervous System

The most important class of medications administered by aerosol are bronchodilators. The timely, appropriate use of inhaled bronchodilators plays an important and often life-saving role in the management of a variety of pulmonary conditions, including asthma and COPD. An understanding of these medications requires a brief review of the autonomic nervous system and airway anatomy and physi-

ology. The autonomic nervous system is divided into two branches, sympathetic and parasympathetic, which innervate a variety of body organs and systems (Fig. 8–3).

Endogenous substances liberated at the ends of presynaptic and postsynaptic fibers act as chemical neurotransmitters to conduct nerve impulses across the synaptic gap to the receptor site. Naturally occurring catecholamines, such as norepinephrine, serve as chemical neurotransmitters that stimulate sympathetic branch α- and β-adrenergic receptors. Drugs that possess the capacity to stimulate sympathetic receptors are classified as **sympathomimetic**.

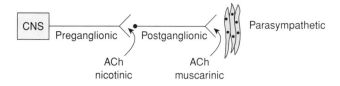

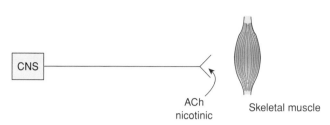

FIGURE 8–3 • Arrangement of the autonomic nervous system, indicating the pharmacology of synaptic junctions. In the sympathetic branch, acetylcholine (Ach) is the neurotransmitter for nicotinic action at the ganglia. Norepinephrine is the neurotransmitter in the postganglionic region. (Witek, TJ, Schachter, EN. *Pharmacology and Therapeutics in Respiratory Care,* Philadelphia: WB Saunders1994:138.)

Those that act by stimulating β-adrenergic receptors are referred to as β_2-adrenergic sympathomimetics, β_2-adrenergic agonists, or simply β_2-agonists; the latter term is used in the remainder of this chapter. Those that act by stimulating α-receptors are referred to as *α-agonists.* Table 8–1 lists common sites of adrenergic receptors and the responses elicited by their stimulation.

β_2-Agonist Stimulation and Bronchodilation

Stimulation of β_2-adrenergic receptors initiates a cascade of biochemical events that ultimately leads to relaxation of bronchial smooth muscle. Figure 8–4 illustrates events leading to β_2-adrenergic receptor stimulation and airway smooth muscle relaxation as currently understood. The beneficial effects of β_2-agonist bronchodilators when taken by inhalation are primarily related to their deposition on the airway mucosa, leading to β_2-adrenergic receptor stimulation. Direct delivery to the lung tissue allows for minimal dosing, a combination of which significantly reduces undesirable side effects, as described earlier. Side effects associated with sympathomimetic β_2-agonist therapy include tachycardia, palpitations, blood pressure changes, nausea and vomiting, tremors, and headache. These side effects are seen more commonly with oral or parenteral therapy but may also occur in patients receiving β_2-agonists by aerosol, particularly with frequent- or high-dose therapy.

Inhaled aerosol medication that is deposited in the oropharynx is absorbed or swallowed, which can lead to systemic side effects. The goal of aerosol bronchodilator therapy is to optimize lower airway deposition and mini-

mize extrapulmonary deposition. As discussed in Chapter 12, the use of holding chamber devices when taking MDI medications contributes to increased pulmonary deposition and reduced extrapulmonary drug delivery in the oropharynx. Instructing patients who experience side effects from aerosol medication administration by SVN or MDI to rinse their mouths out after therapy may prove beneficial.

A variety of commercially available β_2-agonist bronchodilators administered by aerosol inhalation mimic norepinephrine, producing airway smooth muscle relaxation. Table 8–2 lists a number of β_2-agonist bronchodilators commonly used in the United States. The chemical structures of the various β_2-agonists determine their actions. Early catecholamine β_2-agonists, such as isoproterenol, were short-acting, nonspecific drugs with strong β_1-adrenergic receptor agonist properties, which had the potential for significant cardioacceleratory side effects. Through pharmacologic manipulation, noncatecholamine β_2-agonist compounds have evolved that are long-acting and specific to the airway receptors, with negligible cardiac side effects when taken in recommended doses.

Current-generation bronchodilators can be taken orally as a syrup or tablet because they are not susceptible to degradation in the stomach. Extended-release albuterol tablets (Volmax) taken once or twice daily may allow for enhanced compliance and more stable blood levels of bronchodilator. Systemic administration (oral, IV, subcutaneous) of bronchodilators involves a larger dose of medication than that delivered by aerosol because the medication is delivered to the systemic circulation and is susceptible to first-pass elimination by the liver. These two factors combine to produce a greater potential for systemic side effects, such as tremor, tachycardia, palpitations, gastrointestinal upset, anxiety, and headache. The reader is encouraged to review resources such as the *Physician's Desk Reference* (PDR) or product literature specific to each bronchodilator to develop a full understanding of each medication's profile.

One poorly appreciated side effect associated with bronchodilator therapy is alteration in serum electrolytes. This dose-dependent response can manifest with frequent- or high-dose therapy using any of the β_2-agonists as well as the anticholinergic bronchodilators, such as atropine. In a study by Bodenhamer and coworkers,[11] 23 asthmatic patients were treated in the emergency department with a series of nebulized albuterol treatments (range, two to six treatments, each with 2.5 mg albuterol). Serum potassium, magnesium, and phosphate levels decreased significantly, with 57% of patients manifesting hypokalemia during therapy. Gelmont and colleagues[12] found similar hypokalemia-inducing results in a study of metaproterenol and atropine. Hypokalemia and hypomagnesemia are arrhythmogenic in nature. Because hypoxia can also induce cardiac rhythm disturbances, an awareness of the cardiac risks associated with frequent- or high-dose β_2-agonist therapy in acutely ill patients is necessary.

Table • 8–1   PRINCIPAL LOCATIONS OF ADRENERGIC RECEPTORS AND RESPONSES TO THEIR ACTIVATION

Site	Receptor Type	Response
Lung		
Tracheobronchial smooth muscle	Mainly β_2	Relaxation
Bronchial glands	β_2	Increased secretion
Heart		
Sinoatrial node	β_1	Increased heart rate
Atria	β_1 (β_2)	Faster conduction
Bundle of His-Purkinje fibers	β_1	Faster conduction and automaticity
Ventricles	β_1 (β_2)	Faster conduction, increased contractility, increased tendency for automaticity and pacemaker activity
Arterioles		
Abdominal viscera, renal arterioles	α, β_2	α: Vasoconstriction β_2: Vasodilation
Cerebral	α	Mild vasoconstriction
Coronary	α, β_2	α: Vasoconstriction β_2: Vasodilation
Mucosal	α	Vasoconstriction
Pulmonary	α, β_2	α: Vasoconstriction β_2: Vasodilation
Salivary glands	α	Vasoconstriction
Skeletal muscle	α, β_2	α: Vasoconstriction β_2: Vasodilation
Skin	α	Vasoconstriction
Systemic veins	α	Vasoconstriction
Uterine smooth muscle	α, β_2	α: Contraction in pregnancy β_2: Relaxation (nonpregnant)
Stomach	α, β_2	α: Sphincter constriction β_2: Decreased motility and tone
Intestine	α, β_2	α: Sphincter contraction β_2: Decreased motility and tone
Liver	β_2	Gluconeogenesis Glycogenolysis
Pancreas		
Acini	α	Decreased secretion
β cell (islets)	α, β_2	α: Secretion β_2: Increased secretion
Skin		
Sweat glands	α	Increased secretion
Pilomotor muscles	α	Contraction
Fat cells	β_2	Lipolysis
Mast cells	α, β_2	α: Increased mediator release β_2: Decreased mediator release
Eye		
Radial muscle of iris	α	Contraction

Reprinted from Witek TJ, Schachter EN. *Pharmacology and Therapeutics in Respiratory Care.*
Philadelphia: WB Saunders; 1994.

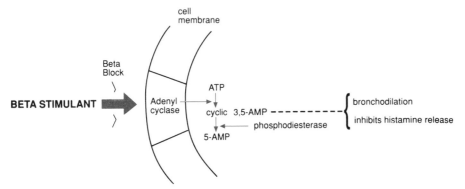

FIGURE 8–4 • The β-receptor agonist pathway. β-Stimulants combine with the β-receptor agonist to activate the enzyme adenyl cyclase in the cell membrane, which catalyzes the conversion of adenosine triphosphate (ATP) to cyclic adenosine monophosphate (AMP). (Rau JL Jr. *Respiratory Care in Pharmacology,* 4th ed. St. Louis: Mosby-Year Book; 1994:118.)

Table • 8–2 COMMONLY USED INHALED β₂-RECEPTOR BRONCHODILATORS

Drug	Method of Administration		Dosing*
Epinephrine (eg, Primatene Mist)	MDI	300 µg/puff	Variable
Racemic epinephrine	SOL	2.25%	0.5–0.25 mL
Isoproterenol	SOL	1 : 200 (0.5%)	0.5–0.25 mL
Isoetharine (eg, Bronkosol)	SOL	1.0%	0.25–0.5 mL
Metaproterenol (eg, Alupent)	SOL	5.0%	0.3 ml ±
	MDI	650 µg/puff	Variable
Terbutaline (eg, Brethaire)	MDI	200 µg/puff	Variable
	SOL	1.0%	Variable
Albuterol (eg, Ventolin, Proventil)	SOL	0.5%	0.5 mL ±
	MDI	90 µg/puff	Variable
	DPI	200 µg/capsule	1 capsule
Salmeterol (eg, Serevent)	MDI	21 µg/puff	2 puffs q 12 h
Pirbuterol (eg, Maxair)	MDI	200 µg/puff	Variable
Bitolterol (eg, Tornalate)	MDI	370 µg/puff	Variable

*Metered dose inhaler (MDI) dosages are listed in this table as variable. Consult PDR for manufacturer-recommended dosages. The term *variable* is used because scientific literature suggest that MDI dosages beyond those recommended by the manufacturer may be administered safely and effectively if the patient is closely monitored and administration is based on clearly defined therapeutic outcome criteria, such as changes in peak expiratory flow rate, symptoms, or development of side effects.
  SOL, solution.

Although the two studies cited did not clearly demonstrate a clinical significance associated with the serum electrolyte changes, care providers should be aware of potential adverse responses to high-dose β₂-agonist or atropine therapy and conduct appropriate close monitoring as warranted. This is particularly important today because clinicians pursue bronchodilator management strategies, such as MDI titrations, whereby patients are medicated at increasing doses, sometimes up to 40 puffs/treatment, to achieve preestablished therapeutic end points.[13] Continuous nebulization and undiluted nebulization of β₂-agonist bronchodilators may also involve doses that exceed traditional levels, necessitating a heightened level of monitoring, to include the use of electrographic monitoring and serial measurement of serum electrolytes when appropriate.

Ironically, the potassium-lowering side effect of β₂-agonists in selected cases may represent a clinical indication for nebulization of a β₂-agonist such as albuterol. Patients on hemodialysis who develop acute, dangerously elevated potassium levels may benefit from IV or aerosol administration of albuterol in an effort to lower potassium rapidly.[14] Institutions in which this practice occurs should have a written policy guiding the clinician in the safe, appropriate administration of aerosolized β₂-agonists for purposes of treating hyperkalemia, particularly within the context of using other traditional systemic pharmacologic interventions to treat acute hyperkalemia, such as IV insulin administration.

Two sympathomimetic drugs bear special mention.

Salmeterol xinafoate (Serevent) became available in MDI form in 1993 and is a highly selective, long-acting β₂-agonist. The drug has slower onset of action relative to other β₂-agonists, with duration reported to last 12 hours or longer. The drug is recommended for use as a preventative, **"controller"** medication, taken as a standard dose of 42 µg

(2 puffs) twice daily with doses taken 12 hours apart, most commonly as part of a therapy regimen that includes inhaled steroids. Studies have shown that salmeterol xinafoate is particularly useful in the management of exercised-induced bronchospasm and nocturnal episodic asthma, conferring prolonged bronchodilation during the sleeping hours, when endogenous corticosteroid levels are at their nadir and when susceptible asthmatic patients experience problems.[15] The use of a controller medication such as salmeterol xinafoate may enhance the quality of life of asthmatic patients through better control of symptoms and an improved sense of well-being.

Because salmeterol xinafoate has a slow onset of action and is used as a controller drug, those who take it should have a second β₂-agonist available for **"reliever"** short-term use. Patients must receive comprehensive education

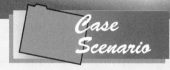

CRITICAL THINKING CHALLENGES

Case Scenario

A 37-year-old asthmatic man visits the nurse practitioner at clinic with complaints of increasing frequency of episodes of wheezing (twice per week), requiring use of albuterol MDI. He also complains of nocturnal coughing that awakens him 3 to 4 nights/week. His current medications include 2 puffs of triamcinolone acetonide (Azmacort, a steroid), b.i.d. and albuterol p.r.n. Is there another medication for which this patient should be evaluated?

Answer: salmeterol xinofoate (Serevent).

CRITICAL THINKING CHALLENGES

Case Scenario

A 14-month-old infant girl is being extubated 2 days after having undergone surgery for repair of a cardiac anomaly. Immediately on removal of the endotracheal tube, the infant exhibits labored breathing, with mild retractions and nasal flaring and an audible, high-pitched crowing noise on inspiration. Her heart rate increases by 40 beats/minute, and her saturation drops from 91% to 84% almost immediately. Is there any respiratory medication that should be evaluated for use in this situation?

Answer: racemic epinephrine.

on the role of salmeterol xinafoate as a prophylactic medication and on the use of their other β_2-agonists, such as albuterol or metaproterenol, for the management of acute bronchospasm. Failure to provide this information places the patient at *increased risk* for inappropriate and inadequate management of what could be a life-threatening asthma attack. There is no pharmacologic reason that patients cannot be prescribed both salmeterol xinafoate and a second β_2-agonist, so long as patient education has occurred regarding appropriate dosing and use in relation to other asthma medications.

Racemic epinephrine possesses both β_2- and α-agonist properties. As shown earlier, α-adrenergic receptor stimulation of mucosal vasculature produces vasoconstriction. This particular action of racemic epinephrine makes it the drug of choice in the treatment of conditions in which upper airway mucosal swelling may occur, such as seen with laryngeotracheal bronchitis (croup) or after extubation. The presence of stridor coupled with other signs and symptoms of airway swelling after removal of an artificial airway may necessitate immediate administration of aerosolized racemic epinephrine. The timely use of this therapy may avert the need for reintubation or, worse, emergency tracheostomy if there is difficulty in securing a patent airway because of swelling. The use of this medication in the treatment of croup requires careful assessment of need and close monitoring of the response to therapy and undesirable side effects.[16,17]

β_2-agonist bronchodilators have come to be viewed as a first-line therapy for the treatment of airway hyperreactivity, particularly in the acute phase, and played a prominent role in the 1991 and 1997 NIH Asthma Guidelines (see Appendix D). Ironically, at the same time that the NIH guidelines were being developed, reports published in scientific journals pointed to data that suggested a relationship between β_2-agonist use and increased mortality in asthmatics. Analysis of statistical data from studies in New Zealand and other countries raised questions about the safety of chronic β_2-agonist bronchodilator use.[18,19] Multiple variables confound the issue of whether a direct correlation between β_2-agonist use and mortality rates exists, not the least of which is the dissimilarity among the various research studies. As a consequence, there is considerable dialogue regarding the exact future role of this class of medications for both acute and chronic management of symptoms. A fundamental shift in thinking has evolved toward a growing role for inhaled antiinflammatory agents (**corticosteroids**) in chronic severe asthma, with a concomitant reduction in reliever β_2-agonist use. Practitioners are encouraged to maintain an awareness of current scientific literature and to incorporate new information into their clinical practice and patient education accordingly.

Leukotriene Modifiers

Leukotrienes are metabolites of arachidonic acid and, in the past, were collectively referred to as *slow-reactive substances of anaphylaxis*. The different leukotrienes that have been identified possess varying degrees of the following four properties, all of which contribute to airflow obstruction in allergic asthma: (1) increased mucus production, (2) airway inflammation and edema formation, (3) bronchial smooth muscle bronchoconstriction, and (4) cellular infiltration. The focus of therapy with leukotriene modifiers is to interrupt the synthesis, action, or both of

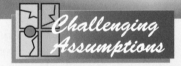

CRITICAL THINKING CHALLENGES

Challenging Assumptions

Americans are particularly enamored of pills and tablets to treat illness. A great deal of emphasis has been placed on a discussion of the central role of inhaled bronchodilators to treat asthma. Is there no magic pill that can be taken orally to control asthma?

If you asked that question during the 1970s, 1980s, and even into the first half of the 1990s, the answer would have been "no way."

The future role of inhaled β_2-agonist bronchodilators changed in 1996, however, with the emergence of a new class of medications to treat airway hyperreactivity. As our understanding of the biophysiology of mediators of bronchoconstriction and airway inflammation evolves, new classes of drugs emerge. Leukotriene modifiers, also referred to as *leukotriene pathway interrupters*, represent the latest type of medications being used in the management of asthma.

these detrimental metabolites of arachidonic acid, as illustrated in Figure 8–5. Zafirlukast (Accolate) functions as a leukotriene receptor antagonist. This medication received Food and Drug Administration (FDA) clearance in 1996 and is marketed as a 20-mg tablet, to be taken twice a day. It acts by blocking receptor response to leukotrienes, preventing or attenuating receptor response. Another leukotriene inhibitor, zileuton (Zyflo) blocks the production of leukotrienes by inhibiting enzymes involved in leukotriene synthesis. Zileuton is supplied as a 600-mg tablet, to be taken four times per day. Montelukast sodium (Singulair) is a leukotriene receptor antagonist introduced in 1998. This once-a-day therapy is taken in the evening as a 10-mg tablet for adults and adolescents 15 years of age or older, and as a 5-mg cherry-flavored chewable tablet for children between the ages of 6 and 14. Montelukast offers the duel advantages of once-a-day dosing, presumably improving compliance with therapy, and FDA approval for use in children as young as 6 years of age.

The second edition of the NIH Asthma Guidelines, published in 1997, suggests the use of leukotriene modifiers as long-term controller drugs in patients 12 years or older with mild persistent asthma, perhaps as an alternative to low-dose inhaled corticosteroids or antiasthma drugs, such as nedocromil. Where zafirlukast and zileuton fit into asthma management protocols in the long term remains to be articulated, pending further research and clinical experience with this class of medication.[20]

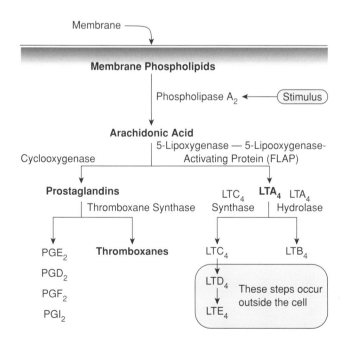

FIGURE 8–5 • The formation of leukotrienes and thromboxanes through arachidonic acid breakdown. (Spector SL. Leukotriene inhibitors and antagonists in asthma. *Ann Allergy Asthma Immunol.* 1995;75[6]:464.)

Anticholinergic and Xanthine Bronchodilators

Anticholinergics

Aerosol therapy with anticholinergic medications can produce bronchodilation by blocking cholinergic receptor activity (see Fig. 8–3). Parasympathetic innervation exists in several generations of large airways, and the balance between sympathetic and parasympathetic activity contributes to overall bronchomotor tone. Increased parasympathetic activity can result from a variety of endogenous or exogenous stimuli, triggering a cascade of biochemical events that produce bronchoconstriction. Certain pulmonary conditions predispose to increased cholinergic activity and thus are preferentially more responsive to the use of anticholinergic bronchodilators, either as a primary therapy or as a complement to β_2-agonist therapy. In COPD, airway hyperreactivity is thought to occur predominantly as a result of abnormal cholinergic tone, thus suggesting a role for anticholinergic medications, as opposed to β_2-agonists, as a first-line therapy. A symposium conducted in 1996 pointed to the continued dialogue regarding the evolving role of anticholinergic bronchodilator therapy in patients with COPD.[21,22]

Atropine was the primary anticholinergic medication traditionally used to treat cholinergic-based bronchoconstriction. Atropine sulfate is available in liquid form for parenteral use in cardiac patients and as a preoperative drug to reduce salivary and mucous secretions. Clinicians have diluted this liquid preparation with normal saline for aerosol delivery by HHN or intermittent positive-pressure breathing (IPPB). Because the drug is not expressly prepared as an aerosol medication, recommended dosages when used by inhalation are not officially available from the PDR. Research studies with atropine suggest an adult dose based on body weight, ranging anywhere from 0.01 to 0.07 mg/kg.[23] Potential side effects associated with atropine use, based on the dosage, frequency, and predisposing factors in individual patients, include tachycardia, urinary retention, dry mouth, drying of pulmonary secretions, and visual disturbances. Atropine therapy is not recommended for use in patients with narrow-angle glaucoma.

Because anticholinergic medications such as atropine are not without significant dose-related side effects, as mentioned earlier, other atropine-like drugs have been developed. The primary anticholinergic atropine-like drug is ipratropium bromide (Atrovent), which is available as a traditional chlorofluorocarbon (CFC)-driven metered dose preparation delivering 18 μg of medication per puff. A dry-powder inhaler (DPI) preparation is also under development. The standard recommended dose of ipratropium bromide by MDI is two puffs four times daily. Ipratropium bromide is also available as a unit dose aerosol preparation, which contains 500 μg per 2.5-mL ampule. Atrovent has the bronchodilator properties of atropine without the many side effects associated with atropine. Most commonly, patients complain of dry mouth or bad taste when using this medication. As with β_2-agonists, proper aerosol administration techniques should be used to optimize drug delivery, including use of a holding chamber when indicated with MDI use. Protocols for the use of β_2-agonists and anticholinergics and for when to use MDI instead of nebulized solution are evolving.

Since anticholinergics produce effects on the autonomic nervous system in a different way than do sympathomimetics, they may be part of a combination therapy to treat airway reactivity. Both types of medications may be combined in a single nebulizer treatment or may be administered sequentially by nebulizer, MDI, or a combination thereof. Combivent is an MDI preparation that combines albuterol (90 µg) and ipratropium bromide (18 µg) in a single puff. Studies suggest that in some patient populations, the combination of ipratropium bromide solution with an inhaled β_2-agonist, such as albuterol, produces greater improvement in FEV_1 than either agent by itself. Howder describes a rationale approach to the clinical use of anticholinergics, either by themselves or in combination with β_2-agonists.[24]

The 1991 NIH Asthma Guidelines were relatively silent on the use of anticholinergics in asthma as compared with the British Asthma guidelines, which suggest a more prominent use in patients not responding to optimal β_2-agonist drug use. A growing body of research on anticholinergic bronchodilator therapy since 1991 led to a clearer role for this class of medications in the 1997 NIH Guidelines. The revised guidelines suggest that medications such as ipratropium bromide have a potential additive benefit when used in conjunction with β_2-agonists in severe exacerbations or when used as an alternative in asthmatic patients who do not tolerate inhaled β_2-agonists.

In 1995, the FDA approved the use of an intranasal ipratropium bromide spray for the treatment of rhinorrhea. An 0.03% ipratropium bromide nasal spray is available for the treatment of allergic and nonallergic perennial rhinitis. Studies have shown that intranasal ipratropium bromide can safely ameliorate the symptoms of nonallergic perennial rhinitis, which include nasal hypersecretion, mucosal swelling, and sneezing, with minor topical side effects[25]; recommended dosage is 2 sprays (42 µg) per nostril twice or three times daily. An 0.06% solution is available in spray form for the treatment of the common cold; recommended dosage is 2 sprays (84 µg) per nostril three to four times per day.

Methylxanthines

A class of drugs known as **methylxanthines** also possess bronchodilating properties. Caffeine and theobromine are two common examples of methylxanthines found in a variety of commonly consumed foods, including coffee, tea, and cocoa. On a historical note, Theodore Roosevelt, who suffered from childhood asthma, was sometimes treated by his mother throughout the night with multiple cups of coffee, until his breathing improved. Clinically, the methylxanthine most commonly associated with the treatment of bronchospasm is theophylline. Theophylline is available in an oral preparation or in the IV preparation aminophylline. Early researchers postulated that theophylline produced bronchodilation by functioning as a phosphodiesterase inhibitor. This inhibition of phosphodiesterase, an enzyme involved in the degradation of intracellular cyclic adenosine monophosphate, would lead to elevated cyclic adenosine monophosphate levels, enhancing sympathetic tone and thus bronchodilation. It has also been suggested that methylxanthines contribute to bronchodilation by functioning as adenosine antagonists, prostaglandin inhibitors, or even antiinflammatories. Although in use for more than 50 years, the exact mechanisms by which these drugs actually affect airway hyperreactivity are complex and remain poorly understood.

Aminophylline is administered intravenously as a loading dose to achieve therapeutic blood levels and then continued as an IV maintenance dose. Loading doses (6 mg/kg or less) and maintenance doses (0.2 to 0.7 mg/kg) are calculated based on ideal body weight but must be adjusted for a significant number of factors that influence the pharmacokinetics of this drug. Traditionally, the goal was to achieve a therapeutic blood level between 10 and 20 µg/mL. Once the patient stabilizes, transition is made to intermittent oral administration of theophylline, preferably using a sustained-release preparation after discharge. Factors such as age, illness, smoking history, concomitant medication use, and even food intake all influence the metabolism and clearance

CRITICAL THINKING CHALLENGES

Shifting Care Plans

A 54-year-old woman with a history of mild persistent asthma was admitted through the emergency department, where she received 7.5 mg/h albuterol by continuous nebulizer plus 4 puffs ipratropium bromide (Atrovent) and 2 puffs triamcinolone acetonide (Azmacort) q 1 h. It is now 18 hours after admission. She has been titrated down to 4 puffs albuterol and 2 puffs Azmacort q.i.d. She continues to receive 4 puffs Atrovent q.i.d. The patient's peak expiratory flow rate is 30% higher than on admission. Her wheezes have diminished, she is taking oral fluids well, and there is a team conference to discuss her discharge. Which medications should be evaluated for discontinuation?

Answer: Atrovent. The postdischarge use of Atrovent should be closely evaluated. If the patient does not normally use this medication at home, and the RCP can demonstrate that a predischarge treatment without Atrovent produces an acceptable positive clinical response, discharge medications might not include Atrovent.

of xanthines. This makes dosing with theophylline preparations difficult and dangerous because the therapeutic index (TI) of this drug is extremely narrow and the side effects potentially fatal. On an outpatient basis, the use of sustained-release once-daily therapy with theophylline preparations such as Uni-Dur help to enhance compliance with medication use, sustain stable therapeutic blood levels, and minimize the risks of undesired side effects. The NIH Asthma Guidelines suggest aiming toward a serum concentration in the range of 5 to 15 µg/mL.

Theophylline and aminophylline were at their height of popularity in the 1970s in the treatment of acute asthma and as maintenance therapy for outpatient use. The measurement of serum concentrations was one of the factors that contributed to the drug's rise in popularity in the 1970s. This was coupled with the recognition that there were other potential benefits of this class of drugs, including improved diaphragmatic muscle function, mucociliary clearance, and respiratory center stimulation. Yet, although xanthines were once considered a first-line therapy for obstructive lung disease, their use waned by the mid-1980s for a number of reasons, not the least of which were their side effects, which ranged from minor to life-threatening problems, even at levels close to or below the high end of the therapeutic range. Nausea and vomiting, headache, nervousness, diuresis, and tachycardia and other more serious arrhythmias, as well as seizures, have been associated with the use of aminophylline and theophylline. Patients on

CRITICAL THINKING CHALLENGES

Shifting Care Plans

A neighbor with a history of asthma complains to you that he is feeling "quite excitable," with a rapid pulse and nausea the past few days. He takes theophylline daily, 2 puffs Alupent b.i.d., and 10 mg prednisone daily. His family practice physician recently wrote a prescription for a new asthma pill, which he has taken for the past 2 weeks. When you ask him the name of the drug, he says, "I'm not sure, I think it begins with a Z." What would you do?

Answer: Confirm the new asthma medication your neighbor is taking. (You confirm it is the new leukotriene modifier Zyflo). Instruct your neighbor to contact his physician *immediately* concerning his theophylline therapy or go to an Emergency Department if his physician is unavailable. Leukotriene pathway interrupters such as Zyflo produce a known drug interaction with theophylline. Clearance of theophylline can be significantly decreased, increasing the drug's half-life and serum blood levels, leading to side effects. This patient needs his theophylline level checked and therapy adjusted accordingly.

methylxanthine therapy must receive accurate dosing, education about the use of these drugs and their side effects, monitoring of blood levels, and appropriate timely intervention when side effects occur.

The future role of methylxanthines remains to be defined as ongoing research looks at the use of this class of drugs in specific populations.[26] The original 1991 NIH Asthma Guidelines recommended considering the introduction of oral methylxanthines in patients with chronic moderate to severe asthma, preferably once optimal β_2-agonist and antiinflammatory therapy have been established, for symptom control. The 1991 guidelines suggested that patients who experience asthma exacerbations and present to the emergency department may be candidates for IV aminophylline therapy after stabilization and admission to the medical facility. The updated 1997 guidelines appear to have eliminated IV aminophylline as a suggested therapy, limiting the use of methylxanthines to chronic outpatient use of oral theophylline.

Antiallergenic Antiasthma Medications

A class of medications exist which act not as bronchodilators but rather as agents that help inhibit the biochemical cascade of events that trigger airway reactivity. The primary mechanism of action of these drugs is thought to be mast cell stabilization, preventing the release of chemical mediators of airway reactivity. Sodium cromoglycate and nedocromil sodium are the two common commercially available medications in this class of antiasthmatic drugs. Although both the chemistry and mechanism of action are different from those of salmeterol xinafoate or the leukotriene modifiers, they share the same classification of controller asthma medications. These drugs do not relieve acute bronchospasm but rather promote airway stability and integrity in an effort to reduce the frequency and severity of asthma exacerbations.

The characterization of patients with asthma demonstrates that a large percentage have ectopic, allergic asthma, with identified allergens. In susceptible asthmatic patients, exposure to the allergens causes an interaction between immunoglobulin E and the allergen on the surface of the mast cell. This interaction causes degranulation of the mast cell and release of mediators, such as histamine, which initiate a cascade of events leading to inflammation and bronchoconstriction. Studies have shown that certain drugs can help preserve the integrity of the mast cell, preventing the release of these mediators. Although this theory is certainly a simplified and incomplete explanation, it helps in the categorization of the antiasthma actions of this class of drugs.

Sodium cromoglycate (cromolyn sodium) is the prototype agent in this class of drugs. This drug is a synthetic compound patterned after a naturally occurring substance called *khellin,* found in a Mediterranean herb. Available since the 1970s, this drug is marketed in several forms. Initially, it was introduced as a powder-filled gelatin capsule, containing 20 mg of medication. The capsule was taken using a special breath-actuated Spinhaler, usually four times daily. Several years later, the drug became available in liquid preparation in an ampule containing 20 mg per 2 mL of purified water and as an MDI preparation that delivered 800 µg/puff; both preparations are recommended in four times/daily dosing. Sodium cromoglycate is also available as a nasal spray preparation for allergic rhinitis, delivering 40 µg/spray. Side effects associated with cromolyn sodium use are predominantly localized, with patients exhibiting cough and gastrointestinal upset.

The role of cromolyn sodium falls into several categories. It may be used for the prophylactic management of atopic asthma, with particular application in the pediatric population. Initiation of therapy requires several weeks of use to determine its beneficial effects. Because cromolyn sodium is not a bronchodilator, it is usually part of a polydrug regimen of β_2-agonists, steroids, and other medications, as needed. Effective management of airway hyperreactivity with this medication, however, may permit a reduction in concomitant drug therapy, including corticosteroids, theophylline, and β_2-agonists. Use of cromolyn sodium is also of value as pretreatment for exercise-induced bronchospasm and as prophylaxis against exposure to environmental triggers of reactivity, such as sulfur dioxide and ozone. The drug has also been shown to block response to antigen challenge in the laboratory setting.

Nedocromil sodium (Tilade) is a more recent antiasthma drug available in the United States that possesses a clinical profile similar to that of cromolyn sodium. Successful use of nedocromil sodium has led to a reduction in wheezing and coughing. The primary reported side effects include unpleasant taste, headache, and gastrointestinal upset. This drug is available as an MDI preparation, with each actuation delivering 1.75 mg of nedocromil sodium; recommended dosing is 2 inhalations four times daily (14 mg/d), perhaps tapered to three times daily or less when the patient is stable.

For the sake of completeness, a third drug that should be mentioned is ketotifen. This oral medication has been shown to possess antiallergic properties similar to those of the inhaled drugs previously described. At present, the drug is not available in the United States. The reader is referred to the NIH Asthma Guidelines for a description of where antiasthma medications fit into the treatment of asthma.

Corticosteroids

Corticosteroids are a second, common type of aerosol medication. Corticosteroids are substances that occur naturally in the human body and that contribute to a variety of biochemical and metabolic activities. The cortex of the adrenal gland is the site of production and secretion of dozens of corticosteroids. These corticosteroids fall into categories, such as glucocorticoids, mineralocorticoids,

and sex hormones. Mineralocorticoids are primarily involved in fluid and electrolyte regulation. Glucocorticoids influence a wide range of metabolic activities that affect total-body homeostasis, including that of the immune system. Cortisol is the predominant glucocorticoid produced by the adrenal gland and plays a major role in multiple physiologic functions. Specific to the respiratory system, glucocorticoids such as cortisol act to inhibit the inflammatory process, regulate β_2-adrenergic receptors, and stabilize vascular permeability.

Because asthma is characterized by mucosal inflammation, it is logical that exogenous steroids would play a valuable role in the management of that condition. Corticosteroids can be administered intravenously, orally, or by aerosol inhalation. With the exception of asthma, the role of steroids in other respiratory conditions is not universally embraced, particularly with respect to at what point they should be introduced relative to other pharmacologic interventions. As the reader can appreciate from discussions of other classes of medications in this chapter, the use of steroids in pulmonary disease is continually evolving as a result of ongoing clinical and laboratory research, resulting in the introduction of newer, more potent corticosteroids. Tables 8–3 and 8–4, taken from the 1997 NIH Asthma Guidelines, illustrate the relative potency of inhalational corticosteroids and their comparative suggested daily dosing.

The use of oral and IV steroids has long been a mainstay of therapy for acute and chronic asthma. In the past, symptom control in chronic asthma often involved the use of oral prednisone or another exogenous glucocorticoid, prescribed to asthmatic patients depending on the severity of the asthma and the clinical expertise of the physician. Patients who presented to the emergency department with an acute attack and who failed to respond to bronchodilators, such as inhaled β_2-agonists or IV aminophylline, received IV glucocorticoids such as methylprednisolone or hydrocortisone. The use of IV steroids required several hours before a response was seen, necessitating ongoing therapy with other agents for symptom management and stabilization until the glucocorticoids "kicked in." After admission to the hospital, the patient was transitioned from IV to oral steroid therapy over the course of several days and often discharged on oral prednisone.

Patients who take oral corticosteroids must do so according to a specific regimen not only to optimize their effects but also to minimize side effects. The use of systemic corticosteroids is not without significant risk, particularly when taken on a continued basis. The administration of exogenous corticosteroids can cause a blunting of adrenal gland function through suppression of the hypothalamic–pituitary–adrenal axis. This complex feedback mechanism interprets the presence of exogenous corticosteroids as a message to "turn off" adrenal gland cortisol production, ultimately leading to adrenal gland dysfunction. A life-threatening condition can occur if the patient is then

Table • 8–3   ESTIMATED COMPARATIVE DAILY DOSAGES FOR INHALED CORTICOSTEROIDS

Drug*	Low Dose	Medium Dose	High Dose
Adults			
Beclomethasone	168–504 µg	504–840 µg	>840 µg
42 µg/puff	(4–12 puffs—42 µg)	(12–20 puffs—42 µg)	(>20 puffs—42 µg)
84 µg/puff	(2–6 puffs—84 µg)	(6–10 puffs—84 µg)	(>10 puffs—84 µg)
Budesonide Turbuhaler	200–400 µg	400–600 µg	>600 µg
200 µg/dose	(1–2 inhalations)	(2–3 inhalations)	(>3 inhalations)
Flunisolide	500–1000 µg	1000–2000 µg	>2000 µg
250 µg/puff	(2–4 puffs)	(4–8 puffs)	(>8 puffs)
Fluticasone	88–264 µg	264–660 µg	>660 µg
MDI: 44, 110, 220 µg/puff	(2–6 puffs—44 µg) *or*	(2–6 puffs—110 µg)	(>6 puffs—110 µg) *or*
	(2 puffs—110 µg)		(>3 puffs—220 µg)
DPI: 50, 100, 250 µg/dose	(2–6 inhalations—50 µg)	(3–6 inhalations—100 µg)	(>6 inhalations—100 µg)
Triamcinolone acetonide	400–1000 µg	1000–2000 µg	>2000 µg
100 µg/puff	(4–10 puffs)	(10–20 puffs)	(>20 puffs)
Children			
Beclomethasone	84–336 µg	336–672 µg	>672 µg
42 µg/puff	(2–8 puffs)	(8–16 puffs)	(>16 puffs)
84 µg/puff			
Budesonide Turbuhaler	100–200 µg	200–400 µg	>400 µg
200 µg/dose		(1–2 inhalations—200 µg)	(>2 inhalations—200 µg)
Flunisolide	500–750 µg	1000–1250 µg	>1250 µg
250 µg/puff	(2–3 puffs)	(4–5 puffs)	(>5 puffs)
Fluticasone	88–176 µg	176–440 µg	>440 µg
MDI: 44, 110, 220 µg/puff	(2–4 puffs—44 µg)	(4–10 puffs—44 µg) *or*	(>4 puffs—110 µg)
		(2–4 puffs—110 µg)	
DPI: 50, 100, 250 µg/dose	(2–4 inhalations—50 µg)	(2–4 inhalations—100 µg)	(>4 inhalations—100 µg)
Triamcinolone acetonide	400–800 µg	800–1200 µg	>1200 µg
100 µg/puff	(4–8 puffs)	(8–12 puffs)	(>12 puffs)

The most important determinant of appropriate dosing is the clinician's judgment of the patient's response to therapy. The clinician must monitor the patient's response on several clinical parameters and adjust the dose accordingly. The stepwise approach to therapy emphasizes that once control of asthma is achieved, the dose of medication should be titrated carefully to the minimum dose required to maintain control, thus reducing the potential for adverse effect.

See Table 8–5 for an explanation of the rationale used for the comparative dosages. The reference point for the range in the dosages for children is data on the safety of inhaled corticosteroids in children, which, in general, suggest that the dose ranges are equivalent to beclomethasone dipropionate 200–400 µg/d (low dose), 400–800 µg/d (medium dose), and >800 µg/d (high dose).

Some dosages may be outside package labeling.

Metered-dose inhaler (MDI) dosages are expressed as the actuater dose (the amount of drug leaving the actuater and delivered to the patient), which is the labeling required in the United States. This is different from the dosage expressed as the valve dose (the amount of drug leaving the valve, all of which is not available to the patient), which is used in many European countries and in some of the scientific literature. Dry-powder inhaler (DPI) doses (eg, Turbuhaler) are expressed as the amount of drug in the inhaler following activation.

improperly withdrawn from pharmacologic therapy with corticosteroids, because the adrenal gland is not producing endogenous cortisol. For this reason, elaborate dosing schedules and tapering formulas must be implemented to ensure that gradual withdrawal allows for the adrenal gland to reestablish secretion of the necessary glucocorticoids.

Major metabolic and physiologic side effects are also associated with chronic exogenous corticosteroid use. Cushing's syndrome, a condition associated with long-term use of oral steroids such as prednisone, is characterized by a constellation of features, including fat redistribution, the development of a moon face and buffalo hump in the upper back; body hair growth (hirsutism); easily bruised skin; and acne. Asthmatic patients who require long-term use of exogenous steroids may also develop osteoporosis as a result of bone calcium loss, placing them at increased risk of fractures. Serious fluid and electrolyte disorders, hyperten-

sion, peptic ulcer, and labile emotions are other side effects associated with systemic corticosteroid therapy.

Inhaled steroids delivered by IPPB and nebulizer were available in the 1960s. In the 1970s, MDI steroids were introduced. Although steroid administration by IPPB and nebulizer is no longer used, it has only been since the late 1980s that MDI use as a primary alternative to systemic steroid therapy in patients with asthma and COPD has been appreciated. Glucocorticoids administered by inhalation developed a more prominent role in the management of asthma with the publication of the NIH Asthma Guidelines in 1991. This report reviewed the scientific information on the pathophysiology of asthma and on the major role that the inflammatory process plays in both early- and late-phase airway reactivity. NIH algorithms for the treatment of asthma illustrate the prominent role that inhaled (MDI) and oral steroids play in the treatment of this condition (see

Table • 8–4   ESTIMATED CLINICAL COMPARABILITY OF DOSES FOR INHALED CORTICOSTEROIDS

Data from in vitro and clinical trials suggest that the different inhaled corticosteroid preparations are not equivalent on a per puff or microgram basis. However, it is not entirely clear what implications these differences have for dosing recommendations in clinical practice because there are few data directly comparing the preparations. Relative dosing for clinical comparability is affected by differences in topical potency, clinical effects at different doses, delivery device, and bioavailability. The Expert Panel developed recommended dose ranges (see Table 8–3) for different preparations based on available data and the following assumptions and cautions about relative doses needed to achieve comparable clinical effect.
- Relative topical potency using human skin blanching
  - The standard test for determining relative topical antiinflammatory potency is the topical vasoconstriction (MacKenzie skin blanching) test.
  - The MacKenzie topical skin blanching test correlates with binding affinities and binding half-lives for human lung corticosteroid receptors (see table below).
  - The relationship between relative topical antiinflammatory effect and clinical comparability in asthma management is not certain. However, recent clinical trials suggest that different in vitro measures of antiinflammatory effect correlate with clinical efficacy.

Medication	Topical Potency (Skin Blanching)*	Corticosteroid Receptor Binding Half-Life (h)	Receptor Binding Affinity
Beclomethasone dipropionate (BDP)	600	7.5	13.5
Budesonide (BUD)	980	5.1	9.4
Flunisolide (FLU)	330	3.5	1.8
Fluticasone propionate (FP)	1200	10.5	18.0
Triamcinolone acetonide (TAA)	330	3.9	3.6

*Numbers are assigned in reference to dexamethasone, which has a value of "1" in the MacKenzie test.
- Relative doses to achieve similar clinical effects
  - Clinical effects are evaluated by a number of outcome parameters (eg, changes in spirometry, peak flow rates, symptom scores, quick-relief β_2-agonist use, frequency of exacerbations, airway responsiveness).
  - The daily dose and duration of treatment may affect these outcome parameters differently (eg, symptoms and peak flow may improve at lower doses and over a shorter treatment time than bronchial reactivity).
  - Delivery systems influence comparability. For example, the delivery device for budesonide (Turbuhaler) delivers approximately twice the amount of drug to the airway as does the metered dose inhaler (MDI), thus enhancing the clinical effect.
  - Individual patients may respond differently to different preparations, as noted by clinical experience.
Clinical trials comparing effects in reducing symptoms and improving peak expiratory flow demonstrate the following:
- BDP and BUD achieved similar effects at equivalent microgram doses by MDI.
- BDP achieved effects similar to twice the dose of TAA on a microgram basis.
  - FP achieved effects similar to twice the dose of BDP and BUD using an MDI on a microgram basis.
  - BUD by Turbuhaler achieved effects similar to twice the dose delivered by MDI, thus implying greater bronchial delivery by the delivery device.

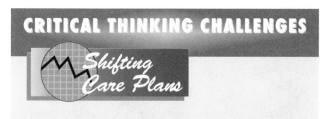

CRITICAL THINKING CHALLENGES
Shifting Care Plans

By the mid-1990s, the use of IV and oral steroid therapy began to wane, with inhaled corticosteroids evolving as a primary management strategy in the treatment of asthmatics. Four reasons for this shift toward the use of inhaled steroids are as follows:

1. An increased understanding of the mechanisms of airway inflammation in asthma

2. The introduction of more potent, long-acting inhaled glucocorticoid medications

3. Advances in MDI and holding chamber technology

4. Emergence of scientific literature, such as the NIH Asthma Guidelines, AARC Aerosol Consensus Statement, and AARC Clinical Practice Guidelines.

Appendix D). A growing body of research points to the early introduction of steroids in the management of asthma, using doses sufficient to achieve the therapeutic goals.

Inhaled steroids possess a high ratio of local to systemic effects, producing negligible systemic side effects as compared with oral steroids. The topical administration of potent inhaled steroids can be highly effective in controlling asthma symptoms, reducing frequency of exacerbations, and improving pulmonary function. The successful transition to inhaled steroids, with a concomitant reduction in systemic steroid use, must be viewed as a major benefit for patients who experienced minor and major systemic problems with oral steroid use. As Tables 8–3 and 8–4 show, the introduction of potent inhaled steroids presents the clinician with an excellent opportunity to manage the most severe asthma in a manner that minimizes oral steroid use.

Numerous clinical trials comparing the relative benefit of inhaled steroids demonstrate that they all clearly confer clinical antiinflammatory benefits when administered at recommended doses. The use of higher doses of inhaled steroids may confer additional benefits, such as a blunting of eosinophilic activity. Ongoing research is needed to identify the extent to which increasing clinical benefits accrue in a dose-dependent fashion, in light of the increased

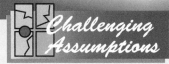

CRITICAL THINKING CHALLENGES

Challenging Assumptions

Patients who take MDI medications often describe it in the following manner: "Well, I take two puffs from a yellow inhaler, then two puffs from a white inhaler with a green tip. When I get tight in my chest, I take a couple of extra puffs from the yellow inhaler. I have a white inhaler that opens up into a tube, but I don't take it very often because I don't think it does any good. I tried it once or twice when I was wheezing, and it didn't do anything."

Have health care providers done the best job they could in educating patients to their medications? *No.*

We have a professional duty to engage in ongoing patient education with our clients. In addition to clinical and technical knowledge, practitioners must possess knowledge and skills in patient education and develop mechanisms to ensure that patients are educated to the medications they rely on for their health and well-being. The patient taking the medication from a "white inhaler that opens up into a tube" clearly does not understand the role of this steroid (Azmacort) as a "controller" drug for chronic management, rather than as a "rescue" drug for acute bronchospasm.

---

potential for systemic side effects. A study by Boe and colleagues[27] failed to demonstrate any statistically significant differences in treatment using 400 µg/d and 1000 µg/d beclomethasone in 128 asthmatic patients. Toogood[28] studied 34 asthmatic patients who were given doses of beclomethasone tapered down from 1600 µg/d, demonstrating symptom control in a dose-dependent fashion. Although multiple variables influenced the findings in these and other studies, some level of controversy exists about whether "more is better than less." This is an important consideration for the practitioner, who may be faced with requests to administer titrated doses or doses that exceed PDR recommendations. Close monitoring of patient response to therapy and an awareness of the heightened risks of dose-dependent systemic side effects must be recognized. The importance of inhaled steroids is illustrated by the emergence of higher-dose MDI steroid preparations, such as Vanceril Double Strength, which contains 84 µg/puff of beclomethasone diproprionate, twice the original dose of 42 µg/puff. The introduction of newer inhaled steroids, such as budesonide and fluticasone, both of which are potent, highly selective, long-acting agents, will certainly have an impact on future steroid dosing strategies.

The administration of inhaled steroids requires adherence to certain principles. The pulmonary antiinflammatory benefits conferred by use of these medications depends on their local deposition on the airway mucosa. Thus, proper administration techniques are critical to optimizing pulmonary effects and minimizing extrapulmonary side effects. Side effects are generally localized; the most serious side effect is the development of an oropharyngeal fungal infection (*Candida albicans,* or thrush), which in large part is related to dosage and delivery techniques. The use of a holding chamber with aerosol MDI steroid therapy has been shown to decrease oropharyngeal deposition significantly, thus reducing the incidence of oral candidiasis. The development of thrush may necessitate discontinuation of that inhaled steroid and the introduction of topical oral antifungal therapy. Other side effects seen with inhaled steroid use include hoarseness, dry and irritated throat, and cough, all of which are self-limited and transient. The introduction of non–CFC-propellant inhalers, and dry powder, breath-actuated inhalers, such as the Turbuhaler, which delivers budesonide, may affect both the efficacy of inhaled steroid therapy and its concomitant side effects (Box 8–2).

A number of nasal steroid preparations are available for the treatment of seasonal allergic rhinitis, estimated to oc-

---

Box • 8–2 STEPS TO TAKE WHEN ADMINISTERING INHALED STEROIDS

1. All propellant-driven inhaled steroids should be administered using a holding chamber. This reduces oropharyngeal deposition, decreasing the risks of oral candidiasis (thrush) and other localized side effects and increasing topical pulmonary deposition.
2. Because inhaled steroids work entirely by topical action, efforts should be made to maximize airway deposition and retention, as follows:

   - Each breath should be taken with a slow, deep inspiration, followed by a 5- to 10-second breath hold, when using propellant-driven metered dose inhaler canisters. (If other types of devices are used, follow manufacturer instructions.)
   - Patient's requiring concomitant aerosol bronchodilator therapy should inhale their bronchodilator first to increase airway caliber for maximal steroid deposition.
   - Patients on concomitant inhaled mucolytic therapy should receive their mucolytic therapy before their inhaled steroids (and bronchodilators). This clears airway secretions, enhancing airway mucosa deposition.
   - After the final steroid inhalation, the patient should rinse the mouth with water to eliminate any residual drug deposited in the oropharynx.

A growing number of asthmatics with allergic rhinitis are being placed on nasal steroids. Why?

Answer: There is a relationship between control of allergic rhinitis and asthma exacerbations.

cur in as many as 30 million Americans. These drugs act as antiinflammatory agents, reducing the nasal inflammation associated with allergic rhinitis. The symptoms of stuffy, runny, itchy nose and sneezing may be treated effectively with a variety of these topically active steroid sprays. Additionally, research suggests that failure to control rhinitis in asthmatic patients may precipitate asthma exacerbations. Fluticasone propionate (Flonase), one of the most recently available antirhinitic drugs, comes a 0.05% aqueous nasal spray. This drug is recommended for use once daily in adults, 1 to 2 sprays per nostril. Systemic side effects have not been reported at the recommended doses, with the most common complaint being topical nasal mucosal irritation.[29] Another recent addition to the family of nasal steroids is budesonide (Rhinocort). Other nasal steroids also available include trimacinolone acetonide (Nasacort) and beclomethasone dipropionate (Vancenase AQ nasal spray or Vancenase Pockethaler nasal inhaler).

Antimicrobial Medications

Antimicrobials are used in the treatment or prevention of infection. A variety of organisms are *pathogenic*, that is, capable of producing disease in humans; the most common of these organisms are bacteria and viruses. Multiple variables determine how a particular microorganism produces infection, how that infection manifests in the body, and how it is diagnosed and treated. In the outpatient setting, prevention or treatment of an infection most often involves the administration of oral antimicrobial medications, although there are occasional exceptions. In the acute or inpatient setting, administration more commonly occurs by IV or oral therapy, in an attempt to produce systemic levels of drug high enough to treat the infection.

The treatment of some pulmonary infections may also include the use of inhaled antimicrobials. Table 8–5 lists a number of selected organisms commonly associated with respiratory infections that might be treated with the inhalation of aerosolized antimicrobials. There is logic in attempting to deliver the drug directly to the site of infection (ie, the lung) in selected pulmonary conditions. The rationale for aerosolizing antimicrobials includes: (1) maximizing pulmonary deposition, (2) augmenting systemic antimicrobial therapy, and (3) avoiding systemic side ef-

Table • 8–5   RESPIRATORY INFECTIONS THAT MAY BE TREATED WITH AEROSOLIZED ANTIMICROBIALS

Organism	Antimicrobial Therapy
Patients With Cystic Fibrosis*	
Gram-negative *Pseudomonas aeruginosa*	Aminoglycosides (gentamicin, tobramycin)
Gram-negative *Staphylococcus aureus*	Aminoglycosides (gentamicin, tobramycin) Kanamycin, polymixin B
Patients With Respiratory Syncytial Virus Pneumonia	
Respiratory syncytial virus	Ribavirin (Virazole)
Patients With *Pneumocystis carinii* Pneumonia	
P. carinii (protozoan)	Pentamidine (NebuPent)
Opportunistic Infections	
Candida albicans (fungal)	Amphotericin B or nystatin

*Insufficient data are available to recommend routine use of aerosolized antibiotics to treat pulmonary infections. Their relative merit appears to derive from their role as a supplement to systemic treatment of persistent colonizing gram-negative organisms in patients with chronic pulmonary conditions that predispose to colonization, such as cystic fibrosis, chronic bronchitis, and bronchiectasis.

fects from oral or IV therapy. Certain conditions predispose to the use of inhaled antibiotics, including CF. Patients with CF have been treated successfully with inhaled gentamicin, tobramicin, and other agents specifically targeted at the gram-negative *Pseudomonas* species that predominates in pulmonary infections. SVN therapy given three or four times daily, often in conjunction with inhaled bronchodilators, can serve to treat an exacerbation effectively, limiting in-hospital stays and allowing for outpatient or home antibiotic therapy. The use of protocol care for patients requiring aerosolized antimicrobials can have a positive impact on both costs and outcome for this patient population. Effective use of outpatient aerosolized antimi-

Medico-Legal Alert #2

The administration of an antimicrobial to a patient who is allergic to that drug may have fatal consequences, producing anaphylactic reaction, respiratory arrest, and death. Under *no* circumstance should an RCP administer aerosolized antibiotics *until* he or she confirmed that the patient does not have a history of allergy to the prescribed drug. Claiming that, "the medical record was not available to check," or "I was too busy to review the medical record," or "the allergy section was not filled out by the nurse," is meaningless. The principle of affirmative duty requires that the RCP act as a patient advocate, ensuring that all care is in the patient's best interest and safety and should include a complete review of the medical record and direct communication with the patient.

crobial therapy has the potential for significant reductions in hospitalizations, with concomitant financial savings.

When administering aerosolized antimicrobials, it would be prudent to minimize exposure of the practitioner to the drug because this class of medications is not without side effects, including hypersensitivity. The use of reservoir nebulizers, such as the Respigard II, is recommended for antimicrobial aerosol medication administration because these devices can decrease environmental levels of drug. The additional costs associated with the use of a reservoir nebulizer system is outweighed by the added measure of safety it provides to care providers and others present during therapy.

Ribavirin

Infants and children who suffer from RSV pneumonia may respond to treatment with the antiviral agent ribavirin (Virazole). Ribavirin acts by cleaving the viral membrane on the RSV cell, preventing cell reproduction. The pathophysiology of RSV includes airway inflammation and hyperreactivity, increased mucus production, atelectasis, $\dot{V}/\dot{Q}$ mismatch, impaired gas exchange, and hypoxemia with or without hypercarbia. Severe cases of lower respiratory tract RSV pneumonia may necessitate intubation and mechanical ventilation. Even mild and moderate cases may cause increased morbidity and mortality if contracted in susceptible infants such as those who are immunocompromised or those who have concomitant cardiac disease.

The American Academy of Pediatrics first issued guidelines on the use of ribavirin in 1987, in an effort to identify appropriate use of this new antiviral agent.[30] Early research data pointed to the efficacy of ribavirin in symptom relief and improvement in pulmonary status.[31,32] Overall benefits of this drug in terms of reducing mortality associated with RSV pneumonia are less clear.[33] Issues such as when to initiate therapy, optimal dosing techniques, and safety contribute to the controversy surrounding this medication. Generally, it was thought that the earlier therapy is started, the more effective it is. Although ribavirin may be initiated without a definitive RSV diagnosis, rapid detection confirming the presence of RSV should occur to justify continuation of the drug. Because this medication is expensive (more than $1000 per day), and is associated with exposure risks to care providers, there is considerable variability nationwide about the frequency of its implementation to treat RSV infection.

Ribavirin is administered using a special aerosol delivery device called a *small-particle aerosol generator* (SPAG-2) nebulizer unit, manufactured specifically for the drug. The drug comes as a 6 g powder in a 100 mL glass vial, which is reconstituted with 300 mL sterile water (not normal saline) to achieve a delivery concentration of 20 mg/mL. Standard therapy involves delivering the solution by the SPAG-2 unit over a period of 12 to 18 hours for a course of 3 to 7 days. Alternative dosing strategies have been proposed because of exposure to the patient and care

provider.[34] The medication is usually delivered using an oxygen hood or mechanical ventilator. A scavenger unit is available for hood use to decrease environmental levels of the drug, thus reducing exposure to the care provider.[35,36] The manufacturer cautions against the use of ribavirin with ventilator patients except in situations in which skilled clinicians are present. The risk of sudden deterioration secondary to precipitate buildup in the ventilator circuit or endotracheal tube necessitates close monitoring and response. Sudden deterioration can also occur during ribavirin therapy from bronchospasm, requiring timely intervention with bronchodilators and manipulation of ventilator parameters.

Special precautions should be followed when using this medication because it has been shown to be teratogenic and embryocidal in some animal species tested. Standards have been established on isolation techniques and care provider exposure levels when the drug is administered in a clinical setting; these are summarized in Box 8–3. A 1988 Centers for Disease Control recommendation stated that women who are pregnant or actively pursuing pregnancy should avoid exposure and that female care providers should receive an alternative patient care assignment. Side effects from exposure include headache, conjunctivitis, rhinitis, nausea, rash, and dizziness. Cough and bronchospasm have been reported in health care providers with a history of reactive airways.

Box • 8–3 HEALTH CARE PROVIDER GUIDELINES DURING RIBAVIRIN ADMINISTRATION

- A screening system should be in place to exempt employees who may have a contraindication to exposure to ribavirin.
- Staff should be trained in proper safety procedures for handling ribavirin before, during, and after delivery.
- Appropriate personal protective equipment should be available and used during ribavirin administration and handling.
- Patients should be in negative-pressure rooms, with the door closed, and warning signs posted for staff and visitors.
- Scavenger systems and ventilator circuit filters should be used as appropriate to reduce airborne level of ribavirin during administration.
- These guidelines are based upon a review of scientific literature, recommendations from State Health Care agencies (ie, Cal/OSHA), the Ribavirin material safety data sheet, and prudent safety measures to minimize exposure to ribavirin. Each institution administering this medication should take into account specific standards or guidelines that may exist for their state.

Medicolegal Alert #3

Only caregivers who have been trained in the proper set-up, administration, and monitoring of ribavirin should be allowed to work with this medication. This is particularly applicable when the medication is administered by ventilator to a patient with an artificial airway in place. The risks of unrecognized airway obstruction or ventilator malfunction attributable to the buildup of drug residue can have fatal consequences for the patient. Clinicians must possess competency in the set-up, use, monitoring, and disposal of this medication before use.

In 1996, the American Academy of Pediatrics issued a statement that limits support for the use of aerosolized ribavirin. A lack of objective data clearly demonstrating the clinical efficacy of this medication has led to a significant decline in the use of ribavirin as a treatment modality for RSV pneumonia. Another factor contributing to its decline has been the introduction of a new drug to treat infants prophylactically who are at risk for developing RSV pneumonia. The polyclonal antibodies in RespiGam may prevent the development of RSV pneumonia in susceptible infants. Administered intravenously once per month prior to and during RSV season, this medication can reduce the likelihood for the infant developing RSV pneumonia and consequently the need for ribavirin.

Pentamidine

Inhaled microbials also have a role in the treatment of *Pneumocystis carinii* pneumonia (PCP). PCP is a pulmonary infection caused by a protozoan organism and is seen most commonly in patients with AIDS. Pentamidine isethionate (NebuPent) is an antimicrobial that possesses antiprotozoon properties. In the late 1980s, pentamidine became popular for PCP treatment or prophylaxis, administered by SVN. It was not uncommon to see pentamidine "puff parlors" set up in hospitals and outpatient clinics, with patients coming in for a monthly prophylactic aerosol treatment. Evolving research into the pharmacologic management of AIDS, including the introduction of protease inhibitors, has led to a relative decline in the use of inhaled pentamidine. Current guidelines for AIDS management relegate aerosolized pentamidine to a secondary role, with limited yet valuable application for PCP prophylaxis in high-risk human immunodeficiency virus–positive patients who have one or both of the following: (1) a history of one or more episodes of PCP, and (2) a peripheral CD4+ (T4 helper or inducer) lymphocyte count of 200 mm^3 or lower.

Pentamidine should be prepared as a 300-mg dose reconstituted in 6 mL of sterile water. Because PCP is an alveolar process, a special nebulizer is recommended, to generate a mass median aerodynamic diameter that maximizes alveolar deposition. The Respirgard II nebulizer contains a one-way valve on the inspiratory limb to optimize particle size, and a filter on the expiratory side to reduce environmental exposure of the medication (Fig. 8–6). No other medication should be mixed in the nebulizer with pentamidine. As with ribavirin, multiple environmental and infection control guidelines have been established to protect the care provider from exposure not only to pentamidine but also to potential pathogenic organisms coughed out from the patient's lungs during therapy, such as tuberculosis bacilli.[37,38] Care providers responsible for administration of pentamidine should receive thorough competency training in the safe, effective administration of this medication. The most common patient side effects are cough and bronchospasm, with some studies reporting a higher incidence in smokers and asthmatic patients.[39] These side effects require that a bronchodilator be immediately available for administration. The potential for bronchospasm necessitates a safety program that ensures timely administration of β_2-agonists or anticholinergics as needed, and some pentamidine administration centers pretreat their patients prophylactically with β_2-agonist bronchodilators.

Other antimicrobials that have been administered on occasion by inhalation include the antifungal drug amphotericin B, to treat opportunistic pulmonary fungal infections, and cephalexin monohydrage (Keflex), to treat chronic bronchitis. Because no published guidelines exist for using these medications by inhalation, their aerosol administration should be avoided unless the institution has established written protocols for their use and they have been approved by the institution's executive medical board and the pharmacy and therapeutic committee. Clear guidelines are required on indications and contraindications, hazards, dosage and frequency of therapy, and expected outcomes.

Future developments will lead to an expanded role for aerosolized antimicrobials. All care providers should be

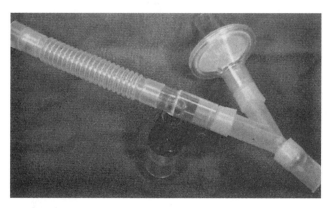

FIGURE 8–6 • Respirgard II small-volume medication nebulizer with one-way valves (for unidirectional gas flow), tubing reservoir, and expiratory particle filter. (Courtesy of Marquest Medical Products, Inc., Englewood, CO.)

aware of the potential side effects and risks associated with the administration of antimicrobials, not only to the patient but also to themselves. Anaphylactic reaction, hypersensitivity reaction, cough, and bronchospasm are side effects that should be planned for, recognized, and managed in a timely manner to ensure the well-being of both the patient and the care provider. As mentioned previously, practitioners should consider using special reservoir nebulizers, which significantly reduce environmental exposure to the antimicrobial aerosol during therapy.

Mucokinetic Agents

Mucokinesis refers to the mobilization of pulmonary secretions. Various agents can be administered to facilitate mucokinetic activity in the lung. These substances can be administered intravenously, by instillation down an artificial airway, or by aerosol inhalation. **Expectorants** are oral preparations used to facilitate removal of pulmonary secretions. These oral drugs act by stimulating the gastropulmonary mucokinetic vagal reflex, which triggers mucous secretions from the bronchial glands located in the airway mucosa. In addition to commercial oral expectorants, most of which contain the chemical guaifenesin, there is evidence to suggest that certain "spicy" food substances promote expectoration. For example, garlic, chili powder, and curry can stimulate rhinorrhea and productive cough, lending nonscientific credence to the folk wisdom of taking chicken soup to treat a cold. Box 8–4 lists a number of substances used to enhance the clearance of pulmonary secretions.

The most common mucokinetic agent is water. Whether taken orally or by inhalation, it represents the default choice for assisting with secretion mobilization. The AARC Clinical Practice Guideline on Bland Aerosol Administration articulates the clinical role of sterile water and hypotonic, isotonic, and hypertonic saline solutions in the diagnosis and treatment of pulmonary conditions in which secretion mobilization might need to be augmented pharmacologically.[40] One of the primary mucokinetic agents available to clinicians for the past 30 years has been *N*-acetylcysteine. The proposed mechanism by which this agent works is disruption of disulfide bonds in nonpurulent sputum. Standard doses of 10% or 20% concentration, diluted with normal saline, are usually administered using a

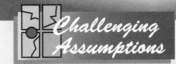

CRITICAL THINKING CHALLENGES
Challenging Assumptions

Truth be told, a paucity of clinical research exists regarding the efficacy of *N*-acetylcysteine; rather, it is most commonly used as a result of habit, having been passed down from generation to generation of pulmonologists (or RCPs) as a valuable therapy "that works with their patients." Other methods that are more cost-effective and less potentially harmful should be attempted before the use of *N*-acetylcysteine. These methods include bland aerosol therapy, systemic hydration with oral fluids, or IV therapy should an IV line be in place. In patients who require secretion mobilization, less expensive and safer techniques should be attempted first, such as lung expansion therapy, positive expiratory pressure, or flutter. The continued use of aerosolized *N*-acetylcysteine in the absence of documented clinical efficacy poses yet another risk—legal liability. Should a patient experience a significant reaction to an aerosol treatment, leading to a negative outcome and lawsuit, one must wonder where the defense attorney would find credible experts to testify to the medical appropriateness of aerosolized mucolytics like *N*-acetylcysteine.

nebulizer. A 1970 study by Rao and associates[41] showed that in 16 patients with obstructive lung disease, administration of a 20% solution led to bronchospastic reactions, adversely affecting pulmonary mechanics and gas exchange. It is therefore recommended that patients with known or suspected hyperreactive airways receive the drug in conjunction with a bronchodilator. A more prudent clinical strategy would be to evaluate whether the drug is clinically indicated at all.

One area in which *N*-acetylcysteine has unique value is in the treatment of overdose with acetaminophen (Tylenol). Metabolic actions of *N*-acetylcysteine, when taken orally, help inactivate byproducts of acetaminophen, reducing the latter drug's toxic effects on the liver. Standard therapy for overdose management is 30 to 40 mL taken orally, perhaps with a cola drink to alleviate the drug's nauseating (rotten-egg–like) taste.

Dornase Alfa

In the early 1990s, Genentech received FDA approval and began marketing the biotechnology drug dornase alfa (Pulmozyme). This drug is cloned from the gene for human DNase. Laboratory and clinical studies demonstrated that dornase alfa hydrolyses extracellular DNA in purulent sputum, producing a thinning effect on sputum.[42] DNA is pro-

---

Box • 8–4 MUCOKINETIC AGENTS

Sterile water or saline solution (isotonic, hypotonic, or hypertonic)
N-acetylcysteine
Dornase alfa (Pulmozyme)
Saturated solution of potassium iodide (SSKI)
Guaifenesin

duced from degenerating leukocytes that accumulate in response to the infectious process in the lung. Initial approval limited dornase alfa use to selected patients with CF who had a forced vital capacity of greater than or equal to 40% of the predicted value. CF is a condition characterized by chronic sputum hypersecretion and colonization with gram-negative organisms, which leads to pulmonary infections, decline in pulmonary function, and repeated hospitalizations. The chronic condition of mucus hypersecretion, plugging, and infection leads to progressive lung tissue destruction, $\dot{V}/\dot{Q}$ mismatch, gas exchange abnormalities, and ultimately respiratory failure and death. The introduction of a pharmacologic agent that can help clear pulmonary secretions, reduce the incidence of infection, and improve lung function may contribute to reducing morbidity and improving the quality of life for many CF patients. Secondary clinical trials with this drug subsequently led to its approval for use in COPD patients, such as those with chronic bronchitis, in whom regular secretion clearance therapy may prove useful. Dornase alfa can be incorporated successfully into bronchial hygiene protocols that include postural drainage therapy, positive expiratory pressure, intermittent percussive ventilation, high frequency chest wall oscillation or Flutter, as an adjunct for secretion clearance.

Pulmozyme is marketed as a single-use ampule containing 2.5 mg in 2.5 mL normal saline. The drug should remain refrigerated until just before use and is delivered using special nebulizer. The clinical trials were conducted using three specific brands of nebulizer: the Hudson T Up-draft II, Marquest Acorn II, and PARI LC Jet+. Although the use of another type of nebulizer is not absolutely contraindicated, the manufacturer recommends use of one of the three aforementioned brands to ensure appropriate delivery. The chemistry of the drug precludes mixing any other substance, such as a bronchodilator, in the nebulizer. For CF patients with hyperreactive airways, it therefore is recommended that the bronchodilator treatment be administered first, either by MDI or nebulizer, followed by nebulization of Pulmozyme. Standard dosing involves administration of dornase alfa once or twice daily. Commonly reported side effects are benign and include voice change and laryngitis.

Cough Management

Although effective mobilization of pulmonary secretions includes the ability to have a strong, effective cough, the presence of a persistent nonproductive cough may be bothersome, affecting activities of daily living and disrupting sleep. Additionally, uncontrolled coughing can contribute to throat irritation, thoracic pain, and even spontaneous rib fracture and pneumothorax. In these situations, patient evaluation may lead to the recommendation that a cough suppressant be used. Narcotic cough suppressants are available, with codeine as a common ingredient. Because of the side effects associated with codeine, however, more commonly a nonnarcotic cough preparation is recommended. The most common ingredient in over-the-counter cough medications is dextromethorphan.

Gas Therapy

More than 50 years ago, Barach pioneered the use of a mixture of helium and oxygen (**heliox**) gas to treat pulmonary conditions exhibiting increased airway resistance, such as asthma. Carbon dioxide gas therapy was commonly used in the 1960s and early 70s due to its vasodilating properties and has gained renewed application in selected children with hypoplastic left-heart syndrome (HLHS). The administration of nitric oxide has gained widespread attention in the 1990s for the treatment of a variety of conditions associated with pulmonary hypertension. Heliox, nitric oxide, carbon dioxide, and various volatile anesthetic gases, all of which involve administration by practitioners, play a valuable role in the pharmacologic management of selected cardiopulmonary disorders. A basic understanding of these gases can broaden the practitioner's arsenal of therapies available to treat patients with cardiopulmonary disorders. Further information on this topic can be found in Chapter 10.

Heliox

Although heliox therapy has fallen into relative disuse since its introduction in the 1940s, its therapeutic benefits have a rationale basis and are employed today in many fa-

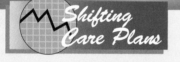

CRITICAL THINKING CHALLENGES

Shifting Care Plans

Patients with cystic fibrosis or chronic obstructive pulmonary disease might benefit from the use of aerosolized dornase alfa (Pulmozyme). The costs of adding this therapy to their daily management regimen range from $3000 to $6000 per year. What variables must be considered in determining whether or not this is cost-effective care?

1. Does the use of Pulmozyme decrease the frequency and or severity of exacerbations?

2. Does the use of Pulmozyme decrease the use of other medications, such as antimicrobials?

3. Is the long-term decrease in the decline of pulmonary function a factor in improving the health (and productivity) of the patient?

Just as with the introduction of leukotriene modifiers, the cost/benefit ratio must be addressed before incorporating new medications into the patient's care plan.

CRITICAL THINKING CHALLENGES

Case Scenario

You are caring for a 12-year-old boy with multiple tracheal tumors. The tumors have produced airway narrowing, leading to mild respiratory distress and compromised gas exchange. For the past 36 hours, you have been administering oxygen and aerosolized racemic epinephrine q 2–4 h to help maintain airway caliber and oxygenation, while the patient undergoes radiation therapy. Suddenly the patient deteriorates, exhibiting hypercarbia, hypoxemia, increased shortness of breath, tachypnea, tachycardia, and labored breathing. The tumors are too low in the trachea to allow the use of an endotracheal tube, and the airway is so narrowed that only a 3.0 tube could be inserted, too small to allow for adequate ventilation of a 130-lb 12-year-old. Are any pharmacologic options available to you?

Answer: Heliox gas therapy, *but*

1. Is it available at your facility?

2. Do you have the proper equipment to administer it?

3. Do you have a policy and procedure governing its proper, safe use?

4. Are your staff competently trained to administer heliox safely and effectively?

cilities across the country.[43] The basic principle behind the use of heliox lies in its low density. The density of air is 1.29 g/L and that of oxygen is 1.43 g/L. A mixture of 80% helium and 20% oxygen has a density of 0.43 g/L, about one third that of oxygen or air. A gas with a lower density requires less driving pressure to generate flow through a tube (Poiseuille's law). Additionally, Graham's law states that gas diffusion is inversely proportional to the square root of its density. The use of a mixture of 80:20 heliox gas would therefore promote more efficient gas flow and diffusion relative to that of an air–oxygen mixture. In patients with selected conditions associated with airway obstruction, the use of a heliox gas mixture can facilitate improved flow, thus reducing the work of breathing and enhancing distribution of ventilation and better $\dot{V}/\dot{Q}$ and gas exchange.[44–47] Patients with upper and central airway tumors or upper airway obstruction secondary to edema, such as occurs after extubation, may benefit from a trial of heliox gas therapy.

Nitric Oxide

Nitric oxide is an unstable gas that occurs naturally in the body as a normal product of biochemical processes. A growing body of literature points to the important role of nitric oxide in a variety of homeostatic processes, one of which is vasomotor tone.[47,48] The presence of endogenous nitric oxide contributes to the delicate balance of vascular tone in both the pulmonary and systemic circulations. Multiple conditions can upset this balance, leading to pulmonary hypertension and its sequelae, including $\dot{V}/\dot{Q}$ abnormalities and hypoxia. The administration of exogenous nitric oxide gas in concentrations ranging from 5 to 80 ppm can help modulate pulmonary vascular tone, reducing pulmonary artery pressure and leading to improved $\dot{V}/\dot{Q}$, gas exchange, and oxygenation. Nitric oxide produces its effects by inhibiting the "constricting" action of Ca^{2+} ions in cells of smooth muscle.

Nitric oxide is administered as a gas, most commonly titrated into the ventilator circuit of critically ill patients. The use of nitric oxide has been shown to be of benefit in a variety of cardiopulmonary conditions, including ARDS and persistent pulmonary hypertension of the newborn.[49] The administration of nitric oxide involves sophisticated technology and meticulous attention to detail because its use can present significant potential risks to the patient. For this reason, close attention must be paid to the set-up and administration of this gas, and users should possess a thorough understanding of its risks and benefits.[50,51]

Carbon Dioxide

Infants born with the congenital heart defect of HLHS rely on the presence of an atrial-septal defect and patent ductus arteriosus for life-sustaining systemic circulation. During the initial period when the condition exists or is being treated with palliative surgeries, the survival of the infant centers on maintaining a delicate balance between the pulmonary and systemic circulations through these shunts. Increases in oxygen or reductions in carbon dioxide levels can lead to unwanted closure of the patent ductus arteriosus (PDA), leading to an imbalance in the pulmonary and systemic circulations, pulmonary flooding, decreased systemic circulation, metabolic acidosis, shock, and death. Consequently, it is sometimes necessary to manipulate the infant's O_2 or CO_2 levels through exogenous administration of either hypoxic gas mixtures (FIO_2 less than 21%) or carbon dioxide gas. Because elevated $PaCO_2$ causes pulmonary vasoconstriction, judicious titration of endogenous CO_2 gas can help manipulate the PDA and control the tenuous homeostasis between systemic and pulmonary blood flow.[52,53] The use of carbon dioxide gas therapy to manage patients with HLHS involves the delivery of known concentrations of CO_2 gas, ranging from 1% to 4%, through the infant's gas administration device or ventilator circuit. The use of premixed cylinders of CO_2 and O_2 is most desirable because the use of pure CO_2 gas in a system would have fatal consequences should the infant be unknowingly exposed to 100% CO_2 by human error or equipment malfunction. A low flow of CO_2 and O_2 gas is titrated into the breathing system, with the use of a CO_2 analyzer (capnometer) to confirm the actual concentration of CO_2 delivery at the patient's airway. Physiologic monitoring of vascular pressures, transcutaneous CO_2, and arterial blood gases guides the clinician in adjusting the level of CO_2 administration to meet the clinical goals. Because of the sophisticated technology involved in this gas therapy and the unstable condition of the infant with HLHS, CO_2 administration is usually confined to tertiary-care newborn and pediatric intensive care units where staff are available with advanced training and competency in this delicate therapy.

Surfactant Replacement Therapy

The presence of surfactant, a surface-active substance naturally found in the alveoli, helps maintain alveolar geometry during exhalation, preventing alveolar collapse. Pulmonary surfactant is produced by the type II pneumocytes of the alveolar cells and is composed predominantly of phospholipids (80% or more), proteins (10% or less), and neutral lipids (10% or less). Pulmonary conditions, such as ARDS and RDS of the newborn, are highlighted by the presence of abnormal levels of or dysfunctional surfactant. The abnormalities associated with surfactant deficiencies include atelectasis, reduced functional residual capacity and compliance, $\dot{V}/\dot{Q}$ mismatch, and shunting. The consequences are impaired gas exchange, hypoxia, and respiratory failure.

Efforts have been made to restore lung function by the delivery of exogenous surfactant. Exogenous surfactants are derived from two primary sources; they are scavenged from mammalian lung (human, bovine, porcine) or produced synthetically. As of 1996, the FDA had approved two brands for clinical use, Survanta and Exosurf, for administration by either aerosol delivery or liquid instillation. Clinical trials of surfactant replacement therapy are ongoing to determine appropriate dosage and timing, delivery techniques, and outcomes data. Studies have shown that the safe, effective delivery of exogenous surfactants can contribute to decreased morbidity and mortality in in-

fants with RDS.[54] The beneficial effects of this therapy in adults with ARDS are less definitive. The dynamics of ARDS, coupled with the technical issues associated with both the drug preparation and delivery technology, have led to a lack of data clearly showing value.[55] Research is ongoing to define more clearly the role of surfactant replacement therapy in pulmonary disease.

Multiple considerations surround the administration of exogenous surfactants, described in a comprehensive review of the topic by Haas and Weg.[54] RCPs play a central role in surfactant replacement therapy because most of these patients require some level of ventilatory support. Risks associated with administration include bradycardia and dramatic changes in oxygenation and lung compliance. Therefore, only knowledgeable, competent clinicians should administer this drug because timely, appropriate interventions must occur in the presence of significant side effects. Surfactant replacement therapy can positively affect both patient outcome and health care costs, through more efficient use of human and equipment resources, decreased morbidity, and decreased length of stay. These factors add value to the role of the RCP as an important member of the critical care team. RCPs are encouraged to consult the AARC Clinical Practice Guideline on Surfactant Replacement Therapy for a better understanding of the clinical application and delivery techniques of this medication.[56]

CLINICAL ADMINISTRATION OF AEROSOLIZED MEDICATIONS

Multiple options are available to the care provider for the delivery of aerosolized pharmacologic agents. The primary considerations are concerned with the medication itself and the desired therapeutic outcomes. Certain drugs may be available only in MDI form or may exist in solution form but have restrictions on their administration, such as described with Pulmozyme. Others may require large-volume delivery, such as with ribavirin, necessitating that specific manufacturer guidelines be followed regarding equipment and delivery techniques. The clinician always should consult the manufacturer's product information first, to determine if any guidelines or limitations exist with respect to the aerosol administration of the medication. Failure to deliver pharmacologic agents appropriately

---

CRITICAL THINKING CHALLENGES

Go Figure

You are asked to administer Survanta to a premature newborn weighing 750 g. The administration dose is 100 mg/kg. Your ampule of Survanta contains 200 mg of medication contained in 8 mL of NaCl. What volume of Survanta will you draw up to deliver?

Answer: Milligram dosage for infant: **75 mg**   (750 g = 0.75 kg × 100 mg/kg)
Volume dosage for infant: **3.0 mL**   (200 mg/8 mL ∞ 75 mg/X)

not only compromises their therapeutic value but could also adversely affect patient morbidity and mortality!

A variety of bronchodilator medications were described previously, many of which can be administered by nebulization. For these drugs, multiple variables play a role in the selection of equipment and delivery techniques. As described previously, the use of medication administration protocols can be effective in optimizing pharmacologic therapy with the desired clinical outcomes achieved in a cost-effective manner. RCPs possess the skills to assess need, select and implement the best delivery strategies, and monitor and adjust therapy based on patient response.

Aerosol administration of bronchodilators in the 1950s involved the use of IPPB devices, which used the application of positive pressure to delivery the medication into the lungs within a pressurized stream of gas. A critical review of IPPB therapy, presented at the Sugerloaf conference in 1974, led to a consensus that most patients could be treated effectively with aerosolized drugs using a hand-held nebulizer, with the patient spontaneously breathing in the medication. By the late 1970s, HHN therapy had replaced IPPB as the default technique for bronchodilator medication administration. MDI, also available since the 1950s, delivers a fixed dose of bronchodilator medication from a canister pressurized with CFC gases serving as propellant gases. In the late 1970s, a new generation of steroid medications were introduced, available only in MDI form. These medications, such as beclomethasone diproprionate, were administered to patients as an MDI "add-on" after HHN therapy with a β_2-agonist bronchodilator. Although second- and third-generation MDI bronchodilator medications were introduced into clinical medicine during the late 1970s and early 1980s, clinical practice combining HHN bronchodilator and MDI steroid by and large continued throughout the early 1980s.

In the late 1980s, several factors contributed to a fundamental shift in the role of MDI toward that of a primary therapy modality: (1) a growing number of potent, long-acting β_2-agonists introduced from Europe, (2) the introduction of spacer and holding chamber technology, (3) clinical research on the efficacy of MDI therapy, and (4) a growing mandate to control costs. The use of spacer devices, such as the Ace or Aerochamber, helped to bring MDI therapy to the forefront as a primary treatment strategy. These devices enhanced MDI drug delivery through improved lung deposition and decreased oropharyngeal deposition, thus reducing side effects. During the latter half of the 1980s and into the 1990s, a growing body of research pointed to the equivalency of MDI to HHN in all types of patient populations, delivered at a fraction of the cost. Publications such as the 1991 AARC Aerosol Consensus Statement, the AARC Clinical Practice Guidelines,[57,58] and the NIH Asthma Guidelines all helped to establish MDI therapy as a primary technique for bronchodilator and steroid administration. By the mid-1990s, a large percentage of hospitals had adopted MDI as the default therapy, often administered within the context of protocol-driven therapy, popular at that time.

As mentioned previously, first-generation MDIs introduced in the mid-1950s used pressurized CFC gases to deliver the medication. The recognized hazardous effects of Freon on the earth's atmosphere (the greenhouse effect) led to a proposed ban on the use of CFC propellants by the year 2000. The pharmaceutical industry responded by pursuing the development of alternatives to CFC-propellant MDIs. Proventil HFA, an MDI preparation of albuterol, uses the non-CFC propellant hydrofluoroalkane (HFA).

The pharmaceutical industry also introduced DPI and BAI devices, such as the Maxair Autohaler, which dispenses the β_2-agonist pirbuterol acetate. BAI devices are activated to deliver the bolus of drug in response to the patient's inspiratory effort and use about two thirds less CFC propellant than do conventional MDIs. Advantages of BAI devices include increased volume of active drug, allowing for longer use of the canister, and no need for a spacer device, both of which may represent cost savings to the patient. Clinical studies have demonstrated that BAI devices provide comparable clinical results to those of conventional MDIs, particularly in specific patient populations such as the elderly.[59]

Albuterol, beclomethasone, and budesonide are examples of medications available in DPI form. A DPI-containing salmeterol xinafoate (Serevent) was introduced in 1998. The Serevent Diskus® contains sixty doses of medication in powder form. Patient breath actuation delivers each dose from the device into the patient's lungs. The Diskus incorporates a built-in counter, which displays the number of doses left in the device, counting down from sixty to zero. In addition to providing the patient with feedback on the number of doses remaining, the counter allows both the patient and the practitioner to document compliance with the daily dosing regimen. DPI preparations of β_2-agonists and steroids have not enjoyed widespread use, owing to technical administration considerations; however, studies have shown that they

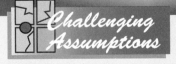

CRITICAL THINKING CHALLENGES
Challenging Assumptions

Are bronchodilator medications delivered by MDI as clinically effective as the same medication administered by aerosol nebulization?

Answer: Yes. A large volume of scientific research points to the equivalent efficacy of bronchodilators delivered by MDI or HHN across the full spectrum of pediatric to geriatric patients. When proper dosing and administration techniques are met, clinical responses are comparable for such measures as pulmonary function, symptom control, exacerbations, emergency room and hospital admission rates, and quality of life indices.

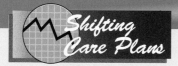 **CRITICAL THINKING CHALLENGES**

Technology has gone well beyond the days of the simple HHN treatment which combined a small dose of medication with normal saline diluent. By the mid-1990s, a variety of techniques existed for the delivery of aerosolized bronchodilators by nebulization (see Box 8–5). These techniques all confer a combination of two potential advantages over standard HHN therapy: (1) increased efficacy, and (2) decreased costs. Financial savings may occur through use of less expensive equipment or more efficient allocation of human resources. In the era of man-

aged care and capitation, aerosol pharmacology has not escaped the keen eye of the bean counters and administrators. The efficient use of supplies and personnel can represent significant savings to institutions engaged in aerosol medication administration. Although beyond the scope of this pharmacology chapter, the reader is encouraged to review the references cited for each of the techniques listed in Box 8–5. Appropriate use of these devices and techniques can benefit patient outcome, resource use, and costs.

possess equivalent efficacy to that of standard MDIs if taken properly. As pharmaceutical companies explore alternative non-CFC propellants, such as HFA, and alternative MDI devices, their application will continue to evolve.[60]

An exciting new area of aerosol research is exploring the use of DPI for treatment of a wide range of nonpulmonary conditions. Inhale Therapeutic Systems (Palo Alto, CA) is developing aerosol medications to treat conditions such as diabetes, osteoporosis, and immune disorders. Special technology allows for the delivery of a single breath of a powdered preparation of insulin deep into the lungs, where it is absorbed into the bloodstream to exert its effects. The potential application of aerosol pharmacology to a whole host of medical conditions promises to expand the role of the RCP far beyond that of treating pulmonary conditions.[61–71]

NONPULMONARY MEDICATIONS RELATED TO THE RESPIRATORY SYSTEM

Cardiovascular Drugs

Respiratory care practitioners are involved in the management of patients who frequently are receiving cardiovascular medications. A knowledge of cardiovascular drugs is

essential, especially for RCPs engaged in critical care. The ability to assess patient needs and apply appropriate respiratory care requires an understanding of the patient's cardiovascular drug therapy. We strongly recommend that all RCPs who work in that environment pursue advanced cardiac life support or neonatal resuscitation program credentialing where the use of these drugs is taught in the context of clinical application.

Cardiovascular drugs fall into several categories, including the following:

Antiarrhythmic agents: Used to alter the electromechanical performance of the heart, such as lidocaine, atropine, and verapamil
Cardiac output agents: Used to strengthen the force of myocardial contraction, such as with digitalis (a cardiac glycoside), or to stimulate the force and frequency of contractions, such as occurs with epinephrine
Blood pressure agents: Used either to reduce (antihypertensives) or elevate blood pressure
Diuretics: Used to increase urine output; may be used in the treatment of hypertension, but are used primarily to promote the elimination of excess vascular volume
Antiangina agents: Used to treat classic chest pain (angina pectoris); the primary class includes nitrates, such as sublingual tablets or transdermal patches containing nitroglycerine

Central and Peripheral Nervous System Drugs

A variety of medications are administered for their direct action on the central or peripheral nervous system. These include skeletal muscle relaxants, sedatives and hypnotics, stimulants and depressants, and analgesics. Practitioners must possess a working knowledge of these classes of drugs because their administration can have a profound influence on respiratory function. Although an in-depth discussion of these drugs is beyond the scope of this textbook, what follows is a brief overview of these classes of medications.

Box • 8–5 NEBULIZATION TECHNIQUES

Continuous nebulization with large-volume nebulizers[61–66]
Hand-held nebulizer therapy with positive expiratory pressure[67–69]
Hand-held nebulizer therapy with heliox gas mixtures[70]
Hand-held nebulizer therapy with a reservoir device (Circulaire)[71]
Hand-held nebulizer therapy without any diluent (full strength)

Skeletal Muscle Relaxants

Skeletal muscle relaxants, referred to as *neuromuscular blocking agents,* fall into two general categories based on their mode of action (see Fig. 8–4). Essentially, both types of drug produce paralysis of skeletal muscle, such as would be necessary during surgery or endotracheal intubation. Nondepolarizing agents exert their paralytic action by competitively blocking acetylcholine receptors at skeletal muscle receptor sites. Unable to respond to endogenous acetylcholine because of the presence of the drug, the patient's skeletal muscle is unable to contract, resulting in paralysis. The classic nondepolarizing drug is curare. Curariform drugs include such agents as tubocurarine and vecuronium. These drugs are administered intravenously, with an onset of action of 1 to 2 minutes and a duration of action of several hours, depending on the dosage.

A drug in this category might be used as a continuous IV infusion to produce paralysis during mechanical ventilation. Newborns on ventilatory support may be paralyzed, to blunt their spontaneous ventilation to reduce O_2 consumption and CO_2 production. Status asthmaticus patients who are difficult to ventilate mechanically might receive a paralyzing agent to decrease dyschronism between spontaneous and mechanical breaths. Succinylcholine (Anectine) is an example of a depolarizing paralytic agent. This medication acts by depolarizing the muscle cells, producing a transient wave of muscle contraction (fasciculation). Once contracted, the muscle is unable to respond further and essentially is in a state of paralysis. Succinylcholine has a short onset of action when given intravenously and a very short duration of action, usually less than 5 minutes. It is an ideal agent to use when performing an intubation.

Both classes of skeletal muscle relaxants obliterate normal respiratory function. The practitioner involved in the care of patients receiving this class of drugs must possess skills in airway management and artificial ventilation to ensure that the patient is ventilated and oxygenated adequately during the period of paralysis. Additional side effects of neuromuscular blocking agents include cardiovascular instability and bronchospasm, both of which must be monitored for and treated in a timely manner.

Analgesics, Respiratory Stimulants, Sedatives, and Hypnotics

Analgesics, respiratory stimulants, sedatives, and hypnotics all act directly on the central nervous system. Analgesics, sedatives and hypnotics may exert an undesirable effect on the respiratory centers in the medulla, leading to respiratory depression. Multiple factors determine to what extent, if any, respiratory function is compromised; these include type of medication, dosage and frequency of administration, and the unique characteristics of the patient. The practitioner should be aware of and monitor for changes in depth and frequency of spontaneous ventilation in a patient receiving drugs in these categories. The prompt recognition of respiratory compromise, coupled with timely appropriate intervention, can prevent a life-threatening respiratory event.

Nicotine Replacement Therapy

Individuals who develop an addiction to nicotine through tobacco use may require nicotine replacement therapy as part of their smoking cessation program. Nicotine is one of the strongest addictive agents known, and the ability to wean oneself from the drug is difficult. A variety of nicotine replacement products are available, including gums,

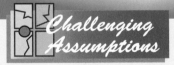

CRITICAL THINKING CHALLENGES
Challenging Assumptions

RCPs can play a valuable role in curbing the use of tobacco delivery systems, not only by becoming involved in smoking cessation programs but also by encouraging teens and others to avoid developing a nicotine addiction habit. Serving as a role model by personally not smoking can send a powerful message to those we treat and to those we come in contact with professionally and socially. Consider the message communicated by an RCP treating a patient while carrying a pack of cigarettes in their lab coat pocket. RCPs must become active advocates for a tobacco-free America.

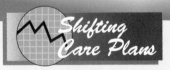

CRITICAL THINKING CHALLENGES
Shifting Care Plans

For cost-containment reasons, efforts are being made to shift patients from brand-name drugs to generic substitutions. Managed care programs may promote formulary restriction on the use of more expensive brand-name medications.

Beware!

Although generic formulations may contain the same type and quantity of medication as the brand name, their biologic activity is not always comparable. A study by Horn and coworkers[73] showed a correlation between formulary restrictions and increased use of health care services in asthmatic patients. RCPs should be vigilant concerning any changes in a patient's pulmonary status that might be related to medication substitutions dictated by their insurance carrier.

transdermal skin patches, and even nasal sprays. No one product has been shown to be more effective than another. Successful tobacco cessation programs are those that combine optimal pharmacologic therapy with effective education and support.

Bupropion HCL (Zyban) was introduced in 1997 as the first non-nicotine therapy for smoking cessation. The drug's mechanisms of action are thought to involve the neurochemical pathways associated with nicotine addiction and nicotine withdrawal. Zyban comes in tablet form, and is taken once or twice a day in a systematic manner over the course of several weeks. Preliminary results of clinical trials are promising, but the long-term role of this smoking cessation medication remains unknown, especially in relation to the use of existing nicotine-replacement drugs. Since Zyban has multiple contraindications and precautions regarding its use, practitioners are encouraged to seek a complete profile on this medication from the manufacturer (Glaxo Wellcome) and consult scientific literature.

A SPECIAL NOTE ON GERIATRIC DRUG USE

The aging of the American population has particular meaning for those who administer medications to the elderly. People older than 65 years take three times as many drugs as do younger people, averaging 13 prescription medications per year. For a variety of reasons, the elderly experience twice as many adverse reactions to medications as do younger people. Multiple physiologic changes alter the pharmacokinetics of drugs in elderly patients. **Polypharmacy**, a condition in which a patient takes a variety of medications in a manner that produces adverse effects, contributes to the challenge facing those who care for geriatric patients. Noncompliance due to physical, psychological, or economic reasons can also contribute to medication "failures." Another consideration is the potential lack of sufficient or ongoing education of elderly patients to the drugs they are taking. Every practitioner should receive specific education in the dynamics of elder care and in the significance of medication use and administration in geriatric patients. Specific knowledge concerning care of the elderly can contribute to better management of chronic illnesses, better health promotion and disease prevention, decreased morbidity and mortality, and enhanced quality of life.

SUMMARY

Respiratory care practitioners play a valuable role in the administration of aerosolized medications for the treatment of pulmonary disorders. Safe, appropriate delivery of inhaled medications requires an in-depth understanding across the entire spectrum of respiratory care academia. RCPs can serve as valuable resources and members of the health care team, as long as they continue to educate themselves about the latest research findings and technology related to aerosol medication administration. Focusing on outcome-oriented care positively affects the quality of care.[72] In addition, appropriate aerosol medication administration contributes to cost-efficient care, adding value to the presence of RCPs in the future health care delivery landscape.

References

1. Goodman LS, Gilman AG. *The Pharmacologic Basis of Therapeutics.* 9th ed. New York: McGraw Hill; 1996.
2. Harvey RA, Champe PC. *Lippincott's Illustrated Reviews: Pharmacology.* Philadelphia: JB Lippincott; 1992.
3. Rau JL Jr. *Respiratory Care Pharmacology.* Chicago: Year Book Medical Publishers; 1995.
4. Witek TJ, Schachter EN. *Pharmacology and Therapeutics in Respiratory Care.* Philadelphia: WB Saunders; 1994.
5. AARC aerosol consensus statement. *Respir Care.* 1991;30(9): 916–921.
6. *AARC Clinical Practice Guidelines.* Dallas: AARC; 1991–1996.
7. *Guidelines for the Diagnosis and Management of Asthma.* Washington, DC: National Asthma Education Program; 1991. US Department of Health and Human Services publication NIH 91–3042.
8. *Highlights of the Expert Panel Report. II. Guidelines for the Diagnosis and Management of Asthma.* Washington, DC: National Asthma Education Program; 1997. US Department of Health and Human Services publication NIH No. 97-4015A.
9. Hess D, Fisher D, Williams P, et al. Medication nebulizer performance: Effects of diluent volume, nebulizer flow, and nebulizer brand. *Chest.* 1996;110:498–505.
10. Loffert DT, Ikle D, Nelson HS. A comparison of commercial jet nebulizers. *Chest.* 1994;106:1788–1793.
11. Bodenhamer J, Bergstrom R, Brown D, et al. Frequently nebulized B-agonists for asthma: Effects on serum electrolytes. *Ann Emerg Med.* 1992;21(11):53–58.
12. Gelmont DM, Balmes JR, Yee A. Hypokalemia induced by inhaled bronchodilators. *Chest.* 1988;94(4):763–766.
13. Fink JB, Cohen NH, Covington J, Mahlmeister MJ. Titration for optimal dose response to bronchodilators using MDI and spacer in ventilated adults; titration for optimal dose response of albuterol using MDI and spacer in non-intubated adults. *Respir Care.* 1991; 36(11):1321–1322. Abstracts.
14. Allon M, Dunlay R, Copkney C. Nebulized albuterol for acute hyperkalemia in patients on hemodialysis. *Ann Intern Med.* 1989; 110:426–429.
15. Palmer JBD, Stuart AM, Shepherd GL, Viskum K. Inhaled salmeterol in the treatment of patients with moderate to severe reversible obstructive airways disease: A 3-month comparison of the efficacy and safety of twice-daily salmeterol (100 mcg) with salmeterol (50 mcg). *Respir Med.* 1992;86(5):409–417.
16. AARC clinical practice guideline: Delivery of aerosols to the upper airway. *Respir Care.* 1994;39(8):803–807.
17. AARC clinical practice guideline: Selection of aerosol delivery device. *Respir Care.* 1992;37(8):891–897.
18. Ernst P, Habbick B, Suissa S, et al. Is the association between inhaled beta-agonist use and life threatening asthma because of confounding by severity? *ARRD.* 1993;148:75–79.
19. Spitzer WO, Suissa S, Ernst P, et al. The use of B-agonists and the risk of death and near death from asthma. *N Engl J Med.* 1992; 326:501–506.
20. Spector SL. Leukotriene inhibitors and antagonists in asthma. *Ann Allergy Asthma Immunol.* 1995;75(1):463–470.
21. Chapman KR (guest ed). Obstructive airways disease: Antimuscarinic bronchodilator therapy. Proceedings of a symposium. *Am J Med.* 1996;100(suppl 1A)15–70S.
22. Bennard SI, Serby CW, Ghafouri M, et al. Extended therapy with ipratropium bromide is associated with improved lung function in patients with COPD. *Chest.* 1996;110(1):62–70.
23. Gross NJ, Petty TL, Friedman M, et al. Dose response to ipra-

tropium bromide as a nebulized solution in patients with chronic obstructive pulmonary disease. *ARRD.* 1989;139(5):1188–1191.

24. Howder CL. Antimuscarinic and B2-adrenoreceptor bronchodilators in obstructive airways disease. *Respir Care.* 1993;38(12): 1364–1388.

25. Druce HM, Spector SL, Fireman P, et al. Double-blind study of intranasal ipratropium bromide in nonallergic perennial rhinitis. *Ann Allergy Asthma Immunol.* 1992;69(1):53–60.

26. Emad A. Effectiveness of adding alternate-day theophylline to the treatment regimen of patients with moderate-to-severe asthma. *Respir Care.* 1996;41(6):520–523.

27. Boe J, Rosenhall L, Alton M, et al. Comparison of dose-response effects of inhaled beclomethasone dipropionate and budesonide in the management of asthma. *Allergy.* 1997;44:349–355.

28. Toogood JH. High-dose inhaled steroid therapy for asthma. *J Allergy Clin Immunol.* 1989;83:528–536.

29. Nathan RA, Bronsky EA, Fireman P, et al. Once daily fluticasone propionate aqueous nasal spray in the effective treatment for seasonal allergic rhinitis. *Ann Allergy Asthma Immunol.* 1991;67(3): 332–338.

30. American Academy of Pediatrics. Ribavirin therapy of respiratory syncytial virus. *Pediatrics.* 1987;79:475–478.

31. Hall CB, McBride JT, Walsh EE, et al. Aerosolized ribavirin treatment of infants with respiratory syncytial viral infection. *N Engl J Med.* 1983;308:1443–1447.

32. Conrad DA, Christenson JC, Waner JL, Marks MI. Aerosolized ribavirin treatment of respiratory syncytial virus infection in infants hospitalized during an epidemic. *Pediatr Infect Dis J.* 1987; 6:152–158.

33. Smith DW, Frankel LR, Mathers LH, et al. A controlled trial of aerosolized ribavirin in infants receiving mechanical ventilation for severe respiratory syncytial virus infection. *N Engl J Med.* 1991;325:24–29.

34. Englund JA, Piedra PA, Jefferson LS, et al. High-dose, short-duration ribavirin aerosol therapy in children with suspected respiratory syncytial virus infection. *J Pediatr.* 1990;117:313–320.

35. Demers RR, Parker J, Frankel LR, Smith DW. Administration of ribavirin to neonatal and pediatric patients during mechanical ventilation. *Respir Care.* 1986;31(12):1188–1195.

36. Kacmarek RM, Kratohvil J. Evaluation of a double-enclosure double-vacuum unit scavenging system for ribavirin administration. *Respir Care.* 1992;37(1):37–45.

37. Montgomery AB, Corkery KJ, Brunette ER, et al. Occupational exposure to aerosolized pentamidine. *Chest.* 1991;100:624–627.

38. Kacmarek RM. Ribavirin and pentamidine aerosols: Caregiver beware! *Respir Care.* 1990;35(11):1034–1036. Editorial.

39. Quieffin J, Hunter J, Schechter MT, et al. Aerosol pentamidine-induced bronchoconstriction: Predictive factors and preventative therapy. *Chest.* 1991;100:624–627.

40. AARC clinical practice guideline: Bland aerosol administration. *Respir Care.* 1993;38(12):1196–1200.

41. Rao S, Wilson DB, Brooks RC, Sproule BJ. Acute effects of nebulization of N-acetylcysteine on pulmonary mechanics and gas exchange. *ARRD.* 1970;102:17–22.

42. Aitken ML, Burke W, McDonald G, et al. Recombinant human DNase inhalation in normal subjects and patients with cystic fibrosis. *JAMA.* 1992;267(14):1947–1951.

43. Curtis J, Mahlmeister MJ, Fink JB, et al. Helium-oxygen gas therapy: Use and availability for the emergency treatment of inoperable airway obstruction. *Chest.* 1986;90(3):455–457.

44. Mantous CA, Hall JB, Melmed A, et al. Heliox improves pulsus paradoxus and peak expiratory flowrate in nonintubated patients with severe asthma. *Am J Respir Crit Care Med.* 1995;151:310–314.

45. Kass JE, Castriotta RJ. Heliox therapy in acute severe asthma. *Chest.* 1995;107(3):757–760.

46. Elleau C, Galperine RI, Guenard H, Demarquez JL. Helium-oxygen mixture in respiratory distress syndrome: A double blind study. *J Pediatr.* 1993;122:132–136.

47. Miller CC, Miller JWR. Pulmonary vascular smooth-muscle regulation: The role of inhaled nitric oxide gas. *Respir Care.* 1992;37:1175–1785.

48. Zapol WM, Rimar S, Gillis N, et al. Nitric oxide and the lung: NHLBI Workshop Summary. *Am J Respir Crit Care Med.* 1994; 149:1375–1380.

49. Hess D, Bigatello L, Kacmarek RM, et al. Use of inhaled nitric oxide in patients with acute respiratory distress syndrome. *Respir Care.* 1996;41(5):424–444.

50. Hess D, Kacmarek RM, Ritz R, et al. Inhaled nitric oxide delivery systems: A role for respiratory therapists. *Respir Care.* 1995; 40(7):702–705.

51. Betit P, Adatia I, Benjamin P, et al. Inhaled nitric oxide: Evaluation of a continuous titration delivery technique for infant mechanical and manual ventilation. *Respir Care.* 1995;40(7):706–715.

52. El-Lessy HN. Pulmonary vascular control in hypoplastic left-heart syndrome: Hypoxic- and hypercarbic-gas therapy. *Respir Care.* 1995;40(7):737–742.

53. Jobes DR, Nicholson SC, Steven JM, et al. Carbon dioxide prevents pulmonary overcirculation in hypoplastic left heart syndrome. *Ann Thorac Surg.* 1992;54:150–151.

54. Haas CF, Weg JG. Exogenous surfactant therapy: An update. *Respir Care.* 1996;41(5):397–414.

55. Weg JG, Balk RA, Tharratt S, et al. Safety and potential efficacy of an aerosolized surfactant in human sepsis-induced adult respiratory distress syndrome. *JAMA.* 1994;272(18):1433–1438.

56. AARC clinical practice guideline: Surfactant replacement therapy. *Respir Care.* 1994;39(8):824–829.

57. AARC clinical practice guideline: Selection of an aerosol delivery device for neonatal and pediatric patients. *Respir Care.* 1995; 40(12):1325–1335.

58. AARC clinical practice guideline: Assessing response to bronchodilator therapy at point of care. *Respir Care.* 1995;40(12): 1300–1307.

59. Chapman KR, Love L, Brubaker H. A comparison of breath actuated and conventional metered dose inhalers inhalation techniques in elderly subjects. *Chest.* 1993;104:1332–1337.

60. Kleerup EC, Tashkin DP, Cline AC, Ekholm BP. Cumulative dose-response study of non-CFC propellant HFA 134a salbutamol sulfate metered-dose inhaler in patients with asthma. *Chest.* 1996; 109:702–707.

61. Colacone A, Wolcove N, Stern E, et al. Continuous nebulization of albuterol (Salbutamol) in acute asthma. *Chest.* 1990;97(3): 693–697.

62. Moler FW, Hurwitz ME, Custer JR. Improvement in clinical asthma score and PaCO$_2$ in children with severe asthma treated with continuously nebulized terbutaline. *J Allergy Clin Immunol.* 1988;81:1101–1109.

63. Montgomery VL, Eid NS. Low-dose β-agonist continuous nebulization therapy for status asthmaticus ion children. *J Asthma.* 1994;31(3):201–207.

64. Levitt MA, Gambrioli EF, Fink JB. Comparative trial of continuous nebulization versus metered-dose-inhaler in the treatment of acute bronchospasm. *Ann Emerg Med.* 1995;26(3):273–277.

65. Reisner C, Kotch A, Dworkin G. Continuous versus frequent intermittent nebulization of albuterol in acute asthma: A randomized, prospective study. *Ann Allergy Asthma Immunol.* 1995;75: 41–47.

66. Reisner C, Lee J, Kotch A, Dworkin G. Comparison of volume output from two different continuous nebulizer systems. *Ann Allergy Asthma Immunol.* 1996;76:209–213.

67. Mahlmeister MJ, Fink JB, Hoffman GL, Fifer LF. Positive-expiratory-pressure mask therapy: Theoretical and practical considerations and a review of the literature. *Respir Care.* 1991;36(11): 1218–1230.

68. Anderson JB, Klausen NO. A new mode of administration of nebulized bronchodilator in severe bronchospasm: PEP. *Eur J Resp Dis.* 1982;63(suppl 119):97–100.

69. Gradwell G, Klein LD, Brosbe G, et al. Emergency room asthma treatment with positive expiratory pressure (PEP effect on hospitalization. *Respir Care.* 1994;39(2):1072. Abstract.

70. Anderson M, Svartgren M, Blyin G, et al. Deposition in asthmatics of particles inhaled in air or helium-oxygen. *ARRD.* 1993;147:524–528.

71. Mason JW, Miller WC, Small S. Comparison of aerosol delivery via circulaire system vs conventional small volume nebulizer. *Respir Care.* 1994;39(12):1157–1161.

72. Wollam PJ, Kasper CL, Bishop MJ, et al. Prediction and assessment of bronchodilator response in mechanically ventilated patients. *Respir Care.* 1994;39(7):730–735.

73. Horn SD, Sharkey PD, Tracy DM, et al. Intended and unintended consequences of HMO cost-containment strategies: Results from the managed care outcomes project. *Am J Manag Care.* 1996;2 (3):253–264.

Resources

1. *Asthma Management in Minority Children: Practical Insights for Clinicians, Researchers, and Public Health Planners.* Washington, DC: US Department of Health and Human Services; 1995. National Institutes of Health–National Heart, Lung, and Blood publication. NIH 95–3675.
2. *Considerations for Diagnosing and Managing Asthma in the Elderly.* Washington, DC; US Department of Health and Human Services; 1996. NAEPP Working Group Report publication. NIH 96–3662.
3. *Asthma Management Kit for Emergency Departments.* NIH 94–2992.
4. *Asthma Management Kit for Clinicians.* NIH 92–2113.
5. *Asthma Management Kit.* Allens & Hanburys, Division of Glaxo, Inc. Research Triangle Park, NC, 27709.
6. *Peak Performance USA: A Program for Managing Asthma in the School.* AARC, Dallas, TX.
7. Allergy and Asthma Network: Mothers of Asthmatics, Inc. Publishes a monthly report, which includes a learning resource center. AANÑMA, 3554 Chain Bridge Road, Suite 200, Fairfax, VA, 22030–2709, 800–878–4403.
8. Asthma and Allergy Foundation of America. 1125 15th Street, NW, Suite 502, Washington, DC, 20005.

APPENDIX A

STANDARD ABBREVIATIONS USED IN DRUG PRESCRIPTIONS

ABBREVIATION	MEANING	ABBREVIATION	MEANING
$\overline{a}$	before	q 6 h	every 6 hours
$\overline{aa}$	of each	q.i.d.	4 times per day (w/a)
a.c.	before meals		
ad lib	as much as desired	q.d.	once per day
b.i.d.	twice a day	q.o.d.	every other day
$\overline{c}$	with	QS	quantity sufficient
cc	cubic centimeter	qt	quart
dil	dilute	$\overline{s}$	without
fl or fld	fluid	sc	subcutaneous
g	gram	sol	solution
gr	grain	p.r.n.	as needed
gtt(s)	drops	Rx	prescription (treat)
h	hour(s)		
hs	at bedtime	tab	tablet
IM	intramuscular	t.i.d.	three times per day
I&O	intake and output	T½	half-life
IV	intravenous	tbsp	tablespoon
kg	kilogram	tsp	teaspoon
L	liter	UD	unit dose
mcg, μg	microgram		
MDI	metered dose inhaler		
mg	milligram		
mL	milliliter		
neb	nebulize/nebulizer		
NPO	nothing by mouth		
N/S	normal saline		
$\overline{p}$	after		
q	every		
q h	every hour		
q 2 h	every 2 hours		

APPENDIX B

DRUG DOSAGES AND CALCULATIONS

Several systems exist for the measurement of medications, including metric, avoirdupois, apothecary, and household. This appendix discusses the metric system and provides several common conversion measurements between metric and household systems.

METRIC

Weight: 1 kg = 1000 g

         1 g   = 1000 mg

         1 mg = 1000 µg

Volume: 1 L   = 1000 mL or 1000 cc

HOUSEHOLD

Weight: 1 lb = 16 oz

Volume: 1 qt = 32 oz
           1 pt = 16 oz

CONVERSIONS

Weight: 1 lb   = 454 g

         1 kg = 2.2 lb

Volume: 1 qt   = 1 L (1000 mL)

         1 gtts =1 minim = 1 drop = 0.0625 mL

         1 tsp = 5 ml   1 tbsp = 15 mL

How many grams does a 6 lb, 12 oz newborn baby weigh? 6.75 lbs $\times$ 454 g = 3065 g (3.065 kg)

How many drops are in a 0.5-mL dose of Bronkosol? 16 drops/mL = 8 drops/0.5 mL

Medication dosages usually are described in one of three ways: weight/weight
                                                      weight/volume
                                                      volume/volume

For respiratory medications, the drug solution usually is a weight per volume mixture.

For example, a 5% solution of albuterol contains 5000 mg (5 g)/100mL solution, meaning that when the drug is bottled, the concentration is 5000 mg of active drug mixed in a 100-mL volume of fluid. Orders for aerosol therapy by hand nebulizer may be written as a milligram dose, "give 2.5 mg albuterol," or as a volume dose, "give 0.5 mL albuterol." Practitioners must be able to perform simple conversion calculations to ensure that the proper dose of medication is administered as ordered.

PROBLEM: The normal dose of a 5% solution of albuterol is 0.5 mL.
                How much albuterol by weight is in 0.5 mL?

To solve this problem, set up an equation of equivalents, as follows:

Step 1: Set up an equivalency: 5000 mg/100 mL = X/0.5 mL

Step 2: Solve for X as follows: 5000 $\times$ 0.5   = 100X

                            2500   = 100X

                            2.5   = X

Therefore, there are 2.5 mg of albuterol in 0.5mL of a 5% solution of albuterol.

PROBLEM: The normal concentration of racemic epinephrine is 2.25%.
                You are asked to administer 11.25 mg to an 8-year-old.
                How much racemic epinephrine will you draw up in your syringe?

Step 1: Set up an equivalency: 2250/100 = 11.25/X

       Solve for X as follows: 2250X   = 11.25 $\times$ 100(1125)

       Divide both sides by 2250:   X   = 0.5

You would draw up 0.5 mL of solution to aerosolize 11.25 mg of medication in your nebulizer treatment.

Try the following five problems on your own.

PROBLEM: How many drops of medication would you give if ordered to administer 0.25 mL?

PROBLEM: You are ordered to administer 3 mL of a 10% solution of medication. You note that the only concentration of medication available is a 20% solution. How much of the 20% solution would you draw up to equal 3 mL of a 10% solution?

PROBLEM: How many milligrams of Bronkosol is in 1.0 mL of a 1% solution?

PROBLEM: How many milligrams of drug in 3 puffs of fluticasone at 110 μg/puff?

PROBLEM: You mix 6 g of ribavirin in 300 mL of sterile water. If you nebulize the ribavirin at 20 mL/h: a. How many mg/h are you delivering? b. How long will the medication last?

Metered Dose Inhaler Protocol

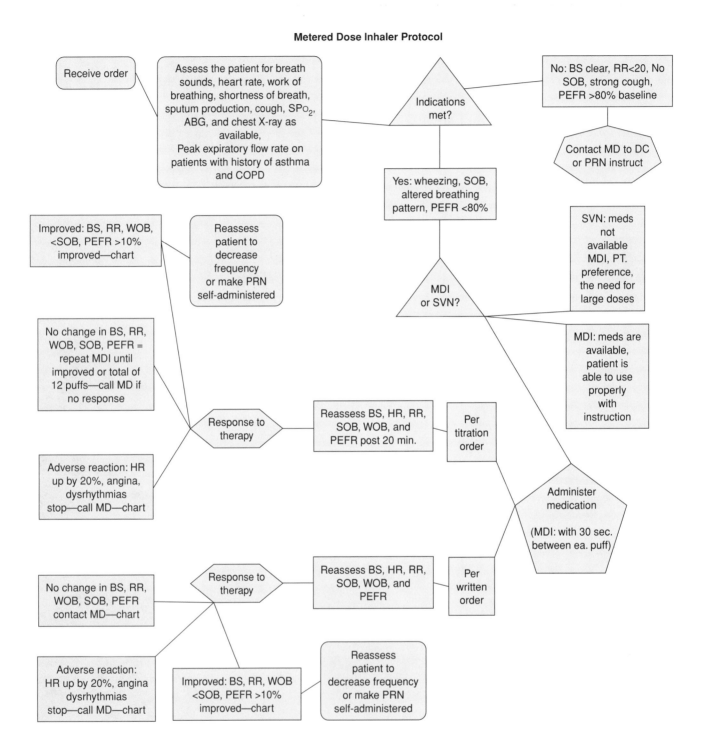

Receive order

Assess the patient for breath sounds, heart rate, work of breathing, shortness of breath, sputum production, cough, SP_{O_2}, ABG, and chest X-ray as available,
Peak expiratory flow rate on patients with history of asthma and COPD

Indications met?

No: BS clear, RR<20, No SOB, strong cough, PEFR >80% baseline

Contact MD to DC or PRN instruct

Yes: wheezing, SOB, altered breathing pattern, PEFR <80%

MDI or SVN?

SVN: meds not available MDI, PT. preference, the need for large doses

MDI: meds are available, patient is able to use properly with instruction

Improved: BS, RR, WOB, <SOB, PEFR >10% improved—chart

Reassess patient to decrease frequency or make PRN self-administered

No change in BS, RR, WOB, SOB, PEFR = repeat MDI until improved or total of 12 puffs—call MD if no response

Response to therapy

Reassess BS, HR, RR, SOB, WOB, and PEFR post 20 min.

Per titration order

Adverse reaction: HR up by 20%, angina, dysrhythmias stop—call MD—chart

Administer medication

(MDI: with 30 sec. between ea. puff)

No change in BS, RR, WOB, SOB, PEFR contact MD—chart

Response to therapy

Reassess BS, HR, RR, SOB, WOB, and PEFR

Per written order

Adverse reaction: HR up by 20%, angina dysrhythmias stop—call MD—chart

Improved: BS, RR, WOB <SOB, PEFR >10% improved—chart

Reassess patient to decrease frequency or make PRN self-administered

Management of Asthma Exacerbation: Emergency Department and Hospital-based Care

Initial Assessment
History, physical examination (auscultation, use of accessory muscles, heart rate, respiratory rate), PEF or FEV$_1$, oxygen saturation, and other tests as indicated

---

FEV$_1$ or PEF ≥50%
- Inhaled β$_2$-agonist by metered dose inhaler or nebulizer, up to three doses in the first hour
- Oxygen to achieve O$_2$ saturation ≥90%
- Oral systemic corticosteroids if no immediate response or if patient recently took oral

FEV$_1$ or PEF ≤50% (Severe Exacerbation)
- Inhaled high-dose β$_2$-agonist and anticholinergic by nebulization every 20 min. or continuously for 1 h
- Oxygen to achieve O$_2$ saturation ≥90%
- Oral systemic corticosteroids

Impending or Actual Respiratory Arrest
- Intubation and mechanical ventilation with 100% O$_2$
- Nebulized β$_2$-agonist and anticholinergic
- Intravenous corticosteroid

Admit to Hospital Intensive Care

Repeat Assessment
Symptoms, physical examination, PEF, O$_2$ saturation, other tests as needed

---

Moderate Exacerbation
FEV$_1$ or PEF 50%–80% predicted/personal best
Physical exam: moderate symptoms
- Inhaled short-acting β$_2$-agonist every 60 min.
- Systemic corticosteroid or increased dose of inhaled corticosteroid
- Continue treatment 1–3 h, provided there is no improvement

Severe Exacerbation
FEV$_1$ or PEF <50% predicted/personal best
Physical exam: severe symptoms at rest, accessory muscle use, chest retraction
- History: high-risk patient
- No improvement after initial treatment
- Inhaled short-acting β$_2$-agonist, hourly or continuous + inhaled anticholinergic
- Oxygen
- Systemic corticosteroid

Good Response
- FEV$_1$ or PEF ≥70%
- Response sustained 60 min., after last treatment
- No distress
- Physical exam: normal

Incomplete Response
- FEV$_1$ or PEF ≥50% but <70%
- Mild to moderate symptoms

Individualized decision re: hospitalization (see text)

Poor Response
- FEV$_1$ or PEF <70%
- PCO$_2$ ≥42 mm Hg
Physical exam: symptoms severe, drowsiness, confusion

Discharge Home
- Continue treatment with inhaled β$_2$ agonist
- Course of oral systemic corticosteroid
- Patient education
  - Review medicine use
  - Review/initiate action plan
  - Close medical follow-up

Admit to Hospital Ward
- Inhaled β$_2$ agonist + inhaled anticholinergic
- Systemic corticosteroid (oral or intravenous)
- Oxygen
- Monitor FEV$_1$ or PEF, O$_2$ saturation, pulse

Admit to Hospital Intensive Care
- Inhaled Inhaled β$_2$ agonist hourly or continuously + inhaled anticholinergic
- Intravenous corticosteroid
- Oxygen
- Possible intubation and mechanical ventilation

Improve

Discharge Home
- Continue treatment with inhaled β$_2$-agonist
- Course of oral systemic corticosteroid
- Patient education
  - Review medicine use
  - Review/initiate action plan
  - Close medical follow-up

APPENDIX D

DOSAGES OF DRUGS FOR ASTHMA EXACERBATIONS IN EMERGENCY MEDICAL CARE OR HOSPITAL

DOSAGES

Medications	Adults	Children	Comments
Inhaled short-acting β_2-agonists			
Albuterol Nebulizer solution (5 mg/mL)	2.5–5 mg every 20 min for three doses, then 2.5–10 mg every 1–4 h as needed, or 10–15 mg/h continuously	0.15 mg/kg (minimum dose, 2.5 mg) every 20 min for three doses, then 0.15–0.3 mg/kg up to 10 mg every 1–4 h as needed, or 0.5 mg/kg/h by continuous nebulization	Only selective β_2-agonists are recommended. For optimal delivery, dilute aerosols to minimum of 4 mL at gas flow of 6–8 L/min
MDI (90 µg/puff)	4–8 puffs every 20 min up to 4 h, then every 1–4 h as needed	4–8 puffs every 20 min for three doses, then every 1–4 h as needed	As effective as nebulized therapy if patient is able to coordinate inhalation maneuver. Use spacer/holding chamber
Bitolterol Nebulizer solution (2 mg/mL)	See albuterol dose	See albuterol dose, thought to be one half as potent as albuterol on a mg basis	Has not been studied in severe asthma exacerbations. Do not mix with other drugs.
MDI (370 µg/puff)	See albuterol dose	See albuterol dose	Has not been studied in severe asthma exacerbations
Pirbuterol MDI (200 µg/puff)	See albuterol dose	See albuterol dose, thought to be one half as potent as albuterol on a mg basis	Has not been studied in severe asthma exacerbations
Systemic (injected) β_2-agonists			
Epinephrine 1 : 1000 (1 mg/mL)	0.3–0.5 mg every 20 min for three doses sq	0.01 mg/kg up to 0.3–0.5 mg every 20 min for three doses sq	No proven advantage of systemic therapy over aerosol
Terbutaline (1 mg/mL)	0.25 mg every 20 min for three doses sq	0.01 mg/kg every 20 min for three doses, then every 2–6 hours as needed sq	No proven advantage of systemic therapy over aerosol

DOSAGES

Medications	Adults	Children	Comments
Anticholinergics			
Ipratropium bromide Nebulizer solution (0.25 mg/mL)	0.5 mg every 30 min for three doses then every 2–4 hours as needed	0.25 mg every 20 min for three doses, then every 2–4 h	May mix in same nebulizer with albuterol. Should not be used as first-line therapy; should be added to β_2-agonist therapy
MDI (18 μg/puff)	4–8 puffs as needed	4–8 puffs as needed	Dose delivered from MDI is low and has not been studied in asthma exacerbations

APPENDIX E

DRUG NAMES

Drugs that pass through the Food and Drug Administration (FDA) approval process and find their way into use have a variety of names by which they are identified. Whether they are a *prescription* drug, such as Valium, which requires the order of a physician or other legally authorized provider such as a nurse practitioner, or an *over-the-counter* (OTC) drug, such as Tylenol, which can be obtained and self-administered without prescription, drugs acquire official names approved by the United States government. Readers who wish to learn more about how drugs become available to the public through the FDA approval process may review a continuing education program entitled, "Molecule to Market: The Drug Development Process," produced by Glaxo Pharmaceuticals.

Brand name: The name is designated by the manufacturers of the drug. For example, Ventolin (Glaxo Pharmaceuticals) and Proventil (Schering Labs Inc.) represent two brand names for the same basic bronchodilator drug (albuterol), although their pharmaceutical compositions may vary. The brand name also may be referred to as the *trade name* or *proprietary name*. Brand names are always written with the first letter capitalized.

Generic name: The name assigned to the drug by the United States Adopted Name Council (USAN). This name usually is referenced to the basic chemical structure of the drug. For example, *albuterol* is the generic name for Ventolin and Proventil, as mentioned previously. The generic name also is sometimes referred to as the *nonproprietary name*. When writing the generic name of a drug, the first letter of the name is not capitalized.

Note: Generic drugs often are less expensive than brand-name medications. The era of managed care and health maintenance organizations has led to a growing effort to have subscribers use less expensive, generic drugs. Conflicting reports have demonstrated varying efficacy between brand and generic drugs in a wide range of medications. RCPs who care for patients taking aerosolized respiratory medications have a duty to determine if any correlation might exist between a deterioration in pulmonary status and the patient's change to a generic respiratory medication.

Official name: The name given to a drug approved for use and added to the United States Pharmacopoeia (USP), the official compendium of approved drugs in the United States. Normally, the official name and the generic name are identical.

Chemical name: The drug's name as it relates to its chemical formula. For example, acetylsalicylic acid is the chemical name for a commonly used drug—aspirin.

DRUG RESOURCES

The **United States Pharmacopeia** (USP) is an official compendium of established drug standards, such as purity, strength of drug preparations, and identifying terminology. Drugs contained in this book have the official label of USP. The American Pharmaceutical Association produces the **National Formulary** (NF), which lists drug formulas and mixtures. Both the USP and the NF have been combined since 1980 into a single publication, produced under the auspices of the United States government.

The **Physician's Desk Reference** (PDR) provides a comprehensive overview of thousands of drugs. Compiled by drug manufacturers and published yearly, the PDR represents a valuable reference for such drug information as indications and contraindications for use, standard doses, routes of administration, and side effects. All RCPs should be able to identify where they can assess a PDR in their workplace because the PDR may need to be consulted as part of the evaluation of the profile of a medication order before implementation. Health care providers *should never* administer a medication for which they lack a comprehensive understanding of actions, indications, contraindications, dosage, and side effects.

DRUG SOURCES

Drugs currently available come from a variety of sources. Early sources of drugs included *animals, plants,* and *minerals. Synthetic* development of drugs from raw materials in laboratories currently serves as the major source of drugs, accounting for about 65% of all drugs manufactured today. *Genetically engineered* medications represent a growing source for drug development. Dornase alfa (Pulmozyme), administered by aerosol inhalation to help mobilize bronchial secretions in patients with cystic fibrosis or chronic obstructive pulmonary disease, is representative of the fast expanding field of genetically engineered drugs.

DRUG TERMINOLOGY AND STANDARD ABBREVIATIONS

Specific terminology is used to describe pharmacologic preparations, routes of administration, and other aspects of medication documentation and prescription writing. Standard abbreviations are used to write prescriptions and document therapy in the patient's medical record. Appendix A lists a number of abbreviations commonly used with all categories of medications. RCPs always should consult the health care facility where they practice to identify any institution-specific list of acceptable abbreviations.

Infection Control and Safety

James B. Fink

Key Terms

aspiration
barrier protection
body substance isolation
condensate
droplet nuclei
effluent
endogenous flora
gastric colonization
iatrogenic complications
isolation procedures
nosocomial infections
nosocomial pneumonia
parenteral exposure
semicritical

Objectives

- Identify sources of risk for transmission of pathogens between patients and care providers.

- Discuss the impact of nosocomial infections on patient mortality and morbidity.

- Understand the rationale for isolation strategies.

- Identify high-risk procedures associated with respiratory care procedures.

- Describe actions that reduce risks associated with respiratory care procedures.

- Identify sources of risk for care providers and actions that can be taken to reduce risk.

Hospitals and health care facilities, by their very nature, serve a greater variety and concentration of sick people than other institutions or businesses. The equation is simple: the more germs in the environment, the greater the risk of transmission between people. Within the population of patients who require respiratory care services, many are at high risk of secondary and superimposed infections.

As health care providers, our goal is to help patients; even when we are unable to help substantively, we have an explicit obligation to "do no harm." Unfortunately, we all too often provide the mechanism by which pathogens are transmitted from one patient to another. Any complications that are associated with the services we provide and that complicate or compromise the patient's well-being are called **iatrogenic complications;** these can range from infections to problems that result from incorrectly administered medications or improperly performed surgical procedures. Infections that the patient did not have when admitted are called **nosocomial infections.** We have an obligation to adopt practices that minimize exposure of patients to dangers that complicate their existing problems.

We also have an obligation to ourselves and our coworkers to reduce avoidable risks. In the health care environment, we are exposed to a wider range of occupational exposures than are workers in many other industries. We are not immune to disease or accidents, and the health care provider's first obligation is to avoid risk of injury and disease. All too often, the health care worker takes the attitude that "it won't happen to me"—a sad epitaph for the worker who contracts hepatitis, tuberculosis, or even human immunodeficiency virus (HIV) in the workplace because of unsafe practices.

INFECTION CONTROL

Many patients develop iatrogenic complications while under our care. Iatrogenic complications are conditions associated with the actions of the health care institution or care provider, rather than the pathology afflicting the patient on admission. Examples of iatrogenic complications range from the administration of the wrong dose of medication to a surgical amputation of the wrong leg. Many iatrogenic complications can be avoided by paying close attention to current orders, care plans, and policies and procedures in the provision of services.

Nosocomial infections are iatrogenic infections that were not in evidence at the time the patient was admitted to the hospital. **Nosocomial pneumonia** is a respiratory tract infection that is acquired in the hospital. This means that the patient did not have evidence of pneumonia on admission to the health care facility or during the incubation period of the causative pathogen (generally, 48 to 72 hours) after admission. Although less than 1% of hospitalized patients develop nosocomial pneumonia, it has been reported in more than 40% of high-risk patients and is associated with mortality rates of up to 50% and an increased length of hospital stay of 4 to 9 days. Nosocomial pneumonia increases the cost of hospital care by more than $1.3 billion each year; we cannot place a dollar value on the pain and suffering for both patients and loved ones (Box 9–1).

Microorganisms invade the lower respiratory tract from a variety of sources. The primary route of transmission of pathogens into an otherwise "sterile" lung appears to be aspiration of oropharyngeal and gastric fluids. About 45% of normal, healthy adults aspirate oropharyngeal secretions during sleep. Risk of **aspiration** is increased with the presence of sedation or depressed consciousness associated with acute and chronic illness. In addition to an increased risk of aspiration, the upper airway of severely ill patients often becomes colonized with gram-negative bacilli. One study demonstrated that patients in intensive care units (ICUs) had a three-fold increase in gram-negative bacteria in dental plaque. **Gastric colonization** occurs when the gastric pH is higher than 4.0, which may occur with antacid therapy. Endotracheal and tracheostomy tubes bypass the normal mechanisms that protect the upper airway from aspiration.

Hospital Practices That Can Reduce Nosocomial Infection

Between 25% and 40% of adult ICU patients acquire infection from cross-transmission among patients.[1,2] These are the infections that can be reduced or eliminated by practices such as effective hand washing and **isolation procedures** (Fig. 9–1). The 40% to 60% of nosocomial infections caused by **endogenous flora** (bacteria found normally in the patient) are not preventable by isolation strategies but may be reduced by good respiratory care practices.

Box • 9–1   RISK FACTORS FOR NOSOCOMIAL PNEUMONIA

- Age >60 years
- Organ dysfunction
- Organ failure
- Underlying pulmonary disease
- Immunocompromise
- Intensive care unit admission
- Mechanical ventilation
- Treatment with broad-spectrum antibiotics
- Stress bleeding prophylaxis
    Antacids
    Histamine-2 blockers
- Aspiration-conducive conditions
    Intubation
    Feeding tubes
    Coma
    Sedation
- Compromised secretion clearance
    Postoperative pain
    Intubation

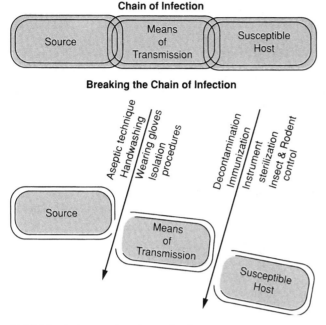

Chain of Infection

Source | Means of Transmission | Susceptible Host

Breaking the Chain of Infection

Aseptic technique
Handwashing
Wearing gloves
Isolation procedures

Decontamination
Immunization
Instrument sterilization
Insect & Rodent control

Source

Means of Transmission

Susceptible Host

FIGURE 9-1 • The chain of infection.

Several types of isolation procedures have been used over the years to reduce cross-contamination. Some of these patient care practices, such as hand washing and sterile catheter insertion, are supported by data from controlled studies, whereas others evolved based on rationalizations that are not supported by empiric data.

Traditionally, isolation precautions were used only with patients suspected of having (or being diagnosed with) certain infectious diseases. These isolation systems attempted to group infection precautions by either the type of infection or the suspected mode of transmission. Once the disease or potential diagnosis was recognized, the patient would be placed in isolation, and a specific set of practices would be set in place. Signs describing the isolation practices were posted outside the patient's room, and carts with the needed supplies were brought to the isolation area for use by the staff caring for the patient.

There are several fatal flaws with traditional isolation practices:

1. If no one recognizes the need for the patient to be isolated, many of the necessary practices to reduce cross-contamination are not put into place.
2. Posting of isolation signs has been associated with reduced compliance with basic infection control procedures outside of the specific patient's isolation. Many of the staff are lulled into a sense of security that if a patient is not in isolation, there is no need to follow even the basics of infection control.
3. Many of the required supplies could only be found on the isolation carts, unavailable for use in care of other patients.

Body Substance Isolation

Body substance isolation is designed to reduce cross-contamination between patients as well as exposure of the care provider to to moist body substances. This practice is based on the assumption that mucous membranes, nonintact skin, and insertion sites for medical devices are likely to have pathogens. All hospitalized patients are put in body substance isolation; other special infection precautions are used only for patients with airborne communicable disease, such as tuberculosis.

Moist body substances are often proteinaceous, sticky, and difficult to remove from hands and skin, and they typically contain the basic ingredients to support pathogen growth as the fluids leave the body (Box 9–2). The goal is to keep body substances off the care provider's skin and clothing, and to avoid these substances moving from one patient to another through contact with the practitioner or with tools, equipment, dishes, laundry, or even furniture that may be shared among patients.

Individual infection prevention practices with known efficacy are listed in Tables 9–1 and 9–2.

Protective Attire

GLOVES

Gloves provide **barrier protection** between the practitioner's hands and the patient. Gloves have been proved to reduce infections and colonization when put on immedi-

---

Box • 9–2 MOIST BODY SITES AND SUBSTANCES

MOIST BODY SITES

- Mucous membranes
- Incision sites
- Body orifices
- Open wounds

MOIST BODY SUBSTANCES

- Blood
- Cerebrospinal fluid
- Secretions
    Sputum
    Saliva
    Sweat
    Tears
- Excretions
    Urine
    Feces
- Exudates
    Pus

Table • 9–1   TYPES OF HAND CARE

	Purpose	Method
Hand washing	To remove soil and transient microorganisms	Soap or detergent for at least 10–15 seconds
Hand antisepsis	To remove or destroy transient microorganisms	Antimicrobial soap or detergent or alcohol-based preparation for at least 10–15 seconds
Surgical hand scrubbing	To remove or destroy transient microorganisms and reduce resident flora	Antimicrobial soap or detergent preparation with brush to achieve friction for at least 120 seconds, or alcohol-based preparation for at least 20 seconds

From *APIC Infection Control and Epidemiology: Principles and Practice*. St. Louis: Mosby-Year Book; 1996.

ately before contact with mucous membranes and nonintact skin. Three types of gloves are in common use.

Examination gloves are not typically sterile and are put on at the time of use, immediately before contact with membranes or articles likely to be soiled.

Sterile gloves are used whenever contact with sterile tissue (or tissue that should be sterile) is anticipated. Sterile gloves should be used with surgical procedures, sterile line insertion, and wound dressing changes. Sterile gloves are packaged individually to maintain sterility while in storage and are designed to allow easy opening and donning without contamination. Should sterile gloves become contaminated from a source other than the initial body site being contacted, they should be removed, the practitioner's hands should be washed, and the gloves should be replaced with new sterile gloves. Figures 9–2 and 9–3 show proper technique for donning and removing sterile surgical gloves. Gloves should also be changed between contacts with different body sites. The practitioner should wear sterile gloves for phlebotomy, arterial puncture, or any procedure that may involve puncture with a used sharps. The gloves help reduce the amount of infectious particles transferred between the practitioner and the patient. Double gloves should be used for procedures involving sharp tools and bloody tissue because two layers reduce penetration of blood to the skin.[3] Latex is stronger than vinyl, although some people have a sensitive or allergic reaction to latex. The practitioner should remove and discard gloves after use and then wash his or her hands. Gloves may develop microscopic tears or pinhole-sized leaks, allowing possible contamination by seepage that is undetectable by sight or feel.

Utility gloves are used for cleaning and performing heavier tasks, such as maintenance and repairs, and not for contact with mucous membranes. They are made of heavier material and designed to be cleaned and reused.

COVER GOWNS

Cover gowns and other protective attire keep the skin and clothing of care providers clean but have not been proved to reduce infection transmission between patients (Fig. 9–4). Cover gowns or aprons are worn when soilage of clothing or bare skin is anticipated with the task to be done. Hair covers keep the practitioner's hair from contaminating the patient and keep blood and fluids off the practitioner's hair. Shoe covers and leg covers keep blood, fluids, and dirt from touching the practitioner's feet and legs.

MASKS AND FACEWEAR

Facewear protects skin and mucous membranes of the face from splattering of the moist body substances. Options include glasses with side shields, goggles, masks, and face shields.

Surgical masks are intended to trap droplets from wearers' exhaled breath and to provide protection against spread of infection. Unfortunately, surgical masks allow as much 100% penetration of particles smaller than 10 μm.

Respirators are breathing devices that filter more than 97% of particles 1 mm or larger and are specified by the Occupational Safety and Health Administration (OSHA) to be worn when caring for patients with suspected, untreated tuberculosis (Fig. 9–5). The National Institute of Occupational Safety and Health (NIOSH) certifies and approves respirators for health care and industry. To be effective, NIOSH-approved respirators must be fit tested, and the employee must be instructed in their proper use. Because this type of filtration respirator can increase the work of breathing during use, employees should receive medical screening before being fit tested to determine whether they have a respiratory or cardiac condition that would place them at risk while using the respirator.

Fit testing requires the employee to be fitted properly with the right-sized respirator, including instruction for proper use. With the respirator in place, the employee is exposed to an aerosol (such as banana oil) and asked to report any taste or smell that permeates the mask. Another method of fit testing involves using a computer-based system that measures normal particulates in the atmosphere and compares that level with levels inside the respirator during the test. During the test, the employee is asked to move the head up and down and side to side and to talk, ensuring a good fit with motion. Fit testing must be repeated annually and with any change in type, style, or size of respirator used by the employee

Employees who cannot use standard respirators either because of the increased work of breathing, facial hair (such as beards), or facial anomalies that keep them from getting a good seal with the respirator may use a positive airway pressure respirator that draws air through a HEPA

Table • 9–2 RECOMMENDATIONS FOR PREPARING HANDS AND CLEANING SKIN BEFORE* NONSURGICAL AND SURGICAL PROCEDURES

Procedure	Example	Hand Washing	Gloves	Preparation of Patient's Skin	Comments
Nonsurgical					
Instruments used in the procedure come in contact with intact mucous membranes	Bronchoscopy; gastrointestinal endoscopy; tracheal suction	Soap and water	Recommended	In general, none is required.	
	Cystoscopy; urinary tract catheterization	Soap and water	Sterile recommended	Antiseptics should be used to prepare the urethral meatus.	
Insertion of a peripheral intravenous or arterial cannula	Intravenous therapy; arterial pressure monitoring	Soap and water or antiseptic	Clean or sterile recommended	Antiseptics should be used; a fast-acting one is desirable; tincture of iodine is preferred, but alcohol is adequate if applied liberally.	Most epidemics of infection associated with arterial pressure monitoring devices appear to be caused by hospital-associated contamination of components external to the skin, such as transducer heads or domes; "endemic" IV-related bloodstream infections are frequently associated with skin flora.†
Percutaneous insertion of a central catheter or wire	Hyperalimentation; central venous and capillary wedge pressure monitoring; angiography; cardiac pacemaker insertion	Antiseptic	Sterile recommended	Antiseptics should be used; a fast-acting one such as tincture of iodine is desirable; "defatting" agents such as acetone are not recommended.	Defatting agents do not appear to decrease infections and can cause skin irritation.
Insertion (and prompt removal) of a sterile needle in deep tissues or body fluids, usually to obtain specimens or instill therapeutic agent	Spinal tap; thoracentesis; abdominal paracentesis	Soap and water or antiseptic	Sterile recommended	Antiseptics should be used; a fast-acting one such as tincture of iodine is desirable.	
Surgical					
Insertion of a sterile tube or device through tissue into a normally sterile tissue or fluid	Chest tube insertion; culdoscopy; laparoscopy; peritoneal catheter insertion	Antiseptic	Sterile recommended	Antiseptics should be used; hair should be clipped with scissors if hair removal is considered necessary.	Efficacy of antiseptic hand-washing products against certain viruses has also been standard.
Minor skin surgery	Skin biopsy; suturing of small cuts; lancing boils; mole removal	Soap and water	Sterile recommended	Antiseptics should be used.	Gloves are usually worn for a short time; thus, antiseptic hand washing is not usually necessary to suppress resident flora for these superficial procedures.
Other procedures (major and minor surgery) that enter tissue below the skin	Hysterectomy; cholecystectomy; herniorrhaphy	Antiseptic	Sterile recommended	Antiseptics should be used after the site has been scrubbed with a detergent; the patient's hair should not be shaved; if necessary, hair may be removed immediately before the procedures; clipping hair or using a depilatory is preferred to shaving.	Hand washing before surgical procedures that enter deep tissue is usually prolonged to ensure that all areas that harbor bacteria are adequately cleaned.

From *APIC Infection Control and Applied Epidemiology: Principles and Practice.* St. Louis: Mosby-Year Book; 1996.

*Hands should also be washed *after* all procedures when microbial contamination of the operator is likely to occur, especially those procedures involving contact with mucous membranes, whether or not gloves are worn.

†Many IV kits contain swabs impregnated with iodophor and alcohol. Each product must be applied for at least 30 seconds and allowed to dry thoroughly. If applied in a cursory manner or with insufficient contact time, these products lose effectiveness.

233

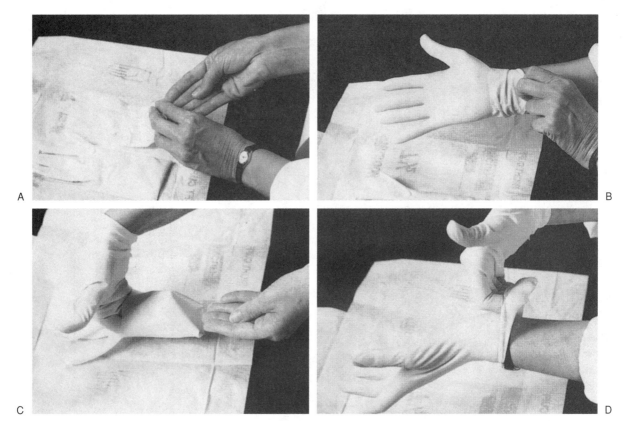

FIGURE 9-2 • Donning surgical gloves. (*A*) Open the prepacked sterile gloves following manufacturer directions. Using the nondominant hand, lift the cuff of the glove for the dominant hand, touching only the inner surface of the cuff. Curl the thumb inward as the hand is inserted. (*B*) Straighten the fingers and pull the glove on with the nondominant hand still just grasping the cuff. (*C*) With the thumb curled, slip the golved dominant hand into the cuff of the remaining glove. (*D*) Unfold the cuff and pull the glove on snugly.

filter and pumps it into a mask or hood at sufficient flow to compensate for any leaks in the system (Box 9–3). Fluid-resistant masks protect the face from splatter.

Infection Control Considerations in Respiratory Care

Patients at the highest risk for respiratory infections are infants and the elderly and patients with severe underlying disease, immunosuppression, depressed sensorium, cardiopulmonary disease, and thoracoabdominal surgery. Respiratory care practitioners and other health care providers may have close contact with many patients in a variety of locations during the course of a work shift. Failure to apply consistently safe hygiene and infection control practices can result in transmission of pathogens to multiple patients in a variety of areas in the facility.

Routes of transmission of pathogens may be from device to patient, from one patient to another, or from one body site to the lower respiratory tract of the same patient by means of hands or devices. Contamination of devices used on the respiratory tract include nebulizers, bronchoscopes, spirometers, oxygen analyzers, laryngoscope blades, and endotracheal tubes. Direct contact with contaminated fluids, hands, and equipment and with airborne droplet nuclei provide the major routes of transmission of pathogens associated with respiratory care.

Contaminated fluids include secretions, saliva, sputum, blood, or condensate in aerosol tubing or a ventilator circuit. Transmission of pathogens in fluid occurs when the fluid moves, flows, or spills from one area to another. Direct contact of fluids or moist substance with hands or equipment is probably the most common mode of transmission. Health care workers' hands are transiently contaminated with *Staphylococcus aureus* and gram-negative bacilli.[3,4] Respiratory syncytial virus infection usually follows inoculation of the conjunctivae or nasal mucosa by contaminated hands.

Airborne **droplet nuclei** are small particles (smaller than 2 to 5 μm in diameter) that may remain suspended in the air for extended periods of time. Particles larger than 0.3 μm are considered capable of carrying pathogens. Droplet nuclei have been shown to remain suspended in room air for hours and to move between room and even floors of a building. Sneezing, coughing, or even talking have been identified as sources of droplet nuclei from pa-

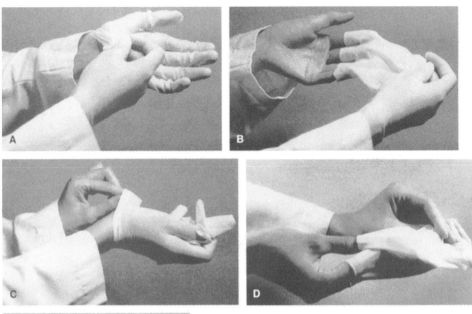

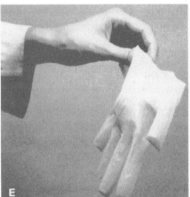

FIGURE 9-3 • Glove removal. (A) The wrist of one glove is grasped with the opposite gloved hand. (B) The glove is pulled inside-out over and off the hand. (C) With the first glove held in the gloved hand, the fingers of the nongloved hand are slipped under the wrist of the remaining glove without touching the exterior surfaces. (D) The glove is then pulled inside-out over the hand so that the first glove ends up inside of the second glove; no exterior glove surfaces are exposed. (E) The contaminated gloves can then be dropped into the proper waste receptacle.

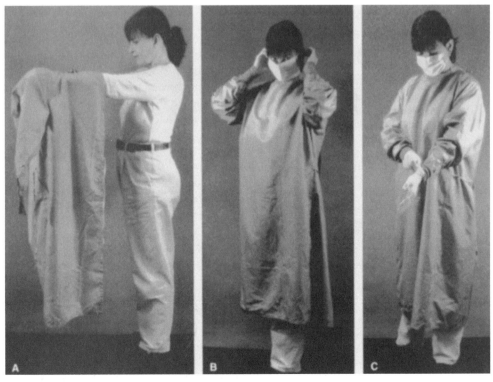

FIGURE 9-4 • Protective clothing. (A) The practitioner slips arms into a protective gown. (B) A mask is applied by slipping the elastic band over the ears. (C) Gloves are put on last and pulled over the gown cuffs.

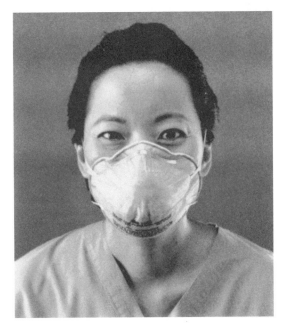

FIGURE 9-5 • Respirator, to be worn when caring for patients with suspected, untreated tuberculosis. (Courtesy of 3M Pharmaceutical, St. Paul, MN.)

tients, whereas nebulizers are a common source from equipment. Molecular water from devices such as passover and wick-type humidifiers cannot carry pathogens.[5]

Nebulizers with a reservoir can allow growth of hydrophilic bacteria that can be nebulized during device use.[6] Gram-negative bacilli, such as *Pseudomonas*, *Xanthomonas*, *Flavobacterium*, and *Legionella* species, and nontuberculous mycobacteria can multiply to substantial concentrations in nebulizer fluid, increasing the risk of acquiring pneumonia.[7] *Legionella* species and other bacteria can multiply to sufficiently large numbers within 24 hours to pose a risk of infection in patients who receive respira-

Box • 9–3 RULES FOR RESPIRATOR USE

MEDICAL SCREENING

History of cardiopulmonary problems
Pulmonary function
Claustrophobia

FIT TESTING

Initially and annually
For each type, size, or model of respirator

INSTRUCTION

Proper use
Cleaning
Storage
Maintenance

tory care.[6] Contaminated aerosols are associated with pneumonias caused by *Legionella* species, *Aspergillus* species, and *Serratia marcesens*. Sterilization or high-level disinfection can eliminate vegetative bacteria from device reservoirs, making them safe for patient use.

Respiratory care devices that touch mucous membranes are classified as **semicritical** according to the system defined by the Centers for Disease Control and Prevention (CDC). When semicritical devices cannot be sterilized (ie, by steam autoclave or ethylene oxide), they should be high-level disinfected. High-level disinfection may consist of pasteurization (submersion in water 75°C for 30 minutes) or use of liquid disinfectants that are approved by the Environmental Protection Agency as sterilants or disinfectants.[8] All equipment to be sterilized or disinfected must be cleaned thoroughly before the sterilization or disinfection process.

Most bacterial nosocomial pneumonias occur by aspiration of bacteria colonizing the oropharynx or upper gastrointestinal tract.[1,2] Intubation and mechanical ventilation alter and bypass first-line defense mechanisms, increasing the risk of aspiration and subsequent infection of the lung. Risk increases with time on the ventilator (up to 1% per day)[3] and is increased by leakage around the endotracheal tube cuff, which allows aspiration of pooled secretions.[10,11]

Unsafe practices or procedures by care providers may increase the incidence of nosocomial infections associated with respiratory care procedures. Failure to identify problems or trends in nosocomial pneumonia or infection rates results in care providers continuing to place patients at risk. Types of problems that have been associated include equipment that may not be handled properly, changed, disinfected, or maintained while in use on and between patients, as well as staff who do not consistently follow hand-washing and standard precaution guidelines.

Identifying problems is the first step in modifying procedures, practices, or devices to reduce the risk of infection. Surveillance should be conducted to identify the incidence of bacterial and aspiration pneumonias in patient populations in which respiratory complications are most likely (eg, patients with mechanically assisted ventilation, those with chronic obstructive pulmonary disease, those who are immunocompromised, and postoperative patients) to determine trends and identify potential problems.[7,12] Data are commonly expressed as rates (such as number of infections per 1000 ventilator days) to facilitate comparison of rates between other units and hospitals and to determine trends.[14]

Routine surveillance cultures of patients or of equipment and devices used to provide respiratory care or pulmonary function testing (PFT) or to administer inhaled anesthesia are not recommended by the CDC.[14]

Most devices are contaminated by the flora of the patient on contact and are not a primary source of infection as long as they are cleaned or disinfected properly between patients. The incidence of infection is much more important than the presence of potential pathogens on equipment.

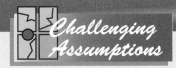

CRITICAL THINKING CHALLENGES

Ventilator Circuit Changes

1. Do not routinely change the ventilator circuit used with an individual patient more frequently than every 48 hours. No maximal length of time has been recommended for use of ventilator circuit between changes when non–aerosol-generating humidifiers are used. Circuit change intervals of less than every 48 hours have been identified as a risk factor for ventilator-associated pneumonia.[14]

2. Wick-type pass-over humidifiers produce no aerosols, and bubble-type humidifiers (used with ventilators) produce insignificant levels of aerosols, posing no significant risk for transmission of bacteria from the humidifier reservoir to patients.[16]

3. Heated humidification systems often operate at temperatures that reduce or eliminate bacterial pathogens. Sterile water is generally used to fill these humidifiers. Tap or distilled water may harbor *Le-*

gionella species, which are more heat resistant than other bacteria.

4. If there is no route of transmission (eg, aerosol or direct movement of fluids) from the heater reservoir to the patient, use of tap water or hospital distilled water should not pose an infection risk. Tap water, distilled water, or sterile water may be used with pass-over or wick-type (non–aerosol-generating) humidifiers.[14] Use sterile water to fill bubble-type humidifiers. Aerosol devices used with ventilator circuits should be filled with sterile fluids only and changed every 24 hours.

5. Sterilize or high-level disinfect circuits, humidifiers, and nebulizers between patients.

6. Closed, continuous-feed humidification systems have not been proved of benefit in reducing infection rates but generally provide more consistent humidification with less interruption of ventilation.

Mechanical Ventilation Devices

Ventilated patients have an increased risk of nosocomial pneumonia on several fronts. Beyond the fact that the patient is ill enough to require mechanical ventilation, the artificial airway is associated with increased opportunity for aspiration of bacteria colonizing the oropharynx and gastrointestinal tract. The respiratory care practitioner should minimize aspiration of secretions (eg, by positioning the patient with the head elevated at 30 degrees except during postural drainage procedures) and avoid total deflation of endotracheal tube cuff on a routine basis.

During the past 30 years, contamination of the ventilator circuit tubing and humidification systems and the frequency of changing these circuits has been linked with ventilator-associated pneumonias. The circuit tubing is contaminated by the patient's secretions in as little as 1 hour, usually with bacteria in secretions that originate from the patient's oropharynx or gastrointestinal tract.

Condensate

Condensate that forms in the inspiratory tubing of the ventilator circuit is often contaminated from patient secretions. Spillage of contaminated condensate (which collects in the ventilator circuit) into the patient's tracheobronchial tree or into a nebulizer reservoir can occur during procedures in which the tubing may be moved (eg, suctioning, repositioning the tubing, changing ventilator circuits, moving the patient) and may increase the risk of infection.[15]

EFFLUENT

Effluent from the ventilator circuit may contain microorganisms that can contaminate the environment, increasing risk of transmission. This can result from condensate spilling onto objects or hands, which then contact other surfaces or patients (Box 9–4).

HEAT–MOISTURE EXCHANGER

Another approach to reduce condensate formation is the use of a heat–moisture exchanger (HME), which provides passive humidification. This device is placed between the ventilator circuit and the patient's airway. HMEs designed to act as bacterial filters have not been proved to reduce ventilator-associated pneumonia significantly over other, less expensive devices. HMEs can increase dead space and resistance to breathing, while providing less humidity than active systems discussed previously, resulting in thick and plugging secretions in some patients. To be effective, 70% of the gas entering the airway must be exhaled through the exchanger; therefore, when leaks exist (eg, bronchopulmonary fistulas or cuffless endotracheal tubes), active humidification systems are more effective.

There is no recommendation by the CDC for preferential use of HMEs over heated humidifiers to prevent nosocomial pneumonia.[14] The respiratory care practitioner should change the exchanger when gross contamination or mechanical dysfunction of the device is present, commonly after 24 hours. Vent circuits are not changed routinely when an HME is being used on a patient.[14]

Box • 9–4   WAYS TO CONTROL CONDENSATE WITH ACTIVE HUMIDIFIERS

- Periodically drain and discard condensate that collects in the tubing of a mechanical ventilator; do not allow to drain toward patient.
- Spillage can be minimized by the use of water traps carefully placed in the inspiratory and expiratory limbs of the ventilator circuits to allow condensate to drain away from the patient by gravity on a continuous basis.
- Microorganisms contaminating condensate can be transmitted by the health care worker's hands.
- Condensate should be treated as contaminated waste and disposed of properly through standard hospital waste stream.
- Heated wire circuits can be used to reduce or eliminate condensate formation in the ventilator circuit.
- Heated wire circuits should be set so that a small amount of condensate forms on the inspiratory limb of the circuit, indicating 100% relative humidity.
- Improper adjustment of a heated wire circuit may result in decreased humidity delivered to the patient, resulting in damage to the epithelium of the respiratory tract and potential occlusion of artificial airways, especially in infants and small children.[17] If the ventilator circuit is hotter than the output of the humidifier, the absolute humidity of gas leaving the humidifier may be lower than that required to maintain the integrity of the airway.

Another potential source of pathogens is medical gas, such as debris and condensed water in compressed air lines, which may pass through the ventilator into the patient's airway. This can be minimized with use of water traps on the incoming gas lines and with filters from between the ventilator and the patient.

The internal mechanisms of ventilators are not considered an important source of bacterial contamination of inhaled air, and routine sterilization of these devices is considered unnecessary.[14]

FILTERS

Use of high-efficiency bacterial filters in the breathing circuit have been advocated on both inspiratory and expiratory limbs of the ventilator circuit. On the inspiratory limb, filters can eliminate particulate contaminants from the inspired gas and theoretically reduce retrograde contamination of the ventilator. There is no substantiation of decreased pneumonias with filter in the inspiratory limb. Filters may change operating characteristics of the ventilator by creating additional resistance in the circuit.

Filters increase turbulence and resistance to gas flow in the ventilator circuit. As the filters become saturated with humidity and water, the resistance may increase even more. Bacterial filters should not be placed between the humidifier and the patient on the inspiratory limb.

Periodically testing reusable filters ensures that resistance is not increased. As particulates build up over time, resistance increases.

Filters on the expiratory limb of the ventilator may help prevent cross-contamination, but their importance in reducing the incidence of nosocomial pneumonia needs further evaluation.

Nebulizers

Nebulizers can become contaminated by the hands of personnel, by contaminated fluid added to the reservoir, by retrograde contamination from the patient, or by inadequate sterilization or disinfection between uses.

Any device that produces aerosols can transmit pathogens and must be changed or cleaned regularly during routine use and consistently between patients to ensure that pathogens in the reservoir do not contaminate the patient.[14]

Nebulizers that are used for treatment of inhaled medication, whether hand-held by the patient or placed in line with a ventilator, can produce bacteria-transporting aerosols.[6] Limited research has been done on infection rates associated with hand-held small-volume nebulizers. Association with nosocomial pneumonia has been rarely documented; in these cases, infection was traced to contaminated medications from multidose vials.[19]

Large-volume nebulizers, mist tents, and hoods should be sterilized or high-level disinfected between patients and after every 24 hours of use on the same patient.

Room humidifiers that create aerosols (eg, vaporizers, spinning disks, and ultrasonic nebulizers) have been associated with development of nosocomial pneumonia secondary to contamination of their reservoirs. The CDC recommends that aerosol-generating room humidifiers not be used unless they can be sterilized or high-level disinfected every 24 hours and filled only with sterile fluids.[13] Wick-type humidifiers, marketed for home use, do not pose the same risk of aerosol transmission of pathogens and may prove to be more cost-effective. Recommendations for the safe use of small-volume nebulizers are provided in Box 9–5.

Suction Catheters

Tracheal suction catheters can introduce microorganisms into the lower respiratory tract. Catheters that are contaminated with microorganisms after being used on a patient's airway may contaminate the immediate environment of the patient. Open-suction systems use a sterile single-use catheter and sterile technique. Breaches in sterile technique, such as allowing the catheter or gloves to contact patient

Box • 9–5 TECHNIQUE FOR USING SMALL-VOLUME MEDICATION HAND-HELD AND IN-LINE NEBULIZERS

1. Sterilize or disinfect nebulizers between patients. Between treatments on the same patient, sterilize, disinfect, or rinse with sterile water and air dry after each treatment.[6,14]
2. Use only sterile fluids and dispense aseptically.
3. If multidose medication vials are used, handle, dispense, and store them according to directions on the vial label or package insert.[14,18]
4. In-line nebulizers should be removed from the ventilator circuit between treatments, then disinfected or rinsed with sterile water and air dried.

skin, secretions, clothing, or objects before suctioning, have been associated with the introduction of pathogens into the lungs. Reusing catheters without proper disinfection is not acceptable practice in the hospital.

If the catheter is to be cleared while suctioning a patient, sterile water should be used. After use, care should be taken to dispose of the catheter properly in normal hospital waste stream.

The CDC offers no recommendation about whether sterile or clean gloves should be used.[14] Clean gloves, right out of the package, have not been shown to be contaminated with the types of pathogens associated with nosocomial infections. Whether clean or sterile, the same care needs to be taken to avoid contaminating the gloves by contacting the patient or environment before suctioning.

Closed-Suction Systems

Insufficient data are available to determine whether multiuse closed-suction catheters are significantly different than single-use catheters in terms of infection risk, oxygenation, and environmental contamination.[20,21,22,23] Sterile fluid should be used to remove secretions from the suction catheter. The suction collection tubing and canisters should be changed between patients.

Resuscitation Bags

Manually operated resuscitation bags may become contaminated from patient secretions and the practitioner's hands.[24,25,26] When the bag valve is visibly soiled with secretions, it should be rinsed clear with sterile water. Resuscitation bags are difficult to dry and clean between uses with the same patient. Microorganisms in secretions left in the bag valve may be sprayed into the lower respiratory tract of the patient with an artificial airway. Bags should be sterilized or high-level disinfected between patients or when still visibly soiled after attempts to rinse clear with sterile water. The exterior of the bag is prone to contamination and may become a reservoir for pathogens. Hands must be washed before and after all contact with equipment or the patient.

Artificial Airways

Box 9–6 describes some of the risks associated with artificial airways. Insertion of oral as opposed to nasoendotracheal tubes significantly reduces the incidence of nosocomial maxillary sinusitis.[29] Tracheostomy should be performed under sterile conditions. Elective tracheostomy should be performed in the operating room. When changing the tracheostomy tube, aseptic technique should be used, the tube should be replaced with one that has undergone sterilization or high-level disinfection.

Immobility and Infection

Immobilization of patients has long been associated with reduced lung volumes and increased pulmonary complications. The most valuable and inexpensive intervention is to turn patients from the supine to lateral position every 2 hours. The sooner a patient gets up and moves around, the faster breathing patterns and lung volumes return to normal. Health care providers should encourage "stir-up" regimens as tolerated.

Box • 9–6 RISKS ASSOCIATED WITH ARTIFICIAL AIRWAYS

- An artificial airway bypasses the upper airway and increases the risk of pulmonary infection.
- Secretions containing oral and gastrointestinal flora often are aspirated into the lung.
- Secretions may collect around the tube above an inflated cuff and be aspirated into the lung along the exterior surfaces of the airway and cuff.[27] Do not routinely deflate the cuff of the endotracheal tube (lavaging the airway with secretions pooled above the cuff) to determine the filling volume of the cuff. Alternative techniques to ensure proper cuff pressure (such as minimal leak or minimal occluding pressure) should be substituted. Endotracheal tubes with double lumens designed to allow suctioning of secretions from above the cuff have been studied,[4] but there is not sufficient data to recommend their use.[14]
- Risk of aspiration is increased with the presence of nasogastric tubes and during tube feedings.[28] When not contraindicated, place patient with head up at 30- to 40-degree angle, especially during and for 1 hour after feedings.[29–30]

Unfortunately, the sicker the patient, the greater is the tendency to maintain the patient in a supine position. Box 9–7 shows a number of excuses that care providers use to justify not turning patients. The bottom line is the perception that it is too much trouble to medicate the patient properly and to get adequate assistance to help reposition the patient every 2 hours. Valid reasons not to move a patient, such as a recent laminectomy or procedure that requires the patient position not to be changed, should be highlighted in the patient's medical record so that the entire team can avoid hurting the patient. General injunctions, especially hearsay that a patient is not being turned because the doctor said so with no supporting documentation in the medical record, should be questioned and challenged with the physician. It is important to differentiate between when the patient needs to be immobilized to avoid complications and when unnecessary immobilization places the patient at increased risk of complications.

Besides turning patients from side to side, it is also of value to know when to raise the head of the bed. Patients receiving mechanical ventilation through a nasogastric or other enteral tube should be positioned with the head elevated at an angle of 30 to 45 degrees, especially during and for 1 hour after tube feedings.[31]

Provision of Oxygen by Mask or Cannula

Three identified sources of infection risk associated with administration of oxygen with devices such as masks and cannulas are (1) contaminated bubble-type humidifiers, (2) contaminated masks or cannulas, and (3) contaminated gas lines. The practitioner should change the tubing and any device, such as cannula or mask, used to deliver oxygen from a wall outlet between patients.

Manufacturer instructions should be followed in the use and maintenance of disposable wall oxygen humidifiers unless data show that modification in their use or maintenance poses no threat to the patient and is cost-effective. This may include use of prefilled bubble-type humidifiers to deliver low-flow oxygen for multiple patients in areas such as emergency departments or postanesthesia recovery rooms.[32,33,34]

The use of bubble-type humidifiers should be restricted to appropriate situations. Humidifiers are not indicated for

oxygen flows less than 4 L/min in adult patients under normal conditions.[35] When operated at flows above 10 L/min, a standard, unheated bubble-type humidifier is less efficient at humidifying gas and may create aerosols that can transmit bacteria from the reservoir of the humidifier.

If the patient is breathing through a normal upper airway, contaminants or bacteria in the gas should pose minimal risk of infection to the lungs. Remember that the nose and upper airway filter out most of the pathogens that are in the air before they reach the lungs. Filters in the gas line between the flowmeter and delivery device have not been shown to reduce the incidence of lung infection.

Diagnostic Testing

PERCUTANEOUS ARTERIAL AND VENOUS BLOOD SAMPLING

Transmission of pathogens from needles and syringes to patients and from needles to care providers can be minimized by the interventions[35] shown in Box 9–8.

TRANSCUTANEOUS OXYGEN ANALYZER

$PtcCO_2$ and $PtcO_2$ levels are measured through intact skin using heated electrodes that can burn the skin, with subsequent risk of increased bacterial colonization and infection of the injured area. This risk of skin burns can be minimized by using the minimal temperature required to make consistent measurements, frequently monitoring the temperatures used, moving the electrode in accordance with the appropriate time interval (every 2 to 4 hours), and fol-

---

Box • 9–7   COMMON EXCUSES FOR NOT TURNING PATIENTS

Turning may cause patient pain.
Moving may pull or split an incision.
Turning may dislodge an access line.
Moving may mess up the monitors.
Patient is resting.
Care provider is resting.
Physician said not to move patient.

Box • 9–8   INTERVENTIONS TO PREVENT PATHOGEN TRANSMISSION

- Perform hand washing and don gloves before prepping patient.
- Perform adequate skin preparation.
- Use sterile equipment.
- Do not precool syringes by submerging in ice water.
- Avoid repeating unsuccessful arterial punctures with the same needle or cannula.
- Handle *all* body fluids as if contaminated; this includes the use of gloves and the proper disposal and transport of specimens.
- Specimens should be placed in a sealed container and then placed in a Zip-lock bag with the biohazard symbol for transport to the appropriate diagnostic laboratory.
- Arterial blood gas samples should be capped (without the needle), labeled as appropriate, and transported to the blood gas laboratory in a Zip-lock bag with the biohazard symbol.
- Avoid recapping needles. If necessary, use one-handed technique to avoid accidental puncture (see Box 9–10).

lowing other manufacturer recommendations. Skin burn injuries should be treated aseptically.

PULSE OXIMETRY

During pulse oximetry, oxygen saturation is measured by passing light through intact skin on the finger, toe, or earlobe. Sensor probes are either a reusable spring loaded clip-on device (attached to the ear lobe or finger) or a wrap-around probe (used on fingers or toes), which uses tape to hold a reusable or disposable probe in place.

Reusable clip-on sensors are difficult to clean and disinfect between patients and may create pressure sores. Probes should be disinfected as thoroughly as possible between patients and their use over broken skin avoided.

Pressure sores at probe site have resulted from pressure of clip-on probes, especially with edematous patients, in as little as 45 minutes. Clip-on probes thus should not be used over edematous areas. The probe site should be checked frequently and the probe repositioned as necessary.

Because the pulse oximeter uses a light-emitting diode, skin burns at the probe site can occur, with subsequent risk of increased bacterial colonization and infection of the injured area. All probes should be repositioned at appropriate time intervals in accordance with the manufacturer's recommendations.

Provision of Pulmonary Function Testing

Pulmonary function testing devices include wedge spirometers, rolling seal spirometers, peak flowmeters, and other devices used to measure the volume or flow of air that a patient can inhale or exhale. Microorganisms can be transmitted to the patient from contact with the mouthpiece, tubing, or nose clips. Surfaces of the device that come into patient contact should be disinfected between uses; mouthpieces and nose clips should be sterilized between patients. Disinfection of the internal components of the PFT device is difficult and not recommended, nor is routine disinfection of the internal machinery of PFT machines between uses.

Inhalation of airborne particles from equipment used on previous patients is theoretically possible. The use of low-resistance, high-efficiency filters between the mouthpiece and the spirometer has been advocated to minimize contamination between device and patient. This filter may also reduce care provider exposure of droplet nuclei generated by the patient during forced expiratory maneuvers.

Sputum Induction for Specimen Collection

Microorganisms can be transmitted to patients from contaminated equipment or solutions in the nebulizer used to induce sputum.[5] Nebulizers should be sterilized or high-level disinfected between patients. All surfaces on equipment that patients would come in contact with during a procedure should be cleaned and disinfected.

Microorganisms can also be transmitted from the patient to the health care provider or other patients in the vicinity in the form of droplet nuclei produced by coughing. Sputum induction should be performed in a private room if possible with six exchanges per hour. The door should be closed. An isolation mask or particulate respirator should be worn by the health care provider in the room during the sputum induction. Visitors should be asked to leave the room during the sputum induction. Engineering and environmental controls should be used if available (eg, isolation booth, HEPA filter treatment station, negative-pressure room). Patient education should occur regarding proper cough covering and protection.

Cleaning and Disinfection of Respiratory Care Devices

Proper cleaning and sterilization or high-level disinfection of reusable equipment is important to reduce infection.[13] Respiratory care devices have been classified as semicritical because they may come into contact with mucous membranes but do not ordinarily penetrate body surfaces.

There is no evidence that low-level contamination of respiratory therapy devices before patient use, such as after high-level disinfection of the device, presents greater risk than does sterile equipment.

All equipment should be cleaned thoroughly. If devices cannot tolerate being sterilized by steam autoclave or ethylene oxide, they can be high-level disinfected by pasteurization at 75°C for 30 minutes or using a liquid chemical disinfectant approved by the Environmental Protection Agency as a sterilant or disinfectant[12] (Table 9–3).

When rinsing is needed after a device has been disinfected, only sterile water should be used. Tap water or locally prepared distilled water may harbor microorganisms that can cause pneumonia.[14]

The CDC recommends that equipment and devices that are manufactured "for single use only" should not be reprocessed unless data show that reprocessing poses no threat to the patient, is cost-effective, and does not change the structural integrity and function of the device.[14]

PERSONAL SAFETY GUIDELINES FOR THE RESPIRATORY CARE PRACTITIONER

Parenteral Exposure to Blood or Other Potentially Infectious Materials

Any health care worker who has a significant **parenteral exposure** to blood or other potentially infectious materials (eg, bloody body fluids, semen, vaginal secretions, body fluids from an unknown source) should report immediately to the employee health department or an equivalent department within the institution or to the emergency department if the employee health department is not open.

Significant exposure is defined as penetration of intact skin or mucous membranes (eg, eye, nose, mouth) by an

Table ● 9–3   CHARACTERISTICS OF ANTISEPTIC (ANTIMICROBIAL) AGENTS

Group and Subgroup	Gram-positive Bacteria	Gram-negative Bacteria	Mycobacterium tuberculosis	Fungi	Virus	Speed of Killing Sensitive Bacteria	Inactivation by Mucus or Proteins	Comments
Alcohols	Good	Good	Good	Good	Good	Fast	Moderate	Optimum strength 70% to 90% with added emollients (eg, glycerine or cetyl alcohol is less drying), not recommended for physical cleaning of skin; good for hand antisepsis and for surgical site preparation
Chlorhexidine: 4% aqueous	Good	Good	Fair	Fair	Good	Intermediate	Minimal	Has persistent effect; good for both hand washing and surgical site or preoperative patient skin preparation; do not use near mucous membranes; toxicity to ears and eyes reported; activity neutralized by non-ionic surfactants
Hexachlorophene: 3% aqueous	Good	Poor	Poor	Poor	Poor	Slow	Minimal	Provides persistent, cumulative activity after repeated use (washing with alcohol reduces persistent action); can be toxic when absorbed from skin, especially in premature infants; good for hand washing but not for surgical site preparation; limited spectrum of antimicrobial activity
Iodine compounds, iodine in alcohol	Good	Good	Good	Good	Good	Fast	Marked	Causes skin "burns," but this is unusual with 1% tincture, especially if it is removed after several minutes; too irritating for hand washing but excellent for surgical site preparation
Iodophors	Good	Good	Fair	Good	Good	Intermediate	Moderate	Less irritating to the skin than iodine; good for both hand washing and surgical site preparation; rapidly neutralized in presence of organic materials such as blood or sputum
Para-chloro-meta-xylenol (PCMX)	Good	Fair*	Fair	Fair	Fair	Intermediate	Minimal	Activity neutralized by nonionic surfactants
Triclosan	Good	Good	Fair	Poor	Good	Intermediate	Minimal	

From APIC Infection Control and Applied Epidemiology: Principles and Practice. St. Louis: Mobsy-Year Book; 1996.
*Activity improved by addition of chelating agent such as EDTA.
Note: Some of these agents, such as iodine or chlorhexidine, are combined with alcohol to form tinctures and are available in the combined formulation.

object that has been contaminated with blood or other body fluid or direct contact of mucous membrane or nonintact skin with blood or other body fluid. Contact of blood or body fluids with *intact skin* is *not* a significant exposure.

Should exposure occur, the incident should be reported and any required reporting forms completed in a timely manner. The employee health or emergency department records the circumstances of the exposure, including the route of exposure and the hepatitis B virus (HBV) and HIV status of the source patient, if known.[36]

Based on the exposure, the employee health or emergency department should offer the employee any screening tests needed. At the employee's request, a blood or serum sample can be collected and saved by the clinical laboratory for later testing. If the source patient can be determined, the patient should be tested for evidence of current infection with HBV and HIV. Based on the incident and the results of the testing, the health care provider should be offered any prophylaxis that may be available. Employees not requiring prophylaxis should be informed. Follow-up testing and counseling should be offered as necessary by the employee health department.

Communicable Diseases

Any employee who has a communicable disease that can be transmitted from person to person in the usual hospital setting should report this fact immediately to his or her direct supervisor or to the employee health department.

Vaccinations

Each fall, many institutions offer all employees influenza vaccinations through the employee health department. This is done for the protection of employees and to prevent employees from transmitting influenza virus to patients or other employees.

Hepatitis B antigen and antibody testing should be offered to determine the need for vaccination. This pretesting is encouraged but is not a requirement for immunization. Practitioners whose testing shows no need for the vaccine should be informed of their results. All employees in direct health care typically can receive the hepatitis B vaccination without prior testing. Follow-up testing may be offered to determine immune response after completion of the vaccine course, but the vaccination, which involves a course of three injections, has such a high success rate that follow-up is no longer mandated in many states. The hepatitis B vaccine typically is offered without cost to the employee.

Safety Requirements

Because many microorganisms can be transmitted through ingestion or by inoculation of mucous membranes, practices that could lead to such transmission are generally prohibited in patient care rooms, clean or soiled holding rooms, and medication rooms.

Administrators and practitioners are responsible for containing their activities of eating, drinking, grooming, and food storage in the proper environments.

Eating, drinking, hair care, and application of cosmetics are universally prohibited in patient care areas and laboratories. Food and beverages are not stored in a refrigerator used for biologic, chemical, specimen, or medication storage.

Body Substance Isolation

Actual or potential contact with the following substances from all patients requires the use of personal protective equipment: blood, semen, vaginal secretions, cerebrospinal fluid, synovial fluid, pleural fluid, peritoneal fluid, pericardial fluid, amniotic fluid, body tissues, and any other body substances containing visible blood.

According to Standard Precautions, personnel are urged to use protective equipment and materials with the following substances: feces, nasal secretions, sputum, sweat, tears, urine, vomitus, and other body fluids. If any of these contain blood, they must be handled with the use of personal protective equipment and materials.

A variety of isolation systems (Box 9–9) have been identified for use with patients with specific clinical symptoms or conditions, as shown in Table 9–4.

Needles, syringes, and other sharps are disposed of in impervious containers located in each patient room or in the area of use. Needles are not recapped, bent, or manipulated before disposal. Intravenous poles are often equipped with resheathers. Single-handed techniques should be used if styrofoam pillows are not provided for resheathing (see Sharps Container section).

There are no special precautions for isolating linen; however, all linen must be wrapped in a fashion that prevents leakage or moisture from escaping.

The trash from all patients in isolation (except granulocytopenic precautions) is considered infectious waste and should be removed by building management in a red bag.

RESTRICTIONS ON PLACEMENT OF ISOLATION PATIENTS

Because of air-circulation patterns, patients who require airborne precaution *cannot* be housed in areas of the hospital where negative-pressure private rooms are not available.

Documentation in the clinical record must identify the type of isolation and precautions initiated and maintained, the reasons for these precautions, and the termination of this care.

Storage and Monitoring of Sterile Supplies

Before use, the care provider should inspect any sterile package for an expiration date and package integrity. If the package is outdated, it is returned for reprocessing. Outdated material from a commercial source and packages that

Box • 9–9   SYNOPSIS OF TYPES OF PRECAUTIONS AND PATIENTS REQUIRING THE PRECAUTIONS

STANDARD PRECAUTIONS

Use Standard Precautions for the care of all patients.

AIRBORNE PRECAUTIONS

In addition to Standard Precautions, use Airborne Precautions for patients known or suspected to have serious illnesses transmitted by airborne droplet nuclei. Examples of such illnesses include the following:

1. Measles
2. Varicella (including disseminated zoster) virus*
3. Tuberculosis

DROPLET PRECAUTIONS

In addition to Standard Precautions, use Droplet Precautions for patients known or suspected to have serious illnesses transmitted by large-particle droplets. Examples of such illnesses include the following:

1. Invasive *Haemophilus influenzae* type b disease, including meningitis, pneumonia, epiglottitis, and sepsis
2. Invasive *Neisseria meningitidis* disease, including meningitis, pneumonia, and sepsis
3. Other serious bacterial respiratory infections spread by droplet transmission, including:
   a. Diphtheria (pharyngeal)
   b. *Mycoplasma pneumoniae* infection
   c. Pertussis
   d. Pneumonic plague
   e. Streptococcal pharyngitis, pneumonia, or scarlet fever in infants and young children
4. Serious viral infections spread by droplet transmission, including:
   a. Adenovirus*
   b. Influenza
   c. Mumps
   d. Parvovirus B19
   e. Rubella

CONTACT PRECAUTIONS

In addition to Standard Precautions, use Contact Precautions for patients known or suspected to have serious illnesses that are easily transmitted by direct patient contact or by contact with items in the patient's environment. Examples of such illnesses include the following:

1. Gastrointestinal, respiratory, skin, or wound infections or colonization with multidrug-resistant bacteria judged by the infection control program, based on current state, regional, or national recommendations, to be of special clinical and epidemiologic significance.
2. Enteric infections with a low infectious dose or prolonged environmental survival, including:
   a. *Clostridium difficile* infection
   b. For diapered or incontinent patients: enterohemorrhagic *Escherichia coli* 0157:H7, *Shigella* species, hepatitis A, or rotavirus infection
3. Respiratory syncytial virus, parainfluenza virus, or enteroviral infections in infants and young children
4. Skin infections that are highly contagious or that may occur on dry skin, including:
   a. Diphtheria (cutaneous)
   b. Herpes simplex virus (neonatal or mucocutaneous)
   c. Impetigo
   d. Major (noncontained) abscesses, cellulitis, or decubiti
   e. Pediculosis
   f. Scabies
   g. Staphylococcal furunculosis in infants and young children
   h. Zoster (disseminated or in the immunocompromised host) virus infection*
5. Viral or hemorrhagic conjunctivitis
6. Viral or hemorrhagic infections (Ebola, Lassa fever, or Marburg virus)

*Certain infections require more than one type of precaution.

---

have been partially opened or otherwise compromised should be returned to the institution's central distribution area.

Used Instrument Trays

After use of an instrument tray, the sharps and needles are placed in a sharps container in the patient room. The tray should be covered with a wrap or towel, carried to the soiled holding room, and placed in covered instrument tray bin.

Infectious Waste and Chemical Spills

Infectious waste should be handled and disposed of in accordance with hospital policy. Infectious waste is defined by hospital policy and is red-bagged for subsequent incineration. Containers filled with body fluids are considered infectious waste.

DOUBLE-BAGGING

Routine double-bagging of isolation laundry and waste has been studied and determined to have no benefit.[27,28] It is of

Table • 9–4   **CLINICAL SYNDROMES OR CONDITIONS WARRANTING ADDITIONAL EMPIRIC PRECAUTIONS TO PREVENT TRANSMISSION OF EPIDEMIOLOGICALLY IMPORTANT PATHOGENS PENDING CONFIRMATION OF DIAGNOSIS***

Clinical Syndrome or Condition†	Potential Pathogens‡	Empiric Precautions
Diarrhea		
Acute diarrhea with a likely infectious cause in an incontinent or diapered patient	Enteric pathogens§	Contact
Diarrhea in an adult with a history of recent antibiotic use	*Clostridium difficile*	Contact
Meningitis	*Neisseria meningitidis*	Droplet
Rash or Exanthems, Generalized, Cause Unknown		
Petechial or ecchymotic with fever	*N. meningitidis*	Droplet
Vesicular	Varicella	Airborne and contact
Maculopapular with coryza and fever	Rubeola (measles)	Airborne
Respiratory Infections		
Cough, fever, or upper lobe pulmonary infiltrate in an HIV-negative patient or a patient at low risk for HIV infection	*M. tuberculosis*	Airborne
Cough, fever, or pulmonary infiltrate in any lung location in an HIV-infected patient or a patient at high risk for HIV infection	*M. tuberculosis*	Airborne
Paroxysmal or severe persistent cough during periods of pertussis activity	*Bordetella pertussis*	Droplet
Respiratory infections, particularly bronchiolitis and croup, in infants and young children	Respiratory syncytial or parainfluenza virus	Contact
Risk of Multidrug-resistant Microorganisms		
History of infection or colonization with multidrug-resistant organisms‖	Resistant bacteria	Contact
Skin, wound, or urinary tract infection in a patient with a recent hospital or nursing home stay in a facility where multidrug-resistant organisms are prevalent	Resistant bacteria	Contact
Skin or Wound Infection		
Abscess or draining wound that cannot be covered	*Staphylococcus aureus*, group A streptococcus	Contact

From *APIC Infection Control and Applied Epidemiology: Principles and Practice.* St. Louis: Mosby-Year Book; 1996.

*Infection control professionals are encouraged to modify or adapt this table according to local conditions. To ensure that appropriate empiric precautions are always implemented, hospitals must have systems in place to routinely evaluate patients according to these criteria as part of their preadmission and admission care.

†Patients with the syndromes or conditions listed below in this footnote present with atypical signs or symptoms (eg, pertussis in neonates and adults may not have paroxysmal or severe cough). The clinician's index of suspicion should be guided by the prevalence of specific conditions in the community as well as clinical judgment.

‡The organisms listed under the column "Potential Pathogens" are not intended to represent the complete or even most likely diagnosis, but rather possible etiologic agents that require additional precautions beyond Standard Precautions until they can be ruled out.

§These pathogens include enterhemorrhagic *E. coli* 0157:H7, *Shigella* species, hepatitis A, and rotavirus.

‖Resistant bacteria judged by the infection control program, based on current state, regional, or national recommendations, to be of special clinical or epidemiologic significance.

greater importance that the laundry be handled safely before it is bagged and when it is processed.

Disinfectant fogging has not been shown to work.

TRASH DISPOSAL

Trash generated during patient care is placed in a plastic-lined waste container in the patient room. Trash generated during patient care that contains blood, such as saturated dressings, drains, and tubes, typically is placed in a red bag.

SHARPS CONTAINERS

Needle sticks are a major source of exposure to many life-threatening pathogens. Safe disposal of needles, sharps, and syringes after use is critical for both practitioner and patient safety.

Sharps containers should be placed conveniently in the vicinity of clinical areas in which needles and syringes are commonly used to permit their safe disposal. Depending on the style of the sharps container, the mailbox slot is pulled open with one hand by pulling one of the tabs on the side of the container toward the user. The needle, syringe, or sharp is inserted horizontally into the slot. The material to be disposed of is dropped into the container by pushing the tab toward the box. It is unsafe to push sharps into any sharps container system, to place them vertically into the system, or to insert fingers into the opening.

A needle unwinder is found at the top of the container to facilitate removal of needles from Vacutainers or oversized

---

Box • 9–10   TECHNIQUE FOR ONE-HANDED NEEDLE

1. Place the sheath on a hard, steady surface. Place your nondominant hand behind your back.
2. Pick up unsheathed needle device with your dominant hand and ease needle into sheath. Hold loosely sheathed needle upright.
3. With your nondominant hand, approach the sheath from below the needle, and gently grasp the outer sheath from the base and pull downward, securing sheath onto the needle.

---

syringes. When the mailbox slot does not move freely, the disposal system is full and must be changed. Once a sharps container is filled, the mailbox slot is secured by pressing it toward the box until it clicks into place. Once secured, filled sharps containers are taken to the soiled holding room for disposal.

Needles should not be recapped, bent, or broken; an exception to this policy may occur when it is imperative that a needle be recapped (Box 9–10).

Box • 9–11   TECHNIQUE FOR CLEANING UP CRITICAL SPILLS

1. Begin cleaning critical spills as soon as possible.
2. Put on gloves. If the spill is large and there is the potential for contamination of clothing, an apron or gown should be worn.
3. Wipe up spill with an absorbent material, such as paper towels; discard these into a plastic-lined wastebasket.
4. Apply hospital disinfectant (eg, Virex) to the area of the spill.
5. Wipe up the hospital disinfectant using an absorbent material, such a paper towels; discard these into a plastic-lined wastebasket.
6. Remove gloves and discard into a plastic-lined wastebasket.
7. Wash hands.
8. If an apron has been worn, remove and discard into a plastic-lined wastebasket.
9. Place plastic waste liner into a "red bag" and carry to soiled holding room.
10. Wash hands.

---

*Critical spills include patient blood, body fluid, excretion, or secretion which has been spilled or splashed into the environment.

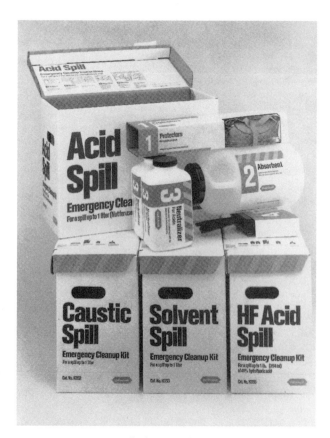

FIGURE 9-6 • Spill clean-up kit. (Courtesy of Mallinckrodt Medical, Inc., St. Louis, MO.)

CHEMICAL SPILLS

Chemical spills present environmental safety concerns. Although safe handing of chemicals, biologic wastes, solvents, and medications can prevent spills, when spills happen, they need to be contained and cleaned up in a safe manner. Each institution should have a spill policy or protocol. Some may use prepackaged kits, such as those shown in Figure 9–6. Box 9–11 illustrates a typical procedure for containing and cleaning up a hazardous spill.

References

1. Schaberg DR, Culver DH, Gaynes RP. Major trends in the microbial etiology of nosocomial infection. *Am J Med.* 1991;91(suppl 3B):72S–75S.
2. Bartlett JG, OKeefe P, Tally FP, et al. Bacteriology of hospital-acquired pneumonia. *Arch Intern Med.* 1986;146:868–871.
3. Larson E. Persistent carriage of gram negative bacteria on hands. *Am J Infect Control.* 1981;9:112–119.
4. Simmons B, Bryant J, Neiman K, et al. The role of hand washing in prevention of endemic intensive care unit infections. *Infect Control Hosp Epidemiol.* 1990;11:589–594.
5. Centers for Disease Control. Guidelines for preventing the transmission of tuberculosis in health-care settings with special focus on HIV-related issues. *MMWR.* 1990;39(RR-17):1–29.
6. Craven De, Lichtenberg DA, Goularte TA, et al. Contaminated medication nebulizers in mechanical ventilator circuits. *Am J Med.* 1984;146:460–467.
7. Pierce AK, Edmondson EB, McGee G, et al. An analysis of factors predisposing to gram-negative bacillary necrotizing pneumonia. *Am Rev Respir Dis.* 1966;94:309–315.
8. Craven DE, Kunches LM, Kilinsky V, et al. Risk factors for pneu-

monia and fatality in patients receiving continuous mechanical ventilation. *Am Review Respir Dis.* 1986;133:792–796.

9. Fagon JY, Chastre J, Domart Y, et al. Nosocomial pneumonia in patient receiving continuous mechanical ventilation: Prospective analysis of 52 episodes with use of a protected specimen brush and quantitative culture techniques. *Am Rev Respir Dis.* 1989;139:877–884.

10. Mahul Ph, Auboyer C, Jospe R, et al. Prevention of nosocomial in intubated patients: Respective role of mechanical subglottic drainage and stress ulcer prophylaxis. *Intensive Care Med.* 1992;18:20–25.

11. Torres A, Aznar R, Gatell JM, et al. Incidence, risk, and prognosis factors of nosocomial pneumonia in mechanically ventilated patients. *Am Rev Respir Dis.* 1990;142:523–526.

12. Favero MS. Principles of sterilization and disinfection. *Anesth Clin North Am.* 1989;7:941–949.

13. Haley RW, Culver DH, White JW. The efficacy of infection surveillance and control program in preventing nosocomial infections in US hospitals. *Am J Epidemiol.* 1985;121:182–205.

14. Department of Health and Human Services, Centers for Disease Control and Prevention. Guidelines for prevention of nosocomial pneumonia. Part 1. Issues on prevention of nosocomial pneumonia—1994. Part 2. Recommendations for prevention of nosocomial pneumonia: Notice of comment period. *Am J Infect Control.* 1994;2:247–292.

15. Craven DE, Goularte TA, Make BJ. Contaminated condensate in mechanical ventilator circuits: A risk factor for nosocomial pneumonia. *Am Rev Respir Dis.* 1984;129:625–628.

16. Rhame FS, Streifel A, McComb C, Boyle M. Bubbling humidifiers produce micro aerosols which can carry bacteria. *Infect Control.* 1986;7:403–406.

17. Myao H, Hirokawa T, Miyasaka K, Kawazoe T. Relative humidity, not absolute humidity is of great importance when using a humidifier with a heating wire. *Crit Care Med.* 1992;20:674–679.

18. AARC. Clinical practice guideline: Humidification during mechanical ventilation. *Respir Care.* 1992;37:887–890.

19. Sanders CV, Luby JP, Johanson WG, et al. *Serratia marcescens* infections from inhalation therapy medications: Nosocomial outbreak. *Ann Intern Med.* 1970;73:15–21.

20. Ritz R, Scott LR, Coyle MB, Pierson DJ. Contamination of a multiple-use suction catheter in a closed-circuit system compared to contamination of a disposable, single-use suction catheter. *Respir Care.* 1986;31:1087–1091.

21. Deppe SA, Kelly JW, Thoi LL, et al. Incidence of colonization, nosocomial pneumonia, and mortality in critically ill patients using Trach Care closed-suction system versus open-suction system: Prospective randomized study. *Crit Care Med.* 1990;18:1389–1393.

22. Mayhall GCG. The Trach Care closed tracheal suction system: A new medical device to permit tracheal suctioning without interruption of ventilatory assistance. *Infect Control Hosp Epidemiol.* 1988;9:125–126.

23. Decker MD, Lancaster AD, Latham RH, et al. Influence of closed suctioning system on ventilator associated pneumonias. Third Annual Meeting of the Society for Hospital Epidemiology of America. 1993:A6. Abstract.

24. Stone JW, Das BC. Investigation of an outbreak of infection with *Acinetobacter calcoaceticus* in a special care baby unit. *J Hosp Infect.* 1986;7:42–48.

25. Thompson AC, Wilder BJ, Powner DJ. Bedside resuscitation bags: A source of bacterial contamination. *Infect Control.* 1985; 6:231–232.

26. Weber DJ, Wilson MB, Rutala WA, Thomann CA. Manual ventilation bags as a source for bacterial colonization of intubated patients. *Am Rev Respir Dis.* 1990;25:232–237.

27. McCrae W, Wallace P. Aspiration around high volume low pressure endotracheal cuff. *Br Med J.* 1981;2:1220–1221.

28. Lee B, Change RWS, Jacobs S. Intermittent nasogastric feeding: A simple and effective method to reduce pneumonia among ventilated ICU patients. *Clin Intensive Care.* 1990;1:100–102.

29. Torres A, Serra-Battles J, Ros E, et al. Pulmonary aspiration of gastric contents in patients receiving mechanical ventilation: The effect of body position. *Ann Intern Med.* 1992;116: 540–542.

30. Rouby J-J, Laurent P, Gosnach M, et al. Risk factors and clinical relevance of nosocomial maxillary sinusitis in the critically ill. *Am J Respir Crit Care Med.* 1994;150:776–783.

31. Torres A, El-ebiary M, Gonzalwz J, et al. Gastric and pharyngeal flora in nosocomial pneumonia acquired during mechanical ventilation. *Am Rev Respir Dis.* 1993;148:352–357.

32. Seto WH, Ching TY, Yuen KY, Lam WK. Evaluating the sterility of disposable wall oxygen humidifiers, during and between use on patients. *Infect Control.* 1990;11:604–605.

33. Golar SD, Sutherland LLA, Ford GT. Multi patient use of prefilled disposable oxygen humidifiers up to 30 days: Patient safety and cost analysis. *Respir Care.* 1993;38:343–347.

34. Henderson E, Ledgerwood D, Hope KM, et al. Prolonged and multi patient use of prefilled disposable oxygen humidifier bottles: Safety and cost. *Infect Control Hosp Epidemiol.* 1993;14: 463–468.

35. Fulmer JD, Snider GL. American College of Chest Physicians—NHLBI: National conference on oxygen therapy. *Chest.* 1984;86:234–247.

36. Centers for Disease Control. Update: Universal precautions for prevention of transmission of human immunodeficiency virus, hepatitis B virus, and other blood borne pathogens in health care settings. *MMWR.* 1988;37:377–388.

Gas Therapy

10

Gerald E. Hunt

Key Terms

anemic hypoxia
circulatory hypoxia
diffusion defect
fixed performance device
histotoxic hypoxia
hypoxemia
hypoxemic hypoxia
hypoxia
transtracheal oxygen
variable performance device

Objectives

- Recall the indications for oxygen therapy.

- Describe the hazards and complications of oxygen therapy.

- Describe the pathophysiologic mechanisms that may produce hypoxemia.

- Recall the four types of hypoxia.

- Describe the role of pressure reduction and regulation devices, flow-regulating devices, and safety indexing systems in the delivery of therapeutic gases from compressed gas systems.

- Calculate duration of gas flow from compressed gas cylinders and liquid oxygen reservoirs.

- Describe the operational characteristics and clinical applications of variable performance (low-flow) and fixed performance (high-flow) oxygen delivery devices.

- Recall the indications and delivery methods of helium–oxygen (heliox) gas mixtures.

The administration of therapeutic gases is one of the fundamental aspects of respiratory care. The safe and efficacious use of medical gas therapy is dependent on the practitioner having a sound understanding of the appropriate indications for the use of a particular therapeutic gas. Knowledge of how medical gases are supplied, the manner in which their flow is regulated, and the devices that serve as the interface for delivery is essential in the provision of quality respiratory care. The ability to monitor the status of oxygen therapy requires that the practitioner be competent in the various techniques of oxygenation assessment. In addition, the practitioner must be well versed in the potential hazards and complications that may be associated with a particular form of medical gas therapy.

INDICATIONS FOR OXYGEN THERAPY

Hypoxemia, as documented by measurement of the partial pressure of oxygen in the arterial blood (PaO_2) or the arterial hemoglobin oxygen saturation obtained by pulse oximetry (SpO_2), is the primary indication for oxygen therapy. In addition to documented hypoxemia, circumstances may exist that indicate a need for oxygen therapy in the absence of immediate documentation. Such situations include severe trauma, myocardial infarction, carbon monoxide poisoning, shock, dyspnea, short-term use for postanesthesia recovery, and acute care situations in which hypoxemia is suspected. Box 10–1 lists the indications for oxygen therapy, as outlined in the American Association of Respiratory Care Clinical Practice Guideline entitled Oxygen Therapy in the Acute Care Hospital.

Documented Hypoxemia

Administration of supplemental oxygen is indicated whenever documented hypoxemia exists. In adults, children, and infants older than 28 days, hypoxemia exists when the PaO_2 is less than 60 mmHg or the arterial oxygen saturation (SaO_2) is less than 90% when breathing room air. In infants 28 days old or younger, hypoxemia is present when the PaO_2 is less than 50 mmHg, the SaO_2 is less than 88%, or the capillary oxygen tension (PcO_2) is less than 40 mmHg.[1]

Hypoxemia can have a profound impact on the amount of oxygen that is delivered to the tissues to meet oxidative metabolic demands. As PaO_2 declines, especially below 60 mmHg, the SaO_2 begins to fall rapidly. To have an appreciation for the consequences of hypoxemia and to understand the rational for oxygen therapy, one must understand how oxygen is carried to the tissues.

Delivery of oxygen to the tissues (DO_2) is the product of the cardiac output (CO) and the arterial oxygen content (CaO_2). Cardiac output, the product of heart rate (HR) and ventricular stroke volume (SV), is a measure of the heart's ability to deliver adequate blood flow to the tissues.

$$DO_2 = CO \times CaO_2$$

$$CO = SV \times HR$$

In situations such as exercise or hyperthermia, in which there is increased oxygen demand by the tissues, the DO_2 may be increased significantly by an increase in the cardiac output. The normal response to hypoxemia includes tachycardia and an increase in stroke volume, in an effort to maintain adequate DO_2.

Arterial oxygen content is a measure of the volume of oxygen (in milliliters) that is carried per 100 mL of blood. Oxygen is transported by the blood in two forms. Under normal circumstances, about 98.5% of the oxygen is bound to hemoglobin for transport. The first portion of the arterial oxygen content equation describes this relationship: the hemoglobin level (g/dL) is multiplied by the oxygen-carrying capacity of hemoglobin (1.34 mL O_2 per 1 g/dL of hemoglobin) and the percentage of oxygen saturation of arterial hemoglobin (SaO_2). SaO_2 is a function of PaO_2 as described by the hemoglobin–oxygen dissociation curve. Using normal values, the portion of the CaO_2 due to transport by hemoglobin is about 19.7 mL O_2/100 mL arterial blood. A small amount of oxygen is transported to the tissues dissolved in plasma. The amount of oxygen dissolved is a function of the PaO_2. About 0.003 mL O_2 is dissolved in the plasma for each 1 mmHg PaO_2. Again, using normal values, the portion of the CaO_2 that is transported in this fashion is about 0.29 mL O_2/100 mL arterial blood.

$$CaO_2 = (15 \text{ g/dL} \times 1.34 \times 0.97) + (0.003 \times 95 \text{ mmHg})$$
$$\approx 20 \text{ mL } O_2/\text{dL arterial blood}$$

Calculation of CaO_2 using normal values: PaO_2 = 95 mmHg, SaO_2 = 97%, hemoglobin = 15 g/dL

Pathophysiology of Hypoxemia

Ventilation–Perfusion ($\dot{V}/\dot{Q}$) Mismatch

Variations exist in the ratio of alveolar ventilation to pulmonary perfusion ($\dot{V}/\dot{Q}$) in different regions of the lung. Overall, the net result of the differing areas of $\dot{V}/\dot{Q}$ is one of about equal matching of ventilation to perfusion. Figure 10–1 represents two idealized lung units with normal ventilation and perfusion. When a situation exists that decreases the amount of ventilation in proportion to perfusion

---

Box • 10–1	INDICATIONS FOR OXYGEN THERAPY

Treatment of documented hypoxemia
Situations in which hypoxemia is suspected
Decreasing the work of breathing
Decreasing myocardial work
Severe trauma

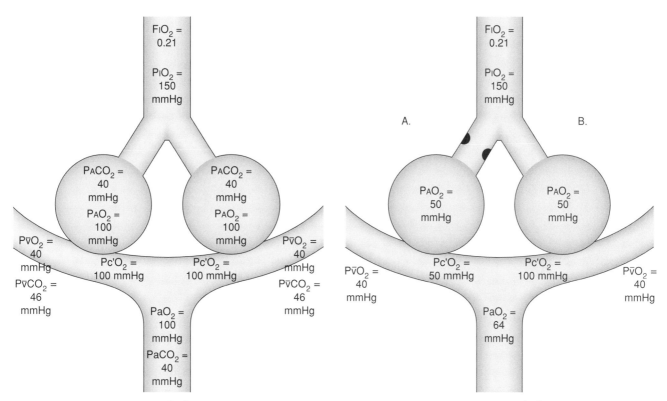

FIGURE 10–1 • Normal $\dot{V}/\dot{Q}$ relationship.

FIGURE 10–2 • Decreased $\dot{V}/\dot{Q}$ relationship.

(low $\dot{V}/\dot{Q}$), hypoxemia results. Figure 10–2 compares an alveolus with normal $\dot{V}/\dot{Q}$ to one with decreased alveolar ventilation. The decrease in ventilation of alveolar unit A has resulted in a situation in which oxygen is removed from the alveolus at a faster rate than it can be replaced by ventilation. As a result of the decreased ventilation, the PO_2 of the pulmonary capillary blood that is in contact with alveolar unit A decreases. The blood from the pulmonary capillary of alveolar unit A mixes with the pulmonary capillary blood of alveolar unit B, resulting in a decrease in PaO_2. Obstructive lung disorders, such as asthma, emphysema, and chronic bronchitis, are examples of pulmonary pathophysiologies that result in a low $\dot{V}/\dot{Q}$.

Hypoxemia that results from $\dot{V}/\dot{Q}$ mismatch can usually be corrected with the administration of small to moderate amounts of supplemental oxygen. Figure 10–3 depicts the effect on PaO_2 of the administration of 40% oxygen to the low $\dot{V}/\dot{Q}$ situation illustrated in Figure 10–2. Elevating the PIO_2 has increased the PAO_2 in alveolar unit A sufficiently to increase the $Pc'O_2$ to a value approaching normal. In this situation, the admixture of blood from the capillary of alveolar unit A does not result in arterial hypoxemia.

Alveolar Hypoventilation

A reduction in alveolar ventilation (VA) results in oxygen being removed from the alveolus at a rate that is faster than it can be replaced by ventilation. If the alveolar-to-arterial oxygen partial pressure difference ($PAO_2 - PaO_2$) is nor-

mal, the decline in PaO_2 is roughly equivalent to the rise in $PaCO_2$ resulting from the decreased VA. Other causes of hypoxemia, such as $\dot{V}/\dot{Q}$ mismatch and shunt, result in an increased $PAO_2 - PaO_2$. Supplemental oxygen corrects the hypoxemia associated with hypoventilation, but the primary therapy should be aimed at increasing the VA. Examples of clinical situations that result in hypoventilation include drug overdose, sleep apnea, and acute exacerbation of chronic obstructive pulmonary disease (COPD). Figure 10–4 illustrates the effect of a decreased VA on PaO_2.

Shunt

When pulmonary capillary blood perfuses a lung unit that is not ventilated, blood that exits the capillary remains deoxygenated. This deoxygenated blood mixes with oxygenated blood from lung units that are both perfused and ventilated. The resulting admixture of deoxygenated blood can produce significant hypoxemia. The magnitude of the decrease in PaO_2 is dependent on the amount of blood that is shunted from right to left. Figure 10–5 illustrates the mechanism of hypoxemia produced by an intrapulmonary right-to-left shunt.

Hypoxemia that is a result of left-to-right intrapulmonary shunting is not easily corrected by the administration of supplemental oxygen. Figure 10–6 depicts the effect on PaO_2 of the administration of 40% oxygen to the intrapulmonary shunt illustrated in Figure 10–5. Elevating the PIO_2 has increased the PAO_2 in alveolar unit A significantly; however,

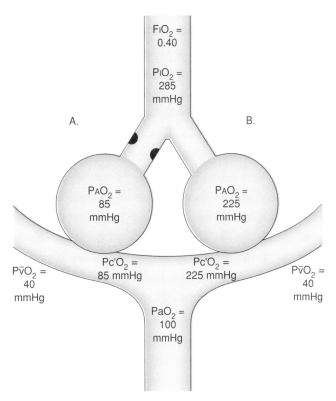

FIGURE 10–3 • Effect of the administration of supplemental oxygen with decreased V̇/Q̇.

owing to the absence of ventilation to alveolar unit B, venous admixture persists, and the PaO_2 is elevated only slightly.

Intrapulmonary shunt may be caused by any process that prevents an alveolar unit from being ventilated. Common examples of clinical situations that result in significant intrapulmonary shunting include acute lobar atelectasis, whole-lung collapse, lobar pneumonia, acute respiratory distress syndrome (ARDS), and cardiogenic pulmonary edema. In addition to the administration of supplemental oxygen, the correction of hypoxemia resulting from interpulmonary shunting requires therapeutic interventions that are aimed at recruiting and stabilizing collapsed alveoli (positive end-expiratory pressure [PEEP] or continuous positive airway pressure [CPAP]), reinflating atelectatic lung (intermittent positive-pressure breathing and incentive spirometry), or improving cardiac performance in cardiogenic pulmonary edema (administration of diuretics and positive inotropic agents).

In addition to intrapulmonary shunting, clinically significant venous admixture may occur through anatomic shunts. Intracardiac defects that result in a right-to-left admixture and vascular lung tumors are examples of anatomic shunts that result in hypoxemia. As is the case with intrapulmonary shunt, the hypoxemia resulting from venous admixture due to anatomic shunting is relatively refractory to the administration of supplemental oxygen. Under normal circumstances, about 2% to 5%

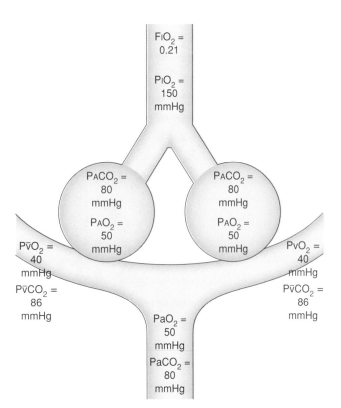

FIGURE 10–4 • Hypoxemia due to hypoventilation.

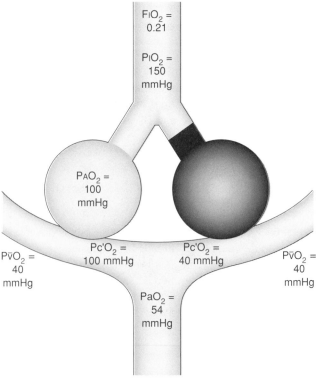

FIGURE 10–5 • Hypoxemia due to left-to-right intrapulmonary shunt.

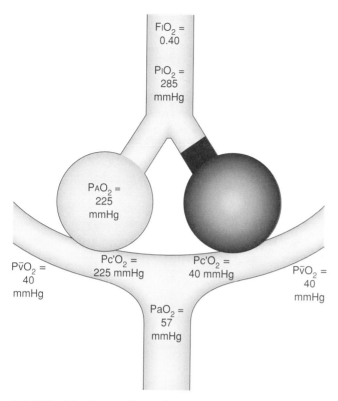

FIO₂ =
0.40

PIO₂ =
285
mmHg

PAO₂ =
225
mmHg

PⱯO₂ =
40
mmHg

Pc'O₂ =
225 mmHg

Pc'O₂ =
40 mmHg

PⱯO₂ =
40
mmHg

PaO₂ =
57
mmHg

FIGURE 10-6 • Effect of the administration of supplemental oxygen with a left-to-right intrapulmonary shunt.

of the cardiac output is shunted to the left side of the heart from a portion of the bronchial circulation and the minor venous drainage of the myocardium (thebesian veins). These normal anatomic shunts are primarily responsible for the difference observed between the calculated (ideal) P_AO_2 and the measured PaO_2 in a young, healthy patient.

Diffusion Defect

Under resting conditions in the normal lung, oxygen diffuses across the alveolar-capillary membrane and reaches equilibrium with the P_AO_2 in about one third of the time required for red blood cell transit through an alveolar capillary. When the cardiac output increases significantly, such as during exercise, the red blood cell transit time through the alveolar capillary may shorten. Fortunately, in the normal lung, the time required for oxygen diffusion remains shorter than the accelerated red blood cell transit time.

A **diffusion defect** results from any pathophysiologic process that increases the barrier between the alveolus and the alveolar capillary. As a result of the thickening of the alveolar-capillary membrane, the time required for oxygen diffusion increases. Under resting conditions, this increased diffusion time may remain less than the time required for red blood cell transit through the alveolar capillary. With severe

thickening of the alveolar-capillary membrane, the time required for oxygen diffusion exceeds the red blood cell transit time, the equilibration of oxygen across the alveolar-capillary membrane does not occur, and hypoxemia is the potential result. Exercise exaggerates the effect of a diffusion defect by decreasing the transit time of the red blood cell. This decreased transit time, in conjunction with the increased time required for oxygen diffusion, results in the two hallmarks of diffusion defects: exercise-induced hypoxemia and severe dyspnea. Examples of diseases that cause diffusion defects are listed in Box 10–2. The use of supplemental oxygen to treat the hypoxemia associated with diffusion defects, especially during exercise, is based on increasing the partial pressure gradient between the alveolus and the alveolar capillary blood, making the transfer of oxygen across the alveolar-capillary membrane more favorable.

Decreased Ambient Partial Pressure of Oxygen

Hypoxemia may result from a reduced partial pressure of oxygen in the atmosphere inspired. The most commonly cited example of this situation is an ascent in altitude. As a person ascends in altitude, the barometric pressure (P_B) decreases steadily. As P_B decreases, so does the partial pressure of oxygen. As an example, at sea level, the P_B is 760 mmHg and the $P_{ATM}O_2$ is about 160 mmHg. At 10,000 feet above sea level, the P_B is 523 mmHg, and the $P_{ATM}O_2$ is about 110 mmHg. When the P_AO_2 is calculated for a person inspiring a PO_2 of 110 mmHg (assuming a P_ACO_2 of 36 mmHg), the resulting value is about 67 mmHg. Luckily, for the person with normal pulmonary function, the resulting arterial hemoglobin saturation (SaO_2) is in excess of 90%.

Clinically, it may appear that decreased $P_{ATM}O_2$ would not play a significant role in the pathogenesis of hypoxemia. This assumption may not be true for a growing popu-

---

Box • 10-2   DISEASES THAT CAUSE DIFFUSION DEFECTS

Conditions that cause interstitial edema*
   Hypoproteinemia
   Left ventricular failure
   High altitude pulmonary edema
Interstitial fibrosis
Sarcoidosis
Asbestosis
Viral interstitial pneumonitis
Collagen vascular diseases
   Goodpasture's syndrome
   Wegener's granulomatosis
   Systemic lupus erythematosus

*Usually not clinically relevant until fluid moves into the alveolus.

CRITICAL THINKING CHALLENGES

Go Figure

A patient with COPD has room air arterial blood gas values at sea level as follows: pH, 7.36; PaO_2, 60 mmHg, $PaCO_2$, 55 mmHg; HCO_3, 30 mEq/L; BE +6 mEq/L. What will this patient's PaO_2 be when traveling on an aircraft pressurized to an altitude of 10,000 feet? During the flight, would this patient qualify to receive supplemental oxygen?

lation of people with COPD. A patient with $\dot{V}/\dot{Q}$ mismatch resulting from COPD or with a diffusion defect derived from pulmonary fibrosis may possess an adequate PaO_2 at or near sea level and not require supplemental oxygen. If this patient, however, travels by automobile to Denver, Colorado (the "mile-high city") or through a high mountain pass, significant hypoxemia may result. In addition to vehicle travel to high elevations, airplane travel may precipitate significant hypoxemia in patients with borderline need for oxygenation. Even though commercial aircraft are pressurized, the pressure maintained can be substantially below P_B and can result in significant hypoxemia in the susceptible patient with COPD. The articles by Krieger,[2] Gong,[3] and Stoller[4] provide detailed discussions of oxygen therapy for cardiopulmonary patients during air travel.

Hypoxia

In contrast to hypoxemia, a lower than normal oxygenation of the arterial blood, **hypoxia** refers to a subnormal oxygen tension at the tissue or organ level. Hypoxia exists when the cellular PO_2 falls below the level necessary to fulfill metabolic demands. Aerobic tissue metabolism requires that a minimum end-capillary PO_2 of 20 mmHg be maintained to prevent the occurrence of anaerobic metabolism.[5] When nonoxidative biochemical pathways are used to produce metabolic energy, the results are the inadequate use of glucose, the formation of lactic acid, and if the anaerobic condition persists, cellular death. Conventionally, hypoxia is subdivided into four categories: hypoxemic hypoxia, anemic hypoxia, circulatory hypoxia, and histotoxic hypoxia.

Hypoxemic hypoxia results from any situation that significantly lowers the PaO_2 and thus decreases the CaO_2. Ascent in altitude, with the attendant decrease in partial pressure of inspired oxygen (PIO_2), suffocation, and any pulmonary pathophysiology that results in a significant reduction in PaO_2 may be the basis for hypoxemic hypoxia. If the hypoxemia is the result of a pulmonary pathophysiology that involves hypoventilation, $\dot{V}/\dot{Q}$ mismatch, or a diffusion defect, the administration of supplemental oxygen may correct the hypoxemia, improve the SaO_2 and resolve the hypoxia. Hypoxemia due to right-to-left shunting may be refractory to oxygen administration alone and may require therapy that is directed at reducing the shunt fraction (eg, CPAP, PEEP).

Anemic hypoxia is caused by a decrease in the circulating erythrocyte mass or the presence of abnormal hemoglobin. Blood loss, anemia, and carbon monoxide poisoning are examples of situations that can significantly lower the CaO_2. The administration of supplemental oxygen in these situations is of little benefit. The PaO_2 may significantly increase, but the CaO_2 remains deficient. Appropriate emergency treatment of carbon monoxide poisoning involves the administration of 100% oxygen. Although the CaO_2 level is not significantly improved initially, the presence of a high PaO_2 dramatically reduces the half-life of carboxyhemoglobin.

Circulatory hypoxia is the result of a decreased cardiac output. Because DO_2 is the product of cardiac output and CaO_2, any situation that results in inadequate tissue perfusion may precipitate a situation in which O_2 consumption ($\dot{V}O_2$) is in excess of DO_2. Cardiogenic shock, hypovolemia, and excessive PEEP are potential causes of circulatory hypoxia.

Histotoxic hypoxia occurs when the tissues are unable to use oxygen despite an adequate cardiac output and CaO_2. The classic example of this form of hypoxia is the poisoning of the intracellular oxidative enzymatic system that occurs with cyanide poisoning.

The effect on PaO_2, CaO_2, and DO_2 of the various forms of hypoxia are summarized in Table 10–1.

Use of Supplemental Oxygen to Reduce Cardiopulmonary Workload

The normal cardiopulmonary response to hypoxemia is an increase in both ventilation and cardiac output. In the hypoxemic patient who is breathing room air, the only way

Table • 10–1   COMPARISON OF THE FORMS OF HYPOXIA

	Hypoxemic	Anemic	Circulatory	Histotoxic
PaO_2	Decreased	Normal	Normal	Normal
CaO_2	Decreased	Decreased	Normal	Normal
DO_2	Decreased	Decreased	Decreased	Normal

that an adequate PaO_2 can be achieved is through hyperventilation, which may impose unacceptable work of breathing. Supplemental oxygen may reduce the elevated ventilatory demand and decrease the work of breathing.

When hypoxemia precipitates a fall in CaO_2, cardiac output increases in an attempt to improve oxygen delivery to the tissues. The added workload placed on the heart increases cardiac oxygen consumption. Hypoxemia may also cause pulmonary vasoconstriction, resulting in pulmonary hypertension and an increase in the work of the right ventricle. In the presence of myocardial infarction or other cardiac dysfunction, the added stress may precipitate added myocardial damage and lower the threshold for dangerous arrhythmias. Supplemental oxygen may increase the CaO_2 sufficiently to reduce the cardiac workload and decrease any pulmonary vasoconstriction mediated by hypoxemia.

Hazards and Complications of Oxygen Therapy

Pulmonary Oxygen Toxicity

Normally, airway irritation, ciliary dysfunction, and decreased mucus clearance occur within the first few hours of breathing an FIO_2 of 1.0. Sore throat, cough, burning substernal chest pain on inspiration, and dyspnea are evident. The resulting tracheobronchitis is reversible and subsides on discontinuance of oxygen breathing.

When the lung parenchyma is exposed to an FIO_2 of 0.6 for a prolonged period of time, cellular damage ensues. Increased intracellular PO_2 results in the formation of excessive cytotoxic free radicals that mediate structural and metabolic changes within the cell. Death of type I and II pulmonary cells is followed by the proliferation of type II cells and a decrease in pulmonary surfactant production. Ultimately, atelectasis, increased alveolar shunt, and changes in alveolar-capillary membrane permeability result in a pulmonary parenchymal injury closely resembling ARDS.

Absorption Atelectasis

Normally, nitrogen makes up about 78% of the alveolar gas. Being metabolically inactive, nitrogen is able to provide stability and maintain alveolar patency. The administration of high concentrations of oxygen (FIO_2 of 0.70) washes out nitrogen from the lung. In areas of poor ventilation, oxygen may be removed from the perfused alveoli more rapidly than it can be replaced by ventilation. Alveoli become reduced in size and ultimately collapse to create atelectasis. Patients with severe airway obstruction, maldistribution of ventilation, or small tidal volumes are at increased risk for the occurrence of absorption atelectasis when breathing high concentrations of oxygen.

Oxygen-Induced Hypoventilation

Spontaneously breathing patients with chronically elevated $PaCO_2$ levels may hypoventilate when exposed to excessive supplemental oxygen. Normally, the drive to ventilate is primarily mediated by the medullary response to CO_2. When CO_2 is chronically retained, such as may be seen in patients with chronic bronchitis, the drive to ventilate may be a function of the hypoxic ventilatory response. As PaO_2 levels fall below 60 to 65 mmHg, a progressively increasing ventilatory stimulus is provoked by stimulation of the peripheral chemoreceptors. Elevating the PaO_2 to more than 65 mmHg in patients who usually ventilate in response to their hypoxemic drive can result in hypoventilation and respiratory acidosis.

Box 10–3 lists patients at risk of developing oxygen-induced hypoventilation as a consequence of receiving excessive supplemental oxygen.[6] Oxygen should never be withheld from a patient because of concern about reducing or ablating the hypoxic drive. Failure to treat severe hypoxemia is potentially life-threatening. When administering supplemental oxygen to a patient at known or suspected risk of oxygen-induced hypoventilation, a target PaO_2 of 55 mmHg (50 to 60 mmHg) should be the goal. Initially, oxygen delivery devices that provide a stable fraction of delivered oxygen (FDO_2), independent of changes in the patient's ventilatory status, should be used. During the initial titration of oxygen, close observation of the patient's level of consciousness, ventilatory parameters (VT and respiratory rate), $PaCO_2$, pH, and PaO_2 are necessary. The ability to support ventilation by endotracheal intubation and mechanical ventilation should be readily available in the event of hypoventilation and respiratory acidosis despite the appropriate administration of supplemental oxygen.

Special Considerations in Neonates

RETINOPATHY OF PREMATURITY

In premature infants, a PaO_2 of more than 80 to 100 mmHg may result in vasoconstriction of the retinal blood vessels. Vascular obliteration results if the hyperoxia is allowed to

---

Box • 10–3 PATIENTS AT RISK FOR OXYGEN-INDUCED HYPOVENTILATION

Patients with a previous history of oxygen-induced hypoventilation

Patients with COPD and chronic CO_2 retention who present with acute respiratory decompensation and worsened hypoxemia

Patients with cor pulmonale and hypoxemia

Patients with sleep apnea syndrome, especially those with hypersomnolence and daytime hypoventilation

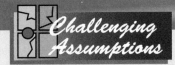

A patient with COPD comes to the emergency department in acute respiratory insufficiency with a pH of 7.30, PaO_2 of 48 mmHg, $PaCO_2$ of 65 mmHg, HCO_3 of 34 meq/L, and BE of more than 8 mEq/L. The patient is severely hypoxic and has evidence of CO_2 retention. The physician expresses concern about giving too much oxygen, assuming that too much oxygen would suppress the patient's hypoxic drive. Should you let the patient die from hypoxia just to be sure that the patient doesn't stop breathing? Absolutely not!

Here are the facts: The strongest single drive to breathing is being awake (afferent sensory). When we go to sleep, our breathing slows down. Normally, the central chemoreceptors monitor the CO_2 or pH and stimulate breathing when the CO_2 rises (secondary to a decrease in alveolar ventilation). If the CO_2 is chronically high, then the central chemoreceptors become less sensitive to changes in CO_2. In such cases, it is hypoxic stimulation of the peripheral chemoreceptors that stimulates breathing during sleep. If a patient with a chronically high CO_2 is too well oxygenated, hypoxia does not stimulate respiration during sleep.

For oxygen to be a problem, the patient would generally need to be: a chronic CO_2 retainer, oxygenated above 55 mmHg, or asleep.

So, if you want to oxygenate above 55 mmHg, keep the patient awake, or closely monitor the patient when she falls asleep. Better to provide ventilatory assistance than to allow the patient to suffer from severe hypoxia.

---

persist. After return to a normoxic state, vasoproliferation of the immature retina ensues. Subsequent retinal detachment and blindness may occur. Although once thought to be the primary cause of retinopathy of prematurity, elevated PaO_2 is now considered one of a number of potential factors, including low birth weight, gestational age, acidosis, hypercarbia, and sepsis, that may interact to influence the development and progression of retinopathy of prematurity. The American Academy of Pediatrics and the American College of Obstetricians and Gynecologists recommend that oxygen supplementation should not result in a PaO_2 of more than 80 mmHg.[7]

UNWANTED CLOSURE OF THE DUCTUS ARTERIOSUS

Increased PaO_2 is one of the stimuli involved in the normal constriction of the ductal smooth muscle after birth. In certain congenital heart lesions, such as pulmonary atresia, tricuspid atresia, and coarctation of the aorta, patency of the ductus arteriosus is necessary for adequate pulmonary or systemic blood flow. Closure of the ductus before surgical palliation or correction usually results in severe hypoxemia and cardiovascular collapse. The goal of supplemental oxygen administration in these situations usually involves maintaining the PaO_2 below the level that initiates ductal constriction yet at a level that provides adequate oxygenation.

ALTERATIONS IN PULMONARY BLOOD FLOW

Before surgical palliation, the balance between systemic and pulmonary blood flow in the single-ventricle heart and hypoplastic left heart syndrome can be labile. Increases in the alveolar oxygen tension and the resultant pulmonary vasodilation may significantly increase pulmonary blood at the expense of systemic blood flow.

Fire Hazard

Oxygen is a nonflammable gas, but its presence greatly accelerates the combustion of flammable materials. Patients receiving supplemental oxygen, their caregivers, and their visitors should be cautioned against smoking, lighting an open flame, or using sparking devices (including sparking mechanical toys and electric razors) in oxygen enclosures or near an open oxygen source. Even though most hospitals enforce a no smoking policy and it is assumed that no one smokes within the building, it remains prudent to post signs indicating that oxygen is in use.

OVERVIEW OF MEDICAL GAS SUPPLY SYSTEMS

Virtually all modern medical facilities have piping distribution systems that supply pressurized gaseous oxygen for use at the bedside. Bulk liquid oxygen that has been vaporized and pressure regulated is commonly the primary source of oxygen, with secondary liquid or compressed gas cylinders as a backup in the event of a primary source failure. Pressurized medical air is frequently obtained by compressing and filtering ambient air on-site. Within the hospital environment, the practitioner may have little or no involvement with medical gas distribution systems beyond plugging in the flowmeter or the ventilator high-pressure hoses.

Because of the easy access to pressurized medical gases, the practitioner may not have the opportunity to develop the knowledge and to practice the skills necessary to use compressed gas cylinders, pressure-reducing valves and regulators, and liquid oxygen systems.

What follows is a brief overview of medical gas supply and regulating systems. The practitioner is encouraged to review the various comprehensive texts on the subject[8–10] to obtain an in-depth review.

Compressed Gas Cylinders

Various medical gases are supplied in cylinders. Gases such as oxygen, helium, and nitrogen can be compressed in a gaseous state into a cylinder. Other medical gases, such as pure carbon dioxide and nitrous oxide, exist as a liquid within the cylinder and evaporate as they are used. Table 10–2 lists medical gases that are commonly available in cylinders and the United States cylinder color code for each. The color coding is used for easy identification of cylinder contents; before use, however, the cylinder label must always be checked to verify the contents. If the cylinder label is unreadable or some doubt exists about the contents of the cylinder, the cylinder must not be used.

Gas cylinders are available in various sizes. Table 10–3 lists the cylinder letter designations and approximate compressed gaseous oxygen content of various-sized cylinders. The most commonly used cylinder sizes are the D, E, G, H and K cylinders (Fig. 10–7). The pressure of full cylinders varies based on the gas that occupies the cylinder. Oxygen cylinders, regardless of their size, have a maximum filling pressure of 2200 psi (2015 psi + 10% overfill). Calculating the duration of gas flow from a compressed gas cylinder requires knowledge of the volume of the cylinder (in cubic feet) and the conversion factor: 1 cu ft = 28.3 L (for oxygen).

$$\text{Conversion factor} =$$

$$\frac{(\text{cubic feet of gas in a full cylinder})(28.3\ \text{L/cu ft})}{2200\ \text{psig}}$$

Example: Conversion factor for an oxygen E cylinder =

$$\frac{(22\ \text{cu ft})(28.3\ \text{L/cu ft})}{2200\ \text{psig}} = 0.28\ \text{L/psig}$$

Table • 10–2 COMMONLY AVAILABLE COMPRESSED MEDICAL GAS MIXTURES AND CYLINDER COLOR CODES

Gas	Color Code
Oxygen (O_2)*	Green (white—international)
Nitrogen (N_2)	Black
Helium (He)	Brown
Carbon Dioxide (CO_2)	Gray
Air	Yellow
Oxygen/carbon dioxide (98%–90% O_2/2%–10% CO_2)*	Gray shoulder, green body
Oxygen/nitrogen (21% O_2/79% N_2)*	Green shoulder, black body
Helium/oxygen (80%–60% He/20%–40% O_2)*	Green shoulder, brown body
Nitrous oxide (N_2O)*	Light blue
Cyclopropane (CH_2)$_3$†	Orange
Ethylene (C_2H_4)†	Red

*Supports combustion.
†Flammable.

Table • 10–3 MEDICAL GAS CYLINDER LETTER CODES AND APPROXIMATE COMPRESSED OXYGEN VOLUMES

	Volume	
Cylinder Size	Cubic feet	Liters
A	2.5	75.7
B	5	151
D	12.6	356
E	22	622
M	106	3000
G	186	5260
H or K	244	6900

Cylinder volume may vary slightly among manufacturers.

Table 10–4 lists the conversion factors for common oxygen cylinders.

The following formula is for calculating the duration of gas flow from an oxygen cylinder:

$$\text{Time remaining in minutes} =$$

$$\frac{\text{cylinder pressure in psig} \times \text{conversion factor}}{\text{gas flow (L/min)}}$$

Example: How long will an E cylinder with 1800 psig last if the oxygen flow to the patient is 6 L/min?

$$\frac{1800\ \text{psig} \times 0.28\ \text{L/psig}}{6\ \text{L/min}} = 84\ \text{min, or 1 h and 24 min,}$$
at a rate of 6 L/min.

In clinical practice, it is prudent to leave 200 psig in the cylinder when calculating the duration of gas flow. In the above example, 1600 psig would be used as the cylinder pressure instead of 1800 psig (1800 psig − 200 psig = 1600 psig). This safety factor is incorporated to account for potential inaccuracies in the measurement of cylinder pressure and actual gas content of a particular cylinder.

The duration of gas flow from cylinders that contain gas stored partially as a liquid, such as carbon dioxide, must be weighed to determine the remaining contents. The pressure within the cylinder remains relatively constant until the cylinder is nearly empty.

Cylinder Safety Systems

Medical gas cylinders are fitted with indexed connections that permit only the attachment of the proper regulator in attempt to prevent inadvertent administration of the wrong gas. The Pin Index Safety System is used on the post valve of small cylinders (sizes AA through E). Two holes are drilled in a specific sequence into the valve body of the cylinder. The regulator yoke has two corresponding pins that fit into the valve body (Fig. 10–8). Gas-specific pin positions are assigned by the Compressed Gas Association. Large medical gas cylinder outlets are indexed using the American Standards Association connection system. This system uses a specific combination of outlet diameter,

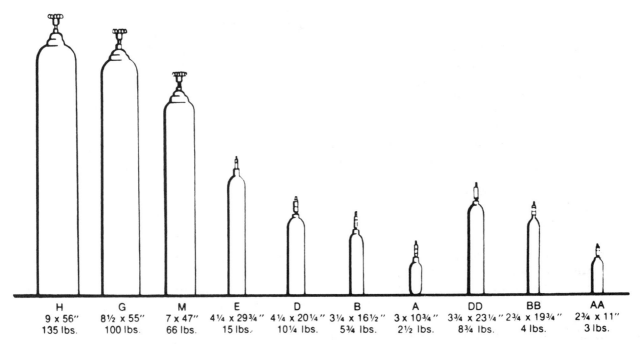

H	G	M	E	D	B	A	DD	BB	AA
9 x 56″	8½ x 55″	7 x 47″	4¼ x 29¾″	4¼ x 20¼″	3¼ x 16½″	3 x 10¾″	3¾ x 23¼″	2¾ x 19¾″	2¾ x 11″
135 lbs.	100 lbs.	66 lbs.	15 lbs.	10¼ lbs.	5¾ lbs.	2½ lbs.	8¾ lbs.	4 lbs.	3 lbs.

FIGURE 10–7 • Letter designations, weights, and approximate dimensions of various gas cylinders. (Ward JJ. Equipment for mixed gas and oxygen therapy. In: Barnes TA, ed. *Core Textbook of Respiratory Care Practice*. 2nd ed. St Louis: CV Mosby; 1994.)

threads per inch, right- or left-handed threads, and internal or external mating nut for each gas (Fig. 10–9). Left-handed threading is reserved for gases that cannot support life, such as pure helium; gas mixtures containing less than 20% oxygen; and carbon monoxide.

Pressure Regulators

Medical gas cylinders require that a high-pressure gas regulator (pressure-reducing valve) be used to reduce the maximum working pressure down to a value that can be used safely by medical equipment. In addition, as the content of a gas cylinder is used, the pressure within the cylinder falls and thus must be regulated to a constant value. Most pneumatically operated medical equipment is calibrated at 50 psig and requires a relatively constant pressure to perform correctly. Single-stage pressure regulators are used for most applications of medical gas therapy. Figure 10–10 illustrates a single-stage pressure regulator. When the pressure in the high-pressure (lower) chamber is greater than the spring tension in the low-pressure (upper) chamber, the diaphragm is horizontal and the pipet valve

closes the communication between the chambers (closed position). When the tension of the spring in the upper chamber is increased by downward movement of the adjustment screw, the diaphragm is displaced downward and pushes the poppet valve away from the communication between the two chambers. Gas flows from the high-pressure chamber, through the low-pressure chamber, and into the outlet. As gas from a cylinder is consumed, the pressure in the high-pressure chamber falls. As the pressure declines, the diaphragm displaces the poppet valve downward, increasing the gas flow into the low-pressure chamber and maintaining a relatively constant outlet pressure.

Pressure regulators may also be classified as adjustable or fixed and as single stage or multiple stage. Adjustable regulator systems allow the practitioner to adjust the main spring tension and thus manually regulate the outlet pres-

Table • 10–4	CONVERSION FACTORS FOR OXYGEN CYLINDERS
Cylinder Size	**Conversion Factor**
D	0.16
E	0.28
G	2.41
H or K	3.14

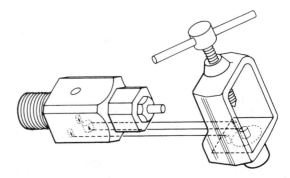

FIGURE 10–8 • Pin index safety system. (Ward JJ. Equipment for mixed gas and oxygen therapy. In: Barnes TA, ed. *Core Textbook of Respiratory Care Practice*. 2nd ed. St Louis: CV Mosby; 1994:382.)

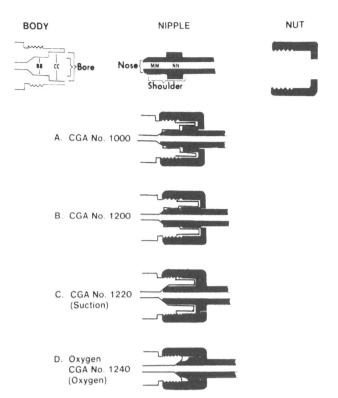

BODY   NIPPLE   NUT

Bore

Nose

Shoulder

A. CGA No. 1000

B. CGA No. 1200

C. CGA No. 1220
(Suction)

D. Oxygen
CGA No. 1240
(Oxygen)

FIGURE 10–9 • American Standards Association connection system. (Dorsch JA, Dorsch SE. *Understanding Anesthesia Equipment.* 3rd ed. Baltimore, MD: Williams & Wilkins; 1994.)

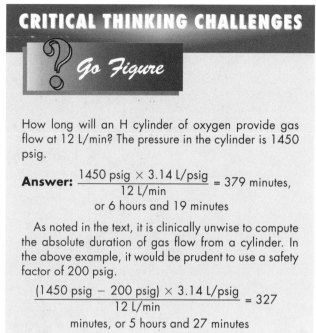

CRITICAL THINKING CHALLENGES

Go Figure

How long will an H cylinder of oxygen provide gas flow at 12 L/min? The pressure in the cylinder is 1450 psig.

Answer: $\dfrac{1450 \text{ psig} \times 3.14 \text{ L/psig}}{12 \text{ L/min}} = 379$ minutes, or 6 hours and 19 minutes

As noted in the text, it is clinically unwise to compute the absolute duration of gas flow from a cylinder. In the above example, it would be prudent to use a safety factor of 200 psig.

$$\frac{(1450 \text{ psig} - 200 \text{ psig}) \times 3.14 \text{ L/psig}}{12 \text{ L/min}} = 327$$

minutes, or 5 hours and 27 minutes

sure. Changes in regulator main spring tension should be made only by an experienced practitioner and must be confirmed by outlet pressure measurement. Fixed-pressure regulators are factory set at a predetermined pressure, usually 50 psig, and generally are not modifiable by the practitioner. Single-stage regulators provide adequate pressure stability for most simple medical gas applications. When more stability in gas pressure is required, regulators may be placed in series to form a multiple-stage regulator. As an example, the first stage of a two-stage regulator may initially regulate the cylinder pressure to 200 psig, with the subsequent stage further regulating the pressure to 50 psig.

Liquid Oxygen Systems

The use of stationary liquid oxygen is the most common method of bulk oxygen storage in the hospital environment. One liter of liquid oxygen vaporizes to produce 860 L of gaseous oxygen at 70°F. Although the practitioner may have little or no direct contact with a hospital's bulk liquid oxygen system, portable liquid systems are in frequent use for interhospital and intrahospital transport and home care.

When a large supply of liquid oxygen is required for transfilling smaller, portable liquid units or for continuous oxygen delivery, a stationary reservoir system is necessary. Stationary reservoir systems are essentially miniaturized

versions of a hospital bulk liquid system. Figure 10–11 illustrates a schematic of a stationary liquid oxygen reservoir. The liquid oxygen is maintained within the Thermos-type vessel at a temperature of −273°F. When in use, the liquid moves up through the withdrawal tube, passes through the warming coils, and vaporizes. The gas then flows through a flow-control valve to the patient. Most liquid reservoir systems operate at about 20 psig. When the reservoir is not in use, ambient temperature causes vaporization to occur, resulting in a buildup of pressure and subsequent venting of the contents. Because of this pressure venting, a liquid oxygen system eventually empties, even if it is not in use.

Portable liquid oxygen reservoirs are transfilled from the larger, stationary reservoirs. Depending on gas flow, a portable unit may provide 8 to 12 hours of oxygen. This longer duration of gas flow, as compared with small oxygen cylinders, can permit patients with a continuous oxygen requirement to be away from their primary oxygen supply for a protracted period of time. In addition to prolonged duration of gas flow, the decreased size and weight of a portable liquid system is ideal for air and ground transport situations. When not in use, portable reservoirs are also subject to loss of content through pressure venting. Portable liquid reservoirs are transfilled from a stationary reservoir system. Care must be exercised when transfilling a portable reservoir because there is a significant danger of freezing exposed skin. Goggles and gloves should always be worn during reservoir transfilling. Figure 10–12 provides examples of various-sized liquid oxygen reservoirs and portable units.

The duration of gas flow from a liquid reservoir requires that the weight of the remaining liquid oxygen be deter-

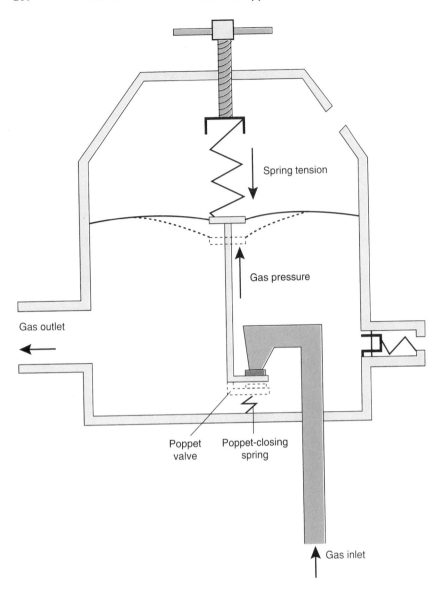

Spring tension

Gas pressure

Gas outlet

Poppet
valve

Poppet-closing
spring

Gas inlet

FIGURE 10-10 • Single-stage regulator. (Dantzker DR, MacIntyre NR, Bakow ED. *Comprehensive Respiratory Care*. Philadelphia: WB Saunders; 1995:501.)

mined. One liter of liquid oxygen weighs 2.5 lb (1.1 kg). As previously noted, 1 L of liquid oxygen equals 860 L of gaseous oxygen.

The following formula calculates the duration of gas flow from a liquid reservoir:

$$\text{gas remaining (L)} = \frac{\text{(liquid weight (lb)} \times 860}{2.5\ \text{lb/L}}$$

$$\text{Time remaining (min)} = \frac{\text{gas remaining (L)}}{\text{flow (L/min)}}$$

Example: a portable reservoir is transfilled with 3 lb of liquid oxygen. How long will the oxygen in this reservoir last if the flow to an oxygen delivery device is 3 L/min?

$$\text{gas remaining} = \frac{3\ \text{lb} \times 860}{2.5\ \text{lb/L}} = 1032\ \text{L}$$

$$\text{Time remaining} = \frac{1032\ \text{L}}{3\ \text{L/min}} = 344\ \text{min}$$

Gas Flow–Regulating Devices (Flowmeters)

Flowmeters allow for the regulation and indication of gas flow. Medical gas delivery systems most frequently regulate gas flow in liters per minute. Low-flow flowmeters are available that permit regulation of flow in increments of millimeters per minute. The operation of the most commonly used medical flowmeters is based on (1) gas flow through a fixed orifice with a variable pressure, or (2) gas flow through a variable orifice with a fixed pressure.

Fixed Orifice Flow Restricter

At a constant pressure across an orifice ($P_1 - P_2$), the flow through an orifice is directly proportional to the square of the diameter of the orifice. If the pressure difference across the orifice is constant, then gas flow through the orifice varies exponentially as the orifice size is changed.

COMPANION STATIONARY

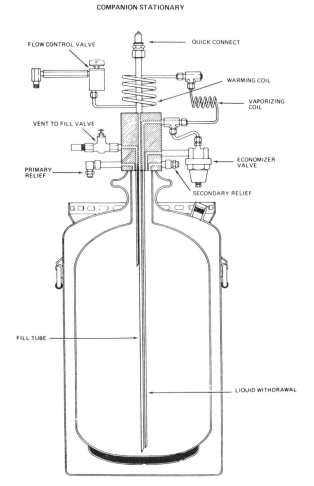

FIGURE 10–11 • Stationary liquid oxygen reservoir. (Courtesy of Puritan-Bennett Corp., Kansas City, MO.)

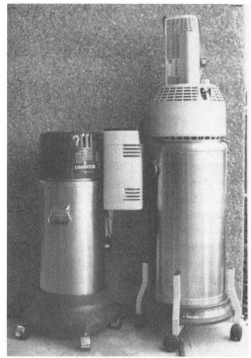

A

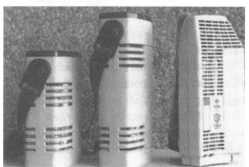

B

FIGURE 10–12 • (*A*) Stationary liquid oxygen reservoirs. (*B*) Portable liquid oxygen units (*Current Status of Oxygen Therapy: Problems in Respiratory Care.* Philadelphia: JB Lippincott; 1990:597.)

Medical gas flow restricters operate based on a fixed 50-psig pressure applied across a fixed orifice (Fig. 10–13). Flow restricters are commonly used to regulate gas flow in home care applications, such as oxygen concentrators, liquid oxygen systems, and compressed gas cylinders. Advantages of flow restricters are ease of operation, stability, and accurate control of gas flow rate regardless of position. Flow restricters may become inaccurate if there is an alteration in the relationship of P_1 to P_2. This is most commonly the result of an inlet pressure that is not 50 psig or the attachment of a device that creates downstream back pressure. Debris lodged in the fixed orifice may alter the diameter and result in an inaccurate flow rate being delivered. Figure 10–14 illustrates an adjustable fixed orifice flow restricter.

Bourdon Gauge

The Bourdon gauge flowmeter is, in actuality, a pressure gauge. The gauge measures the pressure that is applied against a known fixed orifice. Flow through an orifice is directly proportional to the square root of the pressure difference ($P_1 - P_2$) across the orifice.

$$\text{Flow} \propto \sqrt{P_1 - P_2},$$

where P_1 = driving pressure of the source gas through the orifice; and P_2 = pressure downstream of orifice (in most medical applications, this approximates atmospheric pressure).

As P_1 is increased, the flow through the orifice increases. If P_2 is increased, as may occur if a back pressure is created by placing a distal restriction that is smaller than the orifice, the difference between P_1 and P_2 decreases. The decrease in $P_1 - P_2$ across the orifice results in a decrease in flow.

Figure 10–15 illustrates a Bourdon gauge. As noted previously, this is actually a pressure gauge that has been calibrated in units of flow. The gauge is composed of a crooked, hollow copper tube that deforms its shape as pressure is ap-

CRITICAL THINKING CHALLENGES

Go Figure

A stationary liquid oxygen reservoir is providing 2 L/min continuous gas flow to a home care patient. The reservoir, when full, holds 93 lb of liquid oxygen. How long will this reservoir provide gas flow if the content gauge indicates that the reservoir is half full?

Answer: Pounds of liquid oxygen available = 93 lb × 0.5 = 46.5 lb

$$\text{Gas remaining (L)} = \frac{46.5 \text{ lbs} \times 860}{2.5 \text{ lb/L}} = 15{,}996 \text{ L}$$
gaseous oxygen

$$\text{Time remaining (min)} = \frac{15{,}966 \text{ L}}{2 \text{ L/min}} = 7998 \text{ minutes,}$$
or 133 hours and 18 minutes (about 5½ days)

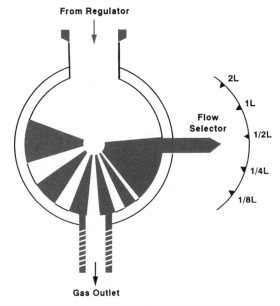

FIGURE 10–14 • Adjustable flow restrictor.

plied. This deformation is translated into a flow reading by a gearing mechanism that alters the position of an indicator on the gauge face. As the practitioner changes the pressure applied to the fixed orifice (P_1) by the adjustment of an upstream pressure regulator, flow through the fixed orifice varies as the square root of the pressure difference.

The Bourdon gauge is useful in transport situations in which a relatively small device that can regulate gas flow over a broad range would be advantageous. In addition, the gauge displays gas flow accurately regardless of position.

The Bourdon gauge indicates incorrect gas flow in any situation that results in creation of back pressure that increases P_2 and results in a decrease in $P_1 - P_2$. Under these conditions, the Bourdon gauge indicates a *higher* flow than actually exists. Situations that can result in back pressure

include partial or complete obstruction of oxygen delivery tubing and attachment of any device that has a smaller orifice than the fixed orifice of the Bourdon gauge. Pneumatic nebulizers and small orifice jet-mixing devices should not be used with a Bourdon gauge if accurate determination of gas flow rate in required. Figure 10–16 illustrates the effect of back pressure and complete orifice occlusion on the accuracy of a Bourdon gauge.

Thorpe Tube Flowmeter

The Thorpe tube flowmeter is the most commonly used flow-regulating device in clinical medicine. The Thorpe tube operates as a fixed pressure, variable-sized orifice device. The flowmeter is composed of a needle valve, a calibrated tapered tube, and a float ball. When the Thorpe tube is attached to a 50-psig gas source and the needle valve is

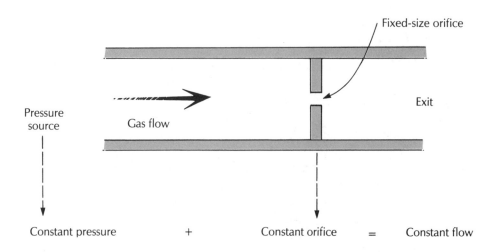

Pressure source

Gas flow

Constant pressure   +   Constant orifice   =   Constant flow

Fixed-size orifice

Exit

FIGURE 10–13 • Flow restrictor. (Eubanks DH, Bone RC. *Principles and Applications of Respiratory Care Equipment.* St Louis: CV Mosby; 1995:23.)

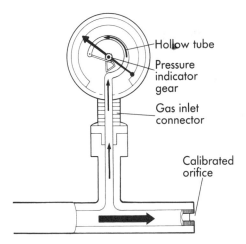

FIGURE 10–15 • Bourdon gauge. (Scanlon. *Egan's Fundamentals of Respiratory Care.* 6th ed. 1995:652.)

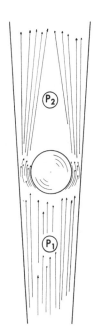

FIGURE 10–17 • The pressure difference (P₁ − P₂) across the float ball of a Thorpe tube. The position of the float ball is determined by a balance between the force created by the flow of gas upward through the variable-sized orifice and the force of gravity (Scanlon. *Egan's Fundamentals of Respiratory Care.* 6th ed. 1995:653.)

opened, gas enters the tube and the float ball moves up. The force of the gas under the float ball opposes the effect of gravity and lifts the float ball. The float ball stabilizes when the force below the float ball (P₁) equals the force of gravity above the float ball (P₂; Fig. 10–17). The tapered tube becomes progressively wider toward the top. Because of this progressive widening, more gas flow is required to lift the float ball higher in the tube.

The *pressure-compensated* Thorpe tube flowmeter is used almost exclusively when regulating medical gases in the clinical environment. The pressure-compensated Thorpe tube is distinguished from the *non–pressure-compensated* device by the placement of the flow-controlling needle valve downstream from the tapered Thorpe tube (Fig. 10–18). Based on this configuration, the entire

Thorpe tube is exposed to a constant pressure of 50 psig. The flowmeter is thus calibrated to operate at 50 psig. Any back pressure that is imposed by the addition of a downstream resistance occurs after the flow-control needle valve. Thus, as long as the back pressure does not exceed 50 psig, the float ball of a pressure-compensated Thorpe tube indicates the actual gas flow. With the flow-control

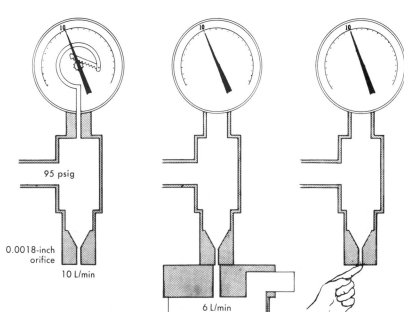

FIGURE 10–16 • Effect of back pressure and complete orifice occlusion on the accuracy of a Bourdon gauge. (Scanlon. *Egan's Fundamentals of Respiratory Care.* 6th ed. 1995:653.)

95 psig

0.0018-inch orifice

10 L/min

6 L/min

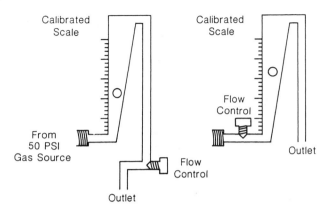

FIGURE 10–18 • Pressure-compensated Thorpe tube flowmeter (*left*) and non–pressure-compensated Thorpe tube flowmeter (*right*).

needle valve closed, the float ball "jumps" when a pressure-compensated Thorpe tube is attached to a 50-psig gas source.

In contrast, the flow-control needle valve of the non–pressure-compensated device is positioned before the tapered Thorpe tube. The flowmeter is calibrated at atmospheric pressure. Gas from a 50-psig source is metered into the flowmeter by adjusting the needle valve. Any back pressure that occurs downstream from the device increases the pressure within the Thorpe tube to a value greater than atmospheric pressure. As long as the back pressure does not exceed 50 psig, gas continues to flow through the device. The added pressure, however, increases the pressure above the float ball, distorting the relationship between $P_1 - P_2$. Under these circumstances, the non–pressure-compensated Thorpe tube indicates a lower gas flow than

that actually being delivered (Fig. 10–19). Fortunately, non–pressure-compensated Thorpe tubes are not currently used for the administration of medical gases. This type of flowmeter is used with medical laboratory equipment and may remain as the gas flow–controlling device on some older respiratory care equipment.

The flow of a gas through an orifice is inversely proportional to the square root of the gas's density.

$$Flow \propto \frac{1}{\sqrt{density}}$$

Based on this relationship, if the pressure remains constant and the orifice size remains fixed, as gas density is decreased, the flow through the orifice increases. This principle explains why flowmeters are manufactured and calibrated for specific gases. As an example, the use of an oxygen flowmeter to regulate a mixture of helium and oxygen (heliox) can give rise to significant inaccuracy if correction for gas density is not incorporated. As an example, the density of oxygen is 1.43 g/L and the density of a 70%/30% heliox mixture is 0.55 g/L. To determine the gas flow of the heliox mixture using an oxygen flowmeter, the above equation relating flow to gas density can be employed.

$$Actual\ gas\ flow = indicated\ flow \times \frac{\sqrt{density\ of\ O_2}}{\sqrt{density\ of\ heliox}}$$

$$= 1\ L/min \times \frac{\sqrt{1.43}}{\sqrt{0.55}}$$

$$= 1.6\ L/min$$

Therefore, when using an oxygen flowmeter to regulate a 70%/30% heliox mixture, each 1 L/min increment of

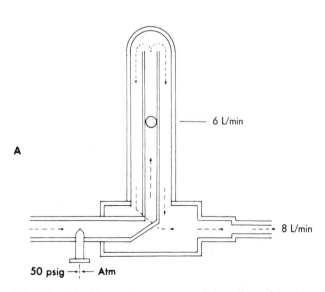

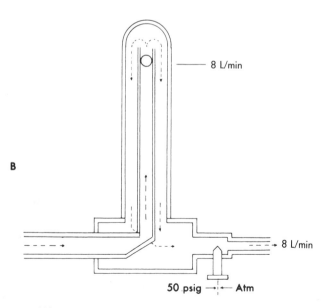

FIGURE 10–19 • Comparison of the effect of back pressure on (*A*) a non–pressure-compensated and (*B*) a pressure-compensated Thorpe tube (Scanlon. *Egan's Fundamentals of Respiratory Care.* 6th ed. 1995:654.)

oxygen displayed on the flowmeter is equal to 1.6 L/min of actual heliox mixture flow.

Oxygen Delivery Devices

A key concept in oxygen therapy is the difference between oxygen *delivered* to the face (or airway) and oxygen *inspired* (actually entering) into the lungs. The fraction of delivered oxygen (FDO_2) is the concentration of oxygen delivered to the airway. The concentration of oxygen that actually enters the lungs is expressed as the fraction of inspired oxygen (FIO_2). The variables that differentiate these two values include the respiratory pattern of the patient (respiratory rate, inspiratory flows, and tidal volumes), delivery device used, flow rates delivered by the device, and proper fit of the device. It is relatively easy to measure the FDO_2 or oxygen as it leaves the device, whereas measurement of FIO_2 is much more obscure, requiring sampling of gas from a well-mixed area, such as the patient's trachea. Often, the best we can do is to calculate or indirectly estimate the FIO_2. See Table 10–5 for different types of oxygen delivery systems.

Consider the case of the nasal cannula running at 2 L/min. The device delivers 100% oxygen ($FDO_2 = 1.0$). If the patient has a minute volume of 6 L/min, then clearly the FIO_2 is less than 1.0 (100% oxygen), but just how much? If the patient inspires the entire 2 L of O_2 with 4 L of room air, the FIO_2 would be 0.47. However, the liter flow of oxygen is continuous, whereas patient inspiration is

cyclical (say with an inspiration/exhalation [I:E] ratio of 1:3), so that the patient is breathing in only 25% of the time and inhaling only 0.5 L/min of oxygen. With a minute volume of 6 L/min, this results in a calculated FIO_2 of 0.28. If the same patient breathes 10 L/min, with the same I:E ratio, calculated FIO_2 is reduced to 0.25. At either minute volume, if the patient has an obstruction between the nose and the hypopharynx, we're back to breathing only room air. Other factors, such as the volume of the patient's nasopharynx (acting as a reservoir) and whether the patient is a nose or mouth breather, will further obscure the relationship of FDO_2 and FIO_2. Table 10–6 lists some of the variables that differentiate FDO_2 from FIO_2.

Oxygen delivery devices are classified as variable performance devices or fixed performance devices based on the differences between FDO_2 and FIO_2. Performance is based on the matching of the flow rate of gas leaving the device with the inspiratory flow rate entering the patient. **Variable performance devices** (also referred to as *low-*

Table • 10–6 VARIABLES THAT DIFFERENTIATE FDO_2 AND FIO_2

	FDO_2	FIO_2
Ability to measure directly with analyzer	Yes	No
Consistently independent of mask fit	Yes	No
Consistently independent of patient effort	Yes	No
Ability to predict accurately with most devices	Yes	No

Table • 10–5 OXYGEN DELIVERY SYSTEMS

Devices	Flow/FDO_2/FIO_2	Required Humidifier	Special Requirements	Hazards
Low-Flow				
Nasal cannula	1/1.0/0.21–0.24	None	Patent nasooropharynx	
	2/1.0/0.23–0.28	None	Devices changed between patients	FIO_2 fluctuates with
	3/1.0/0.27–0.32	None	and when visibly soiled	patient respiratory rate,
	4/1.0/0.29–0.36	None		volumes and flow rates
	5/1.0/0.31–0.40	BH		Skin irritation
	6/1.0/0.33–0.44	BH		
	>6/1.0/0.33–0.44	BH		
Reservoir nasal cannula	0.5–5/1.0/0.22–0.44	None	Requires oximetry testing	
Simple face mask	6–10/1.0/0.30–0.50	BH	Short-term use	Claustrophobia
				Skin irritation
Nonrebreather mask	10–15/1.0/0.60–0.80	BH—sterile H_2O	Short-term use	Suffocation
High-Flow			Within limits: $FIO_2 = FDO_2$	
Jet (Venturi) mask/tc	3–12/0.24–0.40/0.24–40	None	Becomes low flow at FIO_2 of 0.40	
Jet nebulizers (LVN)				**Nebulizers**
Standard-flow	6–12/0.28–0.40/0.28–0.40	Sterile H_2O	Becomes low flow at FIO_2 of 0.40	Infection risk
High-flow	12–14/0.38–0.98/0.38–0.80		Becomes low flow at FIO_2 of 0.80	Bronchospasm
Gas-injection nebulizer	20–120/0.40–1.0/0.40–1.0	Sterile H_2O	Oxygen and air sources required	Fluid overload
Heated humidifier	15/0.40	Sterile H_2O		
Heat moisture exchanger		None	Device is changed daily	Increased work of
				breathing
Blenders	20–120/0.22–1.0/0.22–1.0	WH—sterile H_2O	Expensive equipment	
CPAP/BiPAP	1–13/0.22–0.50/0.22–0.50	WH—sterile H_2O	Oxygen flow >13 affects performance	Not reliable FIO_2 >0.40

BH, bubble diffusion humidifier; CPAP, continuous positive airway pressure; BiPAP, bilevel positive airway pressure; LVN, large-volume nebulizer; WH, wick humidifier.

flow devices) may provide less gas than the patient is breathing in. Any time that the patient's inspiratory flow exceeds the flow from the device, the FIO_2 varies. In contrast, **fixed performance devices** (also referred to as *high-flow devices*) consistently provide a gas flow that meets and exceeds the patient's inspiratory flow rates. Because it is the interface between the patient and device that determines whether the device performance is variable or fixed, the previously used label of a device as low-flow or high-flow is often misleading.

In a variable performance device, the gas flow from the oxygen device is less than the patient's total inspiratory flow rate, requiring the patient to draw in ambient (or room) air in addition to the gas being delivered by the device, reducing the FIO_2. Variable conditions exist any time that the FIO_2 is less than the FDO_2. Some low-flow devices, such as nasal cannulas, deliver 100% oxygen (ie, $FDO_2 = 1.0$), whereas devices such as jet-mixing masks deliver premixed gases with extraordinary precision. With low-flow systems, FIO_2 is variable based on the output of the device and the ventilatory pattern of the patient (ie, tidal volume, respiratory rate, I:E ratio, peak inspiratory flow rates). Table 10–7 demonstrates the effect of changing I:E ratio on the FIO_2 when the FDO_2 is 1.0.

Fixed performance devices are high-flow systems that provide all the gas that the patient breaths in ($FIO_2 = FDO_2$). The designation of a device as high- or low-flow is rarely an absolute. As discussed later, many devices designed as high-flow devices function as low-flow devices under common clinical conditions. It is important for the practitioner to understand the capabilities and limitations of the various oxygen devices in their abilities to meet the patient's clinical needs. Table 10–8 lists the range of FIO_2 commonly available from variable performance oxygen delivery devices.

Nasal Cannula

Nasal cannulas (Fig. 10–20) can provide 22% to 44% oxygen with flow rates up to 6 L/min in adults (depending on ventilatory pattern); but in newborns and infants, flows should be limited to a maximum of 2 L/min. Oxygen sup-

Table • 10–8   RANGE OF FIO_2 FROM VARIABLE PERFORMANCE OXYGEN DELIVERY DEVICES

Device	L/min	FIO_2
Nasal cannula	1	0.21–0.24
	2	0.23–0.28
	3	0.25–0.32
	4	0.26–0.36
	5	0.31–0.40
	6	0.33–0.44
	>6	0.33–0.44
Simple face mask	5–10	0.35–0.50
Partial rebreathing mask	6–10	0.40–0.70
Nonrebreathing mask	10–15	0.60–0.80

plied to adults by nasal cannula at flow rates of less than or equal to 4 L/min need not be humidified.

Nasal cannulas are the most commonly employed devices for the administration of low-flow oxygen. The cannula is light weight, comfortable, relatively unobtrusive, and inexpensive. The cannula consists of two plastic prongs about 1 cm in length, positioned so that each is inserted in one of the two nares. These prongs are attached to a longer piece of small-bore tubing that is attached to an oxygen source.

Once applied to the patient, these prongs are held in place either by tubing that loops over each ear, joining under the chin with a bolo tie–type cinch (lariat style), or by an elastic band that connects both sides of the cannula with a band running across the back of the head. Although the elastic band may be more secure, the lariat-style cannula has the advantage of coming off easily, without throwing the patient off balance, should the patient move beyond the reach of the oxygen tubing.

A primary administration device for short- or long-term therapy, the cannula is also routinely used to provide supplemental oxygen when a patient removes an oxygen mask to eat, drink, or perform oral care. Major advantages of the cannula are that it does not get in the way when talking, eating, or drinking and that it is well tolerated by most patients when sleeping or moving around.

Use nasal prongs that are soft and pliable, curved rather than straight, and rounded or flared at the ends. Position the cannula to direct flow posteriorly rather than upward toward the frontal sinuses. Comfort is the key for any device used with alert patients for prolonged periods of time, and oxygen devices are no exception.

Improper positioning of the cannula can reduce FIO_2. It is easy for a patient to move too far from the oxygen source, accidentally crimp the tubing, or turn and pull the cannula out of position. Make sure that the device is properly positioned, and take numerous opportunities to show the patient or care provider how to take off and properly replace the cannula.

Table • 10–7   EFFECT OF INSPIRATION/EXHALATION RATIO ON FIO_2 with FDO_2 of 1.0*

	Oxygen Delivered		
I : E Ratio	2 L/min	6 L/min	10 L/min
1 : 2	0.26	0.37	0.47
1 : 3	0.25	0.33	0.41
1 : 4	0.24	0.30	0.37
1 : 5	0.23	0.29	0.34

*Simple calculation of FIO_2 based on tidal volume of 500 mL, rate of 20 breaths/min with changing oxygen flow rate.

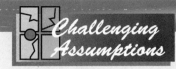

CRITICAL THINKING CHALLENGES

Challenging Assumptions

Oxygen Device Selection for the Severely Hypoxic Patient

Many oxygen delivery devices are rated as being capable of providing FiO$_2$ levels greater than 0.40, including simple masks, nonrebreather masks, and even jet-mixing aerosol devices. In mannikins, we have difficulty demonstrating that any of these devices can reliably provide more than 40% oxygen at patient inspiratory flow rates of 60 L/min. Even when patient inspiratory flows are met, a poorly fitting mask allows ambient air to be inhaled, greatly diluting the inspired oxygen.

The danger lies in assuming that, when you crank up the oxygen from 40% to 80%, the PaO$_2$ or SaO$_2$ should go up, unless there is a massive shunt. This may lead to aggressive attempts to support the patient when the real problem is only that the device is not delivering the amount of oxygen intended.

Consequently, unless you are certain that the oxygen device is delivering 50% more than the patient's peak flow, assume that it will not deliver more than 40% oxygen. When more than 40% oxygen is required to support a patient, consider a high-flow system, such as a blender, high-flow aerosol, or gas-injection nebulizer that is capable of well-exceeding patient inspiratory efforts.

Successful use of oxygen therapy with the nasal cannula requires a relatively clear, unobstructed passage from the nasopharynx to the hypopharynx. Mouth breathers benefit from nasal oxygen. It has been argued that nose breathing may result in a lower FiO$_2$ than mouth breathing under some circumstances. The theory is that the cannula delivers oxygen to the nasopharynx during both inspiration and expiration. During mouth breathing, the nasopharynx serves as a reservoir in which oxygen collects during expiratory cycle. The oxygen is then entrained with the oxygen coming from the cannula during inspiration. In contrast, the nose breather drives oxygen out of the nose during exhalation, reducing the reservoir effect of the nasopharynx. Investigators have reported conflicting support of this concept, but intuitively, the best combination may be to breathe in through the nose and out through the mouth (allowing oxygen to build up in the nasopharynx between inspirations). This may be convenient because it is the way that we instruct patients to breathe during diaphragmatic and relaxation breathing exercises and is a natural pattern for many COPD patients who use pursed-lip breathing (Box 10–4).

Nasal Catheter

The nasal catheter (Fig. 10–21) is a tube (ranging in size from 10F to 14F) placed through the nares, with the distal tip placed into the nasopharynx. Attached to standard oxygen tubing, the nasal catheter is used to deliver low- and medium-flow oxygen to the upper airway. The FdO$_2$ with the nasal catheter is similar to that achieved with the nasal cannula, with oxygen flow rates limited to 8 L/min. Placement of the catheter is determined initially by inserting the catheter, lubricated with a water-soluble solution, into the least obstructed nares, the distance mea-

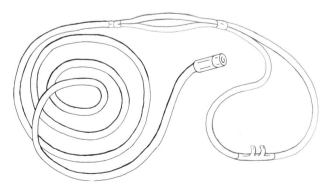

FIGURE 10–20 • Nasal cannula.

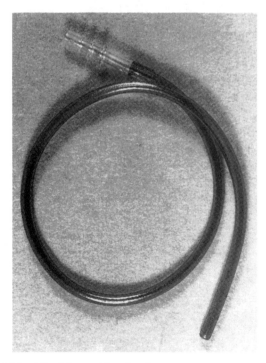

FIGURE 10–21 • Nasal catheter.

Box • 10–4   PROCEDURE FOR APPLYING A NASAL CANNULA

EQUIPMENT

- Oxygen flowmeter or cylinder with regulator or concentrator
- Nipple adapter (oxygen flow <4 L/min) or prefilled humidifier (5–6 L/min or patient complaint of discomfort)
- Nasal cannula with tubing
- Oxygen-connecting tubing and straight connectors, as necessary

EQUIPMENT INDICATIONS

- Patient who requires oxygen administration with desired inspired oxygen levels of 22%–44%
- Nasal cannula: approximate ranges of FIO_2 achieved may vary with extremes in tidal volume, respiratory frequency, and inspiratory flow rates
- May be used in combination with other devices (ie, oxygen or aerosol masks) to supplement that device and further increase FIO_2

EQUIPMENT LIMITATIONS

- Requires patency between nose and pharynx
- May cause irritation of nares, nasal mucosa, and ears from contact with the device
- Oxygen inspired fluctuates with patient respiratory rate, volumes, and flow rates

EQUIPMENT APPLICATION

1. Verify physician order.
2. Wash hands.
3. Identify patient by identification band.
4. Explain to patient the therapy ordered and the goals of the therapy. Instruct in proper use of the device, and caution against fire and safety hazards. Post "no smoking" sign to door of patient's room.
5. Assemble equipment.
6. Attach oxygen flowmeter to oxygen wall outlet (concentrators and cylinders regulators usually have flowmeters built in).
7. Attach nipple adapter or disposable prefilled humidifier to flowmeter.
8. Attach nasal cannula directly to nipple adapter or outlet of humidifier (up to 50 feet of oxygen connecting tubing with straight oxygen tubing connectors may be used between nipple adapter or humidifier and nasal cannula).
9. Turn on the oxygen flowmeter to the prescribed liter flow.
10. Lariat-style cannulas: place the prongs of the cannula into the patient's nares, directing the tubing extending from each side of the cannula over each ear, and adjust the bolo under the chin to provide a firm but comfortable fit (Fig. 10–22).
11. Visually inspect equipment as set up for proper function.
12. Assess patient comfort, and adjust accordingly.
13. Wash hands.

TROUBLESHOOTING

1. Patient complains of discomfort from nasal dryness.
   a. Add humidifier if one is not in use.
   b. Apply topical water-based lotion (eg, K-Y jelly or Nasal Moist gel) to nares (**never use oil- or petroleum-based lotions**).
2. Skin breakdown or irritation occurs in or around nares or at any point that cannula or tubing contacts skin.
   a. Apply topical water-based lotion or Nasal Moist gel or pump to nares or site of irritation (**never use oil- or petroleum-based lotions**).
   b. Remove cannula; consider other device options.
   c. Pad point of irritation with gauze pad or DuoDerm.
3. Patient complains about not getting enough oxygen.
   a. Assess oxygenation (perform pulse oximetry).
   b. Assess system for proper function.
   c. Determine whether patient requires higher liter flow of oxygen with nasal cannula.
   d. Determine whether patient requires change of administration device (eg, mask, aerosol, Venturi mask).
4. Patient's oxygen saturation is <88% or PaO_2 <55 mmHg.
   a. Assess system for proper function.
   b. Determine whether patient requires higher liter flow of oxygen with nasal cannula.
   c. Determine whether patient requires change of administration device (eg, mask, aerosol, Venturi mask).

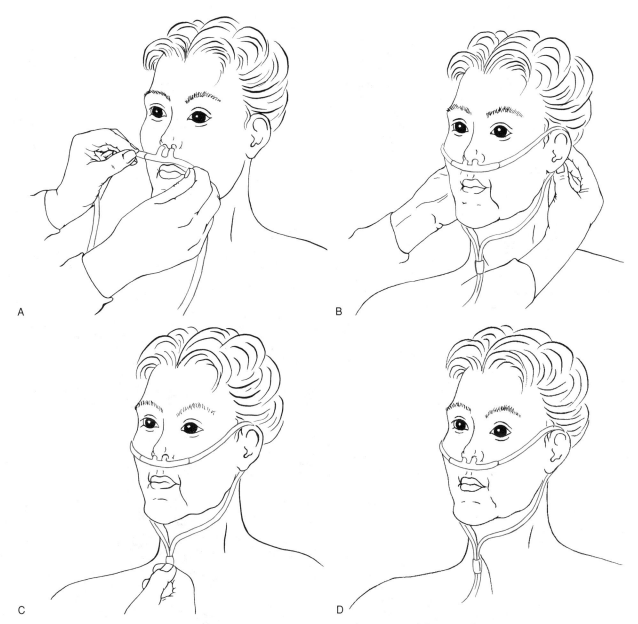

FIGURE 10-22 • Application of a nasal cannula. (A) Place the prongs of the cannula into the patient's nares. (B) Position the tubing extending from each side of the cannula over each ear. (C) Adjust the bolo under the chin to provide a firm fit. (D) Proper placement of a nasal cannula.

sured from the tip of the nose to the earlobe. Care should be taken not to extend the catheter accidentally into the hypopharynx, where it may interfere with the movement of the epiglottis and enter the trachea. Visual inspection through the open mouth with a tongue blade should *not* reveal the catheter extending beyond the tip of the uvula. Once inserted, the catheter is typically taped into position, much as a nasogastric tube. Although textbooks of yesteryear dogmatically recommend changing the site of the catheter every 8 hours to avoid secretion buildup from blocking the tubing, there appears to be little evidence supporting that practice.

Catheters are seldom used in current clinical practice. There may be discomfort and pain on insertion of the catheter, and possible problems include bleeding, irritation of the mucosa, obstruction of the catheter, inadvertent intubation of the trachea, and should the catheter migrate into the esophagus, gastric insufflation.

Oxygen-Conserving Delivery Devices

In the hospital, where piped oxygen is taken for granted and the cost of oxygen is relatively low, wasteful practices such as continuous flow of oxygen into a cannula, whereby less than 25% of the drug is inhaled, have become commonplace. For smaller institutions and for patients who rely on cylinders or liquid oxygen systems in their homes or during travel outside the home, oxygen-conserving devices are available that reduce waste and cost and that extend the time available from a cylinder. Three common devices are available: the reservoir, the pulse-demand device, and the transtracheal oxygen (TTO) catheter.

Reservoir Nasal Cannula

The reservoir nasal cannula device allows the oxygen to collect in a reservoir that is either an integral part of or connected to a cannula. Both the moustache- and pendant-style reservoirs are available (Figs. 10–23 through 10–26). Oxygen savings in terms of cost/benefit ratios of up to 4:1 have been reported when comparing continuous low-flow nasal cannulas to the reservoir device. This savings is realized only if the patient uses a prescribed lower liter flow with the reservoir device. Although some patients may prefer the pendant-style reservoir on aesthetic grounds, the moustache-style device is a more reliable configuration for the patient while in bed, although with either configuration, the nose piece may become dislodged during sleep. Both devices require expiration through the nose (Box 10–5).

Pulse-Demand Valve Device

A pulse-demand valve device is an electronically operated demand valve that uses a flow sensor to detect the onset of inspiration and that releases a preset dose of O_2 through the attached cannula. This device offers the highest oxygen cost/benefit ratio (up to 7:1) and can be attached to any conventional compressed gas cylinder or liquid oxygen system

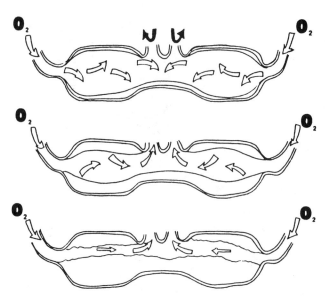

FIGURE 10–24 • During exhalation, oxygen fills an expandable reservoir. During the early phase of inspiration, the patient inspires from the reservoir and from the cannula's continuous gas flow.

(Figs. 10–27 and 10–28). The demand device automatically responds to changes in the patient's respiratory rate. The device replaces the flowmeter attached to a 50-psi outlet or regulator with cylinder or liquid oxygen system. These are relatively expensive, high-technology devices that have some related problems based on the device and strategy of

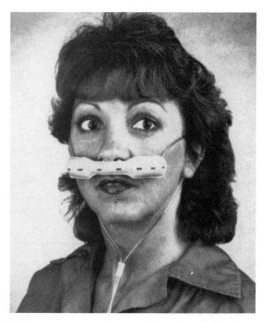

FIGURE 10–23 • Moustache-style reservoir cannula. (Courtesy of Chad Therapeutics, Chatsworth, CA.)

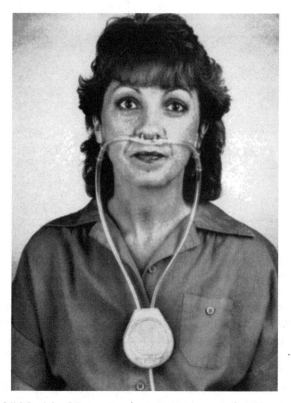

FIGURE 10–25 • Pendant reservoir cannula. (Courtesy of Chad Therapeutics, Chatsworth, CA.)

Box • 10–5 PROCEDURE FOR APPLYING AN OXYMIZER RESERVOIR NASAL CANNULA

EQUIPMENT

- Oxymizer reservoir cannula
- Oxygen-connecting tubing and straight connectors, as necessary

EQUIPMENT INDICATIONS

- Patients who require low-flow oxygen administration with desired inspired oxygen levels of 22%–44%.
- Patients who require oxygen therapy during exercise. Oxygen flow rate range for the Oxymizer is 0.5–5 L/min. Ranges of FIO_2 achieved may vary with extremes in tidal volume, respiratory frequency, and inspiratory flow rates.
- Liter flow prescription with the Oxymizer should be determined by pulse oximetry during rest, exercise, and sleep.
- May reduce cost of oxygen use in domiciliary setting when using liquid oxygen systems and cylinders
- Eliminates need for humidification
- Extends range of FIO_2 beyond nasal cannula within limits of concentrator output.
- Oxymizer comes in two configurations: moustache reservoir model and pendant model.

EQUIPMENT LIMITATIONS

- Large moustache-shaped reservoir cannula may be cosmetically unacceptable to some patients.
- Effectiveness may vary among sleep, rest, and exercise states for any one patient. Prescription should be determined in all three states with use of oximetry.
- Requires patency between nose and pharynx. Do not use when upper airway is bypassed (eg, tracheostomy, stoma).
- May cause irritation of skin on face and ears from contact with the device
- Oxygen inspired fluctuates with patient respiratory rate, volumes, and flow rates.

EQUIPMENT APPLICATION

1. Verify physician order.
2. Wash hands.
3. Identify patient by identification band.
4. Explain to patient the therapy ordered and goals of the therapy. Instruct patient in proper use of the device, and caution against fire and safety hazards. Post "no smoking" sign to door of patient's room.
5. Assemble equipment.
6. Attach oxygen flowmeter to oxygen wall outlet (concentrators and cylinder regulators usually have flowmeters built in).
7. Attach nipple adapter to flowmeter.
8. Attach nasal Oxymizer cannula directly to nipple adapter (up to 50 feet of oxygen connecting tubing with straight oxygen tubing connectors may be used between nipple adapter and Oxymizer cannula).
9. Turn on the oxygen flowmeter to the prescribed liter flow.
10. Place the prongs of the Oxymizer into the patient's nares, directing the tubing extending from each side of the Oxymizer over each ear, and adjust the bolo under the chin to provide a firm but comfortable fit.
11. Visually inspect equipment as set up for proper function.
12. Assess patient comfort and adjust accordingly.
13. Wash hands.

TROUBLESHOOTING

1. White flap valve inside Oxymizer does not move during inspiration.
   a. Replace Oxymizer with new unit.
   b. Perform pulse oximetry.
   c. Consider alternative device.
2. Patient complains of discomfort from nasal dryness.
   a. Consider use of an alternative device with humidifier.
   b. Apply topical water-based lotion (eg, K-Y jelly or Nasal Moist gel) to nares (**never use oil- or petroleum-based lotions**).
3. Skin breakdown or irritation occurs in or around nares or at any point that cannula or tubing contacts skin.
   a. Apply topical water-based lotion or Nasal Moist gel or pump to nares or site of irritation (**never use oil- or petroleum-based lotions**).
   b. Remove cannula; consider other device options.
   c. Pad point of irritation with gauze pad or Duo-Derm.
4. Patient complains about not getting enough oxygen.
   a. Assess oxygenation (perform pulse oximetry).
   b. Assess system for proper function.
   c. Determine whether patient requires higher liter flow of oxygen with Oxymizer.
   d. Determine whether patient requires change of administration device (eg, aerosol or Venturi mask).
5. Patient oxygen saturation is <88% or PaO_2 <55 mmHg.
   a. Assess system for proper function.
   b. Determine whether patient requires higher liter flow of oxygen with Oxymizer.
   c. Determine whether patient requires change of administration device (eg, mask, aerosol, or Venturi mask).

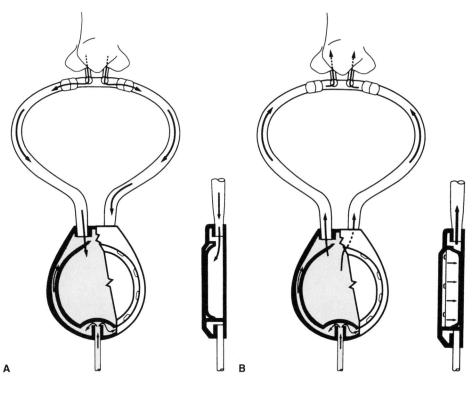

FIGURE 10–26 • As the patient exhales through the nasal prongs, the initial exhaled gas travels down the tubing, pushing the reservoir membrane forward (*A*). Soon after exhalation begins, the flow of oxygen purges the exhaled gases out of the tubing through the nasal prongs, replacing exhaled gas with oxygen. During inspiration, the patient inspires from the tubing, reservoir, and the cannula's continuous gas flow (*B*).

pulsing, such as disconnection, improper placement, poor sensing, and device failure. Pulse-demand devices may be less effective than the reservoirs with some forms of exercise.

Transtracheal Oxygen Catheters

Transtracheal oxygen is administered directly into the trachea by a percutaneous catheter inserted just above the suprasternal notch, allowing the lower airway to act as a reservoir and resulting in an oxygen cost/benefit ratio of up to 3:1 (Figs. 10–29 and 10–30). Beyond benefit as a conserving device, TTO has high aesthetic appeal, with no apparent oxygen appliance in view on the face. The minor surgery required for catheter placement can be done in a physician's office, as can periodic changing of the catheter every 30 to 90 days. TTO provides higher FIO_2 levels than do cannulas at the same flow rate, and up to 50% reductions in oxygen flow may be obtained. Complications, including as bleeding, infection, subcutaneous emphysema, increased secretion production, and displacement or plugging of the catheter, have been reported. Patients receiving TTO at home may continue to receive oxygen by this method in the acute care hospital setting provided that no problems present. If difficulties related to the transtracheal route of administration appear, oxygenation should be ensured by other means.

Oxygen Face Masks

Face masks cover the nose and mouth, with oxygen entering the front of the mask and exhalation escaping to the atmosphere through multiple ports at the side of the mask. These masks are commonly made of clear plastic, with a malleable metal strip positioned across the bridge of the nose to crimp the mask to conform better to the contours of the patient's face. An elastic strap positioned to run over the ears and across the back of the head can be snugged tight through a simple restricted orifice-type clamp located on both sides of the mask. The looser the fit, the more room air enters the airway from around the mask rather than through it.

Three variations of the disposable oxygen mask are the simple mask, the partial rebreathing mask, and the nonrebreathing mask. The simple mask has no reservoir bag, and the exhalation ports are just holes in the mask, so air can pass in or out of the exhalation ports during the respiratory cycle. The partial rebreathing mask has a small bag at the front of the mask attached at the same point at which the oxygen enters. The nonrebreathing mask is the same configuration as the partial rebreathing mask with the addition of one-way valves between the reservoir–oxygen inlet and the mask and on exhalation ports at both sides of the mask.

One should exercise caution with any mask that is placed on an obtunded, sedated, or restrained patient. Oxygen masks are intended to make breathing easier but do not always work that way. Inadequate flow of gas to the mask means that the patient has to work harder to breathe around it. Never leave a patient attached to any tight-fitting mask if the patient cannot remove the mask and is not under direct observation. The worst-case scenario is the patient who vomits into the mask but cannot take it off and either aspirates or asphyxiates. Nasty image? Good, remember it.

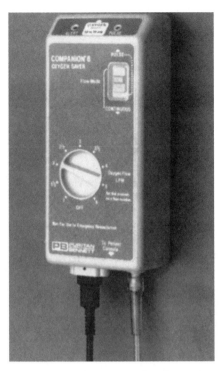

FIGURE 10–27 • Electronic pulse-demand oxygen delivery system. (Courtesy of Puritan-Bennett Corp., Kansas City, MO.)

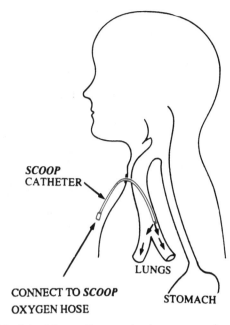

FIGURE 10–29 • Transtracheal oxygen catheter (Courtesy of Transtracheal Systems, Greenwood Village, CO.)

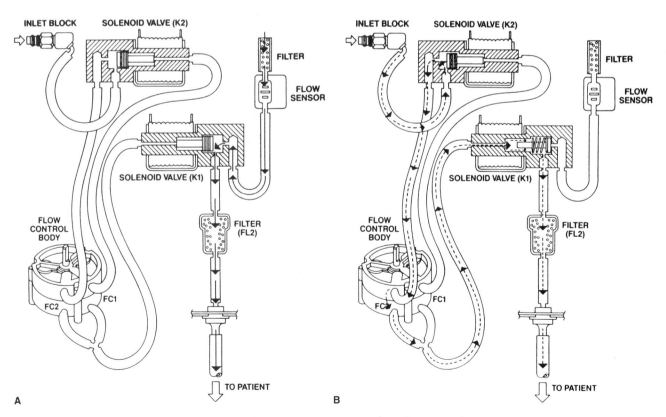

A

B

FIGURE 10–28 • Electronic pulse-demand oxygen system. (*A*) When the patient begins to inspire, gas is drawn through a flow sensor. (*B*) When flow is detected, the solenoid valve opens and delivers a pulsed dose of oxygen. The size of the pulsed dose or flow can be adjusted. (Courtesy of Puritan-Bennett Corp., Kansas City, MO.)

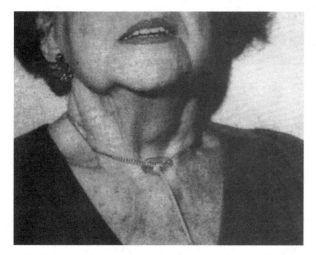

FIGURE 10–30 • Patient with a transtracheal oxygen catheter. (Johnson JT, Ferson PF, Hoffman LA, et al. Transtracheal delivery of oxygen: Efficacy and safety for long-term continuous therapy. *Ann Otol Rhinol Laryngol.* 1991;100: 108.)

Simple Oxygen Mask

Simple oxygen (Fig. 10–31) masks can provide 30% to 50% oxygen at flow rates of 5 to 10 L/min. Flow rates should be maintained at 5 L/min or more to avoid rebreathing exhaled CO_2 that can be retained in the mask. Although these masks are simple and easy to apply, they tend to be uncomfortable, claustrophobic, and hot when used for extended periods of time. Because simple masks and nasal cannulas provide an overlapping range of FIO_2, it makes sense to use the more comfortable, convenient, and less expensive nasal cannula in most situations. The simple mask

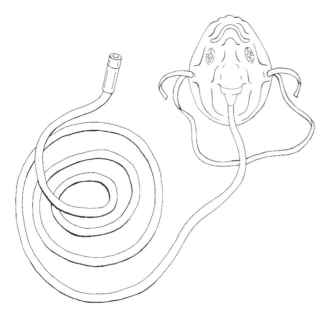

FIGURE 10–31 • Simple mask.

may be the device of choice when the nares are unavailable or particularly sensitive to contact irritation from the cannula (Box 10–6).

Partial and Nonrebreathing Masks

Masks with reservoir bags (partial rebreathing and nonrebreathing) are designed to provide elevated FIO_2 levels. Reservoir masks designed to provide high FIO_2 levels are usually not appropriate for long-term oxygen therapy in or outside of the hospital. These devices are intended to provide short-term elevation in FIO_2 during transport and prehospital care, in the emergency department, and during medical emergencies when hypoxemia is suspected or documented. After the patient is stabilized, if the need for a high FIO_2 continues, oxygen should be administered by a fixed performance device with a known FIO_2.

In practice, both partial and nonrebreathing masks function in a similar manner and provide an FIO_2 of about 0.6 (depending on mask fit and patient respiratory volume, rate, and pattern). The flow rate needs to be sufficient to keep the reservoir bag partially inflated during end inspiration.

In the partial rebreathing mask, there is a direct two-way opening between the mask and the reservoir bag (Fig. 10–32). When the patient breathes in, the bag is partially collapsed. When the patient exhales, the last gas breathed in is the first portion exhaled, filling the reservoir bag. Because the last gas in fills only the anatomic dead space, it is high in oxygen and low in carbon dioxide. Consequently, partial rebreathing masks, when properly used, do not increase CO_2 levels. Figure 10–33 illustrates proper placement of a partial rebreathing mask.

The nonrebreathing mask with one-way valves on both exhalation ports and between the reservoir and the mask are designed to let all inhaled gas come from the reservoir and all exhaled gas go out the exhalation ports to the atmosphere (Fig. 10–34). To operate properly, the nonrebreathing mask must fit snugly against the face and have no leaks. In practice, the disposable nonrebreathing masks that are commonly available rarely provide an adequate seal against the face, and ambient air entrainment is highly likely. In addition, many manufacturers of disposable nonrebreathing masks do not provide one of the expiratory one-way valves that is required for the device to operate in a truly nonrebreathing fashion. The level of leak that is created by the poor facial fit or the absence of the one-way expiratory valve preempts the need for a spring-loaded safety valve to allow patients to breathe ambient air if the oxygen flow to the mask is too low, becomes occluded, or is disconnected.

A tight-fitting mask of this type should deliver 100% oxygen, but in reality, the leak around the mask is virtually always a limiting function, and the FIO_2 achieved is rarely greater than 0.6 at 10 to 15 L/min. Higher FIO_2 is possible,

(text continues on page 276)

Box • 10–6 PROCEDURE FOR APPLYING A SIMPLE MASK

EQUIPMENT

- Oxygen flowmeter or cylinder with regulator
- Prefilled humidifiers
- Simple mask with tubing
- Oxygen-connecting tubing and straight connectors, as necessary

EQUIPMENT INDICATIONS

- Patient who requires emergency or short-term oxygen administration with desired inspired oxygen levels of 35% to 50%
- Simple mask and nasal cannula FiO_2 ranges overlap. The use of a nasal cannula should be considered unless contraindicated.

EQUIPMENT LIMITATIONS

- Primarily used for emergency situations and relatively short-term (<2 h) therapy. Reconsider use within 2 hours of application. If continued oxygen therapy is required, change to a more appropriate long-term device (eg, aerosol mask, Venturi mask, cannula).
- Patient may complain of claustrophobia.
- May cause irritation of skin from contact with the device
- Oxygen inspired fluctuates with patient respiratory rate, volumes, and inspiratory flow rates.
- May pose risk of suffocation in any patient who cannot voluntarily remove a tight-fitting mask
- Will not reliably deliver greater than 50% oxygen

EQUIPMENT APPLICATION

1. Verify physician order.
2. Wash hands.
3. Identify patient by identification band.
4. Explain to patient the therapy ordered and goals of the therapy. Instruct patient in proper use of the device, and caution against fire and safety hazards. Post "no smoking" sign to door of patient's room.
5. Assemble equipment.
6. Attach oxygen flowmeter to oxygen wall outlet (concentrators and cylinders regulators usually have flowmeters built in).
7. Attach disposable prefilled humidifier to flowmeter.
8. Attach simple mask to outlet of humidifier.
9. Turn on the oxygen flowmeter to the prescribed liter flow.
10. Place the mask over the patient's nose and mouth, gently pinching the soft metal at the top of the mask to conform to the patient's nose, and extend the elastic band above the ears across the crown of the head, adjusting band for a snug but comfortable fit (Fig. 10–35).
11. Visually inspect equipment as set up for proper function.
12. Assess patient comfort and adjust accordingly.
13. Wash hands.

TROUBLESHOOTING

1. Patient complains of claustrophobia.
   a. Consider use of Venturi mask (which provides higher flow rates to patients in the same range of FiO_2), or nasal cannula, or aerosol face tent (which does not cover the face).
2. Skin breakdown or irritation occurs at any point that mask or tubing contacts skin.
   a. Apply topical water-based lotion to site of irritation (**never use oil- or petroleum-based lotions**).
   b. Pad point of irritation (eg, gauze pad or Duo-Derm).
   c. Reposition elastic band or device.
   d. Remove mask, and consider other device options.
3. Patient complains about not getting enough oxygen.
   a. Assess oxygenation (perform pulse oximetry).
   b. Assess system for proper function.
   c. Determine whether patient requires higher liter flow of oxygen with nasal cannula.
   d. Determine whether patient requires change of administration device (eg, high flow aerosol mask, Venturi mask).
4. Patient oxygen saturation is <88% or PaO_2 <55 mmHg.
   a. Assess system for proper function.
   b. Determine whether patient requires higher liter flow of oxygen with nasal cannula.
   c. Determine whether patient requires change of administration device (eg, aerosol, Venturi mask).

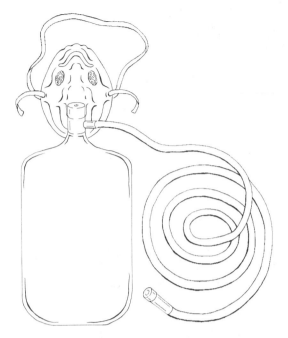

FIGURE 10–32 • Partial rebreathing mask.

depending on mask fit and ventilatory variables. Flow rates of more than 25 L/min, available by flushing the typical flowmeter beyond scale, may be required to provide an FIO_2 of more than 0.80 (Box 10–7).

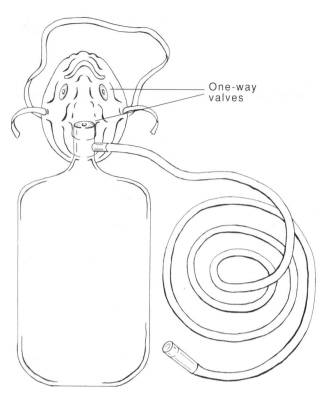

One-way valves

FIGURE 10–34 • Nonrebreathing mask. Note the one-way valves located between the mask and the reservoir bag, and on the expiratory ports.

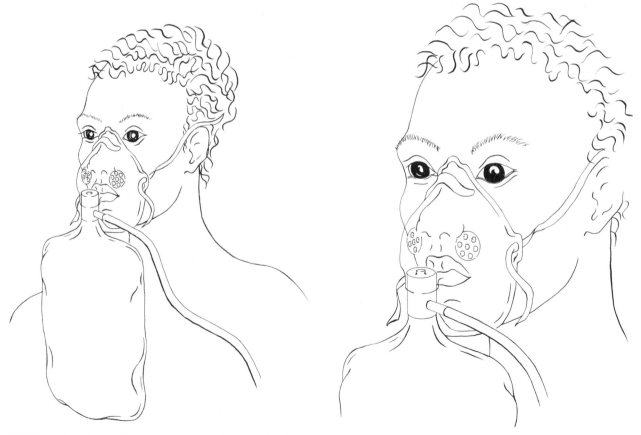

FIGURE 10–33 • Proper placement of a partial rebreathing mask.

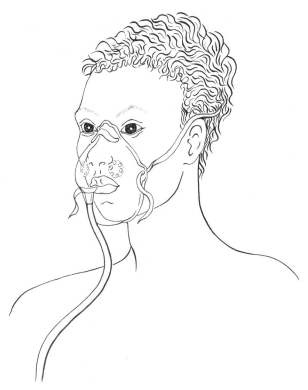

FIGURE 10–35 • Proper placement of a simple mask.

Fixed Performance (High-Flow) Systems

These systems deliver a prescribed gas mixture—either high or low F_DO_2—at flow rates that exceed patient demand, so that F_DO_2 equals F_IO_2.

Jet-mixing (Venturi) Masks

The jet-mixing mask can accurately deliver predetermined oxygen concentrations to the trachea of up to 40%. Jet-mixing masks rated to deliver more than 40% do not deliver flow rates adequate to meet the inspiratory flow rates of most adult patients (peak inspiratory flow of 40 L/min) and especially those in respiratory distress (peak inspiratory flow of more than 80 L/min), as shown in Table 10–9.

Jet-mixing masks and large-volume nebulizers both provide relatively high-flow oxygen delivery using the same general operating principle. Operation is based on the principle of constant-pressure jet mixing.[11] Air is entrained through the viscous shearing interaction between the driving gas (oxygen) and stationary ambient air. The greater the flow of oxygen, the more room air that is entrained. The mixing device is composed of a small orifice fixed opening through which pressurized oxygen is pushed, often at 50 psi. The liter flow of oxygen, the size

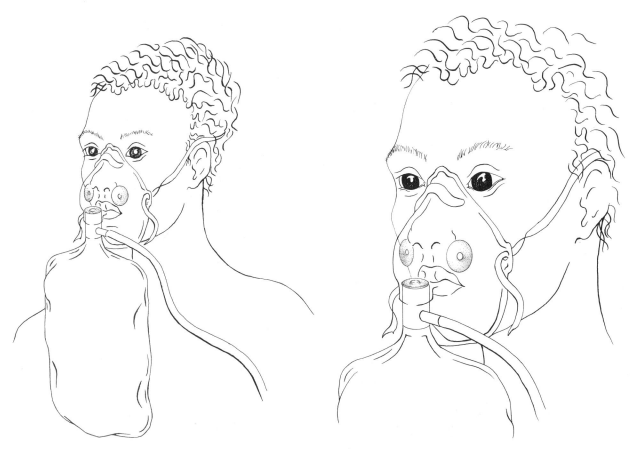

FIGURE 10–36 • Proper placement of a nonrebreathing mask.

Box • 10–7 PROCEDURE FOR APPLYING A NONREBREATHING RESERVOIR MASK

EQUIPMENT

- Oxygen flow meter or cylinder with regulator
- Nipple adapter
- Nonrebreathing reservoir mask, with one-way valves between reservoir bag and mask
- Oxygen-connecting tubing and straight connectors, as necessary

EQUIPMENT INDICATIONS

- Patients who require oxygen administration with desired inspired oxygen levels of >50%
- Liter flow is adjusted to keep reservoir bag from deflating during inspiration (usually 10–15 L/min). This may require adjustments in flow rates based on patient respiratory rate and pattern.
- Liter flow >15 L/min may be required to provide >70% inspired oxygen.

COMPONENTS OF PROPER ORDER

- Physician order for oxygen by nonrebreather mask. (Liter flow is not specified because it is dependent on patient's ventilatory pattern.)

EQUIPMENT LIMITATIONS

- Primarily used for emergency situations and relatively short-term therapy. Reconsider within 2 hours of application and each 24 hours thereafter.
- May cause complaints of claustrophobia. Other high-flow alternatives may be preferable, such as high-flow or blender system.
- May cause irritation of skin from contact with the device
- Oxygen inspired fluctuates with patient respiratory rate, volumes, and inspiratory flow rates
- May pose risk of suffocation on any patient who cannot voluntarily remove a tight-fitting mask
- Will not *reliably* deliver greater than 60%–70% oxygen

EQUIPMENT APPLICATION

1. Verify physician order.
2. Wash hands.
3. Identify patient by identification band.
4. Explain to patient the therapy ordered and goals of the therapy. Instruct the patient in proper use of the device, and caution against fire and safety hazards. Post "no smoking" sign to door of patient's room.
5. Assemble equipment.
6. Attach oxygen flowmeter to oxygen wall outlet (cylinder regulators usually have flowmeters built in).
7. Attach nipple adapter to flowmeter.
8. Attach reservoir mask directly to nipple adapter.
9. Turn on the oxygen flowmeter to the prescribed liter flow >10 L/min, and adjust flow as necessary to keep reservoir bag partially inflated on end inspiration.
10. Place the mask over the patient's nose and mouth, gently pinching the soft metal at the top of the mask to conform to the patient's nose, and extend elastic band above the ears across the crown of the head, adjusting band for a snug but comfortable fit. Place reservoir bag over sheets or bed clothes so that bag can remain inflated (Fig. 10–36).
11. Visually inspect equipment as set up for proper function.
12. Assess patient comfort and adjust accordingly.
13. Wash hands.

TROUBLESHOOTING

1. Patient complains of claustrophobia.
   a. Consider use of high-flow system
   b. Increase flow rate of oxygen into nonrebreathing mask.
2. Skin breakdown or irritation occurs at any point that mask or tubing contacts skin.
   a. Apply topical water-based lotion to site of irritation (**never use oil- or petroleum-based lotions**).
   b. Pad point of irritation (eg, gauze pad or Duo-Derm).
   c. Reposition elastic band or device.
   d. Remove mask, and consider other device options.
3. Patient complains about not getting enough oxygen.
   a. Assess oxygenation (perform pulse oximetry).
   b. Assess system for proper function.
   c. Determine whether patient requires higher liter flow of oxygen.
   d. Determine whether patient requires change of administration device (eg, gas-injection nebulizer or blender.)
4. Patient oxygen saturation is <88% or PaO_2 <55 mmHg.
   a. Assess system for proper function.
   b. Determine whether patient requires higher liter flow of oxygen with addition of nasal cannula.
   c. Determine whether patient requires change of administration device (eg, high-flow system or blender).

of the fixed orifice of the nozzle, and the size of the entrainment ports are important variables that achieve precise gas mixing and delivery of precise FiO_2 with both devices (Box 10–8).

Aerosol masks (Fig. 10–37), face tents (Fig. 10–38), tracheostomy collars (Fig. 10–39), and T-piece adapters (Figs. 10–40 and 10–41) can be used with high-flow supplemental oxygen systems. Table 10–10 lists the range of FiO_2 generally available with various high-flow patient interfaces.

The gas flow can be humidified by a continuous aerosol generator or large reservoir humidifier. Most jet entrainment aerosol generators cannot provide adequate flows at high oxygen concentrations. Another limitation of the entrainment jet nebulizer and jet-mixing mask is that when back pressure develops distal to the jet orifice and entrainment port, less air is entrained and the FiO_2 is increased (Box 10–9).

In the home care setting, high-flow oxygen delivery systems may be impractical if more than 4 L/min are required to drive the device. This may be accomplished with some oxygen concentrators, although the FDO_2 coming from the concentrator may be well below 1.0, resulting in reduced FDO_2 in the delivered gas. Jet nebulizers require too much gas to be powered by an oxygen source outside of the hospital with piped-in gas. In the home setting, they are generally compressor driven with supplemental oxygen bled in at low flows.

When an artificial airway is in place, tracheostomy collars and T-piece tubing adapters may be used with high-flow supplemental oxygen systems. Because the upper airway is bypassed, this gas should be humidified by a continuous aerosol generator or a heated humidifier. The humidifier is preferable because of the greater likelihood of transmission of contagion by the nebulizer.

High-Flow Systems for High-Flow Patients

To provide high-flow oxygen to adult patients in respiratory distress, a total flow of more than 80 L/min may be required. This is best accomplished by using a high-flow blender or a gas-injection nebulizer. Blenders are relatively expensive devices requiring both compressed oxygen and air sources capable of producing precise FDO_2 at flows exceeding 100 L/min. The gas injection nebulizer (GIN) uses two gas inlets that attach to flowmeters: one drives the nebulizer and is limited to maximum flows about 40 L/min; the other inlet is less restricted and can generate flows of more than 80 L/min. If both inlets are attached to oxygen flowmeters, an FiO_2 of 1.0 can be delivered at 120 L/min. Figure 10–42 shows an example of a GIN.

Oxygen Analysis

Many clinical situations call for the analysis of gaseous oxygen to confirm the proper operation of oxygen delivery sys-

Table • 10–9 ENTRAINMENT NEBULIZER FLOW OUTPUTS*

			Total Flow			
FDO_2	Entrainment Ration (Air to Oxygen)	Recommnended Oxygen Flow (L/min)	1 Neb.	2 Neb.	3 Neb.	4 Neb.
0.24	25 : 1	4	104	208	312	416
0.28	10 : 1	4	**44**	88	132	176
0.31	7 : 1	6	**48**	96	144	192
0.35	5 : 1	8	**48**	96	144	192
0.40	3 : 1	8	*32*	**64**	96	128
0.50	1.7 : 1	12	*32*	**64**	96	128
0.60	1 : 1	12	*24*	**48**	72	96
0.70	1 : 0.6	12	*19*	*38*	**57**	76
0.80	1 : 0.3	12	*16*	*32*	**48**	64
0.90	1 : 0.14	12	*14*	*28*	*42*	**56**
1.0	1 : 0	12	*12*	*24*	*36*	**48**

*This table illustrates total flow output from up to four entrainment type nebulizers run at commonly recommended oxygen flow rates in relation to a patient breathing a 40 L/min and 80 L/min. To deliver an FiO_2 >0.60 with a maximum oxygen flow rate of 12 L/min, you would need two nebulizers in tandem to provide high-flow oxygen. In a patient with a peak inspiratory flow of 80 L/min, four nebulizers are required to provide high-flow oxygen. Numbers that appear in bold indicate low-flow device at inspiratory flow rates of 80 L/min. Numbers that appear in bold italics indicate low-flow device at inspiratory flow rates of 40 L/min.

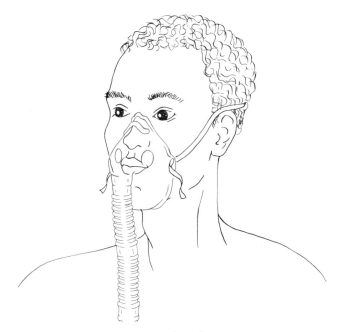

FIGURE 10–37 • Aerosol mask.

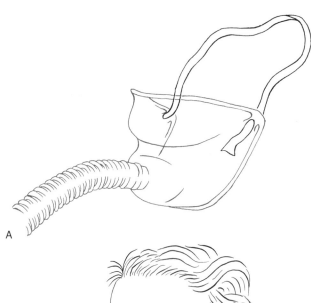

A

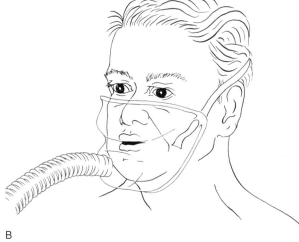

B

FIGURE 10–38 • (*A*) Face tent. (*B*) Proper placement of a face mask.

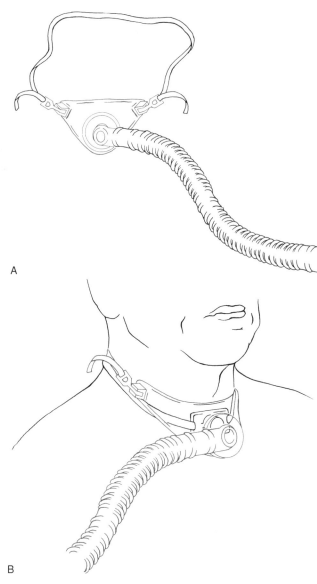

A

B

FIGURE 10–39 • (*A*) Tracheostomy collar. (*B*) Proper placement of a tracheostomy collar.

tems. As an example, the American Academy of Pediatrics and the American College of Obstetricians and Gynecologists in their joint publication[12] recommended that oxygen-enriched environments in neonatal intensive care units be analyzed at least hourly. In addition to confirming proper equipment operation and adjustment, gaseous oxygen analysis can provide important information about the status of a patient's oxygenation. Obviously, a patient who requires 60% oxygen to maintain a PaO_2 of 60 mmHg has significantly worse pulmonary dysfunction than the patient who is adequately oxygenated while receiving 30% oxygen.

Polarographic and Galvanic Analyzers

Clinically, the two most common methods for analyzing gaseous oxygen at the bedside operate using electrochemi-

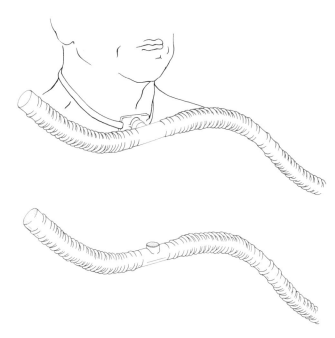

FIGURE 10–40 • T piece attached to a tracheostomy tube.

Table • 10–10 **RANGE OF FiO₂ GENERALLY AVAILABLE WITH VARIOUS HIGH-FLOW PATIENT INTERFACES**

Interface	FiO₂
Aerosol mask	0.21–1.0
Tracheostomy collar	0.21–0.60
Face tent	0.21–0.40
T-piece adapter	0.21–1.0

battery. In the case of the galvanic analyzer, the battery is used to power the display and any built-in alarm systems. Most oxygen analyzers require two-point calibration with known oxygen percentages. The most common calibration points are 21% (room air) and 100% oxygen. Calibration procedures differ based on analyzer type and manufacturer.

Because the actual measurement parameter of polarographic and galvanic analyzers is PO₂, there are a number of situations that may cause inaccurate readings:

- Humid environments. Water vapor exerts a partial pressure and results in a lower O₂% reading if the analyzer is calibrated with dry gas (such as 100% O₂ from a cylinder or wall outlet). If possible, analysis should be performed before any humidification device.
- Water on the electrode membrane. The water creates a barrier to oxygen diffusion.
- Changes in altitude, such as air transport or ground transport over a mountain summit.

(text continues on page 284)

cal cells. Both the polarographic and galvanic electrodes measure PO₂ through a reduction–oxidation reaction that produces an electrical current. Although the measurement parameter is PO₂, the display is in percentage of oxygen. The polarographic analyzer uses a Clark electrode that is adapted for measurement of gaseous oxygen. Polarographic analyzers require a battery to provide current to maintain electrode polarity and to speed the reduction–oxidation reaction. The increased speed of the reduction–oxidation reaction results in a more rapid response time of the polarographic analyzer. The galvanic (fuel cell) analyzer does not require a battery to function. This lack of a charging current in the galvanic electrode results in a slower response time. Most modern oxygen analyzers have a

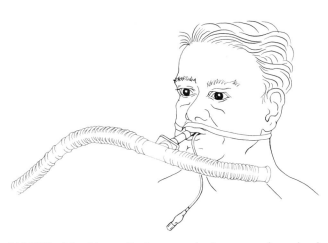

FIGURE 10–41 • T piece attached to an endotracheal tube.

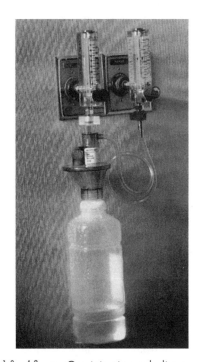

FIGURE 10–42 • Gas injection nebulizer.

Box • 10–8 PROCEDURE FOR APPLYING A JET-MIXING (VENTURI) MASK

EQUIPMENT

- Oxygen flowmeter or cylinder with regulator
- Nipple adapter
- Venturi mask, with adapters
- Patient interface (eg, aerosol mask, tracheostomy collar)
- Oxygen-connecting tubing and straight connectors, as necessary

EQUIPMENT INDICATIONS

- Patients who require oxygen administration with desired inspired oxygen levels of 24%–40% at oxygen liter flowrates of 3–15 L/min
- Patients with unstable ventilatory patterns because, using this device at oxygen concentrations of >40%, the oxygen concentration does not fluctuate based on changes in a patient's respiratory pattern.

COMPONENTS OF PROPER ORDER

- Physician order for oxygen by Venturi mask at FIO_2 desired (0.24, 0.26, 0.28, 0.30, 0.35, 0.40)
- Liter flow is indicated based on FIO_2 and not specified in order.
- Indicate whether nasal cannula should be used when mask is off, such as during meals.

EQUIPMENT LIMITATIONS

- A Venturi mask is a fixed performance device for FIO_2 <40% when running up to 12 L/min on a patient with normal inspiratory flow rates. At FIO_2 >40%, the Venturi mask becomes a variable performance device, incapable of consistently exceeding 40% oxygen delivered.
- May cause irritation of skin from contact with the device

EQUIPMENT APPLICATION

1. Verify physician order.
2. Wash hands.
3. Identify patient by identification band.
4. Explain to patient the therapy ordered and goals of the therapy. Instruct patient in proper use of the device, and caution against fire and safety hazards. Post "no smoking" sign to door of patient's room.
5. Assemble equipment.
6. Attach oxygen flowmeter to oxygen wall outlet (cylinder regulators usually have flowmeters built in).
7. Attach nipple adapter to flowmeter.
8. Attach Venturi mask directly to nipple adapter. If patient has tracheotomy or stoma, remove Venturi mechanism from mask, and attach to trach collar with 22-mm adapter.

9. Turn on the oxygen flowmeter to the liter flow indicated on the Venturi mechanism for the desired percentage. Set the Venturi mask to the prescribed oxygen concentration.
   a. If a variable orifice fixed entrainment device is being used, attach the appropriate color-coded jet (Fig. 10–43).
   b. If a fixed orifice variable entrainment device is being used, rotate the entrainment port to the ordered FIO_2. Be sure that the diluter adapter *snaps* into place (Fig. 10–44).
10. Place the mask over the patient's nose and mouth, gently pinching the soft metal at the top of the mask to conform to the patient's nose. Extend the elastic band above the ears and across the crown of the head, adjusting for a snug but comfortable fit. Place Venturi mechanism over sheets or bed clothes so that air can be entrained (Fig. 10–45).
11. If additional humidity is required, attach the aerosol entrainment collar to the device (Fig. 10–46). Attach the collar to a room air aerosol system using a length of large-bore tubing.
12. Visually inspect equipment as set up for proper function.
13. Assess patient comfort and adjust accordingly.
14. Wash hands.

TROUBLESHOOTING

1. Patient complaints of claustrophobia.
   a. Consider use of a different type of high-flow system.
   b. Increase flow rate of oxygen into Venturi mask.
2. Skin breakdown or irritation occurs at any point that mask or tubing contacts skin.
   a. Apply topical water-based lotion to site of irritation (**never use oil- or petroleum-based lotions**).
   b. Pad point of irritation (eg, gauze pad or DuoDerm).
   c. Reposition elastic band or device.
   d. Remove mask, and consider other device options.
3. Patient complains about not getting enough oxygen.
   a. Assess oxygenation (perform pulse oximetry).
   b. Assess system for proper function.
   c. Determine whether patient requires higher liter flow of oxygen or FIO_2.
   d. Determine whether patient requires change of administration device (eg, high-flow system or blender).
4. Patient oxygen saturation is <88% or PaO_2 <55 mmHg.
   a. Assess system for proper function.
   b. Determine whether patient requires higher liter flow of oxygen with addition of nasal cannula.
   c. Determine whether patient requires change of administration device (eg, high-flow system or blender).

EQUIPMENT

- Oxygen or air flowmeter (high-range flowmeter is used with gas-injection nebulizer (GIN)
- Wall outlet, cylinder with regulator, air compressor
- Large-volume nebulizer (LVN) with distilled water or 0.9% NaCl reservoir
- Aerosol mask, face tent, T-piece adapter, or tracheostomy collar
- Aerosol tubing and connectors, as necessary

EQUIPMENT INDICATIONS

- LVN is indicated for patients who have unstable ventilatory pattern because FIO_2 does not fluctuate based on changes in the patient's ventilatory pattern.
- LVN is indicated for a small subset of patients requiring cool bland aerosol to the airway.
- Three types of LVN are typically available:
  Jet-mixing type standard-flow nebulizer is indicated for FIO_2 levels between 0.28 and 0.40.
  Jet-mixing type high-flow nebulizer is indicated for FIO_2 levels between 0.38 and 0.80.
  GIN is indicated for FIO_2 >0.80.

COMPONENTS OF PROPER ORDER

- Physician order for oxygen by large-volume aerosol should specify FIO_2 desired (0.21, 0.28, 0.35, 0.40, or greater). Liter flow should not be specified.
- Indicate whether nasal cannula should be used when mask is off, such as during meals.

EQUIPMENT LIMITATIONS

- A standard jet-mixing LVN is a high-flow system for FIO_2 <40% when running up to 10 L/min on a patient with normal inspiratory flow rates. At FIO_2 >40%, it becomes a variable performance device, incapable of consistently providing >40% oxygen. The high-flow jet-mixing LVN can provide a reliable FIO_2 up to 80%.
- The GIN is a type of LVN that provides flows >120 L/min at FIO_2 up to 1.0 and that requires two flow sources (two oxygen or one air and one oxygen) to operate. In addition, it requires the use of an oxygen analyzer to verify actual FIO_2 periodically.
- Contact with LVNs may cause irritation of skin.

EQUIPMENT APPLICATIONS

1. Verify physician order.
2. Wash hands.
3. Identify patient by identification band.
4. Explain therapy and goals to patient. Instruct patient in proper use of device; caution against fire and safety hazards. Post "no smoking" sign to door of patient's room.
5. Assemble equipment.
6. Attach oxygen/air flowmeter to appropriate oxygen/air wall outlet (cylinder regulators usually have flowmeters built in).
7. Assemble nebulizer with reservoir bottle.
8. Attach assembled LVN to flowmeter. When using GIN, attach secondary tubing to second flowmeter.
9. Jet-mixing LVN: Set the Venturi mechanism to the prescribed oxygen concentration up to 40% (standard) or 80% (high flow). If room air is ordered, attach LVN to air flowmeter and outlet, and set LVN at either 28% (6–10 L/min) or 40% (10 L/min) setting. For oxygen administration, turn on the flowmeter at or above the liter flow as indicated on entrainment mechanism for the desired percentage.
10. GIN LVN: Attach the primary nebulizer port to oxygen flowmeter if desired FIO_2 is <0.60. If desired FIO_2 is >0.60, attach nebulizer port to air outlet and second port to oxygen flowmeter. Adjust flow of each flowmeter to achieve the ordered FIO_2, and use oxygen analyzer to ensure proper FIO_2.
11. Attach appropriate patient interface (aerosol mask, tracheostomy collar, face tent, or T-piece adapter).
12. Visually inspect set-up for proper function.
13. Assess patient comfort and adjust accordingly.
14. Wash hands.

TROUBLESHOOTING

1. Patient complains of claustrophobia.
   a. Consider use of a different type of high-flow system (eg, GIN system or blended oxygen).
   b. Increase flow rate of oxygen into LVN.
2. Skin breakdown or irritation occurs at any point that mask or tubing contacts skin.
   a. Apply topical water-based lotion to site of irritation (**never use oil- or petroleum-based lotions**).
   b. Pad point of irritation (eg, gauze pad or DuoDerm).
   c. Reposition elastic band or device.
   d. Remove mask; and consider other options (eg, face tent).
3. Patient complains about not getting enough oxygen.
   a. Assess oxygenation (perform pulse oximetry).
   b. Assess system for proper function.
   c. Determine whether patient requires higher liter flow of oxygen or FIO_2.
   d. Determine whether patient requires change of administration device (eg, GIN or blender).
4. Patient oxygen saturation is <88% or PaO_2 <55 mmHg.
   a. Assess system for proper function.
   b. Determine whether patient requires higher liter flow of oxygen with addition of nasal cannula.
   c. Determine whether patient requires change of administration device (eg, GIN or blender).

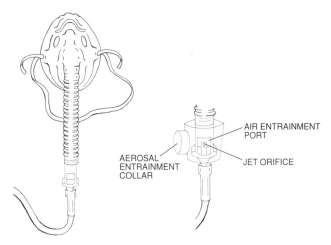

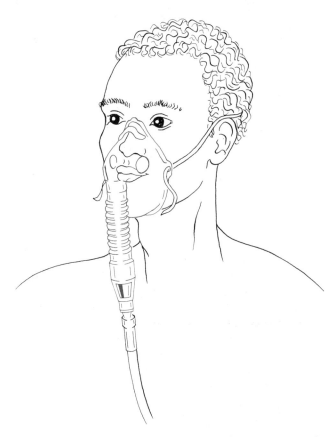

FIGURE 10–43 • Variable orifice fixed entrainment jet-mixing device. Various color-coded jets are available to provide a predetermined FiO$_2$. Unlike most fixed orifice jet-mixing devices, this device can usually provide a high flow at FiO$_2$ levels of more than 0.40 because of the large jet orifice.

- Changes in system pressure, such as placement in a high-pressure ventilator circuit with PEEP.
- Large changes in temperature.

FIGURE 10–45 • Proper placement of a jet-mixing mask.

Helium–Oxygen Therapy

The use of low-density gas mixtures may be of benefit to patients with various forms of obstructive airway disease, including (1) acute upper airway obstruction, such as luminal compression or viral croup; (2) acute asthma; and (3) acute exacerbation of COPD. Helium is about seven times lighter than air and has a density of 0.1758 g/L, as compared with atmospheric air and oxygen, with densities of 1.293 g/L and 1.43 g/L, respectively. A reduction in gas

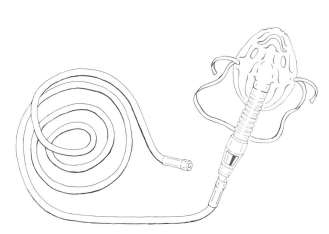

FIGURE 10–44 • Fixed-orifice variable-entrainment jet-mixing device. The entrainment collar is rotated into position to provide a predetermined FiO$_2$.

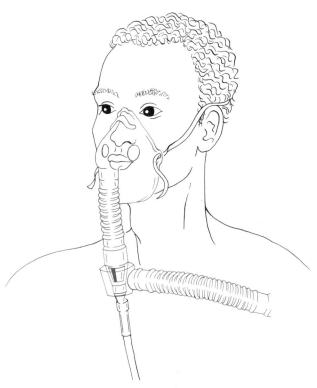

FIGURE 10–46 • Jet-mixing mask with aerosol entrainment adapter in place.

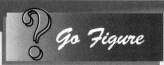

You have set up a large-volume nebulizer to provide oxygen delivery to a patient. You note that the maximum oxygen flow that will go through the jet is 12 L/min. With the nebulizer entrainment collar set at 40% oxygen, what is the approximate total gas flow from the device?

To answer this question, you need to know the oxygen/air mixing ratio for 40% oxygen. A simple and easy-to-remember method for determining the oxygen/air mixing ratio and calculating total flow is known as "tic-tac-flow."

Step 1. Draw a tic-tac-toe outline, and label the upper left O_2 and the upper right *Air*.

O_2	Air

Step 2. Insert 20 for *Air* and 100 for O_2.

O_2	Air
100	20

Note: When calculating oxygen/air mixing ratios for oxygen percentages of 35% and less, use 21 for *air* rather than 20 in the upper right hand corner.

Step 3. Insert the desired oxygen percentage in the center box. In this case, we want to know the ratio for 40% oxygen.

O_2	Air
100	20
40	

Step 4. On the diagonal, compute the absolute difference (no negative numbers) between the center number and the values for O_2 and *air*.

O_2	Air
100	20
40	
20	60

Step 5. To create an oxygen/air ratio, divide the value calculated for *air* by the value calculated for O_2.

$$\frac{60}{20} = 3$$

In this example, the oxygen/air mixing ratio for 40% oxygen is 1 : 3. In other words, one part oxygen mixed with three parts air creates a mixture with an oxygen percentage of about 40%.

To answer the original question, the total flow from an entrainment nebulizer set at 40% oxygen, with an oxygen flow of 12 L/min through the jet, would be calculated as follows:

12 oxygen
+ (3 × 12) air
= 48 L/min total flow of 40% oxygen

Let us expand on this situation. Your patient is currently maintaining an adequate PaO_2 on 40% oxygen delivered by large-volume entrainment nebulizer. You have calculated the total flow at 48 L/min. Over the next 2 hours, the patient's rate and depth of respiration have increased significantly. The PaO_2 is now less than acceptable. Based on this turn of events, you increase the oxygen percentage to 50% by adjusting the air entrainment collar. The oxygen flow to the jet remains at its maximum of 12 L/min. Twenty minutes later, you reassess the situation and note that the patient's rate and depth of respiration have increased even more and that the PaO_2 is less than the previous assessment. What happened? What should you do?

Increasing the oxygen percentage in the face of worsening hypoxemia and increased work of breathing seems like the right thing to do. However, the device used to deliver the supplemental oxygen is no longer appropriate. Compute the total flow available from the entrainment nebulizer now that it is set at 50% oxygen:

O_2	Air
100	20
50	
30	50

$$\frac{50}{30} = 1.7$$

The oxygen/air mixing ratio for 50% oxygen is 1 : 1.7.

12 oxygen
+ (1.7 × 12) air
= 32 L/min total flow of 50% oxygen

Set at 40% oxygen, the device supplied adequate gas flow for the patient under the prevailing conditions. However, the patient's condition changed, and his rate and depth of respiration increased. Under these conditions, the patient's inspiratory demands exceeded the gas flow delivery of the device. As can be seen from the above calculations, increasing the oxygen percentage reduced the total flow available to the patient and actually made the hypoxemia worse. In this situation, changing the oxygen delivery device to one capable of high-flow, such as a gas-injection nebulizer, would have been appropriate.

CRITICAL THINKING CHALLENGES

Go Figure

A patient is receiving an 80%/20% mixture of heliox at 10 L/min by a tight-fitting nonrebreathing mask. The gas is being regulated by an oxygen flowmeter. The gas mixture is being delivered from an H cylinder with a current pressure of 1200 psig (a full H cylinder of 80%/20% heliox contains about 6040 L of gas at 2200 psig). About how long will this cylinder last at 10 L/min gas flow?

Answer: Corrected gas flow = 10 L/min × 1.8 = 18 L/min

$$\text{Cylinder contents} = \frac{6{,}040 \text{ L}}{2200 \text{ psig}} = 2.75 \text{ L/psig}$$

$$\text{Duration of gas flow} = \frac{1200 \text{ psig} \times 2.75 \text{ L/psig}}{18 \text{ L/min}}$$

$$= 183 \text{ minutes, or 3 hours}$$

density may significantly reduce the work necessary for ventilation. After implementation of heliox therapy, a patient may exhibit significant reduction in the clinical signs that indicate increased work of breathing and impending respiratory failure. The use of heliox mixtures is adjunctive. If the therapy is interrupted and the patient returns to breathing an oxygen–air mixture, the low-density benefit of the heliox mixture is lost immediately. Therapy that is directed at the primary problem should always accompany heliox administration.

The most common commercially available heliox mixtures are 80% helium/20% oxygen and 70% helium/30% oxygen. The density of a 70%/30% mixture is 0.554 g/L, and the density of the 80%/20% mixture is 0.429 g/L. Because of the altered density of heliox mixtures, specially calibrated flowmeters are required for accurate regulation of gas flow. In the absence of such flowmeters, an oxygen flowmeter may be used with the following mixture conversion factors:

$$80\% \text{ He}/20\% \text{ O}_2 = 1.8$$

$$70\% \text{ He}/30\% \text{ O}_2 = 1.6$$

The reading on the oxygen flowmeter is multiplied by the appropriate conversion factor to determine the actual heliox mixture flow.

When administered to patients breathing spontaneously, heliox mixtures must be delivered by tight-fitting nonre-breathing mask (all one-way valves must be in place). Because of its low density, helium escapes from any place that a leak is present. If additional oxygen is necessary to maintain an adequate SpO_2 or PaO_2 in the patient who is breathing spontaneously, only the minimum amount necessary should be added to prevent further dilution of the heliox mixture. Below about 70% helium, the low-density property of the mixture is lost.[13]

Heliox mixtures may be administered to patients receiving mechanical ventilation. This, however, is a tricky enterprise and should not be undertaken without prior bench study and a carefully developed administration procedure. Many modern mechanical ventilators use flow sensors, such as large-orifice pneumotachometers or vortex-shedding devices, to measure and control delivered tidal volume. Less dense heliox mixtures cause these flow sensors to measure incorrectly and could potentially result in a significant increase in tidal volume. If the decision is made to use heliox mixtures in conjunction with mechanical ventilation, the use of a pressure-limited breath type would be prudent.

References

1. American Association for Respiratory Care. Clinical practice guideline: Oxygen therapy in the acute care hospital. *Respir Care.* 1991;36(12):1410–1413.
2. Krieger BP. Travel for the technology dependent patient with lung disease. *Clin Pulmonary Med.* 1995;2:1–9.
3. Gong H. Air travel and oxygen therapy in cardiopulmonary patients. *Chest.* 1992;101:1104–1113.
4. Stoller JK. Travel for the technology-dependent individual. *Respir Care.* 1994;39(4):347–360.
5. Landis EM, Pappenheimer JR. Exchange of substances through the capillary walls. In: Hamilton WE, ed. *Handbook of Physiology: Circulation,* vol 2, chap 29. Washington DC: American Physiological Society; 1963.
6. Pierson DJ. Indications for oxygen therapy. *Probl Respir Care.* 1990;3:549–562.
7. American Academy of Pediatrics, American College of Obstetricians and Gynecologists. *Guidelines for Perinatal Care.* 2nd ed. Elk Grove, IL: American Academy of Pediatrics;1988:246–247.
8. Langenderfer R, Branson RD. Compressed gases: Manufacture, storage and piping systems. In: Branson RD, Hess DR, Chatburn RL, eds. *Respiratory Care Equipment.* Philadelphia: JB Lippincott; 1995.
9. Branson RD. Gas delivery systems: Regulators, flowmeters and therapy devices. In: Branson RD, Hess DR, Chatburn RL, eds. *Respiratory Care Equipment.* Philadelphia: JB Lippincott; 1995.
10. Ward JJ. Medical gas therapy. In: Burton GG, Hodgkin JE, Ward JJ, eds. *Respiratory Care: A Guide to Clinical Practice.* 4th ed. Philadelphia: JB Lippincott; 1997.
11. Sacci R. Air entrainment masks: Jet mixing is how they work. *Respir Care.* 1979;24:928.
12. American Academy of Pediatrics and the American College of Obstetricians and Gynecologists. *Guidelines for Perinatal Care.*4th ed. Elk Grove IL: American Association of Pediatrics; 1997.
13. Youttsey JW. Oxygen and mixed gas therapy. In: Barnes TA, ed. *Core Textbook of Respiratory Care Practice.* 2nd ed. St Louis: CV Mosby; 1994.

11

Humidity

James B. Fink

Key Terms

absolute humidity
active humidifier
convection
dew point
evaporation
humidifier
humidity
hydrophobic
hygroscopic
isothermic saturation
  boundary
moisture output
passive humidifier
pass-over humidifier
relative humidity
water content
wick humidifier

Objectives

- Identify indications for humidity therapy.

- Compare and contrast methods of providing humidity to meet specific goals.

- Describe the role of the normal airway in providing and reclaiming heat and humidity.

- Identify physiologic consequences of inadequate humidification.

- Discuss advantages and limitations of available humidification devices.

- Evaluate strategies for meeting humidification requirements.

Humidity is the presence of molecular water in gas. Humidity therapy is the addition of molecular water to gas that is delivered to a patient. This water, in inspired gas at the correct temperature, is essential to a healthy respiratory tract. Administration of dry medical gas, especially when the upper airway is bypassed, is a hazard for heat and water loss that may result in structural damage of the airway.[1] When the airway is exposed to cold dry air from the ambient environment, motility of the cilia is reduced, whereas airway irritability, mucus production, and thickening of secretions are increased.[2] Damage to tracheal epithelium has been demonstrated within 2 hours of administration of dry gases through an endotracheal tube, whereas gases at 60% **relative humidity** at body temperature have been shown to produce no damage.[3] For premature and small infants, providing heat and humidity to dry cold gas is a critical factor in thermal regulation.

The normal airway is a remarkably efficient air-conditioning system, which conditions gas during both inspiration and expiration. The nose is perhaps the best example of an active **humidifier**, adding heat and humidity to gas on inspiration.[4] The nasal mucosa has the greatest concentration of mucous glands in the airway and is particularly vascular, providing a rich source of heat and water and capable of supplying nearly 1 L/d of fluid to inspired air (in adults). The respiratory mucous layer is kept moist by secretions from mucous glands and goblet cells and by transudation of fluid through cell walls. Heat is transferred from capillary beds close to the surface of the mucosa. The turbinates and conchae provide a convoluted path for gas to travel, creating turbulent flow and a large surface area for contact with respiratory gases. This large surface area not only gives up a large amount of heat and moisture to inspired gas but also efficiently recovers both heat and water on exhalation. The mucosa lining the sinuses, trachea, and bronchi also assist in heating and humidifying inspired gas.

ISOTHERMIC SATURATION BOUNDARY

On inspiration, the airway heats and humidifies gas so effectively that by the time inspired gas reaches the lung parenchyma, it is fully saturated to 100% relative humidity at body temperature. The point at which this occurs for air entering the respiratory tract is called the **isothermic saturation boundary** (ISB).[5] The ISB is normally around the third generation of the airways, about 5 cm below the carina. Below the ISB, there are no fluctuations in temperature or relative humidity, whereas above the ISB, temperature and humidity increase on expiration and decrease on inspiration. The active work of humidity control occurs in the airway above the ISB, so that mucus production, ciliary function, and airway irritability vary with shifts in the ISB.[6] When the ISB shifts down the respiratory tract, the increased demands on the mucosa to provide additional water to inspired air can result in thicker secretions with increased plugging. Reduced airway temperature can result in reduced ciliary activity within 10 minutes, and recovery can take several weeks.

Bypassing the upper airway eliminates the body's most efficient mechanisms for retaining heat and humidity.[7] The ISB shifts down the airway as a result of factors such as decreased environmental temperature and humidity, mouth breathing, increased tidal volume, and bypassing the upper airway with insertion of an artificial airway (eg, tracheotomy or endotracheal intubation). Although the ISB never decreases to the level of the respiratory bronchioles and alveoli, the recruitment of less efficient airways, usually above the ISB, dramatically changes their mucosal characteristics in both the short and long term. On expiration, the airway above the ISB, which was cooled during inspiration, extracts heat and moisture, recycling them for the next inspiration.

CLINICAL INDICATIONS FOR HUMIDITY THERAPY

Maintaining Normal Physiologic Conditions

The primary goal for humidity therapy is to provide adequate humidification and heat to inspired gas to approximate normal inspiratory conditions as gas passes through the airway. Heat and humidity ensure normal operation of the mucociliary transport system with administration of dry medical gases and delivery of the bypassed upper airway. Humidity is also used (with less supporting empiric data) for the treatment of hypothermia, reactive airway response to cold air, and thick secretions.

Administration of Medical Gases

Even when room air is being breathed through an artificial airway, extrinsic humidification of the inspired gas should be ensured. The loss of the humidifying capabilities of the upper airway causes the ISB to shift toward the lower airways. This is important when differences between ambient and tracheal temperatures of >10°C exist and the burden of regulating heat and water falls on the more distal airways less accustomed to providing humidification.[3]

When medical-grade gases are processed for storage or delivery to patients, all possible water vapor is removed. Administration of dry gases to the normal airways can result in substantial heat and water loss from the airway, which can cause patient discomfort. Exposure of the lower respiratory tract to dry gas can result in structural damage to the lung. As the airway is exposed to cold dry air from the ambient environment, ciliary motility is reduced, airways become more irritable, mucus production increases, and pulmonary secretions become thick and encrusted in the airways.

Goals for Humidity Therapy

The goal for humidity therapy is to condition gas to approximate normal inspiratory conditions at the point that the gas enters the airway. Proper humidification minimizes the shift of the ISB toward the smaller airways.

To accomplish this goal, gas delivered to the nose or mouth should be heated and humidified to room conditions equivalent to 22°C at 50% relative humidity (absolute humidity, 10 mg/L), whereas gas delivered to the trachea through an endotracheal tube or tracheotomy tube should be 32° to 35°C at 100% relative humidity (absolute humidity, 36 to 40 mg/L).[7]

Secondary Goals: Heated Humidity

The delivery of warmed, humidified gas to the airway has been advocated to prevent and treat a variety of pathologic conditions. Heated, humidified inspired gas is advocated for the treatment of hypothermia; airway hyperactivity associated with breathing cold, dry gases; and prevention and treatment of thick, tenacious pulmonary secretions.[4]

NEONATES

For premature and newborn infants, a neutral thermal environment should be maintained with adequate warmth and humidity to minimize insensible heat and water loss. Adequate heat and humidity provided to low-birth-weight infants has been associated with reduced incidence of pneumothorax and reduction in severity of chronic lung disease, as compared with infants breathing colder and dryer inspired gas.[8]

HYPOTHERMIA

Delivery of warm, humidified gases has been used to treat hypothermia. Because humans expend a considerable quantity of heat to condition inspired air and exhale a portion of that heat, the body loses considerable heat through normal ventilation. For the hypothermic patient, rewarming and reduction of further heat loss can be facilitated in part by heating the inspired gases.[9] Use of heated humidity reduces the time required for patients to return to normal body temperature.

AIRWAY HYPERREACTIVITY TO COLD INSPIRED GAS

Many patients react with severe bronchospasm to breathing cold inspired gas. For example, there is evidence that some asthmatic patients have increased airway resistance when breathing cold air.[10] This effect has also been noted with preterm neonates.[11] The bronchospasm is most likely caused by a shift of the ISB to more distal airways, with associated stimulation of mast cells in those areas. This response can be reduced by warming the inspired gases and by providing gas humidified with more than 20 mg/L of water at 23°C.[4]

Treatment of Thick Secretions

Humidification of inspired gas has been advocated in patients with thick, tenacious secretions, whether or not they have intact upper airways. This practice is highly suspect based on available evidence. No studies have reported a benefit of external humidifiers in improving the character and mobilization of thick secretions. The most effective method for improving the character of pulmonary secretions is systemic hydration. Nonetheless, humidification has been advocated for the patient with tenacious secretions that are difficult to clear.[12,13] Based on the available evidence, when patients with artificial airways have thick or tenacious secretions, humidity therapy should be used judiciously to reduce any humidity deficit in the airway while measures are taken to optimize systemic hydration.

In addition to humidification, aerosol therapy with bland solutions, such as distilled water and hypertonic saline, is used to stimulate cough as well as secretion production. Such therapy has been widely used for diagnostic sputum induction.[13–15]

Secondary Goals: Cool Humidity

The use of cool (colder than room temperature) humidified gases, often with bland aerosols, is advocated in the treatment of upper airway inflammation due to croup, epiglottitis, and postextubation swelling.[14,15] The cool temperature is thought to promote localized peripheral vasoconstriction, reduce swelling, and relieve the discomfort associated with upper airway inflammation.

HUMIDITY

Humidity is defined in terms of the **water content** in air. The actual content or amount of water in a given volume of air is called the **absolute humidity** and typically is expressed in milligrams of water per liter (mg/L) of gas.

Relative humidity is the content of water vapor expressed as a percentage of the maximal capacity of vapor that can be held at the same temperature. Relative humidity is calculated by dividing the amount of water in the air (content) by the capacity (amount of water vapor that a gas can hold at any given temperature) of the air to hold water when totally saturated at a given temperature.

The greater the temperature of a gas, the greater is its capacity to hold water vapor. Table 11–1 shows the capacity of air to hold water at 100% saturation across a range of temperatures. As temperature decreases, so does capacity. The **dew point** is reached when the capacity becomes less than content, and water condenses and "rains out" of the gas.

The lower the temperature, the more water condenses from the air. As the temperature rises, the same absolute humidity results in a decreasing relative humidity. Above

Table • 11–1   WATER CONTENT AS A FUNCTION OF TEMPERATURE

Temperature		Content (mg/L)
°C	°F	
0	32	5
10	50	9
15	59	13
20	68	17
25	77	23
30	86	30
35	95	40
37	98.6	44
40	104	51
45	113	66
50	122	83

20°C, the temperature–humidity curve becomes steeper, allowing a large quantity of water to be exchanged with small changes in temperature.

Two mechanisms of heat exchange are involved in conditioning inspired air: **evaporation** and **convection.** Latent heat of vaporization is the heat lost by evaporation. Energy is required for the water to change from a liquid to a vapor state. Convection is the heat transfer from the mucosa to the inspired air. Although both evaporation and convection cool the mucosa, heat lost as a result of evaporation of water is a bigger factor than is heat lost as a result of convection.

Humidity by the Numbers

The specific heat of air is 1008 J/kg. The specific heat of water is 4200 J/kg, more than four times greater than that of air. Latent heat of vaporization (and latent heat of condensation) of water is 2450 J/kg. Water acts as a heat reservoir in the respiratory tract because of differences in energy requirements between heat of evaporation and heat of convection. Under normal conditions, about 250 mL of water and 1470 J of heat are lost from the lung each day. About 495 mL of water and 28,468 J of heat are required to change

CRITICAL THINKING CHALLENGES

Go Figure

On a hot summer day, the temperature is 37°C with 80% relative humidity, which means the water content, or absolute humidity, is 36 mg/L. As the sun goes down and the air cools, at what temperature does the dew form?

room air from its usual temperature of about 24°C and its usual relative humidity of 50% to alveolar conditions. To accomplish this, 245 mL of water and 27,000 J of heat must be reclaimed and returned to the upper respiratory tract every day.[6]

PHYSIOLOGIC CONTROL OF HEAT–MOISTURE EXCHANGE

Normal heat–moisture exchange within the airways is a complex mechanism.[5] During normal inspiration, turbulent flow of inspired gases ensures adequate contact of air with the mucosa. As inspired gas warms, water vapor is transferred to it by evaporation of fluid from the mucosal lining, resulting in humidity being added to the inspired gas through the latent heat of vaporization. Warming and humidification continue until the inspired gas is fully saturated at body temperature. The latent heat of vaporization remains as water vapor and does not contribute to warming of gases. Loss of latent heat of vaporization causes the mucosa to cool. At the end of inspiration, the temperature of the nasal mucosa is ≈31°C because of loss of heat by turbulent convection and loss of latent heat of vaporization.[15]

During normal exhalation, heat is transferred to the cooler tracheal and nasal mucosa by convection. As gases cool, they hold less water vapor; condensation occurs, causing water to accumulate on the tracheal surfaces, where it is reabsorbed by the mucus. Heat is transferred back to the mucosa, resulting in warming and rehydration. Latent heat and water are held until the next inspiration.

During normal breathing, air flow in the nose is turbulent, and heat is transferred by turbulent convection over the turbinates and conchae and by direct contact of air with the respiratory mucosa. When breathing through the mouth, air flow is more laminar, requiring heat transfer by radiation. Because air is a poor conductor of heat, the mouth is less efficient than the nose in heating inspired air.

The nose has extraordinary heat and humidity maintaining abilities and also functions as an organ of thermoregulation. Under conditions in which the environmental temperature is greater than body temperature, blood flow to the turbinates increases, and heat is lost through the nose. Nose breathing is more effective than mouth breathing. Primiano and colleagues[16] measured temperature and water vapor continuously at the oropharynx during oral and nasal breathing of room air at 22°C with a relative humidity of 15% to 39%. At the pharynx, the temperature difference between inspired and expired gas was 4°C during nose breathing and 7°C during mouth breathing. Inspired gas increased 5°C during mouth breathing and 9°C during nose breathing. During inspiration with nose breathing, the relative humidity was 95% at the oropharynx, whereas during mouth breathing, it was 75%. On exhalation, the relative humidity was 95% at the pharynx and 90% at the airway opening. These data suggest that the normal airway is capable of conditioning inspired gas to add humidity with nose or mouth breathing; however, more heat and moisture are lost with exhalation by the mouth than by the nose.

The upper airway and lungs also protect the airway by filtering particulates from inhaled gas as it travels to the lung parenchyma. The upper airway filters out most particles larger than 10 µm. The nose offers more efficient filtering than does the mouth. Further filtration occurs at the larynx and at more distal levels within the tracheobronchial tree.

The upper airway functions best under normal physiologic conditions. When presented with cold dry inspired gases, the ISB is shifted further down the respiratory tract and ciliary function and mucus production are compromised. The lower gas temperature further down in the airways results in reduced ciliary activity within as few as 10 minutes. Once compromised, ciliary function can take several weeks to recover. Respiratory secretions become thicker, contributing to mucous plugging and inability to maintain normal bronchopulmonary hygiene.

DEVICES USED FOR HEAT–MOISTURE EXCHANGE

A humidifier is a device that adds molecular water to gas, whereas a nebulizer produces an aerosol or suspension of particles in gas. Some humidifiers create aerosols, whereas some nebulizers add humidity to gas.

Active humidifiers are classified according to the method of contact between the water and gas. Humidifier types include bubble humidifiers, **pass-over humidifiers**, and jet nebulizers. Heat–moisture exchangers (HME) are passive humidifiers.

Humidifiers: Principles of Operation

Active humidifiers add water and some add heat to the inspired gas.[17–22] **Passive humidifiers** use the heat and moisture that is exhaled by the patient to humidify inspired gas. The active addition of heat greatly improves the effectiveness of humidifiers.

Unheated humidifiers should meet the American National Standards Institute (ANSI)[20] recommendation that a fluid output of at least 10 mg/L be provided by the humidifier. This is thought to be the lowest acceptable humidity level necessary to minimize mucosal damage to the upper airway under a variety of use environments. In addition, the 10 mg/L of water provides about 50% relative humidity at 22°C ambient conditions, enhancing the dissipation of static electricity and reducing the risk of fires. The ANSI also recommends that heated humidifiers have a water output level of at least 30 mg/L (100% relative humidity at 30°C). This level of humidity for patients who have bypassed upper airways is considered to the minimum level necessary to avoid mucosal damage and inspissation of se-

cretions. The ECRI, a research institute that evaluates biomedical devices,[21] recommends that humidifiers have an absolute humidity output of 37 mg/L of water for inspired gas (85% relative humidity at body temperature or 100% relative humidity at 34°C.)[21]

Heated-water humidifiers are the system of choice for humidification during intubation, tracheostomy, and long-term mechanical ventilation in the widest variety of settings. HMEs have a similar role with a limited subset of these patient populations. Common types of active humidifiers are listed in Box 11–1.

Application of Active Humidifiers

Bubble Humidifiers

Bubble humidifiers are commonly used unheated with simple oxygen administration devices (eg, cannulas, catheters, simple masks, reservoir rebreathers, high-concentration venturi masks) to bring gas to ambient levels of humidity. The dry medical gas is directed into a water-filled reservoir where the stream of gas is broken up (diffused) into bubbles, which gain humidity as they rise through the water (Fig. 11–1). Designs incorporate a tube directing gas beneath the surface of the water, with small holes or a diffuser made of plastic foam, sintered metal or mesh, breaking the stream of gas into small bubbles.

Bubble humidifiers usually are not heated for use with simple oxygen delivery devices. They are most efficient at 5 L/min or less and produce water vapor contents ranging between 10 and 20 mg/L. The higher the flow rate through a bubble humidifier, the lower is the vapor content secondary to reduced temperature of the reservoir. Commercially available bubble humidifiers are capable of humidifying dry medical gas to an absolute humidity between 20 and 13 mg/L, with flow rates of 2 to 10 L/min. When flow rates more than 10 L/min are required, other humidifying device options should be considered.[22,23]

Box • 11–1 COMMON TYPES OF ACTIVE HUMIDIFIERS

Bubble humidifiers: The gas flow is diffused into small bubbles of gas that pass through heated water. Evaporation takes place along the surface area of the bubble.

Pass-over humidifiers with or without wicks: Water vaporizes at the interface where gas contacts the surface of heated water or water-saturated absorbent blotter or wick.

Jet nebulizers: The fluid is broken up into small particles that pass through the gas. Evaporation takes place along the surface of the particle.

Medical Gas Conditions

Temperature	22°C
Relative Humidity	0%
Absolute Humidity	0 mg/L

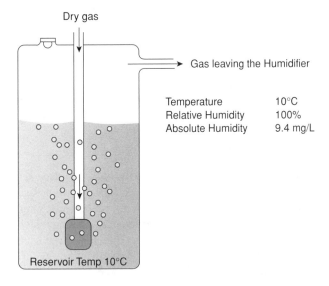

Dry gas

Gas leaving the Humidifier

Temperature	10°C
Relative Humidity	100%
Absolute Humidity	9.4 mg/L

Reservoir Temp 10°C

Room Conditions

Temperature	22°C
Relative Humidity	50%
Absolute Humidity	10 mg/L

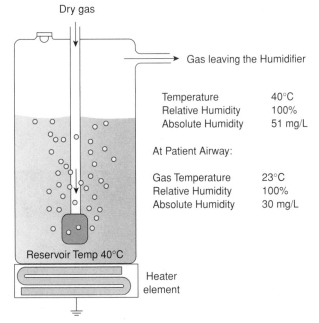

Dry gas

Gas leaving the Humidifier

Temperature	40°C
Relative Humidity	100%
Absolute Humidity	51 mg/L

At Patient Airway:

Gas Temperature	23°C
Relative Humidity	100%
Absolute Humidity	30 mg/L

Reservoir Temp 40°C

Heater element

Electrical outlet

FIGURE 11-1 • The temperature and relative and absolute humidity of medical gas, ambient air at normal room conditions, and gas leaving an unheated bubble-type humidifier. Note that the unheated reservoir actually cools to below room temperature as a result of evaporation and adiabatic expansion of the compressed gas.

These devices, at moderate flow rates of less than 10 L/min, can be applied safely for extended single patient use without risk of infection.[24]

The American College of Chest Physicians[25] recommends eliminating the use of simple bubble humidifiers with flow rates of 4 L/min or less. They maintain that adding humidity to low-flow medical gases is not supported by any objective criteria. Eliminating the use of humidifiers for low-flow oxygen reduces costs for routine administration. The cost savings, however, do not warrant withholding humidifiers from patients who experience discomfort associated with nasal dryness or irritation during medical gas administration. All patients receiving low-flow gas should be monitored for complaints of dryness or irritation; when either exists, additional humidification should be considered. Topical application of water-based lubricants to the nostrils may be a reasonable first step in response to complaints of dryness, followed by addition of a humidifier if the complaints continue.

Because unheated bubble humidifiers are most efficient when used with gas flow rates of 5 L/min or less, and because it is unnecessary to humidify low-flow oxygen at rates 4 L/min or less, the functional range of these devices is limited.

The higher the flow rate, the lower is the temperature of the reservoir as a result of cooling from evaporation and the adiabatic effect of the compressed gas expanding in the humidifier. Although heating the reservoir may improve the efficiency of these units, these devices generally are connected to small-bore tubing that would be quickly obstructed by condensate as the humidified gas cools en route to the patient. The condensate in the tubing counteracts the efficiency gained by heating with this configuration (Box 11–2).

To protect against obstructed or kinked tubing, low-flow, unheated bubble humidifiers have a pressure relief valve with an audible alarm that triggers when pressures of 2 psi or 40 mmHg develop in the humidifier. The alarm indicates that the flow of gas from the device has been interrupted, and the humidifier is protected automatically by a gravity or spring-loaded valve that releases pressures above 2 psi. The pop-off valve should resume normal position automatically when pressures return to normal.

Heated bubble humidifiers have been used with ventilated and intubated patients for many years. These units must accommodate much greater flow rates than the devices used for low-flow oxygen, ranging from 10 to 120 L/min, and incorporate tubing of at least 22 mm internal diameter, reducing resistance to flow. Ribbed aerosol tubing between the humidifier and the patient is also 22 mm in internal diameter, allowing condensate to be trapped in the ribs and minimizing the tendency of condensate to pool at the lowest part of the tubing, occluding the path of the gas to the patient.

At high flow rates, bubble humidifiers produce aerosols that can transmit or carry bacteria, including *Pseudomonas*

1. Obtain appropriate equipment:
   a. Oxygen flowmeter
   b. Bubble humidifier
   c. Oxygen delivery device
2. Attach flowmeter to 50-psi outlet.
3. Assemble humidifier. Using aseptic technique, fill with sterile water for inhalation if device has not been prefilled.
4. Attach humidifier to flowmeter. Avoid cross-threading the plastic fitting because it is attached to the flowmeter.
5. Turn on the gas flow to the appropriate level. Occlude the humidifier outlet and verify that the safety pop-off valve is functioning. Failure of the pop-off valve to function may indicate a loose connection at the flowmeter, a loose reservoir, or a malfunctioning pop-off valve.
6. Attach the oxygen delivery device, and apply to the patient.

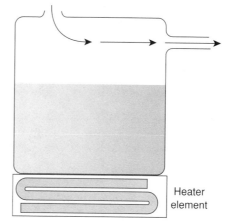

aeruginosa, from the reservoir of the humidifier to the patient. The aerosol droplets carry the bacteria; the molecules of water cannot carry bacteria. Any device that produces aerosols, therefore, must be changed or cleaned regularly during routine use and consistently between patients to ensure that pathogens in the reservoir do not contaminate the patient.[14]

Pass-over Humidifiers

Pass-over humidifiers direct gas over the surface of a body of water (Fig. 11–2). Pass-over **wick humidifiers** incorporate a wick of absorbent paper or cloth that draws water from the reservoir, saturating the fabric or paper, which then contacts the gas stream. The pass-over humidifier uses a **hydrophobic** barrier that allows water molecules to cross from the water reservoir into the gas stream.

Jet Nebulizers

Jet nebulizers use a jet of compressed gas that passes through a restricted orifice, creating a low-pressure area near the tip of a narrow tube and drawing fluid from a reservoir, which is then sheared or shattered into droplets by the airstream (Fig. 11–3). Jet nebulizers incorporate a large reservoir designed with baffles to minimize aerosol from leaving the humidifier, using the aerosol in the device to maximize surface contact with the gas.

Jet nebulizers used as humidifiers can deliver between 26 and 35 mg/L of water when unheated; when heated, they

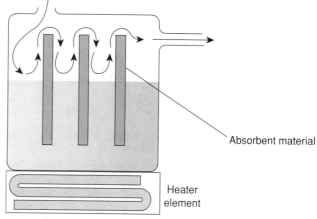

FIGURE 11–2 • In a simple pass-over humidifier, the point of contact between dry gas and the water bath is limited to the surface area of the water. When absorbent wick material is used, the heat and water from the water bath are drawn up through the wick, increasing the surface area available for contact.

can deliver 33 to 55 mg/L of water.[26–28] Although jet nebulizers can increase water content, they pose an increased risk of infection from bacteria that might colonize the reservoir. Consequently, these devices should always be filled with sterile fluids or medications that are changed daily[29]; residual fluids from the reservoir should be discarded before refilling. Jet nebulizers used as humidifiers are identical to the large-volume nebulizers described later. No data support the use of jet nebulizers over any other type of heated humidifier.

Heated Humidifiers

When providing supplemental oxygen to either intubated or nonintubated patients, supplemental humidity should usually be provided using a heated humidifier. A variety of such devices are available. Selection of a heated humidifier should be based on key factors as identified by ANSI stan-

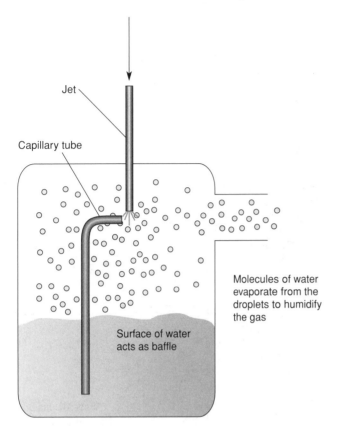

FIGURE 11–3 • In the jet-type humidifier, gas enters through a restricted orifice jet, which is directed across a capillary tube, creating a pressure differential that draws water from the reservoir and shears the water into aerosol particles. The jet also extends air flow into the surface of the water, providing direct contact with gas, and acting as a baffle for large particles. Aerosol provides a much greater total surface area, in addition to the surface of reservoir, for evaporation to occur.

dards,[20] American Association of Respiratory Care Clinical Practice Guidelines,[29] and reports from the ECRI.[21]

Reservoir and Feed Systems

As the inspired gases are humidified, water must be added to the humidifier. Although this is a simple concept, the methods used to refill humidifiers range from the primitive to sublime. At best, the system used to replace the water in the humidifier should ensure continuity of therapy and minimize disruption of ventilatory support for patients who require mechanical ventilation. Continuous-feed systems provide the most consistent replacement and are desirable because they allow replenishment of water without operator intervention. These systems often rely on gravity, usually with a pole-mounted reservoir external to the humidifier mechanism.

Continuous-feed systems include flotation controls and level-compensated reservoirs. With the flotation systems, a float is lifted with the water level in the humidifier, occlud-

ing the flow of water when a predetermined level is reached, much like a common household toilet.

In level-compensated systems, an external reservoir is aligned horizontally with the humidifier, maintaining relatively consistent water levels across the external reservoir to the humidifier chamber (Fig. 11–4).

A hydrophobic barrier incorporates a membrane that separates the gas from the heated water, allowing water molecules to pass through the membrane. The humidifier cannot overfill unless the barrier is disrupted or broken.

Intermittent-feed systems can be as simple as pouring a bottle of water into the humidifier. More commonly, a tube is extended from the water reservoir to a water-feed device that must be manually opened to refill the humidifier.

The Marquest chamber pour-type system permits filling from an internal level reservoir without interruption (Fig. 11–5). This gravity-based water-feed system requires manual filling but uses a valve that is closed before the humidifier is opened and filled, which avoids disconnecting or interrupting humidifier operation.

Intermittent-feed systems have major disadvantages when compared with continuous feed systems. As the water level in a manual feed systems falls, ventilator circuit compliance changes. Because gas is less compressible than water, changing water volume in a fixed-volume container alters the compressible volume in both the humidifier and ventilator circuit. As a result, when the water level changes during use, so does the delivered tidal volume. This problem is of greatest concern when the device is used as part of the circuit for mechanically ventilated infants and chil-

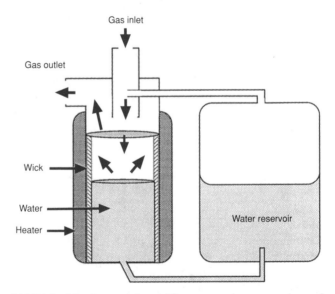

FIGURE 11–4 • A humidifier system that uses a heated wick to produce water vapor. The water level is controlled by the water level in the external reservoir. (Fink J, Cohen N. Humidity and aerosols. In: Eubanks DH, Bone RC, eds. *Principles and Applications of Cardiorespiratory Care Equipment.* St. Louis: Mosby-Year Book;1994.)

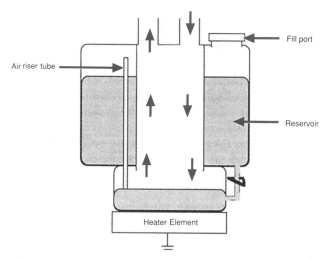

FIGURE 11-5 • The Marquest SCT 2000 humidifier has a pass-over humidifier that incorporates a reservoir that surrounds the humidifier chamber. The reservoir can be filled without interrupting ventilation. (Fink J, Cohen N. Humidity and aerosols. In: Eubanks D, Bone R, eds. *Principles and Applications of Cardiorespiratory Care Equipment.* St. Louis: Mosby-Year Book;1994.)

dren. In addition, open reservoirs are considered more susceptible to contamination. Finally, the humidifier chamber can become empty if not checked regularly, and devices that do not have alarms indicating low water levels may pose a risk to the patient.

Heating Systems

To improve water output, the water in the humidifier should be heated. As the temperature of the gas is increased, the gas can carry a greater volume of water. Heated-water humidifiers are particularly useful for patients with bypassed upper airways and for those receiving mechanical ventilatory support. Active humidifiers use electricity to heat the water or gas.

Heating elements, as shown in Figure 11–6, may include the following:

• A heating plate located under the reservoir
• A curved, often flexible element that is wrapped around the humidifier chamber
• A yolk or collar between the water reservoir and the active mechanism of the nebulizer
• A plate or rod that is immersed into the water reservoir
• A set of heated wires heating an absorbent wick

All heaters have controllers that regulate electric power to the heater element. Units that are not servo-controlled monitor the temperature of the heater, providing power to the heater element based on the setting of the temperature control knob. The patient's airway temperature does not influence the temperature of the heater.

Servo-controlled units monitor the temperature of gas delivered to the patient, adjusting the power to the heating elements based on temperature monitored by a thermistor probe placed downstream from the humidifier, at or near the patient airway connection. When the set temperature of the heater is greater than the distal temperature, the controller applies more power to the heater. As the distal temperature nears or exceeds the set temperature, power is reduced. Thermistor probes at the airway are best placed in the inspiratory limb of the ventilator circuit far enough from the patient so that exhaled gas is not detected. These probes should not be placed inside heated environments, such as isolettes, where the surrounding air temperature fools the heater into thinking it can reduce or stop adding heat to the humidifier.

All heaters should have alarms and alarm-activated heater shut-down devices. Each individual heater has distinct advantages and disadvantages regarding performance, cost, safety, and ease of use that should be taken into account when selecting a system.

Condensation

A problem with actively heating humidifiers is that, once heated and humidified, gas cools as it passes through tubing en route to the patient. As the gas cools, its ability to hold water vapor is reduced, and condensation (rain-out)

CRITICAL THINKING CHALLENGES

Shifting Care Plans

A tracheotomized patient in the medical intensive care unit has been breathing room air through an HME attached directly to the trach. You enter the room to check the patient and find that the patient is coughing and dislodges a plug of mucus into the HME. What should you do to correct the problem?

A common answer is to place the patient on active humidification (heated water) applied to a trach mask. The trach mask is designed to surround the area of the trach, allowing humidified gas to be inhaled, while providing a loose fit that allows secretions to drain clear of the tube and collar.

Another option may be to train the patient to remove the HME when coughing and to collect the expelled secretions on a tissue for disposal. For patients who are acclimatizing for a permanent stoma, this builds confidence in their ability to deal with their own secretion clearance and creates less of a mess than does secretions dripping from the trach onto the patient's neck or bed clothes.

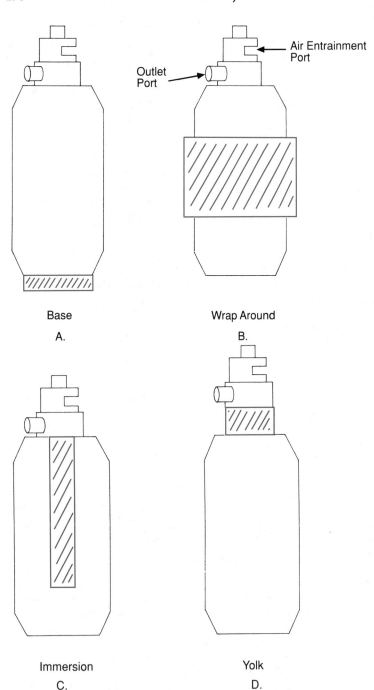

Outlet Port

Air Entrainment Port

Base

A.

Wrap Around

B.

Immersion

C.

Yolk

D.

FIGURE 11–6 • Four methods for heating humidifiers include electrical heating elements located at the base of the device (*A*), wrapped around the body of the humidifier (*B*), inserted into the water reservoir (immersion) (*C*), and placed between the reservoir and the device outlet (yolk) heating gas in transit to the patient (*D*).

occurs. The amount of condensate is proportional to the temperature differential and is affected by the ambient temperature, gas flow, selected patient airway temperature, and the length, diameter, and thermal mass of the tubing between the humidifier and the patient.

To ensure that gas delivered is 35°C by the time it reaches the patient, the gas may be heated to 50°C at the humidifier.[30] At that temperature, the gas contains more than 80 mg/L of water. As the gas cools to 35°C at the patient connection, it can hold less than 40 mg/L of water, and more than half of the total water leaving the humidifier

condenses in the tubing before reaching the patient. In addition to the direct cost of the wasted water that rains out of the system, the tubing must be drained frequently to avoid blockage by the pooling condensate or inadvertent lavaging or "drowning" of the patient when the tubing is moved by pouring the condensate into the airway.

Condensate is contaminated frequently with bacteria from the patient's sputum.[14] This contamination can occur within the first hour after placing the patient on the ventilator. The combination of bacteria, heat, moisture, and secretions in the ventilator circuit creates an effective incubator for growing bacteria. Tubing should be positioned so that the drainage is away from the patient's airway to avoid accidental lavage of the airway.

Condensate also poses a risk to the care provider; when the circuit is disconnected, the practitioner can be sprayed with contaminated fluid in the eyes or other mucous membranes. When heated humidifier systems are used, universal infection control practices must be observed, using gloves and goggles as splash guards to minimize risk of exposure to contaminated secretions, and condensate should always be treated and disposed of as contaminated waste.[29]

Water traps may be placed in both the inspiratory and expiratory limbs to facilitate drainage of condensate from the ventilator circuit, reducing the obstruction to gas flow in the circuit. The water trap should be located at a dependent point in the circuit, so that condensate drains into the trap by gravity. The water traps selected should minimize changes in circuit compliance and allow emptying without disrupting ventilation of the patient (Fig. 11–7).

The most efficient way to reduce condensation during active humidification is to keep it from forming by maintaining a constant temperature of the gas within the circuit. Several mechanisms have been used to accomplish this, including increasing the thermal mass of the circuit, using a coaxial circuit with the inspiratory limb surrounded by the expiratory limb of the circuit, or adding heated wires to the circuit. Increasing the passive thermal mass of the circuit serves to insulate the gas inside the tubing from the cool ambient air outside. This is done by using thicker-walled tubing or by wrapping the tubing with insulating material. These systems tend to reduce temperature drop in the inspiratory limb but fail to eliminate significant condensate formation.

An alternative is to surround the inspiratory limb of the circuit with the expiratory limb in a coaxial manner. This technique uses the patient's warm exhaled gas as a heated air bath surrounding the inspiratory limb. This principle is the basis of the Baines anesthesia circuit but has limited application for ventilator circuits used for long-term support because of concerns about potential increases in imposed airway resistance and work of breathing.

A more practical method to minimize condensation is to place heated wires into the inspiratory and expiratory tubing of the ventilator circuit to heat the gas and reduce the temperature differential between humidifier and patient. Most heated wire circuits use dual servo-controls, with one temperature probe monitoring the temperature of gas leaving the humidification chamber and the other placed at or near the patient airway (Fig. 11–8). The humidifier operates at a lower temperature when heated wire circuits are used (32° to 36°C) than it does with conventional circuits (45° to 50°C) to deliver the desired temperature to the airway. The reduction in condensate in the tubing results in lower sterile water use, reduced need for drainage of the tubing, and less infection risk for both patients and practitioners.

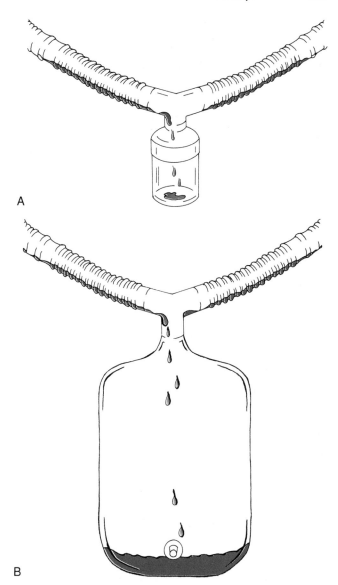

A

B

FIGURE 11–7 • A major problem with heated humidification is the formation of condensate in the connecting tubing. To minimize this problem, large-bore ridged tubing is used. The ribs catch and hold condensate, reducing pooling at the low point of the tubing. Placement of a trap (A) or drain (B) at the low point of the circuit prevents condensate from obstructing the tubing.

Many humidifiers with heated wire capability include a relative humidity control that regulates the temperature differential between humidifier and circuit. With these systems, the temperatures do not reliably reflect absolute or relative humidity; only the temperature differential between the two sites is monitored. If the humidifier is cooler than the gas in the inspiratory limb, the absolute humidity remains the same, whereas relative humidity is decreased. Under these circumstances, the circuit has no condensate, so the practitioner cannot be certain that the gas is being humidified. Similarly, when the humidifier is minimally hotter than the gas in the circuit, the relative humidity in-

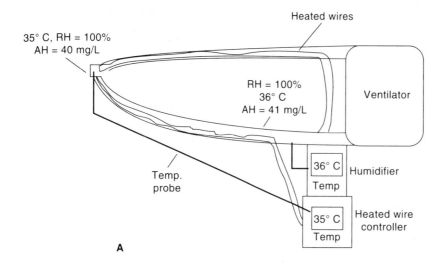

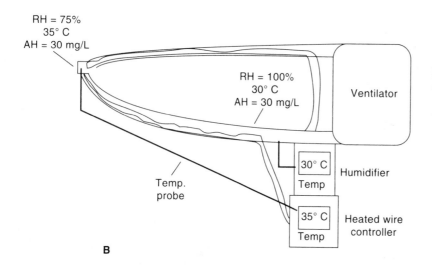

FIGURE 11–8 • A heated wire circuit operates best when the temperature proximal to the heater is higher than that at the airway, producing a small amount of condensation (*A*). When the airway temperature is greater than or equal to the humidifier temperature, no condensate forms (*B*). Condensate is a visual indicator that the system is operating properly. AH, absolute humidity; RH, relative humidity; Temp, temperature probe. (Fink J, Jue P. Humidity and aerosol therapy. In: Barnhart S, Czervinske M, eds. *Perinatal and Pediatric Respiratory Care.* Philadelphia: WB Saunders;1995.)

creases or stays the same, with minimal reduction in absolute humidity; little or no condensate forms in the circuit. To ensure that the inspired gas is being humidified, the temperature differential should be adjusted to the point that a few drops of condensation form near the patient's airway connector. This minimal condensate is the most reliable indicator that gas is fully saturated. If no condensate is visible, the gas relative humidity may be anywhere between 99% and 0%, and clinicians have no way to know without access to a reliable hygrometer.

When using heated wire circuits for infants who are in an isolette or other thermal-neutral environment, care must be taken regarding placement of the thermistor in the circuit. When the sensor measuring the patient's airway temperature is within the thermal-neutral environment, the probe senses the warm ambient temperature and reduces or shuts down power to the heated wires. This results in increased rain-out in the circuit and significant reductions in humidity delivered to the patient. When using heated

wire circuits under these circumstances, the sensor probe in the inspiratory limb must be located outside of the heated environment to allow the heated wire controller to maintain the desired temperature and water content of inspired gases.

The Respiratory Wick Humidification System® (Anamed) humidifies the gas while en route within the inspiratory limb of the ventilator circuit. This is accomplished with a cloth wick and wire heating elements that run parallel in the inspiratory limb of the disposable ventilator circuit, ending with a disposable internal thermistor probe placed just before the patient wye. A water pump is used to prime the circuit by pressurizing a soaker hose within the wick. A wick well positioned at the lowest point of the circuit collects excess water and acts a reservoir to keep the wick wet. The manufacturer claims that the wick needs to be primed only once every 2 to 4 hours. The heated wire controller has a single connection, and the use of the internal probe reduces the potential for leaks secondary to loose or disconnected probes. To reduce work of breathing for the patient's inspiratory efforts, the inspiratory limb tubing has a 2-mm greater internal diameter than the standard adult circuits.

Heat–Moisture Exchanger

The HME is classified as a passive humidifier and has been referred to as an "artificial nose." Like the nose, the HME captures exhaled heat and moisture and uses it to heat and humidify the next inspiration. Unlike the nose, it is a passive humidifier that does not add heat or water to the system. The role of the HME is to conserve heat and moisture from expired gas and to return them to the patient during the next inspiration. The ideal HME should add minimal dead space, weight, and resistance to the airway; incorporate standard connections; and operate at 70% efficiency (defined as the ratio of the absolute humidity of exhaled gas to the humidity returned to the patient by the HME).[30]

Heat–moisture exchangers have been in clinical use for four decades and work in one of three ways.

In condenser humidifiers, the condenser element is usually constructed of metallic gauze, corrugated metal, or parallel metal tubes to provide high thermal conductivity. On inspiration, air cools the condenser to room temperature. On exhalation, the saturated gas cools as it enters the condenser and the water rains out while the temperature of the condenser is increased. On the next inspiration, cool dry air is warmed by the condenser by evaporation of water from the surface. Condenser humidifiers are usually only about 50% efficient under ideal conditions.

Hygroscopic condenser humidifiers contain materials with low thermal conductivity, such as paper, wool, or foam, impregnated with a hygroscopic chemical, such as calcium chloride or lithium chloride. During exhalation, warm saturated gas precipitates water on the cool condenser element while water molecules bind to the salt without transition from vapor to liquid state. During inspiration, the lower water vapor pressure in the inspired gas liberates water molecules from the hygroscopic compound without a decrease in temperature due to vaporization. The efficiency of these devices can be as high as 70%.

Hydrophobic condenser humidifiers (Fig. 11–9) use a water-repellent element with a large surface area and low thermal conductivity, which means that heat from conduction and latent heat of condensation is not dissipated. During exhalation, the condenser temperature rises to about 35°C. On inspiration, cool gas and evaporation cool the condenser down to about 10°C. This large temperature shift results in more water condensed in the humidifier on exhalation, which is used in humidifying the next inspiration. These devices are about 70% efficient. Hydrophobic humidifiers can also act as efficient microbiologic filters.

The efficiency of HMEs decreases as tidal volume, inspiratory flow, or FIO_2 increase.[30] Resistance through the

HME is also important. When the HME is dry, resistance across the device is minimal. After several hours of use, however, the resistance may increase as water is absorbed onto a hygroscopic HME.[31,32] The increased work of breathing imposed by the HME may not be well tolerated, particularly for patients with underlying lung disease who already experience increased work of breathing.

Heat–moisture exchangers are considered bacteriostatic. HMEs eliminate condensation from the ventilator circuit and reduce the role of the circuit as a potential source of infection. Several authors have shown that the hydrophobic condenser humidifier prevents contamination of ventilator circuits and does not produce aerosols that could carry bacteria.[33] Other researchers evaluating a number of HMEs were not able to confirm their safety with respect to nosocomial infection risk, demonstrating that many of the devices produced or passed aerosols that carry bacteria. Of the Siemens, Engstrom, Pall, and Portex hydrophobic condenser humidifiers, only the Pall humidifier satisfactorily removed spores from the gas stream. Hedley and colleagues[34] concluded that the pleated membrane filter provides a wider margin of safety than either the hygroscopic or composite devices. The value or role of the HME as a filter, in terms of patient and health care provider safety, has yet to be substantiated. It is clear that the HME generally forms a barrier between the patient and the ventilator

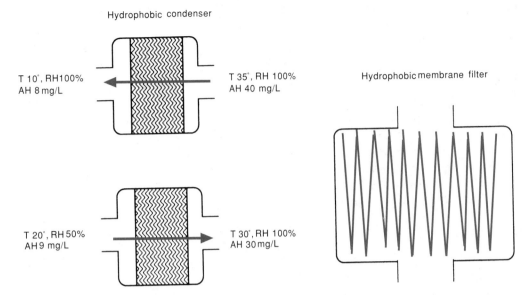

Hydrophobic condenser

T 10°, RH 100%
AH 8 mg/L

T 35°, RH 100%
AH 40 mg/L

Hydrophobic membrane filter

T 20°, RH 50%
AH 9 mg/L

T 30°, RH 100%
AH 30 mg/L

FIGURE 11-9 • Hydrophobic condenser HME (left) during expiration (top) and inspiration (bottom). A hydrophobic membrane filter is shown on the right. AH, absolute humidity; RH, relative humidity. (Scanlon C, Spearman C, Sheldon R. *Egan's Fundamentals of Respiratory Care.* 6th ed. St. Louis: Mosby-Year Book;1995.)

circuit, or outside world, that impedes the passage of bacteria and droplet nuclei.

Heat–moisture exchangers provide an inexpensive alternative to humidifiers when used for short-term ventilation of adult patients who do not have complex humidification needs, such as might be required for a brief period of time in a postoperative recovery room or emergency department, during transport, or to complete a radiologic procedure. Other researchers, such as Weber and Dreyfuss, advocate the use of properly selected HMEs in virtually all patient situations.

An HME device appropriate for the individual patient, based on size and tidal volume, should be selected (Fig. 11–10). Table 11–2 itemizes dead space, measured output, and materials used in several available HMEs. HMEs come in a variety of shapes and sizes, as demonstrated in Figure

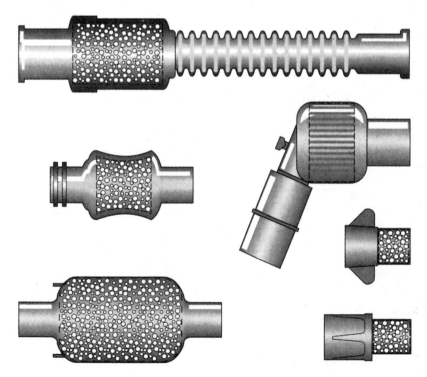

FIGURE 11-10 • Heat–moisture exchangers are available in a variety of shapes and sizes. (Fink J, Jue P. Humidity and aerosol therapy. In: Barnhart S, Czervinske M, eds. *Perinatal and Pediatric Respiratory Care.* Philadelphia: WB Saunders;1995.)

Table • 11–2 CHARACTERISTICS OF VARIOUS HEAT–MOISTURE EXCHANGERS

Device	Type	Moisture output (mg/L H$_2$O)(Vt × f)			Resistance (cm H$_2$O/L/s)		Dead Space (mL)
		500 × 20	1000 × 10	1000 × 20	Before	After	
Aqua H	HCH	31.2	28.3	27.1	0.9	1.2	84
Aqua FH	HCHF	31.8	29.1	27.1	1.62	1.78	87
ARC	HCH	32.0	31.4	30.4	0.7	1.1	89
ARCF	HCHF	32.4	32.0	30.6	2.0	2.2	86
Edith	HCH	30.6	30.0	28.9	1.48	1.54	82
Engstrom 500	HCH	26.7	25.1	24.9	1.60	1.8	19
Engstrom 1000	HCH	27.4	26.1	25.8	2.0	2.1	29
Engstrom 1500	HCH	29.1	28.4	26.5	3.5	3.67	40
FloCare "L"	HCH	30.4	27.1	25.6	1.6	1.78	32
Gibeck HVF	HCHF	32.1	30.8	29.7	2.2	2.36	58
Hygrobac	HCHF	32.5	31.0	29.4	1.9	2.08	92
Hygrobac S	HCHF	29.6	28.0	26.8	2.4	2.57	48
Hygroster	HCHF	33.2	31.9	30.6	2.5	2.7	94
Intersurgical	HCHF	25.4	22.6	21.8	2.2	2.3	65
Intertech 2841	HCH	28.5	27.0	25.5	1.75	1.84	36
Intertech HEPA	HMEF	24.8	23.6	21.1	1.6	1.79	78
Pall	HMEF	24.9	21.2	19.6	2.2	2.38	90
Portex 600	HCH	25.2	24.6	22.4	2.7	2.86	10
Portex 1200	HCH	27.2	26.4	25.1	1.3	1.5	33
Vital Signs HCH	HCH	30.8	28.5	28.1	2.3	2.44	48
Vital Signs HCHF	HCHF	29.7	28.0	26.9	2.5	2.67	58

Modified from Branson RD, Davis K. Evaluation of 21 passive humidifiers according to the ISO 9360 standard: Moisture output, dead space, and flow resistance. *Respir Care.* 1996;41(8):736–743.
HCH, hydroscopic condenser humidifier; HCHF, HCH with filter; HMEF, heat–moisture exchanger with filter.

Box • 11–3 HEAT–MOISTURE EXCHANGER CONTRAINDICATIONS AND HAZARDS

CONTRAINDICATIONS

Presence of thick, copious or bloody secretions
Presence of a large leak around an endotracheal tube, such as might occur with a large bronchopleurocutaneous fistula or leaking endotracheal tube cuff. If the exhaled tidal volume is less than 70% of the delivered tidal volume, incomplete rebreathing will minimize the humidification that can be accomplished with the HME
Body temperature of less than 32°C
Minute ventilation of greater than 10 L/min

HAZARDS

Hypothermia
Underhydration
Impaction of pulmonary secretions
Increase in resistive work of breathing through the HME
Mucous plugging of the airways
Hypoventilation due to increased added dead space[36]

11–10. Several HME devices have been designed for application of low-flow oxygen in patients with bypassed upper airways.

Branson and Davis[35] evaluated the **moisture output** of 21 passive humidifiers using testing methods specified in 1988 by the International Standards Organization, ISO 9360. They classified the devices that used physical mechanisms as HMEs and those that used both chemical and physical principles as hygroscopic condenser humidifiers (HCHs), adding to either device that incorporated a filter the designation "F." Table 11–2 presents the results of their study measuring moisture output, resistance, and dead space for each device over a 2-hour period.

Table • 11–3 TOTAL GAS FLOW

FIO$_2$	Air/Oxygen Ratio*	Total Flow	
		10 L/min	15 L/min
0.24	25.0 : 1	260	390
0.30	8.0 : 1	90	135
0.35	4.6 : 1	56	84
0.40	3.2 : 1	42	63
0.60	1.0 : 1	20	30
0.70	0.6 : 1	16	24
0.80	0.34 : 1	13.4	20
0.9	0.14 : 1	11	16
1.0	0 : 1	10	15

*Liters of Air/liters of oxygen = $\dfrac{1.0 - \text{FIO}_2}{\text{FIO}_2 - .21}$

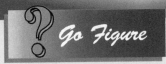

CRITICAL THINKING CHALLENGES

Go Figure

A patient has an inspiratory flow rate of 60 L/min, and the doctor orders an FIO_2 of 0.60. A Venturi nebulizer with a maximal oxygen liter flow of 15 L/min will provide only 30 L/min of gas at 60% oxygen. What FIO_2 will the patient inspire?

Heat–moisture exchangers are contraindicated in a variety of clinical situations.[29] Box 11–3 lists HME contraindications and hazards. HMEs must be removed from the patient circuit during aerosol administration, unless the metered dose inhaler or small-volume nebulizer is placed between the HME and the patient. Placement of the nebulizer between the HME and endotracheal tube has been shown to reduce effective delivery.

BLAND AEROSOL THERAPY

Bland aerosol therapy is used to provide humidity to the airway. When used in conjunction with bland solutions, such as saline, bland aerosol therapy is used for therapeutic

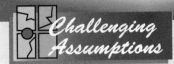

CRITICAL THINKING CHALLENGES

Challenging Assumptions

Jet mixing (Venturi) masks are frequently supplied with an entrainment port collar that allows for the addition of humidity to the entrained ambient air. Is the addition of humidity to a jet mixing mask generally necessary? Let us take a look at the common situation: A jet mixing mask is set to deliver 35% oxygen with an oxygen flow rate of 10 L/min. According to Table 11–3, the air/oxygen mixing ratio is 4.6 : 1, providing a total flow of 56 L/min. The amount of ambient gas entrained is 4.6 times greater than the dry oxygen. If the entrained ambient air contains 10 mg/L of water (22°C at 50% relative humidity), the addition of anhydrous oxygen reduces total water content to about 8.2 mg/L. To put this into perspective, refer to Table 11–1, which shows that 8.2 mg/L is greater than the water content with 50% relative humidity at 20°C (68°F), a pleasant fall day. Would you need additional humidity under such conditions? Not likely.

Box • 11–4   PROCEDURE FOR INITIATION OF COOL OR HEATED AIR-ENTRAINMENT NEBULIZER

1. Obtain appropriate equipment:
   a. Oxygen flowmeter
   b. Nebulizer
   c. Large-bore corrugated tubing
   d. Drain bag
   e. Appropriate patient interface—aerosol mask, face tent, tracheostomy collar, or T-piece
   f. Oxygen analyzer
   g. Thermometer (heated aerosol)
   h. Heating device (heated aerosol)
2. Attach flowmeter to 50-psi outlet.
3. Assemble nebulizer. Using aseptic technique, fill with sterile water for inhalation if device has not been prefilled.
4. Attach nebulizer to flowmeter. Avoid cross-threading the plastic fitting because it is attached to the flowmeter.
5. Attach large-bore corrugated tubing to the nebulizer.
6. Position tubing to allow a dependent loop and cut in the drain bag. The drain bag should be in the lowest position (see Fig. 11–7).

7. Attach the patient interface.
8. Turn on the gas flow to the nebulizer and adjust the entrainment collar to the appropriate FDO_2 - Verify the FDO_2 with the oxygen analyzer and adjust the entrainment collar as necessary to obtain the FDO_{2+}.
9. Ensure adequate gas flow from the device and apply to patient. Confirm adequate gas flow by observing the aerosol escaping from the patient interface. The aerosol should not disappear completely during inspiration. If total flow remains inadequate, as demonstrated by complete disappearance of the aerosol during inspiration, increase the oxygen flow to the nebulizer. If total flow continues to be inadequate and oxygen flow is at maximum, change the device to an injection nebulizer or a high-flow heated humidifier.
10. If a heated aerosol is clinically indicated, add the appropriate heating device to the nebulizer. Place a thermometer close to the patient interface, and verify a safe operating temperature.

Table • 11–4   RELATIVE ATTRIBUTES OF COMMON HUMIDIFICATION SYSTEMS

Attribute	Bubble Unheated	Pass-over Heated	Nebulizer Unheated	Nebulizer Heated	HME
Output (mg/L)	15–20	30–50	15–30	20–40	19–32
Temperature (°C)	10–20	30–40	10–20	22–28	22–30
Flow limitation	Yes	No	Yes	Yes	Yes
Retains body heat	No	Yes	No	Yes	Yes
Infection risk	No	No	Yes	Yes	No
Potential overheating	No	Yes	No	Yes	No
Potential overhydration	No	No	Yes	Yes	No
Potential underhydration	Yes	No	Yes	No	Yes
Increased work of breathing	Yes	No	Yes	Yes	Yes
Potential electric hazard	No	Yes	No	Yes	No

HME, heat–moisture exchanger.

and diagnostic purposes. Large-volume pneumatic nebulizers, ultrasonic nebulizers, and mist tents are commonly used for these purposes.

Large-Volume Nebulizers

Large-volume pneumatic nebulizers, with reservoir volumes greater than 100 mL, are commonly used to aerosolize solutions such as normal saline (0.9% NaCl), half-normal saline (0.45% NaCl), and distilled water, for prolonged periods. These devices have also been used to provide continuous administration of active medications, such as bronchodilators (see Chap. 12).

Large-volume nebulizers with bland solutions are indicated primarily to provide humidification of medical gases for patients with bypassed upper airways, as treatment of upper airway inflammation using cold mist for local vasoconstriction, and to induce sputum production, usually for diagnostic purposes.

There are no data to support the use of bland aerosols as a method to hydrate the dehydrated patient. Fluid administration by the oral or intravenous route is better with less risk. For delivery of humidified inspired gases, large-volume nebulizers offer little advantage over alternative methods such as heated wick humidifiers.

Most large-volume nebulizers use the 50-psig gas source regulated by a flowmeter. The total gas flow delivered through large-volume nebulizers is dependent on the design of the delivery system. Venturi entrainment is used with most of these units to provide the desired FIO_2 level using oxygen as a gas source and air entrainment. Oxygen flow through the flowmeter generally is limited to less than 15 L/min. Total flow is dependent on the flow rate of driving gas and the selected FIO_2 (the aperture size through which air is entrained). Any back pressure in this Venturi system (eg, mask continuous positive airway pressure) reduces total flow and increases the FIO_2.

Most large-volume pneumatic nebulizers are high-flow devices, intended to provide enough flow to meet and exceed patient inspiratory flow rates. The high flow rates are generated with the entrainment of room air and with flow of gas from the high-pressure gas source. Table 11–3 shows the total gas flow developed at various FIO_2 levels at oxygen flows of 10 L/min and 15 L/min with no back pressure. As the required FIO_2 increases, the flow provided from the nebulizer decreases because of less air entrainment.

Table • 11–5.   DEVICE SELECTION CRITERIA

Clinical Indication	Therapeutic Goals	Humidity Device Options Indicated
Medical gas delivery		
Intact upper airway	Ambient temp and RH	
Low flow, <4 L/min		None
8–4 L/min		BU
>8 L/min		PH, NU, NH
Jet mixing <45%		None
Bypassed upper airway	Carinal temp and RH	PH, NH, HME
Thermoregulation	Body temp	PH, NH
Cold air asthma	Carinal temp	PH, NH, HME
Thick secretions	Carinal temp, high RH, reduce humidity deficit	PH, NH with systemic hydration
Tracheal edema stridor	Cool for vasoconstriction	NU

BU, bubble unheated; PH, pass-over heated; NU, nebulizer unheated; NH, nebulizer heated; HME, heat–moisture exchanger.

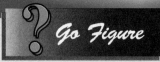

CRITICAL THINKING CHALLENGES

Go Figure

Based on Tables 11–4 and 11–5, determine the best humidity device options for the following patients:

Patient A: 60-year-old emphysema patient receiving oxygen by nasal cannula at 3 L/min

Patient B: 48-year-old patient with chronic bronchitis receiving 5 L/min with a jet mixing (Venturi) mask at 35% oxygen

Patient C: 28-year-old postoperative patient with an endotracheal tube in place in the surgical intensive care unit, not expected to require the tube for more than 24 hours

Patient D: 72-year-old woman with chronic obstructive pulmonary disease and thick secretions who requires mechanical ventilation in the respiratory intensive care unit

Patient E: 30-week gestational age preterm infant in an isolette who requires 24% oxygen

When the patient's inspiratory flow becomes exceedingly high, as can occur with severe tachypnea, the nebulizer may not provide enough flow to provide the desired inspired oxygen concentration.

Additional nebulizers, connected in tandem, may meet the patient's inspiratory flow rate and keep the patient from breathing room air from around the oxygen delivery device. To provide a FIO_2 of 0.9, the four nebulizers required to exceed a patient's inspiratory flow rate of 60 L/min become unwieldy and expensive. In these clinical situations, high-flow nebulizers, such as the Gas Injector (Vital Signs) or closed dilution (Pegasus) nebulizers, or a heated humidifier with a blender should be used (Box 11–4).

DEVICE SELECTION

With so many different devices capable of providing humidity to inspired gas, how does the clinician match the right tool to the task at hand? The first step is to determine the therapeutic goals for the patient. Using Tables 11–4 and 11–5, let us revisit the clinical indications and therapeutic goals associated with humidity therapy. The primary indication was to condition gas to approximate normal conditions for the point of entry into the airway.

References

1. Shelley MP, Lloyd GM, Park GR. A review of the mechanisms and the methods of humidification of inspired gas. *Intensive Care Med.* 1988;14:1–9.
2. Ingelstedt S. Studies on the conditioning of air in the respiratory tract. *Acta Otolaryngol.* 1956;131(Suppl):1.
3. Chalon J, Loew DAY, Malbranche J. Effects of dry air and subsequent humidification on tracheobronchial ciliated epithelium. *Anesthesiology.* 1972;37:338–334.
4. Walker JEC, Wells RE Jr, Merrill EW. Heat and water exchange in the respiratory tract. *Am J Med.* 1961;30:259–267.
5. McFadden ER Jr, Pichurke BB, Bowman HF, et al. Thermal mapping of the airways in humans. *J Appl Physiol.* 1985;2:564–570.
6. Kapadia FN, Shelley MP. Normal mechanisms of humidification. *Recent Advances in Humidification: Problems in Respiratory Care.* Philadelphia: J.B. Lippincott 1991.
7. Chatburn RL, Primiano FP. A rational basis for humidity therapy. *Respir Care.* 1987;32(4):249–243.
8. Tarnow-Mordi WO, Reid R, Griffiths P, et al. Low inspired gas humidity and respiratory complications in very low birth weight infants. *J Pediatr.* 1988;114:438.
9. Anderson S, Herbring BG, Widman B. Accidental profound hypothermia. *Br J Anaesth.* 1970;42:653.
10. Wells RE, Walker JEC, Hickler RB. Effects of cold air on respiratory airflow resistance in patients with respiratory-tract disease. *N Engl J Med.* 1960;263:268.
11. Greenspan JS, Wolfson MR, Shaffer TH. Airway responsiveness to low inspired gas temperature in preterm neonates. *J Pediatr.* 1991;118(3):443–445.
12. Shapiro BA, Kacmarek RM, Cane RD, et al. *Clinical Application of Respiratory Care.* 4th ed. St. Louis: Mosby-Year Book; 1991: 57–73.
13. Kacmarek RM. Humidity and aerosol therapy. In: Pierson DJ, Kacmarek RM, eds. *Foundations of Respiratory Care.* New York: Churchill Livingstone; 1992:793–824.
14. Fink J. Aerosol and humidity therapy. In: Scanlan C, Spearman B, Sheldon R, eds. *Egan's Fundamentals of Respiratory Care.* 6th ed. St. Louis: Mosby-Year Book; 1995.
15. Ward JJ, Helmholtz HF. Applied humidity and aerosol therapy. In: Burton GG, Hodgkin JE, Ward JJ, eds. *Respiratory Care: A Guide to Clinical Practice.* 3rd ed. Philadelphia: JB Lippincott; 1991: 355–396.
16. Primiano FP Jr, Montague FW Jr, Saidel GM. Measurement system for water vapor and temperature dynamics. *J Appl Physiol.* 1984;56:1679–1685.
17. Gray HSJ. Humidifiers. In: Shelly MP, Branson RD, MacIntyre NR, eds. *Problems in Respiratory Care: Recent Advances in Humidification.* 1991;4(4):423–434.
18. Fink J, Cohen N. Humidity and Aerosols. In: Eubanks DH, Bone RC, eds. *Principles and Applications of Cardiorespiratory Care Equipment.* St. Louis: Mosby-Year Book; 1994.
19. Sara C, Currie T. Humidification by nebulization. *Med J Aust.* 1965;1:174–179.
20. American National Standards Institute. American national standards for nebulizer and humidifiers. *ANSI.* 1979;Z-79.9.
21. ECRI. Heated humidifiers. *Health Devices.* 1987;16(7):223–250.
22. Darin J, Broadwell J, MacDonnell R. An evaluation of water-vapor output from four brands of unheated prefilled humidifiers. *Respir Care.* 1981;27:41.
23. Klein EF, Shah DA, Shah NJ, et al. Performance characteristics of conventional prototype humidifiers and nebulizers. *Chest.* 1973; 64:690–696.
24. Seigel D, Romo B. Extended use of prefilled humidifier reservoirs and the likelihood of contamination. *Respir Care.* 1990;35:806–810.
25. American College of Chest Physicians—NHLBI. National conference on oxygen therapy. *Respir Care.* 1984;29:922.
26. Darin J. The need for rational criteria for the use of unheated bubble humidifiers. *Respir Care.* 1982;27 (8):945–947. (Editorial)
27. Mercer TT, Goddard RF, Flores RL. Output characteristics of several commercial nebulizers. *Ann Allergy.* 1965;23: 314–326.
28. Hill TV, Sorbello JG. Humidity outputs of large-reservoir nebulizers. *Respir Care.* 1987;32:225–260.
29. AARC. Clinical practice guidelines: Humidification during mechanical ventilation. *Respir Care.* 1992;37(8):887–890.
30. Shelly MP. Inspired gas conditioning. *Respir Care.* 1992;37(9): 1070–1080.

31. Ploysongsang Y, Branson D, Rashkin MC, Hurst JM. Effect of flowrate and duration of use on the pressure drop across six artificial noses. *Respir Care*. 1989;343:902–907.
32. Nishimura M, Nishijima MK, Okada T, et al. Comparison of flow-resistive work load due to humidifying devices. *Chest* 1990; 97:600–604.
33. Cadwallader HL, Bradley CR, Ayliffe GAJ. Bacterial contamination and frequency of changing ventilator circuitry. *J Hosp Infect*. 1990;15:65–72.
34. Hedley RM, Allt-Graham J. A comparison of the filtration properties of heat and moisture exchangers. *Anaesthesia*. 1992;47(5): 414–420.
35. Branson RD, Davis K. Evaluation of 21 passive humidifiers according to the ISO 9360 standard: Moisture output, dead space, and flow resistance. *Respir Care*. 1996;41(8):736–743.
36. Fink J, Jue P. Humidity and aerosol therapy. In: Barnhart S, Czervinske M, eds. *Perinatal and Pediatric Respiratory Care*. Philadelphia: WB Saunders; 1995.

Aerosol Drug Therapy 12

James B. Fink • Rajiv Dhand

Key Terms

baffle
geometric standard
    deviation (GSD)
holding chambers
median mass aerodynamic
    diameter (MMAD)
micron
nebulizer
particle aging
respirable range
spacers
therapeutic index

Objectives

- Define aerosols and discuss their use in drug delivery.

- Identify the primary indications for aerosol therapy.

- Differentiate between the various types of aerosol devices and key factors affecting their performance.

- Relate the physical properties of aerosols to their penetration and deposition in the human lung.

- Compare and contrast aerosol delivery devices according to their principles of operation.

- Select appropriate aerosol devices for the drug being used and for the targeted site of drug delivery.

- Select the appropriate aerosol device for specific clinical situations.

- Identify hazards and contraindications associated with aerosol therapy.

- Perform effective aerosol administration.

- Understand key elements in teaching patients to self-administer aerosol therapy.

Aerosols are commonly used to deliver medications to the lungs, throat, and nose. Both the upper and lower respiratory tracts provide an ideal route for administration of therapeutic agents. In many cases, aerosols are a superior delivery method in terms of efficacy and safety when compared with the systemic administration of the same drugs used to treat pulmonary disorders.[1] Aerosols deliver drug directly to the airway, resulting in therapeutic action at the site of delivery with relatively low systemic doses and minimal systemic side effects; thus, aerosol delivery is described as having a high **therapeutic index**. Aerosols are generated by **nebulizers** in a variety of sizes and shapes, utilizing various physical principles. This chapter reviews small-volume nebulizers (SVNs) and large-volume nebulizers (pneumatic and ultrasonic), metered dose inhalers (MDIs), and dry-powder inhalers (DPIs) and describes how these devices might best be used to administer medications to the airway.

Aerosol therapy is used to deliver pharmacologically active agents to the airway. The indication for any aerosol is based on the need for the drug and the targeted site of delivery. Table 12–1 lists the wide variety of drugs and the current clinical indications for aerosol drug delivery.[1,2]

Table • 12–1   DRUGS AND CLINICAL INDICATIONS FOR AEROSOL DRUG DELIVERY

Clinical Indication	Drug
Nasal Delivery	
Allergies	Steroids
Osteoporosis	Calcium
Migraine	Ergotamine
Human immunodeficiency virus–related neuropathy	Peptide T
Bone disease	Calcitonin
Diabetes	Insulin
Hormone deficiency	Growth hormone
Immunization	Vaccines
Postoperative pain	Butorphanol
Lung Delivery	
Asthma	Steroids
Chronic obstructive pulmonary disease, bronchiectasis	Cromolyn sodium
Chronic bronchitis	Ipratropium
Bronchiolitis	β-agonists
Parenchymal disease	
Respiratory syncytial virus	Ribavirin
Pneumocystis	Pentamidine
Sarcoidosis	Antiprotease
Dyspnea	Morphine
Diabetes	Insulin
Fungal infection	Amphotericin
Cystic fibrosis	Aminoglycoside
	Antibiotics, amiloride
	Dornase α, β-agonist
	Uridine triphosphate
Intractable cough	Lidocaine
BPD	Antibiotics, furosemide
Bronchopulmonary dysplasia	Dornase

Adapted from Dolovich M. *Physical principles underlying aerosol therapy. J Aerosol Med.* 1989:2(2);171–186; and ODonohue WJ. *Guidelines for the use of nebulizers in the home and in domicillary sites. Chest.* 1996;109:814–820.

PHYSICS OF AEROSOL DELIVERY

An aerosol is a suspension of solid or liquid particles in gas that can vary in shape, density, or size. Aerosols exist all around us as pollens, spores, dusts, smoke, smog, fog, mists, and viruses[3] (Fig. 12–1). Although aerosols appear to be made of particles that are so much smaller than our nose and mouth, most of the aerosols that we can see are too big to deliver medication effectively to our lungs. The ability of aerosols to travel through the air, enter through the airways, and deposit in the lungs is largely based on particle size or mass. An aerosol can be made up of consistent particles that have a similar shape and size (monodisperse) or a wide variety of shapes and sizes (heterodisperse). Monodisperse aerosols are typically created by sophisticated processes, primarily for the laboratory. Most aerosols found in nature and used in respiratory medicine are heterodisperse.

We characterize an aerosol in terms of the **mean mass aerodynamic diameter** (MMAD), which describes the mean size of the particles in **microns** (µm), and the **geometric standard deviation** (GSD), which describes the range of sizes of particles in an aerosol. Unlike the standard deviation, which is added to or subtracted from the mean to reflect a distribution, the GSD is divided into or multiplied by the median to reflect distribution and may actually be a larger number than the MMAD. The greater the MMAD, the larger is the median particle size; the greater the GSD, the more heterodisperse is the aerosol. The importance of these characteristics will become clearer as we describe the mechanisms of deposition and operation of specific types of nebulizers.

Mechanisms of Aerosol Deposition

Deposition of inhaled particles in the airway and lung is caused by impaction resulting from inertia, sedimentation due to gravity, and diffusion due to brownian movement. The relative importance of each factor is dependent on the size, shape, location, and motion of the particle.

Inertial impaction is the deposition of particles when they collide with a surface. This is the primary mechanism for deposition of particles larger than 5 µm in diameter. Inertia is the tendency for an object with mass that is in motion to remain in motion. The larger the particle, the greater is the mass, and the greater is the inertia keeping that particle in motion. When a particle with mass is traveling in a stream of gas and that stream is diverted by a turn in the airway, the inertia of the particle tends to keep it on the initial trajectory (or path), so that instead of making the turn, the particle collides with the surface of the airway. This impaction results in the particle depositing on the surface of the airway. The higher the inspiratory flow of gas, the greater is the inertia of the particles, and the greater is the tendency for even small particles to impact in and deposit in the larger airways. Consequently, turbulent flow, complex convoluted passageways, bifurcation of the airways,

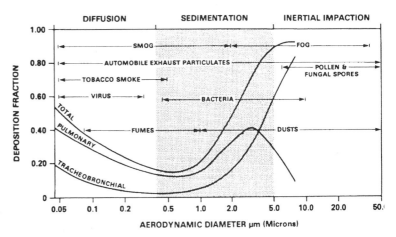

FIGURE 12-1 • Particle deposition. Chart demonstrating the range of particle diameters over which diffusion, sedimentation, and inertial impaction occur, as well as the range of particle diameters of some commonly encountered aerosols. (Adapted from Newhouse MT, Dolovich M: Aerosol therapy in children. In *Basic Mechanisms of Pediatric Respiratory Disease: Cellular and Integrative.* Toronto: BC Decker; 1991.)

and inspiratory flows greater than 30 L/min increase the impaction of particles larger than 2 μm in the larger airways. Most particles larger than 10 μm deposit in the nose or mouth at normal inspiratory flow rates. Particles between 5 and 10 μm tend to deposit in proximal airways before reaching bronchioles 2 mm in diameter.

Gravitational sedimentation occurs when the aerosol particles lose inertia, their movement on a trajectory begins to slow, and they settle out of suspension because of gravity. The greater the mass of the particle, the faster it settles. Gravitational sedimentation increases with time, affecting particles as small as 1 μm. Sedimentation is the primary mechanism for deposition of particles 1 to 5 μm in the central airways (most larger particles impact en route). Breath holding for 4 to 10 seconds after inhaling an aerosol increases the residence time for the particles in the lung, extending the time to allow deposition by gravitational sedimentation, especially in the last six generations of the airway. A 10-second breath-hold has been reported to provide optimal particle deposition compared with other breath-holding times.[4,5] This may increase the deposition of the aerosol inhaled in the individual breath by as much as 10%.

Diffusion, or brownian movement, is the primary mechanism for deposition of particles smaller than 3 μm into the lung parenchyma. As gas reaches this region of the lung, gas flow and inertia for particles is reduced to a no-flow state. Aerosol particles "bounce around" with the other molecules and deposit on contact with the structural surfaces.

Deposition of particles ranging in size from 1 to 3 μm is divided between the central and peripheral airways.[6] Optimal deposition of particles smaller than 3 μm is believed to occur when inspiratory flow is less than 60 L/min and inspiratory volume is greater than 1 L.

Under the best circumstances, inhaling medical aerosols results in less than 20% of the drug dispensed by the nebulizer actually being deposited in the lungs. Aerosols are targeted for delivery to the lung by using nebulizers that produce particles that are the right size for optimal delivery to the desired part of the airway or lung. Aerosol droplets with an MMAD of 1 to 5 μm have a better chance of depositing in the lung than do larger or smaller particles and

CRITICAL THINKING CHALLENGES

Go Figure

An aerosol has an MMAD of 2.8 and a GSD of 2.0. What is the range of particle sizes within 1 standard deviation?

MMAD/GSD = Small

2.8 μm/2 μm = 1.4 μm

MMAD × GSD = Large

2.8 μm × 2 μm = 5.6 μm

CRITICAL THINKING CHALLENGES

Challenging Assumptions

When a single breath containing an aerosol is inhaled, the larger the breath, the more aerosol that enters the lungs, and the greater the opportunity for deposition of the aerosol in the lung from that single breath. When this breath is held for up to 10 seconds, even greater opportunity for deposition exists. Increased deposition is often equated with greater delivery of aerosolized drugs and improved clinical response. The correlation of tidal volume to clinical response has not been well established, however, and there is mounting evidence that tidal volume or ability to hold the breath is not a reliable criterion to differentiate between available aerosol delivery systems (eg, SVN versus MDI with holding chamber).

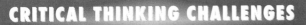

are referred to as being in the **respirable range**. Most particles 10 μm or larger are filtered out by the nose, whereas particles larger than 5 μm tend to impact in the upper airway. The depth of penetration of a particle into the bronchial tree is inversely proportional to the size of the particle, down to 1 μm. Particles smaller than 1 μm, however, are so light and stable that a large proportion do not deposit in the lungs. Aerosols with an MMAD of 0.8 to 2 μm are targeted to the lung parenchyma, whereas particles smaller than 0.8 μm often are exhaled. Particles smaller than 1 μm represent a very small volume of medication (compared with larger particles).

Aerosol particles often change size because of evaporation or hygroscopic properties. Because these changes occur as a factor of time and exposure of the aerosol to environmental conditions, the process is referred to as **particle aging**. The rate of particle growth is inversely proportional to the size of a particle, so that small particles grow faster than larger particles. Rate of particle aging is dependent on the composition of the aerosol, the initial size of the particle, the time in suspension, and external conditions to which the particle is subjected. Small particles get even smaller when inhaled with relatively dry ambient gas at room temperature. As the inspired air is heated en route to the lungs, the capacity of the gas to hold water increases, and evaporation of water from the aerosol particles to the surrounding gas reduces the size of the particles. Aerosols of water-soluble materials (especially salts) introduced into a humidified environment (ie, a ventilator circuit) may absorb water and grow because of hygroscopic properties. In short, most particles change with age as a result of changes in temperature and humidity encountered en route to the lungs.

The only reliable way to determine the output of a nebulizer is by measuring it in the laboratory. The unaided human eye cannot see particles smaller than 100 μm (equivalent to a median-sized grain of sand). The cloud we see in the output of a nebulizer is largely the defraction of light as it passes through the particles (rather than the particles themselves). A nebulizer that produces an optimal particle size may get a less-than-enthusiastic reception from clinicians "looking" for effective aerosol production. The gold standard for characterizing an aerosol by particle size is the staged impactor, such as the Anderson. The impactor has multiple stages with different-sized holes, stacked one above the other, designed to draw the aerosol through the stack at a specified flow rate. Large particles passing through the holes impact in the plate placed beneath the specific stages, with smaller particles traveling with the gas flow, passing on to the next stage. Analysis of the weight or amount of drug deposited on each stage permits computation of respirable fraction (for particles smaller than 5 μm) and the MMAD and GSD for the aerosol being characterized.

The output of a nebulizer, without particle sizing, can be measured by collecting the aerosol that leaves the nebu-

lizer on filters placed at the outlet, and measuring either weight or direct assay of drug deposited on the filter.

In vivo deposition of aerosol in the lungs has been measured by radioactive tagging of the aerosol. A scanner (used in nuclear medicine) is then used to measure the distribution and intensity of radiation across the lungs. Another indirect method of determining drug delivery to the lung is analysis of the amount of drug detected in the blood or urine.

FACTORS AFFECTING AEROSOL DRUG DELIVERY TO PATIENTS

Dosing of aerosolized medication to the lung is, at best, an imprecise science.[7] Ideally, the goal of administration of any medication is to deliver a known quantity of drug to the patient to achieve the desired clinical effect. When a specific dose of a drug is given with an intravenous injection, we know how much of the dose entered the patient's circulatory system. With aerosols, a dose of medication placed in a nebulizer may result in little or no drug reaching the desired site of action in the lungs. To optimize the delivery and clinical effectiveness of aerosol therapy, it is important to understand patient, environmental, and equipment factors that affect delivery of aerosol.

Patient-Related Factors

The following patient-related factors affect aerosol drug delivery:

- Breathing pattern and inspiratory flow rate
- Mouth versus nose breathing
- Airway caliber and patency
- Patient age
- Patient education

Patient Breathing Pattern and Inspiratory Flow Rate

High inspiratory flow rates are associated with greater deposition of drug in the upper airways due to impaction. Encouraging the patient to take slow deep breaths should result in more drug entering the lungs. Although higher flow rates result in less drug entering the lung, the high flow rates may result in improved or at least different distribution of drug that does enter the lungs, providing preferential distribution of gas to the larger airways and non–gravity-dependent areas of the lung. Low respiratory rates and large tidal volumes are associated with improved drug delivery, providing longer time before exhalation of aerosols that have been inhaled into the lung, and increasing the time for gravitational sedimentation of aerosol. Rapid respiratory rate (tachypnea) is associated with higher inspiratory flow rates (increasing impaction in upper airways) and reduced residence time of drug within the lung, allowing less opportunity for deposition from sedimentation. This becomes of greater significance in patients with reduced functional residual capacity (FRC) and expiratory reserve volume, in whom there is less lung volume available to act as a reservoir for aerosol to deposit between tidal breaths.

Inhalation by Mouth Versus Nose

The nose is a much more effective filter than is the mouth, filtering most particles larger than 10 μm. Nose breathing, along with better filtering and humidification of inhaled gas, accounts for 50% of airway resistance with normal breathing. Mouth breathing provides less effective filtration and humidification, allowing larger particles to pass to the hypopharynx, with less airway resistance. With mouth breathing, the narrowest point in the airway is at the larynx, where impaction of larger particles occurs. For particles in the respirable range 5 μm, the difference between nose and mouth breathing on lower respiratory tract deposition is less clear. Lippman[8] demonstrated that with mouth breathing, about 30% of 3-μm particles enter the lung, whereas with nose breathing, about 25% of 2.5-μm particles reach the lower respiratory tract (Fig. 12–2), suggesting that breathing through the nose may still allow reasonable deposition of aerosols in the 2.5-μm respirable range.

Because inhalation through the mouth is believed to allow more respirable particles to deposit in the lower respi-

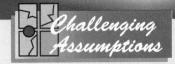

CRITICAL THINKING CHALLENGES
Challenging Assumptions

When might nose breathing be an advantage during aerosol administration?

Inhaled steroids. Aerosolized steroids are targeted to both the nose (allergic rhinitis) and the lungs (asthma and chronic obstructive pulmonary disease). Oral inhalation of inhaled steroids is associated with opportunistic yeast infections, secondary to deposition of large particles in the pharynx, leading to recommendations that patients gargle after oral administration. This has not been a problem with nasal administration of the same preparations (with the doses prescribed).

The problem with gargling is that the area of greatest deposition in the upper airway with mouth breathing is the larynx, an area that is virtually impossible to rinse effectively by gargling without gagging.

Nose breathing would filter out the larger particles, allowing therapeutic deposition of aerosol to the nose, while smaller particles pass through to provide an adequate lung dose, reducing undesirable oral deposition.

Note: DO NOT TRY THIS AT HOME, KIDS! This might make some sense but has yet to be studied adequately to ensure efficacy.

ratory tract than does inhalation through the nose, some clinicians believe that whenever possible, aerosols should be delivered with a mouthpiece. This well-meant desire to provide optimal drug delivery should be tempered by a number of considerations:

- Masks that cover both the nose and mouth during aerosol administration, held in place by an elastic head strap (Fig. 12–3), are generally more comfortable and require less effort for the patient during prolonged aerosol administration.
- Mouthpieces require the patient to hold the nebulizer in position, necessitating the effort of sealing lips around the mouthpiece.
- Mouthpieces have a smaller cross-sectional area than does an open mouth, increasing the work of breathing during severe bronchospasm.

The choice of mask or mouthpiece should involve consideration of patient comfort as well as aerosol deposition, especially when the patient is primarily mouth breathing (as is often the case with asthmatic patients during moderate to severe bronchospasm). Normally, during states of increased work of breathing, patients begin breathing through the mouth, bypassing the nose and reducing the anatomically imposed work of breathing through the upper airway by 50%. In such cases, the patient continues to

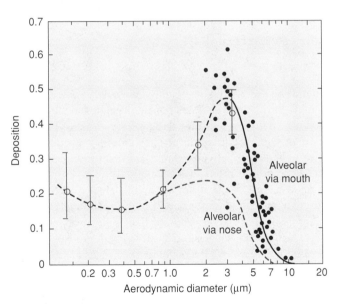

FIGURE 12–2 • Experimental data on deposition in the alveolar region with mouth and nose breathing. Deposition is expressed as fraction of mouthpiece inhalation versus aerodynamic diameter. Breathing 2- to 3-μm particles through the mouth resulted in 35% alveolar deposition, whereas nose breathing yielded 20%. (Lippman M: Regional deposition of particles in the human respiratory tract. In: Lee DHK, Falk HL, Murphy SO, Geiger SR (eds): *Handbook of Physiology: Reaction to Environmental Agents.* Bethesda: American Physiological Society; 1977.)

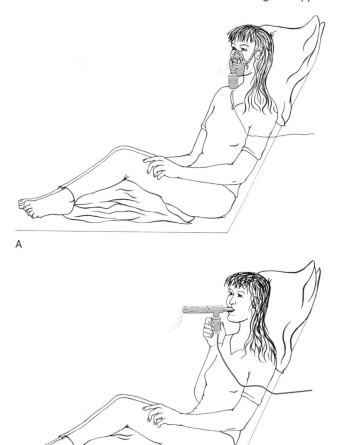

A

B

FIGURE 12-3 • Patients receiving aerosol therapy via mask (*A*) and mouthpiece (*B*). Note preferred patient positioning in an upright or semirecumbent position.

breathe by mouth until airway resistance is reduced (along with the need for a bronchodilator). For these patients, aerosol delivery by mask allows minimal airway resistance and optimal drug delivery with mouth breathing.

Airway Caliber and Patency

The smaller the airway caliber, the greater is the amount of aerosol that deposits in the airway as a result of inertial impaction before reaching the desired target (site of action) within the lungs. This is a key factor in treating patients with severe bronchospasm, airway inflammation, mucosal edema, and other forms of airway obstructions, including mucous plugs, airway collapse, and tumors. Patients who need aerosol therapy the most are often those with small or obstructed airways. In these clinical situations, efforts should be made to remove or relieve the obstruction; administration of larger doses of drug may be required from the nebulizer (to the face) to deliver an adequate dose (to the lung) to achieve therapeutic objectives.

Patient Age

Every patient is different. Small infants are obligate nose breathers; have tiny airways, small inspired volumes, and high respiratory rates; and are unable to cooperate to achieve ideal drug delivery (ie, with breath holding). Older children may be unable or unwilling to cooperate with aerosol administration, fighting against attempts to give an effective treatment. A child does not have a predicted peak inspiratory flow rate of 60 L/min (required to operate a dry powder inhaler [DPI]) until the age of 6 years. Asthmatic patients in acute bronchospasm may have high inspiratory flow rates, with long expiratory times secondary to air trapping. Elderly patients may not be able to manipulate devices physically or to understand or cooperate with techniques to optimize aerosol delivery. Actuation of the aerosol device during inspiration is mandatory with some nebulizers, particularly metered dose inhalers (MDIs). Poor patient coordination drastically reduces the delivered dose of medication.

Patient Education

The patient's ability to understand the therapy and its goals affects the therapeutic efficacy of any treatment significantly. Whenever possible, patients should understand the basic administration techniques, be able to keep track of dosing requirements, recognize undesirable side effects, and understand options and actions that reduce or eliminate those effects.

Environmental and Other Factors

Humidity

Humidity affects both wet and dry aerosols. Droplets of solutions can either evaporate or grow, depending on the water content and temperature of the gas around them. Powders used in DPIs often clump or aggregate in high humidity, thereby reducing delivered doses. Different formulations of the same drug can have substantially different characteristics. Albuterol, as an example, is available in three basic formulations: solution for nebulization, MDI, and DPI. Albuterol sulfate is a salt solution that is hygroscopic, with aerosol particles increasing in size when exposed to increased humidity. In MDIs, albuterol particles are milled to 1-μm particles and covered with surfactants, making the drug hydrophobic. In DPI formulations, the albuterol particles are also milled, but the filler material mixed with the albuterol may be affected by humidity, and clumping when exposed to more than 50% relative humidity.

Temperature

Temperature affects the making of aerosols, aging of aerosol particles, and the patient's response to aerosols. The ambient and device-operating characteristics of nebulizers can result in changes in the amount and concentration of medication nebulized. Evaporation of solutes, solvents, preservatives, and propellant may be affected by temperature, causing changes in the MMAD of the aerosol as it travels from the nebulizer to the patient's airways. The colder the aerosol, the greater is the chance that it will invoke a defensive response from the patient's airway, such as stopping inspiration (cold Freon effect) when the cold air hits the back of the throat, or increasing airway resistance.

Equipment

Equipment that requires electricity, extensive storage space, or considerable effort to transport may limit the availability of some aerosol delivery devices. For instance, nebulizers that are driven by electric compressors do not lend themselves to use during hikes through the woods.

Drug Formulation

The drug formulation can influence drug delivery. Almost any solution can be nebulized, but the physical characteristics of the solution can affect particle size and nebulizer output. Formulations of dry powders are limited to only a few preparations. MDIs have a greater variety of available formulations, but incorporating new drugs into MDIs is a lengthy process requiring years to develop and even longer to gain regulatory approval; therefore, the newer drugs are not always available in the most desirable or therapeutically optimal form.

HAZARDS OF AEROSOL THERAPY

Although aerosol therapy is a valuable clinical tool when properly applied, certain hazards and adverse effects are associated with its use. The primary hazard associated with aerosol therapy is reaction to the medications being administered. Foremost among the hazards that are not medication specific is the risk of infection. Other hazards include reactivity of the airways, systemic effects of bland aerosols, and the potential for too much or too little of the prescribed drug to reach the site of action (Box 12–1).

Box • 12–1   HAZARDS OF AEROSOL THERAPY

Infection
Airway irritation
Systemic effects
  Fluid overload
  Medication
Administration variability
  Too much
  Too little

Infection

Aerosol generators have long been identified as a contributing factor in nosocomial infections.[9–12] The organisms most commonly associated with contamination of aerosol generators are gram-negative bacilli, particularly *Pseudomonas aeruginosa*. Nosocomial infection by *Legionella pneumophila* (the cause of the highly virulent legionnaires' disease) have been reported.[12]

Nebulizers spread bacteria by the airborne route as droplet nuclei. Contaminated medications from multidose vials have been implicated in contamination of nebulizers with pathogens such as *Serratia marcescens* and *Burkholderia cepacia*.[13] In addition, patients may contaminate a nebulizer with pathogens from their oral secretions during aerosol therapy, which may proliferate in a damp nebulizer between treatments.[14] In subsequent treatments, those pathogens are suspended in droplet nuclei that can reach deep into the airways, infecting the lungs. Most nosocomial pneumonias are associated with normal flora in the mouth that are not normally found in the lungs. Exhaled aerosols may place other patients and the practitioner at risk of exposure to airborne pathogens and second-hand exposure to medications. This can be reduced or eliminated through use of one-way valves and filters on the expiratory limb of the nebulizer set-up (Fig. 12–4).

Various procedures have been recommended for reducing contamination and infection for respiratory care equipment. Guidelines from the Centers for Disease Control recommend that nebulizers be sterilized between patients, replaced frequently with disinfected or sterile units, and rinsed with sterile water (not tap or simple distilled water) every 24 hours. More detail on procedures for infection control are provided in Chapter 9.

Airway Irritation and Reactivity

Cold and high-density aerosols can cause reactive bronchospasm and increase airway resistance, especially in patients with preexisting respiratory disease.[15] Acetylcysteine, antibiotics, steroids, cromolyn, ribavirin, and distilled water have been associated with increased airway resistance and bronchospasm during aerosol administration. Administration of bronchodilators before administration of these agents may reduce the risk of increased airway resistance.

Based on this knowledge, the potential for inducing bronchospasm should always be considered a possibility when giving high-density bland aerosols or nebulized drugs to which the airway may be sensitive.[16] Monitoring patients for reactive bronchospasm should include peak flow measurements (or FEV_1/FVC) before and after therapy, auscultation for adventitious breath sounds, observation of the patient's breathing pattern and overall appearance, and communication with the patient during therapy.

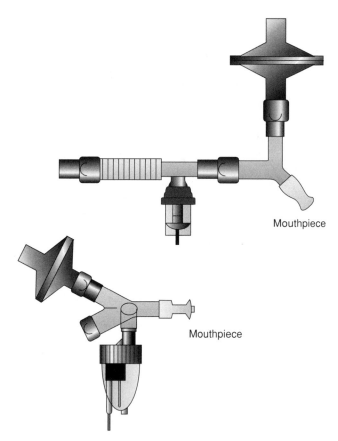

Mouthpiece

Mouthpiece

FIGURE 12–4 • Nebulizers using a combination of one-way valves and filters. One-way valves direct flow of gas to and from the patient, whereas filters collect exhaled aerosols before release to the atmosphere.

Pulmonary and Systemic Effects

Given the rapid absorption of fluid that can occur through the lung, even bland aerosols present potential risks. Excess water can cause overhydration, and excess normal saline has the potential to cause fluid and electrolyte imbalances and hypernatremia.[17] Inhalation of water aerosols for as little as 72 hours may result in focal tissue abscesses, localized inflammation, weight gain, increased respiratory rates, and decreased serum osmolarity. Aerosolized normal saline (0.9%) administered over the same period may result in atelectasis and pulmonary edema.[18] These data suggest that indiscriminate use of continuous bland aerosol therapy should be avoided, especially in infants (Box 12–2).

A related problem is when the patient exhibits difficulty in evacuating mobilized secretions. Care should always be taken to ensure that patients are capable of clearing secretions once they are mobilized by aerosol therapy. Properly directed coughing techniques, controlled deep breathing, and postural drainage should accompany aerosol therapy to promote clear airways. For patients unable to clear secretions adequately, mechanical tracheobronchial aspiration or fiberoptic bronchoscopy may be indicated.

Box • 12–2   PATIENTS AT HIGHEST RISK FOR FLUID OVERLOAD FROM AEROSOLS

Infants
Those patients with:
   fluid retention
   electrolyte imbalances
   diagnosed atelectasis
   pulmonary edema

Drug Delivery per Prescription

Unlike other routes of drug administration, aerosol therapy results in great variations in drug delivered to desired sites of action. Inattention to technique, device, and patient variables can result in drastically reduced drug delivery to the lung. Unless in attendance at the time of administration, the physician prescribing the therapy is unable to determine how the patient took the treatment or responded to the therapy and consequently assumes, *unless told otherwise,* that the therapy was effective. This underlies the need to ensure optimal aerosol delivery and to monitor and communicate patient response to the responsible physician.

Another potential hazard is administering too much medication or a greater concentration of medication than was specified in the physician's prescription. Drug concentration can change during the course of therapy. When dry gas or electricity that generates heat is used to create aerosols, the resulting evaporation removes water from the solution. This results in changing the ratio of solute to solvent, and the concentration of drug increases in the nebulizer reservoir over time, exposing the patient to increasingly higher concentrations of the agent during the course of therapy. This phenomenon occurs in both jet and ultrasonic nebulizers[18] and may be significant when medications are being nebulized for periods longer than 30 minutes.

EQUIPMENT CONSIDERATIONS

Nebulizers produce an aerosol or suspension of particles (each particle composed of many molecules) in gas. Humidifiers add molecular water to gas. Some humidifiers create aerosols, and some nebulizers also add humidity to gas. Nebulizers have been employed to humidify gas, and humidifiers or vaporizers have been used to administer anesthetic agents. The discussion in this chapter is confined to the clinical use of aerosol therapy to administer medications; nebulizers used primarily for humidification are explored in Chapter 11.

AEROSOL GENERATORS

The most common types of aerosol devices used for medical drug delivery are jet nebulizers, MDIs, DPIs, and ultrasonic nebulizers.

Types of Aerosol Generators

Jet Nebulizers

Gas-driven pneumatic (jet) nebulizers have been in clinical use for more than 100 years. The oldest commercially available pneumatic aerosol-generating device still used today is the squeeze bulb atomizer. Most of the more commonly used jet nebulizers require a relative high-pressure gas source, such as a portable compressor, compressed gas cylinder, a 50-psi wall outlet that uses either oxygen or room air. Common to all of these devices is a stream of gas driven under pressure through a restricted orifice (jet). The gas stream leaving the jet passes over the opening of either a capillary tube or fluid-conducting conduit, the base of which is immersed in solution. The jet stream produces an area of low pressure that draws the solution from a reservoir up the capillary tube. As the solution is sucked into the direct path of the gas jet stream, it is sheared from the tip of the tube by the jet stream, producing droplets. The stream of gas directs the droplets to impact against a **baffle**. A baffle is any surface the aerosol stream contacts that permits the larger particles to impact, leaving suspension (Fig. 12–5).

Within the limits of the design of the nebulizer, the higher the gas pressure or flow rate to the nebulizer, the smaller is the particle size generated. Since smaller particles carry less drug, the smaller the particle size generated by the nebulizer, the longer is the time required to deliver the same volume of medication. Nebulizers delivering similar density but smaller-sized particles require more time to deliver the same dose of medication.

Particle size tends to be inversely proportional to gas flow through the jet. For this reason, hand-bulb atomizers with relatively low gas pressure produce larger particles than nebulizers operating from compressed gas sources.

Effects of Nebulizer Design

Design characteristics of jet nebulizers affect the size and density of particles generated. Factors include the size of the jet orifice, the size of the capillary tube, the proximity of the orifice and tube to each other, the driving pressure, and the flow rate of the gas.

The nasal spray pump is the most common device used for nasal aerosol administration of sympathomimetic, antimuscarinic, antiallergic, and antiinflammatory drugs. The spray pump generates lower internal pressures than do pneumatically powered nebulizers targeting the lung, producing larger particles that are better targeted for nasal de-

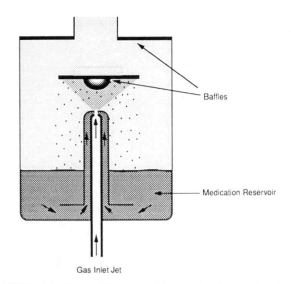

FIGURE 12–5 • Diagram of basic nebulizer. Gas driven through the inlet jet draws medication from the reservoir and creates an aerosol, which is directed against a baffle. The three baffles in this diagram are the primary baffle (which the stream of gas with aerosol is directed toward) and two secondary baffles (the walls of the nebulizer and the surface of the medication.) (Eubanks: *Principles and Applications of Cardiorespiratory Care Equipment*. St. Louis: Mosby–Year Book; 1994.)

position. Deposition with the nasal spray pump is mostly in the anterior nose, with clearance to the nasopharynx. Puffs containing 100 μL appear to deposit more medication than 50-μL puffs, and deposition occurs to a greater surface area with a 35-degree spray angle than with a 60-degree angle.

Entraining a secondary gas as well as the medication into the jet stream also affects aerosol output, density, and particle size characteristics.

Baffles, surfaces that remove aerosol particles from suspension by inertial impaction, are critical elements in the design of the nebulizer and delivery system. Baffles are used to produce optimal-sized particles by allowing large particles to impact in the baffle surface, leaving smaller particles in suspension. Baffles can be the internal walls of the nebulizer, an object placed in line with the jet gas flow, the surface of a one-way valve, or the internal walls of a spacer or drying chamber. Well-designed baffle systems add to the efficiency of jet and mechanical nebulizers by allowing large particles removed from suspension to coalesce and return to the reservoir to be renebulized. Baffling can also occur unintentionally, affecting the aerosol output and deposition. Unintentional baffles can be created by the angles within the aerosol tubing, interfaces with other devices outside of the aerosol generator, and surfaces of the upper airway itself. Large particles that are not baffled by the nebulizer or connecting tubing are deposited in the nose or upper airway. Although baffles affect all types of aerosol generators, they are of greater importance in jet nebulizers because of the inertia developed by the jet stream creating the aerosol (Box 12–3).

Dead volume is the residual volume of medication that remains in the nebulizer after the nebulizer runs dry (Fig. 12–6). Dead volume can vary from 0.5 to 1.5 mL and may represent more than 50% of the total dose of drug placed in the nebulizer. The greater the dead volume, the more drug is wasted, and the less efficient is the delivery system. The proportion of drug nebulized by an SVN increases as diluent is increased. Typical SVNs deliver more drug as an aerosol when the volume in the nebulizer is 4 mL, as opposed to 2 mL, with a constant flow rate of 6 to 8 L/min. This has not been shown to correlate with differences in clinical response at varying diluent volumes and flow rates.[19] When a nebulizer begins to sputter, the medication output is sharply reduced. Nebulizer treatments should end at the point that the nebulizer begins to sputter.

Many of the commercially available SVNs function only when kept in an upright position, and many allow the medication to be inadvertently poured out of the nebulizer when not kept in an upright position.

Humidity and temperature affect the performance of SVNs, particle size, and the concentration of drug remaining in the nebulizer. Evaporation of water and adiabatic ex-

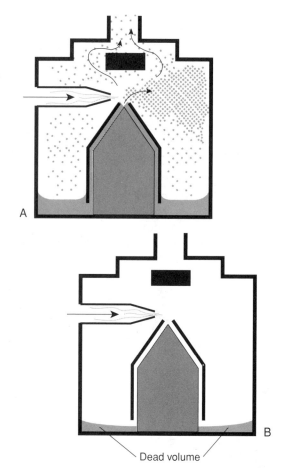

FIGURE 12–6 • Jet nebulizer showing normal operation (*A*) and the medication that is trapped in the nebulizer (*B*). The volume of trapped medication can be as large as 1.5 mL.

pansion of gas can reduce the temperature of the aerosol to as much as 5°C below ambient temperature. As gas warms to room temperature, the particle size is reduced. The aerosol particles entrained into a warm, fully saturated gas stream, such as a ventilator circuit, may increase in size.

SMALL-VOLUME NEBULIZERS (SVNs)

Small-volume nebulizers deliver the medication effectively only when used properly. Inadequate fill volumes, inappropriate pressures, and improper positioning can result in failure to deliver effective aerosol therapy.

Because the nose is such an efficient filter of particles larger than 5 μm, clinicians have long recommended that aerosol be inhaled through the mouth. Nose-breathing filters out large particles and deposits more medication in the upper airway. Despite these theoretical differences, there appears to be no difference in clinical response between treatments given by mouthpiece or by mask when the patient is mouth breathing. Determination of whether the method of delivery is by mask or mouthpiece should be made based on patient preference and comfort.

Box • 12–3   FACTORS THAT AFFECT PERFORMANCE OF SMALL-VOLUME NEBULIZERS

Nebulizer design
  Brand
  Tolerances in manufacturing within lots
  Baffles
    Internal
    One-way valves
    Angles en route to patient
  Residual volume
  Position dependency
  Reservoirs or extension
  Trigger ports
  Use of vents—entrained gas
Gas source—wall, cylinder, compressor
  Pressure
  Gas density
  Flow rate through nebulizer
  Humidity
  Temperature
Characteristics of drug nebulized
  Viscosity
  Surface tension
  Homogeneity
  Volume fill

The ventilatory pattern does influence deposition of aerosols into the lower respiratory tract from SVNs; in most situations, however, normal tidal breathing is encouraged during a treatment. Slow inspiratory flow rates appear to improve deposition. Deep breathing and breath holding during continuous nebulizer therapy do not appear to augment the deposition of drug, as compared with tidal breathing alone.[20]

The terms *continuous nebulization* and *intermittent nebulization* are used in two contexts. In the first, continuous nebulization refers to generating aerosol continuously throughout the patient's respiratory cycle, whereas intermittent nebulization describes generating aerosol only during inspiration. Producing aerosol continuously throughout the patient's respiratory cycle is not an efficient way to deliver medication to the patient because aerosol that is produced between inspirations is largely lost to the atmosphere. For example, a patient who takes a deep breath, with a 10-second breath hold, achieves better particle deposition during that one breath but misses the opportunity to inhale any of the aerosol produced between inhalations.

Nebulizers that actuate on demand, or in coordination with inspiration, are more efficient in delivering the medication nebulized. Intermittent nebulization may increase the treatment time by as much as four-fold for the same volume of medication in the nebulizer but also delivers a comparable increase in medication.

A standard bronchodilator treatment with an SVN often consists of 0.5 mL (2.5 mg) of albuterol with 2 mL of 0.9% NaCl by continuous nebulizer and requires 10 to 20 minutes

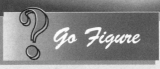

CRITICAL THINKING CHALLENGES
Go Figure

A patient with a tidal volume of 500 mL has an inspiratory time of 1 second and an I/E ratio of 1 : 4 receiving a continuous nebulizer treatment of 4 mL normal saline with 2.5 mg of albuterol at an oxygen flow rate of 8 L/min. What is the patient's respiratory rate, minute volume, and FiO_2? What percentage of the medication (or gas) leaving the nebulizer is inhaled?

If the patient begins 10-second inspiratory holds, what will happen to the respiratory rate, minute ventilation, and percentage of medication inhaled? What happens to the FiO_2?

to nebulize all the medication. If the patient has a normal inspiration/exhalation ratio of 1:3, then 25% of the aerosol leaving the nebulizer is inhaled, and 75% of the drug leaving the nebulizer is not inhaled, passing on to the atmosphere. Breath holding marginally increases deposition of an individual breath, but the decrease in the total amount of medication inhaled with continuous nebulization would be far greater. Under these conditions with continuous nebulization, the standard dose consists of 25% of the aerosol that leaves the nebulizer. With intermittent nebulization,

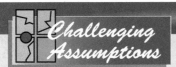

CRITICAL THINKING CHALLENGES
Challenging Assumptions

Do Small-Volume Nebulizer Treatments Add Humidity to the Lungs?

Many clinicians advocate the use of SVNs to add humidity to the lungs. Based on the calculations below, these expectations just don't hold water (at least enough water).

Normally, when we breathe through the nose, the inhaled gas is 85% saturated at body temperature (37 mg/L of water). Mouth breathing is much less efficient in warming and humidifying the inhaled gas in reclaiming heat and humidity during exhalation. When we ask patients to breathe from a nebulizer through a mouthpiece to improve deposition to the lung, we increase the amount of heat and water exhaled.

Question: A standard dose of 0.5 mL of albuterol is mixed with 2 mL of normal saline and placed in an SVN with a dead volume of 0.5 mL. During a 10-minute treatment with 8 L/min O_2, what is the humidity (mg/L) of gas leaving the nebulizer? What is the relative humidity at BTPS?

2 mL = 2000 mg of fluid in 80 L of oxygen (0 mg/L)
Absolute humidity = 2 mL/80 L = 25 mg/L
Capacity at BTPS is 44 mg/L
Relative humidity = absolute humidity/capacity = 25/44 = 57% relative humidity

Using a compressor with 50% relative humidity at room temperature (10 mg/L), the inhaled humidity is 35 mg/L (84% relative humidity BTPS).

Conclusion: SVNs driven by either oxygen or compressed air provide less humidity in the inspired air than the normal level of humidification of gas entering the trachea during normal nose breathing. Less humidity in and more humidity out makes an SVN incapable of meeting the therapeutic objective of adding humidity to the airway. There is no empiric basis to support SVN treatments with normal saline or distilled water to provide humidification.

aerosol is produced only on inspiration, and the same inhaled dose can be achieved with only 25% of the drug volume leaving the nebulizer—same time, less drug.

Providing continuous nebulization also refers to generating aerosol continuously over several hours, with a higher dose of medication, as opposed to administering multiple intermittent standard dose aerosol treatments of 10- to 20-minute duration. This practice is explored later in this chapter.

Intermittent nebulization, using a patient-controlled finger port to direct gas to the nebulizer only during inspiration, provides greater opportunity to deposit more drug in the lung with deep breaths and breath holding. It does, however, increase the duration of treatment by three to five times the normal continuous administration time and requires considerably more patient hand–breath coordination than does continuous nebulization. Drug delivery with continuous nebulization can be enhanced significantly by the use of a reservoir that holds aerosol generated during exhalation. The simple addition of a 50-mL tube as an expiratory reservoir to a nebulizer has long been used to improve drug delivery with SVNs (Fig. 12–7). The Circulaire (Fig. 12–8) uses a larger reservoir bag of 150 mL. The reservoir allows small particles to remain in suspension during exhalation, to be inhaled with the next breath, whereas larger particles "rain out," resulting in greater overall deposition.

Many commercial SVNs are available, with wide variance in design and performance; variability in performance has been seen even among SVNs of the same design.[21] Care should be taken to evaluate the SVN being used. Manufacturers should provide hard data on performance of the nebulizer when operated under different conditions, including with using 100% wall oxygen, compressors, and ventilators. The optimal technique for use of SVNs is described in Box 12–4.

LARGE-VOLUME NEBULIZERS

Large-volume nebulizers can also be used to administer bronchodilators and active medications to the lungs. Large-volume nebulizers are particularly useful when traditional dosing strategies are ineffective in treating severe bronchospasm. In the treatment of acute exacerbations of asthma with bronchodilators, a variety of methods are used to optimize treatment. When the patient with airway obstruction does not respond to standard dosage and frequency of the bronchodilator, the dose may be increased and the treatment administered as frequently as every 15 minutes. An alternative to frequent SVN treatments is to provide continuous nebulization, using a large-volume nebulizer with adequate solution to operate continuously and deliver a controlled rate of medication for an extended period of time. The continuous therapy ensures that the drug not only is delivered frequently enough to optimize

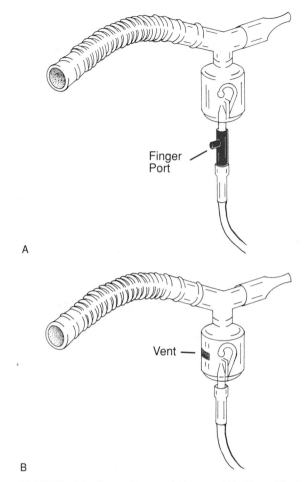

FIGURE 12-7 • Two nebulizers. (*A*) Closed nebulizer with a finger-operated activator valve. Flow is directed to the nebulizer when the finger port is covered by the patient's finger during inspiration and to the atmosphere when the port is released. Gas flow is limited to the flow entering the nebulizer through the inlet jet. (*B*) A vented nebulizer that entrains room air with the jet of compressed gas driving the nebulizer. Note the extension of the exhaust port that also acts as a reservoir of aerosol awaiting the next breath.

bronchodilation but can also be delivered without interruption of aerosol administration to the patient. The bronchodilator can even be delivered while the patient sleeps.

Vortran's High Output Extended Aerosol Respiratory Therapy (HEART) nebulizer (Fig. 12–9) has been used to provide continuous aerosol therapy with bronchodilators and other medications. This nebulizer has a 240-mL reservoir and produces particles between 3.5 and 2.2 µm MMAD. The actual output and particle size vary based on the pressure and flow rate at which the nebulizer operates.[22] A problem with the use of a large-volume nebulizer for continuous treatment is that the concentration of drug increases when used for periods that exceed several hours because of evaporation. The patient receiving continuous bronchodilator therapy must be monitored closely for signs of drug toxicity.

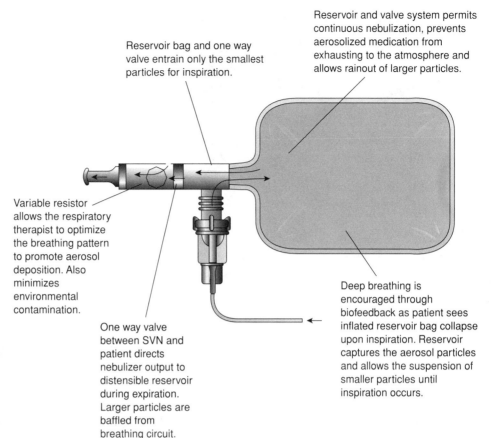

Reservoir bag and one way valve entrain only the smallest particles for inspiration.

Reservoir and valve system permits continuous nebulization, prevents aerosolized medication from exhausting to the atmosphere and allows rainout of larger particles.

Variable resistor allows the respiratory therapist to optimize the breathing pattern to promote aerosol deposition. Also minimizes environmental contamination.

One way valve between SVN and patient directs nebulizer output to distensible reservoir during expiration. Larger particles are baffled from breathing circuit.

Deep breathing is encouraged through biofeedback as patient sees inflated reservoir bag collapse upon inspiration. Reservoir captures the aerosol particles and allows the suspension of smaller particles until inspiration occurs.

FIGURE 12–8 • The Circulaire combines one-way valves, a reservoir, and an expiratory filter to improve the safety and effectiveness of small-volume nebulizer (SVN) therapy. (Courtesy of Westmed, Tucson, AZ.)

Another method for continuous delivery of bronchodilator by large-volume nebulizer is use of an intravenous infusion pump to drip premixed bronchodilator solution into a standard SVN (Fig. 12–10). The high cost and low availability of infusion pumps are disadvantages, but this method appears to be capable of providing a dose each hour that is equivalent to treatments every 15 minutes by SVN using standard dosing[23–31] (Box 12–5).

Metered Dose Inhalers

Metered dose inhalers are the most commonly prescribed method of aerosol delivery in the United States. These devices are pressurized canisters containing a drug, often in the form of a micronized powder, suspended in a mixture of two or more propellants (eg, Freon) along with a dispersal agent. MDIs are the most widely used form of aerosol

---

Box • 12–4   OPTIMAL TECHNIQUE FOR SMALL-VOLUME NEBULIZER USE

1. Assemble apparatus.
2. Mix medication per prescription and add to nebulizer.
3. Ensure that fill volume is between 4 and 6 mL.
4. If SVN is operated continuously, add 50 mL of tubing or other reservoir.
5. Attach gas source, providing adequate gas flow to operate within specification of the nebulizer being used.
6. Position patient in an upright position, sitting or reclining.
7. Through mouthpiece or mask, encourage patient to breathe through mouth.
8. Through artificial or bypassed upper airway, ensure

that nebulizer is positioned appropriately and not placing undue pressure on the airway.

9. Encourage patient to take normal comfortable breaths, with occasional deep breaths, maintaining low inspiratory flow rates.
10. Periodically tap nebulizer to return impacted particles to the reservoir.
11. Assess patient for comfort, adverse effects, and response throughout treatment.
12. When SVN begins to sputter or stops nebulizing, remove from patient and either clean or disinfect, replace, or rinse with sterile water and air dry, properly storing between treatments.

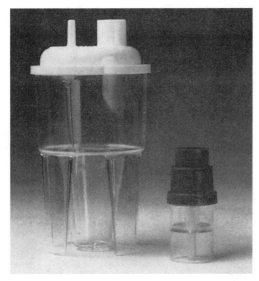

FIGURE 12–9 • The HEART nebulizer is a large-volume nebulizer designed for delivery of medications to the lower respiratory tract. (Courtesy of Vartran.)

Box • 12–5   TECHNIQUE FOR USE OF HIGH-DOSE CONTINUOUS NEBULIZER

1. Assemble equipment (HEART nebulizer, Figs. 12-9 and 12-22; or SVN, Figs. 12-10 and 12-20).
2. Mix and add medication to nebulizer.
3. Apply to patient with mask or adapter to artificial airway.
4. Instruct patient to relax and breathe quietly through the mouth.
5. Monitor patient for adverse effects and clinical response.
6. Ensure that patient has continuous alarmed monitor for heart rate.
7. When patient has achieved desired therapeutic effect, evaluate for switch to lower dose, then periodic therapy.
8. Transfer patient to lower dose.
9. Discontinue continuous therapy.
10. Dispose of excess medication and sterilize or dispose of aerosol equipment

---

device for administration of bronchodilators, anticholinergics, and steroids; more formulations of these drugs are available for use with MDI than for use with other types of nebulizers.

A variety of chemical dispersal agents are used to improve drug delivery by keeping the drug in suspension (Fig. 12–11). The most common dispersal agents are surfactants, such as soya lecithin, sorbitan trioleate, and oleic acid, which help to keep the drug suspended in the Freon and lubricate the valve mechanism. The dispersal agents are present in quantities equal to or greater than the quantity of drug to be administered. The high concentration of the dispersal agent has clinical significance; some patients develop severe cough or wheezing that is caused by the propellant or surfactant, so care must be exercised when initiating therapy by MDI.

Of the spray that comes out of the MDI, 60% to 80% (by weight) consists of the chlorofluorocarbons (CFCs), and < 1% is active drug. The large quantity of CFCs or Freon is also of clinical importance because adverse reactions to CFCs have been reported (when administered in much larger doses than encountered with even aggressive therapy). Freon toxicity would require MDI actuation with more than 20 consecutive breaths. Anecdotal cases of adverse responses to Freon have been reported in adults and children.[32–36]

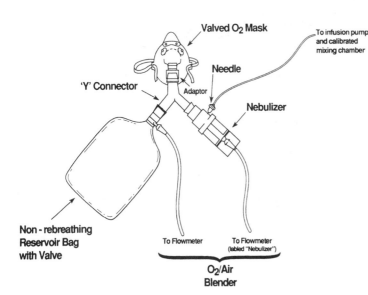

FIGURE 12–10 • Adaptation of a small-volume nebulizer with a needle permitting an infusion pump to allow continuous injection of medication into the nebulizer. Blended oxygen is used to provide a precise FiO$_2$, directed to the nebulizer, and a reservoir from a standard nonrebreathing bag with one-way valve; both are attached to a valved O$_2$ mask (also from a standard nonrebreather oxygen mask). (Moler FW, Johnson CE, Laanen CV, et al: Continuous versus intermittent nebulized terbutaline: Plasma levels and effect. *Am J Respir Crit Care Med.* 1995;151–602.)

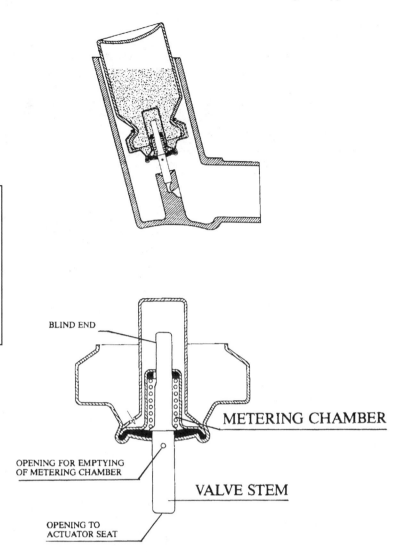

MDI CONTENTS

- drug in suspension or solution
  +
- surfactant (sorbitan trioleate (Span 85)
           or Lecithin
           or oleic acid)
  or co-solvent (ethanol)
  +
- chlorofluorocarbons (F11, F12, F113, F114)
  +
- flavouring agents
  +
- preservatives

BLIND END

METERING CHAMBER

OPENING FOR EMPTYING
OF METERING CHAMBER

VALVE STEM

OPENING TO
ACTUATOR SEAT

FIGURE 12-11 • (*Top*) Longitudinal view of a metered dose inhaler (MDI) with actuator and list of the contents of the MDI. (*Bottom*) Diagram of the metering chamber from MDI. As the MDI is depressed, the cylinder is pushed down one valve stem so that the opening on the stem enters the metering chamber, allowing the contents to pass through to the opening in the actuator seat. (Courtesy of 3M Pharmaceuticals.)

The output volume of MDIs varies from 30 to 100 μL, which contains 50 μg to 5 mg of drug, depending on the drug administered.[3,36] Most MDIs use a 50-μL metering chamber to control drug delivery. Increasing the volume of the chamber does not necessarily improve drug delivery because more of the additional drug is lost at the actuator mouthpiece as a result of the lower rate of evaporation of the greater amount of propellant released.[3]

Aerosol production from an MDI takes about 20 msec. Aerosolization of the liquid released from the MDI canister begins as the propellants vaporize, or "flash," leaving the actuator in a "plume," and continues as the propellant evaporates. The velocity of the liquid spray leaving the MDI is about 15 m/s. The speed falls to less than half the maximum velocity within 0.1 second as a cloud develops and moves away from the actuator orifice.[37] The particles produced from the flashing of propellants are initially 35 μm and rapidly decrease in size as a result of evaporation as the plume of particles moves away from the nozzle[38] (Fig. 12–12).

Because of the velocity and dispersion of the jet fired from the MDI, about 80% of the dose leaving the actuator impacts and deposits in the oropharynx, especially when the canister is fired from inside the mouth.[3,38] Manufacturers of MDIs can alter designs to adjust the particle size delivered by the device to influence drug targeting and subsequent absorption.[39]

DELIVERY CHARACTERISTICS

The MMAD of the aerosol produced by most MDIs is between 3 and 6 μm,[40] with a deposition in the lung of about 10% to 20%.[41,42] As much as 80% of the dose is deposited in the mouth; this may be a factor in systemic absorption as

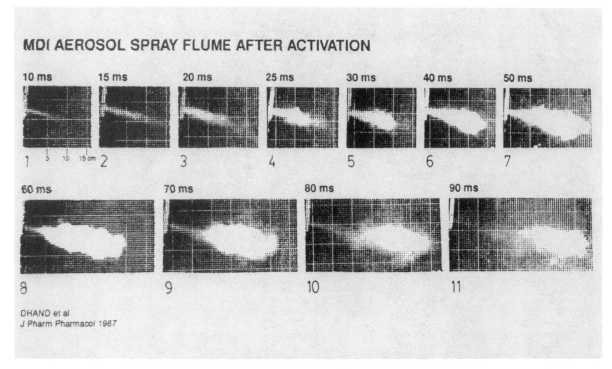

MDI AEROSOL SPRAY FLUME AFTER ACTIVATION

DHAND et al
J Pharm Pharmacol 1987

FIGURE 12–12 • High-speed photography of plume development from a metered dose inhaler after actuation. (Dhand R, Malik SK, Balakrishian M, Verma SK. High speed photographic analysis of aerosols produced by metered dose inhalers. *J Pharm Pharmacol,* 1988;40:429–430.)

opposed to direct aerosol delivery to the lung because the MDI delivers a significant amount of drug to the mucous membranes of the mouth and stomach. Unfortunately, the actual amount of drug delivered to an individual patient is unpredictable because of significant interpatient variability.[39] A number of studies have documented the clinical efficacy of MDIs.[43–46] MDIs have been demonstrated to be at least as effective as other nebulizers used for drug delivery. As a result, they are often the preferred method for delivering bronchodilators to spontaneously breathing as well as intubated, ventilated patients.[47,48]

The MDI has become a common method by which to deliver drugs to the lung. The device is available to administer all commonly used bronchodilators and steroids. The successful administration of medications by MDI is technique dependent. The patient must coordinate actuation of the MDI with early inspiration. The usual recommended method of delivery is to have the patient exhale slowly to residual volume before inspiration and to close the lips tightly around the MDI actuator. Actuating the MDI immediately after beginning a breath with a slow inspiratory flow (less than 30 L/min) and ending with a breath hold of 10 seconds is reported to optimize lung deposition.[49–51]

Investigators have shown increased deposition in the lung when the MDI is placed 4 cm from an open mouth position[42,51,52] (Fig. 12–13). This technique improves lung deposition while decreasing oral deposition. The lung volume at which the aerosol is inhaled, beginning at resid-

ual volume, functional residual capacity, or 80% of total lung capacity, apparently does not significantly affect the amount of aerosol deposited in the lung or the clinical response to the bronchodilator.[53] It is possible that, for patients with unstable airways, exhaling to residual volume could result in closure of airways and reduction of distribution of the next inhaled breath of aerosol to the lung. If true, the preferred technique might be normal exhalation to functional residual capacity before inspiration and actuation of the MDI (Box 12–6).

Oral deposition of drug delivered by MDI, as with small-volume jet and ultrasonic nebulizers, can account for as much as 80% of the dose of the drug being nebulized. This medication is then swallowed and absorbed in the gastrointestinal tract or is absorbed by the mucous membranes, producing greater systemic side effects.

The worst commonly reported side effect of oral deposition with MDI is increased oral thrush or opportunistic yeast infections associated with the use of inhaled steroids. Rinsing the mouth after steroid administration is recommended to reduce effects of oral deposition. Unfortunately, the greatest amount of drug deposits at the point of greatest turbulence en route to the lower respiratory tract (the larynx), which cannot be reached effectively by gargling (most people tend to gag when gargling that far back in their throat).

Twenty-four to 67% of previously instructed patients use improper MDI inhalation technique. This appears to correlate with findings that as many as 65% of physicians

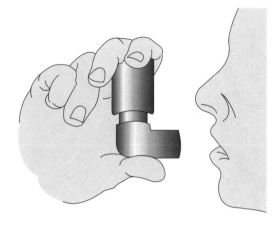

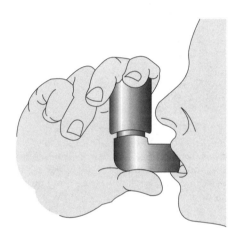

FIGURE 12–13 • Illustration of open- and closed-mouth techniques for MDI administration, without accessory device. Open-mouth technique reduces oropharyngeal deposition.

1. Warm MDI to hand or body temperature.
2. Assemble apparatus (make sure there are no objects or coins in device that could be aspirated or obstruct outflow).
3. Shake canister vigorously.
4. Hold canister upright, placing actuator 4 cm (two fingers) away from open mouth (aimed directly into mouth); an alternative is to place actuator between lips, but this increases oral deposition.
5. After a normal exhalation, begin to inspire slowly (< 30 L/min) while actuating MDI.
6. Continue inspiration to total lung capacity.
7. Hold breath for 10 seconds.
8. Wait 1 minute between actuations.

and nurses involved in outpatient instruction of patients with MDI were unable to perform more than four of seven steps of MDI administration properly.[54] Proper patient instruction is essential even though time-consuming, requiring 10 to 28 minutes for initial instruction. Repeated instruction improves performance but must occur several times.[55–57] Even with the best instruction, some patients, especially infants, young children, and patients in acute distress, may be unable to coordinate proper administration; under these circumstances, accessory devices such as holding chambers should be considered.

ACCESSORY DEVICES

Accessory devices have been used with MDIs to reduce oropharyngeal deposition and to reduce or eliminate the need for hand–breath coordination. These devices have markedly improved the therapeutic efficacy of MDIs and have broadened their usefulness in acute and critical care environments. Accessory devices have been critical to making MDIs consistently equivalent in clinical effect to SVNs.

Spacers and holding chambers are the most common and effective accessory devices for use with MDIs. Spacers provide space between the MDI and the patient for the aerosolized medication, or plume, to expand and for the CFCs to evaporate before reaching the oropharynx, allowing the larger particles leaving the MDI to impact in the walls of the device, reducing oropharyngeal deposition.[58] Inexpensive spacers include homemade options, such as an open-ended, straight tube (eg, an empty tube from a toilet paper roll); small plastic bag; length of aerosol tubing; or even a modified bleach or milk bottle. More sophisticated, commercially available devices, such as the Optihaler, have been better studied and shown to provide a similar dose to the lung as optimal technique with MDI alone, but with much less oral deposition (Fig. 12–14). This effect is less certain with the previously described homemade spacers. Even with a spacer, MDIs require considerable coordination of actuation with breathing pattern. Exhalation immediately after actuation clears the aerosol from the spacer device, wasting the dose to the atmosphere. The open-air type of spacer (eg, Synchronizer) does not contain the aerosol at all, depending entirely on coordinated patient technique for drug delivery.[59]

Holding chambers are similar to spacers in that they allow the plume to develop and reduce oropharyngeal deposition with the addition of a valve or enclosure that holds the aerosol. Holding chambers permit the aerosol to be drawn from the chamber on inspiration, preventing the remaining aerosol in the chamber from being cleared on exhalation. The use of the chamber permits patients with small tidal volumes to empty aerosol from the chamber with successive (usually three) breaths. Using a holding chamber, the patient can exhale into the mouthpiece or

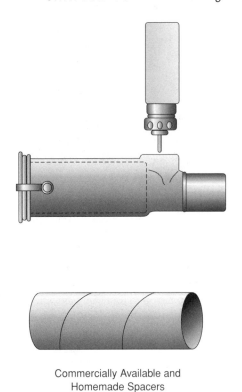

Commercially Available and
Homemade Spacers

FIGURE 12–14 • Two spacer devices that reduce oral
pharyngeal deposition. (*Top*) Commercially available Optihaler. (*Bottom*) Commonly available toilet paper roll. Neither
device ensures dose delivery with poor hand–breath coordination.

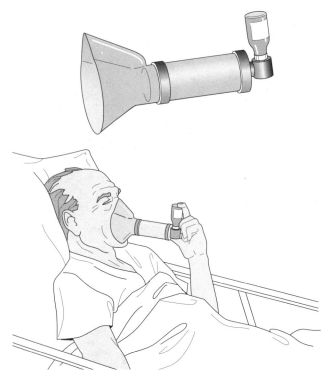

FIGURE 12–15 • Holding chambers are spacers that
use a one-way valve to hold aerosol in the chamber between
inspirations, to minimize the loss of dose inhaled because of
poor hand–breath coordination. (*Top*) Patient uses a holding
chamber with mask. (*Bottom*) Three chambers with one-way
valves and indicators to signal patient when inspiratory flow
rate is too high for optimal deposition. (*Bottom*, Fink J, Cohen N: Humidity and aerosols. In: Eubank D, Bone R: *Principles and Applications of Cardiorespiratory Care Equipment.*
St. Louis: Mosby–Year Book; 1994.)

mask as the MDI is actuated, without blowing away much
of the medication (Fig. 12–15). The InspirEase uses a collapsible bag, rather than a one-way valve, to contain the
aerosol.

Spacers and holding chambers improve the use of MDIs
for delivery of bronchodilators and inhaled steroids. Spacers and holding chambers tend to reduce oral deposition,
reduce bad taste of medication, and reduce the cold Freon
effect that causes many children to stop inhalation with
MDI actuation (when the cold discharge reaches the back
of the throat). Medication delivered to the lower respiratory tract with reduced oropharyngeal deposition results in
a greatly improved therapeutic index. Both accessory
devices provide comparable advantages for the patient
who *can* coordinate MDI discharge with optimal breath
control.[60]

So why would a patient need a holding chamber rather
than a spacer? Many patients, with repeated training, can
demonstrate good technique and hand–breath coordination
when they are feeling well. Unfortunately, when the
breathing becomes difficult, the hand–breath coordination
can suffer, resulting in less drug being delivered to the airway at the very time it is needed the most. Figure 12–16
shows results from an in vitro comparison of a simple tube
spacer to a valved holding chamber with actuation of the
MDI synchronized to the beginning of inspiration, 1 second before inspiration, and actuation during exhalation.

The valved holding chamber protected the patient from
losing drug dose, due to poor hand–breath coordination,
better than did the spacer. We provide all of our moderate
and severe asthmatic patients with holding chambers for
their MDIs and teach them to use the MDI both ways. Patients are instructed to use the holding chamber with the
MDI whenever they feel short of breath. Many of these patients find that they get much better relief from the MDI
with holding chamber than from the MDI alone. It is not
uncommon for patients who have been "abusing" the MDI
with minimal relief to come to the emergency department
and have their airways cleared with the addition of the
holding chamber.

Holding chambers with masks that cover the patient's
nose and mouth are available for use with infants, children,
and adults with excellent results (see Fig. 12–15). These
units allow effective administration of aerosol from MDI to
patients who are unable to use a mouthpiece device because
of their size, age, coordination, or mentation.[60–62] The use of
the MDI with a holding chamber is at least as effective a
method of delivering drugs as is the use of SVN.[63–65]

The use of the holding chamber is particularly helpful
when administering steroids because deposition of drug in

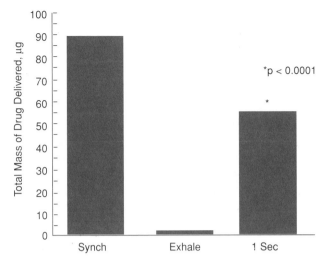

A: Tube Spacer

*p < 0.0001

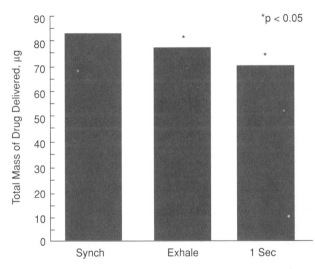

B: Valved holding chamber

FIGURE 12–16 • Comparison of tube spacer with valved holding chamber during dysynchrony.

*p < 0.05

Box • 12–7 OPTIMAL TECHNIQUE FOR USE OF METERED DOSE INHALER WITH HOLDING CHAMBER

1. Warm MDI to hand or body temperature.
2. Assemble apparatus (make sure there are no objects or coins in device that could be aspirated or obstruct outflow).
3. Shake canister vigorously and hold upright.
4. Place holding chamber in mouth (or place mask over nose and mouth), encouraging patient to breathe through mouth.
5. Instruct patient to breathe normally. Actuate MDI at the beginning of inspiration and instruct patient to continue to breathe through the device for three breaths. (*Note:* Larger breaths with breath holding may be encouraged in a patient who can cooperate, but this has not been shown to increase clinical response to inhaled bronchodilators.)
6. Allow 30 to 60 seconds between actuations.

MDI canister is spring loaded in preparation for firing by cocking a lever at the top of the unit. A vane is moved when the patient-generated flow is more than 20 to 60 L/min, causing the canister to be pressed down into the actuator, firing the MDI. This device addresses hand–breath coordination problems with bronchodilator administration, but it remains unclear whether it requires use of a spacer or holding chamber to reduce pharyngeal deposition. The Autohaler can be breath actuated only. Thus, during acute exacerbation of asthma, the patient may not be able to generate sufficient flows to actuate the MDI. Patients with possible periodic severe airway obstruction should have a

the mouth is largely eliminated and systemic side effects can be minimized.[66,67] Even with a holding chamber, respirable particles containing drug settle out and deposit within the device. This is about the same amount as would normally settle in the patients mouth and is seen as a white buildup within the chamber. This drug in the chamber or spacer poses no risk to the patient but may be rinsed out periodically (ie, once a week). Interestingly, after washing out a chamber or spacer, it is less effective for the next few puffs, until the electrostatic charge on the walls of the chamber is once again reduced to normal. Use of standard dish soap reduces this static charge. Consequently, routine cleaning is not recommended in the optimal technique (Box 12–7).

The Autohaler is another device designed to reduce the need for hand–breath coordination in MDI administration by flow-triggered actuation of an MDI in response to patient inspiratory effort. As shown in Figure 12–17, the

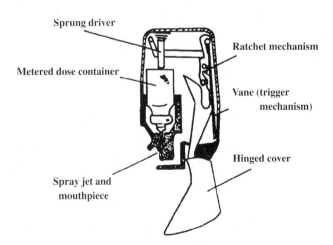

FIGURE 12–17 • Autohaler (3M) uses a spring-loaded mechanism with a vane-trigger mechanism. When patient inhales, the vane is moved, allowing the metered dose canister to be pressed down and actuated. The spring must be reset after each puff. (*Respir Care.* 1991;36[11].)

manually operated MDI or nebulizer available to provide bronchodilator resuscitation. The ability to fire the MDI manually, independent of patient's ability to generate specific flow rates, would allow broader application for the breath-actuated MDI in patients who experience periodic life-threatening increases in airway obstruction. The Autohaler is currently available only with pirbuterol, a β-adrenergic receptor bronchodilator that is similar to albuterol.

The association of CFCs with degradation of the earth's atmosphere and ozone layer has resulted in an international treaty banning the use of CFCs. An exception was made for use of CFCs in MDIs because of the prolonged process required for regulatory approvals of new MDIs using other propellants. HFAs are more environmentally friendly and provide comparable drug bioavailability. Due to differences in actuator designs, use of third-party actuator devices may reduce the respirable drug available from a MDI.

Dry-Powder Inhalers

Dry-powder inhalers are another form of MDI. Inhalation of drug in a crystalline or powder form has become increasingly popular because this delivery system is relatively inexpensive, does not depend on the use of CFCs, and does not require the hand–breath coordination required for use of MDIs. Aerosols of dry powder are created by drawing air though an aliquot of a powder (Fig. 12–18).

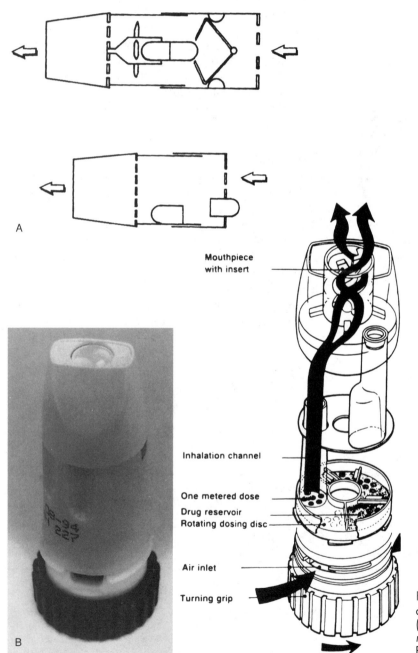

A

Mouthpiece with insert

Inhalation channel

One metered dose

Drug reservoir

Rotating dosing disc

Air inlet

Turning grip

B

FIGURE 12–18 • Four types of dry-powder inhalers available in the United States. ([A], Scanlon: *Egan's Fundamentals of Respiratory Care.* 6th ed., St. Louis: Mosby–Year Book; 1995.)

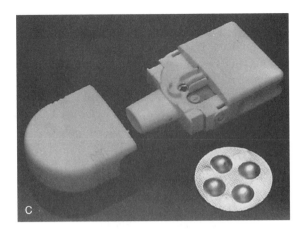

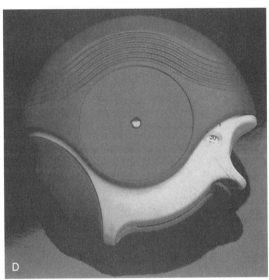

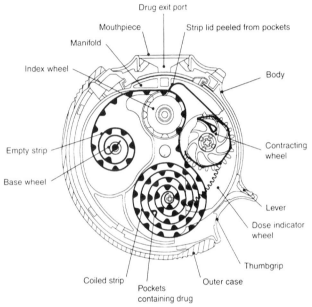

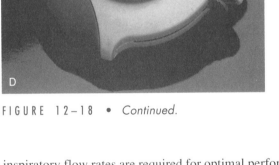

FIGURE 12-18 • *Continued.*

High inspiratory flow rates are required for optimal performance and results in pharyngeal impaction of carrier while drug is inhaled. The clinical efficacy of drugs delivered by DPI appears to be similar to that of MDIs, particularly when the MDI is used without an accessory chamber.[68]

A variety of factors influence drug delivery by DPI. DPIs are breath actuated, and relatively high inspiratory flow rates are required to release the powder as respirable particles.[69,70] The required high inspiratory flow rates required for use of DPIs make them unsuitable for use by small children and patients who cannot achieve flow rates of 0.5 to 1 L/s or greater. DPIs usually are restricted to use for prophylactic and maintenance therapy. They are not acceptable for use during an acute bronchospastic episode and generally are not recommended for infants and children younger than 6 years (because normal inspiratory flow rates for children younger than 6 years is below operating threshold).[71] For maintenance therapy, however, DPIs are preferred by many adults and older children.

Although hand–breath coordination is not as important an issue with DPIs as with MDIs, coordination in use of the device can influence drug delivery. Exhalation into some device can result in loss of drug delivered to the lung. Some devices require assembly, which can be cumbersome or difficult for some patients.

High humidity can also affect drug availability from DPIs. The hygroscopic powder clumps when exposed to high humidity, creating larger particles that are inhaled less effectively. Drugs delivered by DPI are carried in lactose or glucose. The drug particle size ranges from 1 to 2 μm, whereas the carrier has a particle size of about 20 to 25 μm. Most of the carrier impacts in the oropharynx, where it can cause irritation. DPIs may not be reliable when used by patients with artificial airways, either endotracheal or tracheotomy tubes.

Several DPIs use individual doses administered as gelatin capsules that are punctured before inhalation (Spinhaler, Rotohaler) or individual blister packets of drug

---

Box • 12–8   TECHNIQUE FOR USE OF DRY-POWDER INHALER

1. Assemble apparatus.
2. Load dose—insert and open capsule.
3. Exhale slowly to functional residual capacity.
4. Seal lips around mouthpiece.
5. Inhale rapidly (more than 60 L/min breath-hold not necessary).
6. Repeat process until capsule is empty.
7. Monitor adverse reactions.
8. Assess beneficial effects.

(Diskhaler). The Turbohaler, Diskhaler, and Diskus inhaler provide multidose preloaded powder systems with up to 200 doses of drug (Box 12–8).

Ultrasonic Nebulizers

An ultrasonic nebulizer uses a piezoelectric crystal vibrated at a high frequency (greater than 1 MHz) to create an aerosol. The crystal transducer, composed of substances such as quartz-barium titanate, converts electricity into sound. The beam of sound is focused in the liquid above the transducer, creating waves in the liquid immediately above the transducer. If the frequency is high enough and the amplitude of the signal strong enough, the oscillation waves crest, disrupting the surface of the liquid and creating a "geyser" of droplets.

Large-volume ultrasonic nebulizers usually have the transducer built into an apparatus that includes multiple electronic components (Fig. 12–19). These devices include relatively inexpensive medication cups for individual patient use, eliminating the need to sterilize the entire apparatus between patients, with a bath of water serving as a couplant between the transducer and the medication being nebulized. The medication cup, with a flexible diaphragm on the bottom, is seated into a couplant chamber filled with enough water to allow a firm water seal between transducer and cup. This water conducts the sound energy to the diaphragm or cup bottom, which in turn vibrates the medication to produce an aerosol. The water used as couplant must be changed regularly and the unit cleaned to minimize contamination from direct physical contact with the nebulizer and medication cups between treatments.

Ultrasonic nebulizers tend to have higher outputs (0.5 to 7 mL/min) and higher mist density than conventional jet nebulizers. The particle or droplet size (MMAD) delivered by an ultrasonic nebulizer is related to the frequency at which the crystals vibrate. The frequency usually is specific to the device selected and rarely is adjustable by the user. The particle size is inversely proportional to frequency. For example, the DeVilbiss Portasonic operates at a frequency of 2.25 MHz and produces an MMAD of 2.5 µm, whereas the DeVilbiss Pulmosonic operates at 1.25 MHz and produces a less respirable particle range of 4 to 6 µm. The greater the amplitude, the greater the output from the nebulizer, up to the limit of the device design. Increases in amplitude beyond the specified upper limit do not improve device output.

Particle size and aerosol density are also affected by the source and flow of gas that conducts the aerosols from the nebulizer to the patient. If the nebulizer is producing a steady output of particles, the greater the flow of gas through the chamber, and the more dilute are the same number of particles in the larger volume of gas. The faster the flow of gas, the greater is the chance that large particles will be driven out of the nebulizer before they can coalesce with other particles and settle out, increasing both particle size and output. Low flow rates are associated with smaller particles and higher density of mist. High flow rates yield larger particles and less density. Unlike jet nebulizers, the temperature of the solution placed in the ultrasonic nebu-

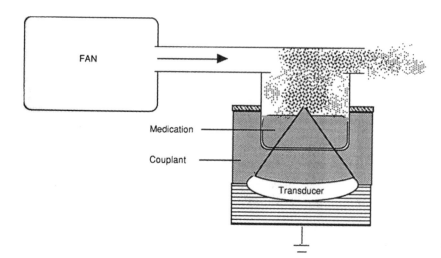

FIGURE 12–19 • An ultrasonic nebulizer uses electricity to vibrate a transducer at high frequency, producing ultra–high-frequency sound waves that disrupt the surface of the medication, creating an aerosol. In larger units, water, an excellent conductor of sound, is used as a couplant between the transducer and the medication in a thin plastic cup. A fan may be used to propel the aerosol from the chamber to the patient. (Eubank D, Bone R: *Principles and Applications of Cardiorespiratory Care Equipment.* St. Louis: Mosby-Year Book, 1994).

lizer increases during use. As the temperature increases, the drug concentration rises, increasing the likelihood of undesired side effects.

The larger commercial units use low-flow blowers, which can deliver either air or other compressed gases by a flowmeter. A blender can be added to the delivery system to control the delivered gas concentration more precisely. Aerosol tubing, a mask, or a mouthpiece can be used to administered the ultrasonically nebulized solution.

Smaller ultrasonic nebulizers have been designed for individual patient use. They may not use water-filled couplants between transducer and medication. Medication is placed directly into the manifold in direct contact with the transducer. The transducer is connected by cable or connector to a power source, often battery-powered, to increase portability. The small nebulizers that incorporate the transducer manifold at the patient's airway rely on the patient's inspiratory flow rate to draw the aerosol from nebulizer to the lung.

Many different ultrasonic nebulizers are available. The particle size and output from the nebulizers vary considerably among devices; some are capable of producing particle sizes up to 12 μm.

The primary use of the ultrasonic nebulizer is to induce sputum for diagnostic purposes. Small-volume ultrasonic nebulizers have been promoted for bronchodilator therapy in nursing homes or other extended care facilities as an alternative to pneumatically driven SVNs. Most small-volume ultrasonic nebulizers have less dead space than do SVNs, reducing the need for a large quantity of diluent to ensure drug delivery. The contained portable power source adds convenience and mobility. Both these advantages of the ultrasonic devices, however, are outweighed by their high cost, which can be up to 10 times the cost of pneumatic SVNs and 100 times the cost of treatment with MDIs or DPIs. In fact, the primary limitation of the use of ultrasonic nebulizers is their cost, which ranges from $150 to more than $1000.

Ultrasonic nebulizers have also been used to administer undiluted bronchodilators to patients with severe bronchospasm.[72] Because these nebulizers have minimal dead space, the treatment time is shortened. Use of undiluted bronchodilator is typically included in the manufacturer's product dosing information found in the *Physician's Desk Reference*. Because the ultrasonic nebulizer manifold is expensive, some practitioners have suggested a technique that entails using a one-way valve between the medication chamber and mouthpiece so that multiple patients can be treated consecutively without concern about infection. It is yet to be confirmed that a simple one-way valve manifold is adequate protection against contamination of the medication chamber; in addition, contact with infectious secretions on the outside of the nebulizer manifold could result in transmission of pathogens from one patient to another.[73]

The use of ultrasonic nebulizers is associated with a number of potential complications, including overhydration, bronchospasm, infection, and disruption of the drug structure when used to administer medications.[74,75] Over-

hydration can result from the large fluid output from the nebulizers and their potential to deliver small particles to the lung parenchyma directly. Overhydration is of greatest risk after prolonged treatment of newborns, small children, and patients with fluid and electrolyte imbalances. In addition to overhydration of the patient, pulmonary secretions can swell after treatment with an ultrasonic nebulizer.

Bronchospasm can also occur after treatment with an ultrasonic nebulizer. The delivery of cold high-density aerosols has been associated with increased airway resistance and irritability in a number of patients. In addition, sterile water administered through the ultrasonic nebulizer is known to be more irritating than normal saline.[76]

Medications administered by ultrasonic nebulizer can become more concentrated during treatment because the solvent evaporates at a faster rate than the drug. Ultrasonic nebulizers have been known to disrupt the structure of medications. Nebulizers with an acoustic output of greater than 50 watts/cm² cause changes in the structure of aerosolized medications. If the power output of the nebulizer is 50 watts/cm² or less and the aerosol output is less than 2 mL/min, the nebulizers are reported to be safe when used to deliver medications.[77]

Device Selection to Administer Bronchodilators (and Other Drugs) to the Lungs

Metered dose inhalers with holding chambers are the most convenient, versatile, and cost-effective way to deliver aerosol and should be the first choice for delivery when the required drug formulation is available (Fig. 12–20). DPIs are a viable alternative with the subset of medications available for patients who can generate the required flow rates. Because delivering multiple doses makes administration more time-consuming, SVNs or continuous nebulizers are a viable alternative in patients with that need. Table 12–2 presents a comparison of devices used to deliver bronchodilators to the lungs.

Selection of the appropriate aerosol delivery device is largely dependent on the drug to be delivered, the volume of output required, and the intended site of action. Particles smaller than 1.8 μm are targeted to the lung parenchyma, and devices such as the SPAG or a well-baffled SVN may be the nebulizer of choice in these cases. Bland aerosols with MMADs larger than 5 μm may best be targeted by bland aerosols to the upper airway, 1 to 5 μm particles used for sputum inductions, and 2 to 10 μm particles (by heated bland aerosol) to treat a bypassed upper airway (Table 12–3).

In the current economic environment, none of us can ignore the costs of the aerosol delivery strategy chosen. Table 12–4 presents the costs of aerosol therapy using MDI with holding chamber and SVN, evaluated in terms of initial costs, individual treatments, initial treatment, and daily costs for every-4-hour treatments for 7 days. Although the MDI with holding chamber has the higher initial set-up costs, the costs at the end of day 1 are comparable between

Aerosol Device Selection

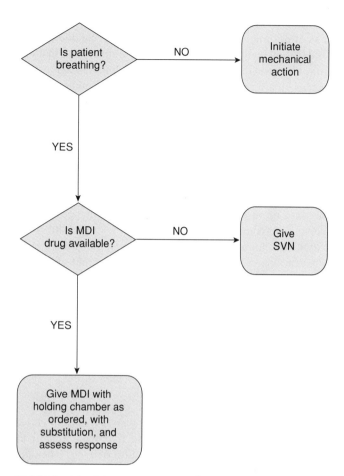

FIGURE 12–20 • Decision-making tree for device selection between metered dose inhaler (MDI) and small-volume nebulizer (SVN).

Table • 12–3 EFFECT OF PARTICLE SIZE ON AEROSOL DELIVERY DEVICE SELECTION

Device	MMAD	GSD
Jet Nebulizers		
Respirgard II	0.93	1.8
Centimist	1.1	2.2
Aerotech II	2.0	2.5
Fan JET	4.3	2.5
Vortran HEART	3.5–2.2	1.8–2.1
MedicAid Sidestream	2.75–3.0	
Devilbiss 646		
6 L/min	6.0	
12 L/min	3.7	
Ultrasonic Nebulizers		
FISO Neb	5.0	2
Green Machine	>12.0	
Portasonic	1.6	2.2
Pulmosonic	4.2	2.3
DeVilbiss 900	2.8	2.1

Device	MMAD	Output
Metered dose inhalers	2.4	100–250 g/breath
Rotahaler	2.6	100–250 g/breath
Jet nebulizer	2–5	0.25–0.4 mL/min
Baffled jet nebulizer	0.25–4.0	0.1–1.0 mL/min
Ultrasonic nebulizer	1.6–12	6 mL/min
Hydrosphere	1.2–4	7 mL/min

MMAD, mean mass aerodynamic diameter; GSD, geometric standard deviation.
Adapted from Fallot, *Respir Care*. 1991;36(9):1011.

therapies, and the MDI with holding chamber gains a clear cost advantage after the first 24 hours.

SPECIAL CONSIDERATIONS

Bronchodilator Resuscitation

Patients often arrive at the emergency department with severe exacerbation of asthma or acute bronchospasm.

Table • 12–2 COMPARISON OF CHARACTERISTICS OF TYPES OF NEBULIZERS FOR ADMINISTRATION OF MEDICATIONS TO THE LUNG

Characteristic	MDI With Holding Chamber	SVN	DPI	USN	MDI Alone
Flow independent	+++	+++	−	+++	−
Volume independent	+++	+++	−−	+++	−
Coordination independent	+++	+++	+	++	−
Low oral deposition	+++	−	−	−	−
Ease of use	+++	+++	+++	++	++
Portable	+++	+	+++	+	+++
Quick to administer	+++	+	+++	+	+++
Low cost	++	−	++	−−	+++
Low infection risk	+++	−−	+++	−−	+++
Effective with:					
Severe asthma	+++	+++	+	+	+
Small children	+++	+++	−	++	−
Ventilators	++++	++	−−	+++	−
Unusual medication	−−	+++	−−	+	−−

MDI, metered dose inhaler; SVN, small-volume nebulizer; DPI, dry-powder inhaler; USN, ultrasonic nebulizer; +, positive characteristic; −, negative characteristic.

Table • 12–4   COMPARATIVE COSTS OF BRONCHODILATOR DELIVERY FOR INDIVIDUAL TREATMENTS

Itemization	Metered Dose Inhaler	Small-Volume Nebulizer	
Equipment	$4.00 (chamber)	$1 (neb - changed daily)	
Medication	$6.00 (200 puffs)		
Cost/treatment	$0.12 (4 puffs)	$0.28 (albuterol + NS) standard $0.56 ($\times 2$) and $1.40 ($\times 5$)	
Personnel			
Time	2 min @ $20/h	5 min	10 min
Cost	$0.66	$1.65	$3.30
Cost/treatment (time and medication)	$0.78	$2.21	$4.70
First treatment set-up (equipment, medication, and 30 min staff time)	$20.00	$11.56	$12.40
Daily treatment costs (time, medication, and equipment)	$3.96*	$14.26	$29.20
Cumulative costs, q 4 h treatment			
Day 1 (with set-up)	$23.33	$22.61	$35.90
Day 2	$27.29	$36.87	$65.10
Day 3	$31.25	$51.13	$94.30
Day 5	$39.17	$79.65	$162.70
Day 7	$47.09	$108.17	$221.10

*Medication for first 9 days is included in startup cost.

These patients typically were taking their β-agonist before presentation to the emergency department and fail to respond to a standard dose of β-agonist from either SVN or MDI in the emergency department. A common response is to order another nebulizer treatment with a standard dose of bronchodilator and to continue ordering treatments at high frequency until the patient responds. This strategy may require several hours of delay in giving the patient relief and hours of additional staff time in treating the patient.

Several alternative strategies of bronchodilator resuscitation have been advocated, including high-dose MDI treatment, high-dose continuous nebulizer treatment, and administration of undiluted bronchodilators. It is important to remember that bronchodilators *relieve* symptoms, and the goal is to provide the patient with relief of respiratory distress, with the greatest improvement in airflow in the shortest period of time and with a minimum of toxic side effects while waiting for the steroids to "kick in."

A standard SVN treatment with 2.5 mg of albuterol takes about 10 minutes to administer. When the patient fails to respond, end-on-end treatments may be ordered until the airway is cleared. A patient with severe exacerbation of asthma may receive up to six treatments in 1 hour, or a nebulizer dosage of 15 mg of albuterol in 1 hour. Papo and colleagues[78] described a method of continuous nebulization (Fig. 12–21) in which a Harvard pump is adjusted to inject an albuterol and saline mixture into an SVN. A blender and humidifier are incorporated to control oxygen concentration with a high level of humidity. These investigators found that continuous nebulization in children, as compared with SVN, reduced the duration of hospital stay ($P < 0.04$), duration of therapy, and therapist time ($P < 0.001$) and provided greater re-

duction in asthma score within 1 hour of therapy (Fig. 12–22). Moler and associates[79] described an SVN system using an infusion pump to fill the nebulizer continuously and a valved oxygen mask and reservoir bag (see Fig. 12–10).

A less equipment-intensive approach incorporates the use of a large-volume nebulizer, such as the HEART nebulizer, as shown in Figure 12–23. A 20-mL bottle of albuterol solution is mixed with 180 mL of 0.09% NaCl, and dose is regulated roughly by the flow rate driving the nebulizer (for example 10 L/min delivers 10 mg/h and 15 L/min

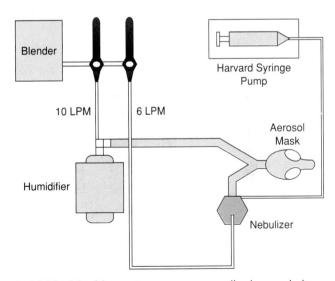

FIGURE 12–21 • Device using a small-volume nebulizer to deliver continuous nebulization. (Papo MC, Frank J, Thompson AE: A prospective, randomized study of continuous versus intermittent nebulized albuterol for severe status asthmaticus in children. *Crit Care Med.* 1993;21[10]:1479–86.)

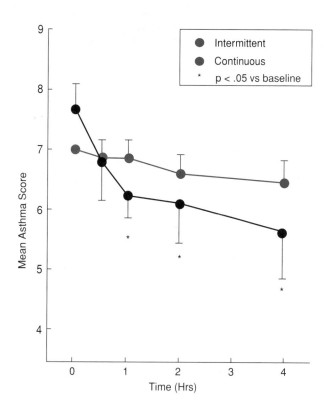

Large Volume (Heart) Nebulizer

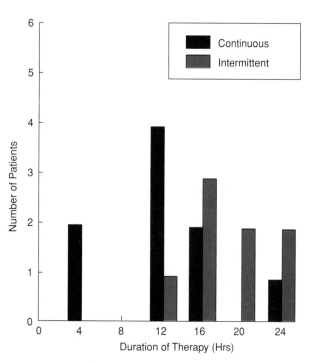

With 20 ml of albuterol solution
and 180 ml of NS

10 LPM = 10 mg/hr.

FIGURE 12–23 • Diagram of setup with HEART nebulizer.

FIGURE 12–22 • Data comparing intermittent with continuous nebulization of bronchodilators with a mean asthma score during the first 4 hours of administration (*A*) and the duration of aerosol therapy required by each patient (*B*). (Papo MC, Frank J, Thompson AE: A prospective randomized study of continuous versus intermittent nebulized albuterol for severe status asthmaticus in children. *Crit Care Med.* 1993;21[10]:1479–1486.)

at 15 mg/h). Patients are placed in monitored beds with electrocardiogram and pulse oximeter. If treatment extends beyond 3 hours, serum potassium should be monitored, with repetition every 4 hours. Lin and colleagues[80] studied the effects of such dosage levels and found minimal toxicity when used in the treatment of acute exacerbation of asthma.

In a double-blind, randomized, placebo-controlled study, high-dose MDI treatment (24 puffs/h) or 15 mg/h of albuterol by HEART nebulizer was administered to 40 adult patients for 3 hours in the emergency department of an urban tertiary-care medical center.[81] Most patients in both treatment arms presented with peak flows that were less than 25% of predicted value and experienced 100% to 300% improvement in peak flows or FEV_1/FVC within the 3-hour treatment period (Fig. 12–24). Forty percent of the patients did not require therapy for the full 3 hours, and more than 60% of the patients were discharged home with no readmission within 78 hours. None of the patients required intubation and mechanical ventilation secondary to the asthma. The investigators concluded that treatment by high-dose MDI with holding chamber and by continuous nebulization of albuterol were equally safe and effective.

If we accept the premise that all of these methods of high-dose administration of albuterol have similar clinical effectiveness and safety, the choice of method should be based on other criteria. Cost, quick response to care, patient comfort, and education consistency should be considered. Figure 12–25 presents an algorithm for bronchodilator resuscitation; Table 12–5 shows the relative costs of the three methods.

Continuous Neb - % Baseline

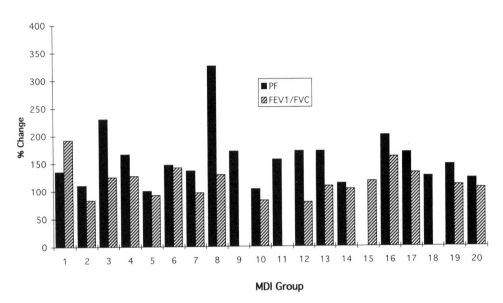

MDI Group

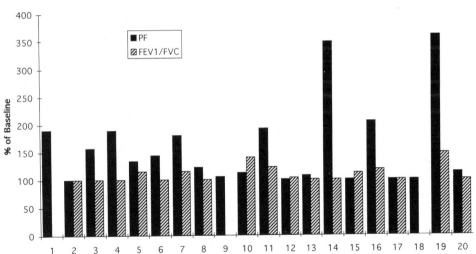

FIGURE 12-24 • Changes from baseline for patients treated with high-dose bronchodilator therapy by continuous nebulizer and metered dose inhaler (MDI) with holding chamber. There was no statistical difference between treatment groups. (Levitt MA, Gambrioli EF, Fink JB: Comparative trial of continuous nebulization versus metered-dose inhaler in the treatment of acute bronchospasm. *Ann Emerg Med.* 1995;26[3]:273–277.)

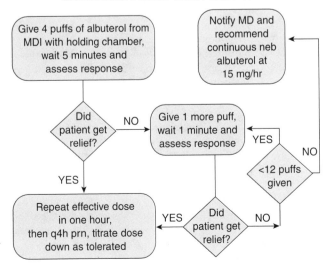

FIGURE 12-25 • Algorithm for bronchodilator resuscitation.

Table • 12–5   COMPARATIVE COSTS OF BRONCHODILATOR DELIVERY DURING ACUTE EXACERBATION FOR 3 HOURS OF TREATMENT

Itemization	Continuous Nebulizer*	Metered Dose Inhaler	Small-Volume Nebulizer
Equipment	$10 (HEART nebulizer)	$6.00 (spacer)	$1 (neb)
Medication	$9.50[†]	$6.00[‡]	$2.67[§]
Personnel			
Time	20 min 1st h + 10 min/h	45 min 1st h + 15 min each hours 2 and 3	15 min ×9 treatments
Cost	$13.33	$25.00	$45.00
Total costs	$32.83	$37.00	$48.67

Results: Continuous nebulizer and MDI with holding chamber are comparable in total costs as well as efficacy. Increased equipment and medication costs with continuous nebulizer are offset by reduced time required by the care giver at the bedside. Labor costs for each of the first 3 hours drive SVN administration costs to more than 150% of continuous nebulizer or MDI with holding chamber, with no greater clinical benefit.

*All patients on continuous nebulizer should be monitored closely during administration. Costs of electrocardiogram and pulse oximetry have not been added.

†Medication costs for continuous nebulizer include 20 mL of albuterol solution mixed with 180 mL of 0.9% NaCl.

‡Reflects costs of an MDI canister containing 200 doses of 90 g of albuterol ($0.03/puff). The actual medication cost of 72 actuations over 3 hours is $2.16.

§SVN costs are calculated with three 15-min treatments each hour, for a 3-hour period.

Aerosol Administration to Intubated Patients

Use of Small-Volume Nebulizers During Mechanical Ventilation

Aerosol administered by SVN to intubated and ventilated patients tends to deposit more of the aerosolized medication in the tubing of the ventilator circuit, resulting in less medication delivered to the patient. Deposition in the lungs of ventilated patients during normal conditions has been measured as 1.5% to 3%.[82–84]

A number of factors have been shown to affect delivery of SVN during controlled mechanical ventilation (CMV).

These factors include humidity and temperature of inhaled gas, tidal volume, respiratory rate, duty cycle, inspiratory flow patterns, choice of nebulizer, and whether the nebulizer cycles during inspiration only or continuously (Fig. 12–26). When all of these factors are optimized, as much as 15% of the aerosol can reach the patient's lung,[85] with treatments requiring 40 minutes. McPeck and coworkers[86] have demonstrated that ventilators have a wide variety of output flows to drive nebulizers during CMV, which can greatly affect aerosol output.

When delivering medication by SVN to intubated, mechanically ventilated patients, the clinician must identify the most appropriate location for the nebulizer. Hughes and

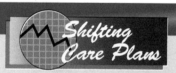

CRITICAL THINKING CHALLENGES

Rationale for an Algorithm

Metered dose inhaler with holding chamber is the fastest way to administer albuterol; 2 to 4 puffs are equivalent to a 2.5-mg SVN dose. More than 80% of the response to albuterol occurs within the first 5 minutes. We give 4 puffs, wait 5 minutes, then give 1 puff per minute up to 12 puffs (see Fig. 12-25). If the patient does not break open, we set up continuous nebulization at 15 mg/h in a monitored bed, with electrocardiogram and pulse oximeter.

One of the advantages of this approach is the educational consistency for the more than 90% of patients who respond to the MDI with holding chamber after abusing the MDI for several hours before admission without relief. If the patient does not respond after the equivalent of three to six standard doses of albuterol in the 17 minutes required for 12 puffs with either reduced distress or a toxic response, the continuous nebulizer provides a less

labor-intensive and more comfortable method for receiving the medication.

Patients who do respond to the MDI with holding chamber are given follow-up treatment at the initial dose in 1 hour and then every 4 hours and as needed. The dose is evaluated by titration after each treatment. Patients receiving more than 4 puffs of albuterol should be treated by a trained respiratory care practitioner and reevaluated at 24-hour intervals.

Note: Bronchodilators relieve symptoms but do not fix the primary problem of inflammation causing the acute airway obstruction. High doses of β-agonists may be appropriate for resuscitation, but doses and frequency of administration should be reduced as soon as possible. Patients should be evaluated for reduced dosage with each treatment after initial resuscitation.

Ventilator Related

- Mode of ventilation
- Tidal volume
- Respiratory rate
- Duty cycle
- Inspiratory waveform
- Breath triggering mechanism

Device Related—MDI

- Type of spacer or adapter used
- Position of spacer in circuit
- Timing of MDI actuation

Patient Related

- Severity of airway obstruction
- Mechanism of airway obstruction
- Presence of dynamic hyperinflation
- Spontaneous ventilation
- Disease process

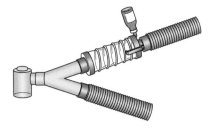

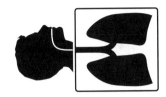

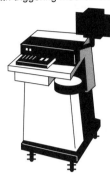

Circuit Related

- Size of endotracheal tube
- Type of humidifier
- Relative humidity
- Density/viscosity of inhaled gas

Device Related—Neb

- Type of nebulizer used
- Fill volume
- Gas flow
- Cycling—inspiration vs continuous
- Duration of nebulization
- Position in the circuit

Drug Related

- Dose
- Aerosol particle size
- Targeted site for delivery
- Duration of action

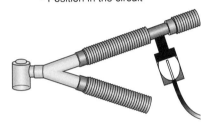

FIGURE 12-26 • Variables affecting aerosol deposition during mechanical ventilation.

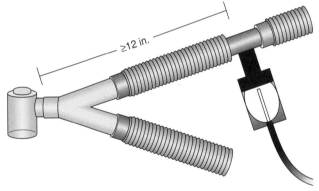

Nebulizer placement:
Inspiratory line ≥ 12 inches from wye
Remove nebulizer from circuit between treatments

Nebulizer selection:
1–2 μm MMAD at operating pressure
Fill volume: ≥ 4 mL

Dose:
200%–500% of standard dose
Nebulizer flow for optimal output:
6–8 L/min at 50 psi
Nebulizer time —40 minutes or until neb is dry

Ventilator parameters to optimize delivery with SVN:
Low peak inspiratory flow
Sine or ramp vs square inspiratory waveform
Duty cycle ≥ 0.30
Breath triggering: Pressure vs flow sensing

Cautions:
Adjust volumes for nebulizer flow
Adjust alarms before and after SVN treatments
Properly store, clean, or replace SVN between treatments

FIGURE 12-27 • Proper nebulizer placement in a ventilator circuit.

Saez[87] found that the optimal placement of the nebulizer is in the inspiratory limb at the manifold of the ventilator circuit, about 18 inches from the patient wye. They demonstrated that the worst position for the nebulizer was between the patient and the wye connector of the circuit, particularly when using continuously nebulized medication, because the drug that is nebulized after inspiration is driven down the expiratory limb of the ventilator circuit and lost to the patient.

Figure 12–27 illustrates proper nebulizer placement as well as a variety of factors, such as nebulizer selection, dose, flow, treatment time, and ventilator parameters, that influence and optimize aerosol delivery from a SVN during CMV (Box 12–9).

Box • 12–9 OPTIMAL TECHNIQUE FOR USE OF SMALL-VOLUME NEBULIZER WITH MECHANICAL VENTILATION

1. Assess need for medication.
2. Establish dose to compensate for decreased delivery, possibly two to five times the dose given to nonventilated patients.
3. Place drug in nebulizer to a fill volume of 4 to 6 mL.
4. Place SVN in inspiratory line (12 to 18 inches from the patient wye).
5. Remove heat–moisture exchanger from between SVN and patient; use alternative form of humidification.
6. Consider placing filter in expiratory limb of the ventilator circuit to avoid loading expiratory flow transducer with medications.
7. Set gas flow to nebulizer at 6 to 8 L/min.
   a. Use ventilator nebulizer compressor if it meets flow needs of the nebulizer used and cycles on inspiration; *otherwise:*
   b. Use continuous flow from external 50-psi source, and adjust volume or pressure limit to compensate for additional flow during treatment.
8. Turn off flowby or continuous flow while nebulizing.
9. Tap nebulizer periodically until all medication is nebulized.
10. Remove nebulizer from circuit, rinse with sterile water and run dry, store in clean bag between treatments, or replace between treatments.
11. Return ventilator and alarms to previous settings.
12. Monitor patient for adverse response.
13. Assess outcome.

Use of Metered Dose Inhalers in Intubated, Ventilated Patients

Spacers are used to optimize drug delivery by MDI to intubated, mechanically ventilated patients. Although a variety of styles are sold (Fig. 12–28), chamber-style devices are designed to allow an aerosol plume to develop before the bulk of the medication contacts the surface of the chamber or ventilator tubing, providing more aged, stable particles to enter the lungs. The use of the chamber-style device may result in less impaction of the medication on the walls of circuit tubing or airway than occurs with the other devices used with ventilated patients (Fig. 12–29).

One question that arises frequently when using drugs delivered by MDI to ventilated patients is the dose of drug required. Many studies have suggested that the dose of drug delivered per puff from the MDI is less when administered to the ventilated patient than that delivered to the nonintubated, spontaneously breathing patient. Fuller and colleagues,[84] using the AeroVent chamber to deliver medication by MDI to intubated, ventilated patients, demonstrated a 5.5% deposition of drug delivered by MDI, compared with 1.5% deposition of drug delivered by SVN (Fig. 12–30).

It may be reasonable to assume that all intubated or ventilated patients receive a significantly smaller percentage of medication in the lung than nonintubated patients and that to deliver comparable amounts of medication, larger doses (up to 10-fold) may be required. A number of studies

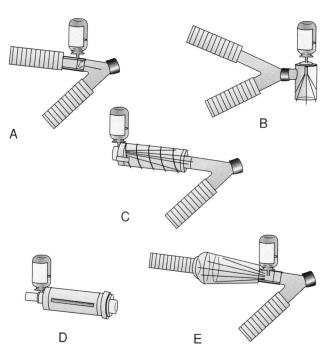

FIGURE 12–28 • Variety of metered dose inhaler (MDI) adapters used during mechanical ventilation. (*A*) Inline low-volume adapter. (*B*) Elbow or swivel adapter. (*C*) Collapsible chamber-style adapter. (*D* and *E*) Rigid chamber-style adapters.

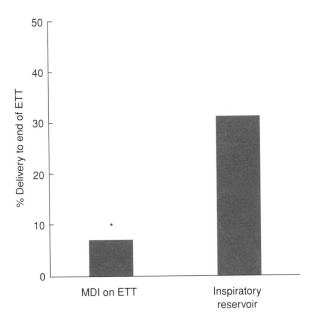

* p < 0.01

FIGURE 12-29 • Comparison of in vivo delivery of albuterol from a metered dose inhaler (MDI) with holding chamber and a small-volume nebulizer to patients receiving mechanical ventilation with a heated and humidified ventilator circuit. ETT, endotracheal tube.

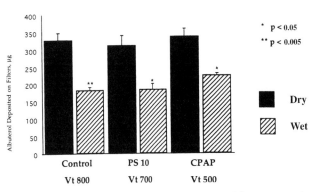

FIGURE 12-31 • Effect of heated humidification on deposition of albuterol to 12 puffs of albuterol with three modes of ventilation compared with similar experiment under dry (0% relative humidity at ambient temperature) conditions. The symbols * and ** indicate a significant difference between the dry and wet measurements with each mode of ventilation. (Scanlon: *Egan's Fundamentals of Respiratory Care.* 6th ed., St. Louis: Mosby–Year Book, 1995.)

have demonstrated that a larger dose is required to achieve the same therapeutic end point for medications delivered by MDI to intubated patients than to nonintubated patients.

Because the specific dose required is unpredictable, several years ago we attempted to titrate the dosage of bronchodilator delivered to ventilated patients using an MDI, usually with albuterol, and to incorporate a chamber spacer

(AeroVent) adapter.[88] Doses were administered in groups of 10 puffs administered twice, followed by 5 puffs administered up to five times, at intervals of at least 5 minutes and with individual puffs given at 1-minute intervals. The patient's response was monitored to determine clinical response and onset of side effects. If the patient demonstrated no side effects but continued to show clinical signs of increased airway resistance, repeated doses were administered by the protocol until the desired clinical response was achieved or toxicity developed. Using this technique, only 60% of adult patients demonstrated a significant response to the bronchodilator when given up to 40 puffs. Adverse reactions (tachycardia or premature ventricular contractions) occurred in only 4 of 120 patients; all were

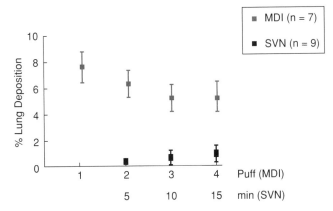

FIGURE 12-30 • Comparison of lung deposition during mechanical ventilation between metered dose inhaler (MDI) and small-volume nebulizer (SVN). (Fuller HD, Dolovich MB, Posmituck G, et al: Pressurized aerosol versus jet aerosol delivery to mechanically ventilated patients: Comparison of dose to the lungs. *Am Rev Respir Dis.* 1990;141: 440–444.)

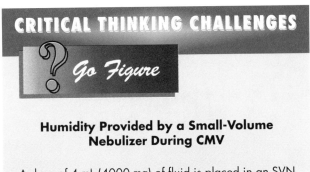

Humidity Provided by a Small-Volume Nebulizer During CMV

A dose of 4 mL (4000 mg) of fluid is placed in an SVN (with a dead volume of 0.5 mL) in the inspiratory limb of a ventilator circuit. The humidifier is turned off to improve aerosol deposition for the 40 minutes required to nebulize all the medication. If the patient has a minute volume of 10 L/min, what is the absolute humidity that will be delivered to the end of the patient's endotracheal tube? What is the relative humidity at body temperature?

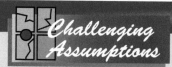
Small-Volume Nebulizer by Ventilator

It has been demonstrated with both MDI and SVN that the presence of heat and humidity during (CMV) reduces aerosol delivery to the lung by about 40% compared with dry conditions. This has resulted in some short-sighted recommendations to turn off the humidifier during aerosol administration to improve deposition. The reason we add heat and humidity to the airway during CMV is to produce the normal conditions for inspired gas when breathing through an intact upper airway (40 mg/L of water). Compressed air and oxygen used during CMV in acute care facilities is bone dry. Prolonged exposure of the lower respiratory tract to cold dry air may result in problems far worse than the need for additional aerosol delivery to achieve the desired clinical response.

As calculated in the previous *Go Figure!,* an SVN provides an absolute humidity of 8.75 mg/L and a relative humidity of less than 20% at BTPS. This is far too little humidity (and heat) to provide to an airway for a 20-40-minute treatment. An even greater risk is the tendency for the practitioner *not* to turn the humidifier back on after the treatment, subjecting the patient to cold dry air for hours.

Conclusion: Turning off the humidifier to administer SVN treatment during CMV subjects the patient to room temperature gas with less than 20% of the humidity usually found at the carina. We recommend keeping the humidifier on and increasing the dose by 40%.

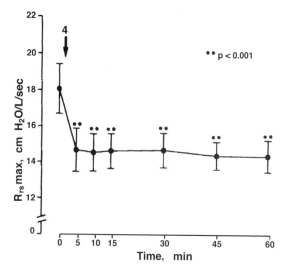

FIGURE 12-32 • Changes in airway resistance for patients with chronic obstructive pulmonary disease during mechanical ventilation, with humidity, after 4 puffs of albuterol using a chamber-style adapter. (Duarte AG, Dhand R, Reid R, Fink JB, Fahey PJ, Tobin MJ, Jenne JW. Serum albuterol levels in mechanically ventilated patients and healthy subjects after metered-dose inhaler administration. *Am J Resp Crit Care Med* 1996; 154:1658-1663.)

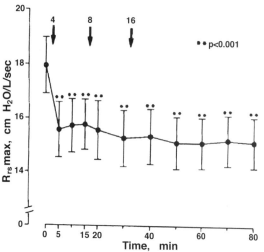

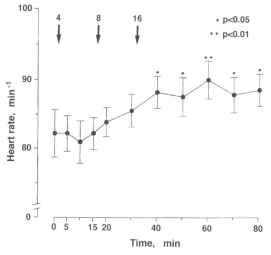

FIGURE 12-33 • Response to titrated doses of 4, 8, and 16 puffs of albuterol from a metered dose inhaler with a chamber-style adapter during CMV of patients with chronic obstructive pulmonary disease. (*Top*) Additional puffs after 4, did not result in a further reduction in airway resistance (that was significant). (*Bottom*) 16 puffs resulted in a significant increase in heart rate. (Duarte AG, Dhand R, Reid R, Fink JB, Fahey PJ, Tobin MJ, Jenne JW. Serum albuterol levels in mechanically ventilated patients and healthy subjects after metered-dose inhaler administration. *Am J Resp Crit Care Med* 1996; 154:1658-1663.)

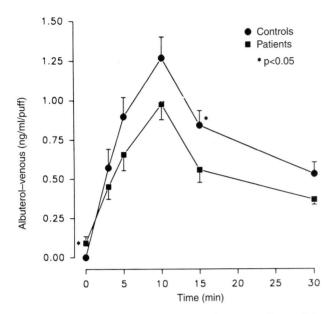

FIGURE 12-34 • Comparison of serum albuterol levels, per puff, with controls (normal volunteers using metered dose inhaler with holding chamber with optimal technique, and patients with chronic obstructive pulmonary disease on mechanical ventilation using chamber-style adapter. (Duarte AG, Dhand R, Reid R, Fink JB, Fahey PJ, Tobin MJ, Jenne JW. Serum albnterol levels in mechanically ventilated patients and healthy subjects after metered-dose inhaler administration. *Am J Resp Crit Care Med* 1996; 154:1658–1663.)

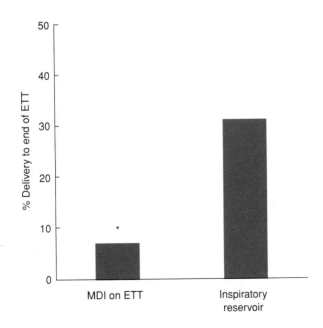

* p < 0.01

FIGURE 12-35 • Proper metered dose inhaler (MDI) placement in ventilator circuit. ETT, endotracheal tube.

minor and required no treatment. This evaluation suggested that more medication is required for clinical improvement of ventilated patients and that the higher doses are usually well tolerated, with minimal adverse reaction.

Effective delivery of aerosol with MDI in the ventilator circuit can vary from 2% to 40% in in vitro models. Fink and coworkers[89] demonstrated a variety of factors, including mode of ventilation, spontaneous volumes, flow patterns, and humidity. Using an in vitro model, spontaneous volumes of 500 mL resulted in greater deposition than an 800-mL control machine breath in a humidified circuit. Figure 12–31 shows the effect of humidity and modes of ventilation on aerosol delivered from an MDI with cham-

---

Box • 12–10 TECHNIQUE FOR ADMINISTRATION OF METERED DOSE INHALER IN VENTILATOR CIRCUIT

1. Assess need for medication.
2. Establish ventilator dose of 4 puffs (for bronchodilators with standard dose of 2 to 4 puffs) for stable chronic obstructive pulmonary disease patients. Higher doses may be required for treatment of acute exacerbation.
3. Adjust ventilator as follows:
   Leave humidifier on (remove heat–moisture exchanger from between MDI and patient).
   To optimize delivery:
   Ensure VT (500 mL).
   Decrease peak inspiratory flow rate, as tolerated.
   Use ramp or sine wave flow patterns.
   Increase TI/TTOT to about 0.30.
   Turn off continuous flow-through circuit.
4. Shake MDI and warm to hand temperature.
5. Place MDI in chamber-style adapter in ventilator circuit in inspiratory limb at wye or between elbow and endotracheal tube.
6. Actuate MDI at beginning of inspiration.
7. Wait about 15 seconds between actuations (no need to shake between puffs, up to a total of 8 actuations).
8. If patient can take a spontaneous breath (500 mL), coordinate actuation with beginning of deep spontaneous breath and encourage breath-hold for 4 to 10 seconds.
9. After administering total dose, collapse or remove chamber from the circuit, replace exchanger, and return all ventilator parameters to pretreatment settings.
10. Monitor for adverse response.
11. Assess outcome.

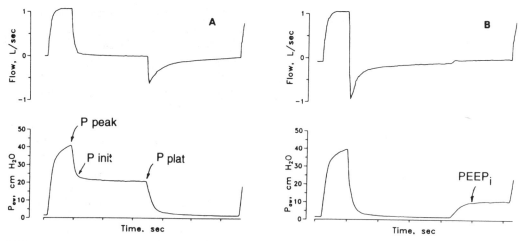

FIGURE 12-36 • Waveforms depicting key parameters for monitoring patient response to inhaled bronchodilators. Resistance commonly is determined by difference in peak airway pressure (P peak) and plateau pressure (P plat). (A) Following a rapid airway occlusion, the airway pressure falls to an initial pressure (P init) that is a considerably higher value than that at the plateau measured 2.5 seconds later. The difference between P peak and P init reflects the ohmic resistance of the airways. PEEP$_i$, positive end-expiratory pressure. (Dhand et al. AJRCCM 151:1827-1833)

ber-style adapter to the lower respiratory tract of a spontaneously breathing lung model.

Dhand and colleagues[90] demonstrated measurable responses in controlled, lightly sedated patients with chronic obstructive pulmonary disease (COPD) during CMV with a heated ventilator circuit, with 10 puffs of albuterol (using a chamber-style adapter), whereas Manthous and associates[91] reported no measurable response with up to 100 puffs (using an elbow-style adapter).

Dhand[92] later demonstrated that during mechanical ventilation of COPD patients using heated humidification, 4 puffs of albuterol with a chamber-style adapter resulted in significant reduction in airway resistance (Fig. 12-32), and as the dose was increased to 8, 16, and 24 puffs, further reductions in airway resistance were not significant (Fig. 12-33). Duarte and coworkers[93] compared serum albuterol levels of ventilated COPD patients in a humidified ventilator circuit with those of nonintubated normal volunteers using optimal technique with MDI and holding chamber and with 4-second inspiratory holds. On a puff-to-puff basis, the ventilated patients had about 66% of the serum levels found in the normal subjects (Fig. 12-34). If 4 puffs of MDI albuterol with a chamber-style spacer in a humidified ventilator circuit provides an adequate decrease in airway resistance, recommendations to turn off humidifiers during aerosol administration to increase the percentage of deposition might not be worth the risk of adverse effects.

These factors are considered in the recommended technique for MDI administration during mechanical ventilation itemized in Table 12-5. Figure 12-35 illustrates proper MDI chamber placement as well as a variety of factors, such as nebulizer selection, dose, flow, treatment time, and ventilator parameters, that influence and optimize aerosol delivery from an MDI during CMV (Box 12-10).

Assessing response to bronchodilators in normal patients usually is based on forced expiratory maneuver, which may not be possible during mechanical ventilation, in which exhalation is typically passive. During CMV, we determine bronchodilator response during inspiration. Based on our work, an acceptable compromise for accurately assessing the response to bronchodilators during mechanical ventilation is the use of a 2-second inspiratory occlusion with sedation of the patient, which allows the ventilator to cycle without artifact (Fig. 12-36).

References

1. Dolovich M. Physical principles underlying aerosol therapy. *J Aerosol Med.* 1989;2(2);171-186.
2. O'Donohue WJ. Guidelines for the use of nebulizers in the home and it domicillary sites. *Chest.* 1996;109:814-820.
3. Newhouse MT, Dolovich M. Aerosol therapy in children. In: *Basic Mechanisms of Pediatric Respiratory Disease: Cellular and Integrative.* BC Decker; 1991.
4. Heyder J, Gebbart J, Rudolf G, Stahlhofen W. Physical factors determining particle deposition in the human respiratory tract. *J Aerosol Sci.* 1980;11:505-515.
5. Newman SP, Bateman JRM, Pavia D, Clarke SW. The importance of breath-holding following the inhalation of pressurized aerosol bronchodilators. In: Baran D, ed. *Recent Advances in Aerosol Therapy: First Belgian Symposium on Aerosols in Medicine.* Brussels, 1979:117-122.
6. Yu CP, Nicolaides P, Soong TT. Effect of random airway sizes on aerosol deposition. *Am Ind Hyg Assoc J.* 1979;40:999-1005.
7. Svedmyr N. Clinical advantages of the aerosol route of drug administration. *Respir Care.* 1991;36(9):922-930.
8. Lippman M. Regional deposition of particles in the human respiratory tract. In: Lee DHK, Falk HL, Murphy SO, Geiger SR, eds. *Handbook of Physiology: Reaction to Environmental Agents.* Bethesda: American Physiological Society; 1977.
9. Pierce AK, Edmondson EB, McGee G, et al. An analysis of factors predisposing to gram-negative bacillary necrotizing pneumonia. *Am Rev Respir Dis.* 1966;94:309-315.
10. Pierce AK, Sanford JP, Thomas, GD, Leonard JS. Long-term eval-

uation of inhalation therapy equipment and the occurrence of necrotizing pneumonia. *N Engl J Med.* 1970;282(10):528–531.

11. Rhame FS, Streifel A, McComb C, Boyle M. Bubbling humidifiers produce microaerosols which can carry bacteria. *Infect Control.* 1986;7:403–406.

12. Kaan JA, Simons-Smit AM, McLaren DM. Another source of aerosol causing nosocomial legionnaires' disease. *J Infect.* 1985; 11:145–148.

13. Hamill RJ, Houston ED, Georghiou PR. An outbreak of *Burkholderia cepacia* respiratory tract colonization and infection associated with nebulized albuterol therapy. *Ann Intern Med.* 1995; 122:762–766.

14. Christopher KL, Saravolatz LD, Bush TL, Conway WA. The potential role of respiratory therapy equipment in cross infection: A case study using a canine model for pneumonia. *Am Rev Respir Dis.* 1983;128:271–275.

15. Cheney FW, Butler J. The effects of ultrasonically produced aerosols on airway resistance in man. *Anesthesiology.* 1968;29: 1099.

16. Ziment I. Respiratory pharmacology and therapeutics. Philadelphia: WB Saunders; 1978.

17. Lyons HA. Use of therapeutic aerosols. *Am J Cardiol.* 1969;12:462.

18. Stehlin CS, Schare BL. Systemic and pulmonary changes in rabbits exposed to long-term nebulization of various therapeutic agents. *Heart Lung* 1980;9:311–315.

19. Hess D, Horney D, Snyder T. Medication-delivery performance of eight small-volume, hand-held nebulizers: Effects of diluent volume, gas flowrate and nebulizer model. *Respir Care.* 1989;34: 717–723.

20. Zainuddin BM, Tolfree SEJ, Short M, Spiro SG. Influence of breathing pattern on lung deposition and bronchodilator response to nebulized salbutamol inpatients with stable asthma. *Thorax.* 1988;43:987–991.

21. Alvine GF, Rodgers P, Fitzsimmons KM, Ahrens RC. Disposable jet nebulizers: How reliable are they? *Chest.* 1992;101:316–319.

22. Raabe OG, Lee, JIC, Wong GA. A signal actuated nebulizer for use with breathing machines. *J Aerosol Med.* 1989;2(2):201–210.

23. Colacone A, Wolkove N, Stern E, et al. Continuous nebulization of albuterol (salbutamol) in acute asthma. *Chest.* 1990;97: 693–697.

24. Moler FW, Hurwitz ME, Custer JR. Improvement in clinical asthma score and PaCO₂ in children with severe asthma treated with continuously nebulized terbutaline. *J Allergy Clin Immunol.* 1988;81:1101–1109.

25. Portnoy J, Aggarwal J. Continuous terbutaline nebulization for the treatment of severe exacerbations of asthma in children. *Ann Allergy.* 1988;60:368–371.

26. Robertson C, Smith F, Beck R, Levison H. Response to frequent low doses of nebulized salbutamol in acute asthma. *J Pediatr.* 1985;106:672–674.

27. Schuh S, et al. High- versus low dose, frequently administered nebulized albuterol in children with severe acute asthma. *Pediatrics.* 1989;83:513—518.

28. Rebuck AS, Chapman KR, Abboud R, et al. Nebulized anticholinergic and sympathomimetic treatment of asthma and chronic obstructive airway in the disease in the emergency room. *Am J Med.* 1987;82:59–64.

29. Ba M, Thivierge RL, Lapierre JG, et al. Effects of continuous inhalation of salbutamol in acute asthma. *Am Rev Respir Dis.* 1987; 135:A-326. (Abstract)

30. Amado M, Portnoy J, King K. Comparison of bolus and continuously nebulized terbutaline for treatment of severe exacerbations of asthma. *Ann Allergy Clin Immunol.* 1988;81:318. (Abstract)

31. Amado M, Portnoy J. A comparison of low and high doses of continuously nebulized terbutaline for treatment of severe exacerbations of asthma. *Ann Allergy.* 1988;60:165. (Abstract)

32. Des Jardins T. Freon-propelled bronchodilator use as a potential hazard to asthmatic patients. *Respir Care.* 1980;21(1)50–57.

33. Breeden CC, Safirstein BH. Albuterol and spacer-induced atrial fibrillation. *Chest.* 1990;98:762–763.

34. Silverglade A. Cardiac toxicity of aerosol propellants. *JAMA.* 1972;222(7);827–828.

35. Moren F. Aerosol dosage forms and formulations. In: Moren F, Newhouse MT, Dolovich MB, eds. *Aerosols in Medicine: Principles, Diagnosis and Therapy.* Amsterdam: Elsevier; 1985: 261–287.

36. Hallworth GW. The formulation and evaluation of pressurized metered deose inhalers. In: Ganderton D, Jones T, eds. *Drug Delivery to the Respiratory Tract.* Chichester, UK: Ellis Horwood; 1987:87–118.

37. Dhand R, Malik SK, Balakrishan M, Verma SK. High speed photographic analysis of aerosols produced by metered dose inhalers. *J Pharm Pharmacol.* 1988;40:429–430.

38. Wiener MV. How to formulate aerosols to obtain the desired spray pattern. *Soc Cos Chem.* 1958;9:289–297.

39. Newman SP. Aerosol generators and delivery systems. *Respir Care.* 1991;36:939–951.

40. Kim CS, Trujillo D, Sackner MA. Size aspects of metered-dose inhaler aerosols. *Am Rev Respir Dis.* 1985;132:137–142.

41. Newman SP, Pvia D, Moren F, et al. Deposition of pressurized aerosols in the human respiratory tract. *Thorax.* 1981;36:52–55.

42. Dolovich M, Ruffin RE, Roberts R, Newhouse MT. Optimal delivery aerosols from metered dose inhalers. *Chest.* 1981;80 (suppl):911–115.

43. Jenkins SC, Heaton RW, Fulton TJ, Moxham J. Comparison of domicilliary nebulized salbutomol and salbutomol from a metered-dose inhaler in stable chronic airflow limitation. *Chest.* 1987;91:804–807.

44. Cissik JH, Bode FR, Smith JA. Double-blind crossover study of five bronchodilator medications and two delivery methods in stable asthma: Is there a best combination for use in the pulmonary laboratory? *Chest.* 1990;90 (4):489–493.

45. Shim CS, Williams MH Jr. Effect of bronchodilator administered by canister versus jet nebulizer. *J Allergy Clin Immunol.* 1984; 73:387–390.

46. Mestitz H, Coplan J, McDonald C. Comparison of outpatient nebulized vs metered dose inhaler terbutaline in chronic airflow obstruction. *Chest.* 1989;96:1237–1240.

47. AARC. Clinical practice guidelines: Selection of aerosol delivery device. *Respir Care.* 1992;37(8):891–897.

48. Faculty and Working Group: American Association for Respiratory Care. *Aerosol Consensus Conference Statement—1991. Respir Care.* 1991;36:916–921.

49. Newman SP, Pavia D, Clarke SW. Simple instructions for using pressurized aerosol bronchodilators. *J R Soc Med.* 1980;73:776–779.

50. Riley DJ, Liu RT, Edelman NH. Enhanced response to aerosolized bronchodilator therapy in asthma using respiratory maneuvers. *Chest.* 1979;76:501–507.

51. Grainger JR. Correct use of aerosol inhalers. *Can Med Assoc J.* 1977;116:584–585.

52. Woolf CR. Correct use of pressurized aerosol inhalers. *Can Med Assoc J.* 1979;121:710–711.

53. Riley DJ, Weitz BW, Edelman NH. The responses of asthmatic subjects to isoproterenol inhaled at differing lung volumes. *Am Rev Respir Dis.* 1976;114:509–515.

54. Guidry GG, Brown WD, Stogner SW, George RB. Incorrect use of metered dose inhalers by medical personnel. *Chest.* 1992; 1010(1):31–33.

55. Crompton GK. Problems patients have using pressurized aerosol inhalers. *Eur J Respir Dis.* 1982;119(suppl):101–104.

56. De Blaquiere P, Christensen DB, Carter WB, Martin TR. Use and misuse of metered-dose inhalers by patients with chronic lung disease: A controlled randomized trial of two instruction methods. *Am Rev Respir Dis.* 1989;140:910–916.

57. Allen SC, Prior A. What determines whether an elderly patient can use a metered dose inhaler correctly? *Br J Dis Chest.* 1986; 80:45–49.

58. Kim CS, Eldridge MA, Sackner MA. Oropharyngeal deposition and delivery aspects of metered-dose inhaler aerosols. *Am Rev Respir Dis.* 1987;135:157–164.

59. Tschopp JM, Robinson S, Caloz JM, Frey JG. Bronchodilating efficacy of an open-spacer device compared to three other spacers. *Respir Care.* 1992;37:61–64.

60. Lee N, Rachelefsky G, Kobayashi RH, et al. Efficacy and safety of albuterol administered by power driven nebulizer (PDN) versus metered dose inhaler (MDI) with Aerochamber and mask in infants and young children with acute asthma. *Am Acad Pediatr.* 1990;Nov: (Abstract)

61. Kraemer R, Frey U, Sommer CW, Russi E. Short-term effect of albuterol, delivered via a new auxiliary device, in wheezy infants. *Am Rev Respir Dis.* 1991;144:347–351.

62. Conner WT, Dolovich MB, Frame RA, Newhouse MT. Reliable salbutamol administration in 6- to 36-month old children by means of a metered dose inhaler and aerochamber with mask. *Pediatr Pulmonol.* 1989;6:263–267.

63. Madsden EB, Bundgaard A, Hidinger KG. Cumulative dose-response study comparing terbutaline pressurized aerosol administered via a pear shaped spacer and terbutaline in a nebulized solution. *Eur J Clin Pharmacol.* 1982;23:27–30.

64. Hodder RV. Metered dose inhaler with spacer is superior to wet nebulization for emergency room treatment of acute severe asthma. *Chest.* 1988;94(suppl):52S.

65. Dolovich M, Chambers C, Mazza M, Newhouse MT. Relative efficiency of four metered dose inhaler (MDI) holding chambers (HC) compared to albuterol MDI. Presented at American Lung Association American Thoracic Society 1992 International Conference at the Symposium on Aerosol Delivery Systems.

66. Salzman GA, Pyszczynski DR. Oropharyngeal candidiasis in patients treated with beclomethasone dipropionate delivered by metered-dose inhaler alone and with Aerochamber. *J Allergy Clin Immunol.* 1988;81:424–428.

67. Toogood JH, Baskerville J, Jennings B, et al. Use of spacer to facilitate inhaled corticosteroid treatment of asthma. *Am Rev Respir Dis.* 1984;129:723–729.

68. Pederson S. How to use a rotohaler. *Arch Dis Child.* 1986;61:11–14.

69. Pederson S, Hansen OR, Fuglsang G. Influence of inspiratory flowrate upon the effect of a Turbuhaler. *Arch Dis Child.* 1990; 65:308–310.

70. Engel T, Heinig JH, Madsen F, Nikander K. Peak inspiratory flowrate and inspiratory vital capacity of patients with asthma measured with and without a new dry powder inhaler device (Turbuhaler). *Eur Respir J.* 1990;3:1037–1041.

71. Hansen OR, Pederson S. Optimal inhalation technique with terbutaline Turbuhaler. *Eur Respir J.* 1989;2:637–639.

72. Ballard RD, Bogin RM, Pak J. Assessment of bronchodilator response to a β-adrenergic delivered from an ultrasonic nebulizer. *Chest.* 1991;100:410–415.

73. Chatburn RL, Lough MD, Klinger JD. An in-hospital evaluation of the sonic mist ultrasonic room humidifier. *Respir Care.* 1984;29:893–899.

74. Doershuk CF, Mathews LW, Gillespie CT, et al. Evaluation of jet type and ultrasonic nebulizers in mist tent therapy for cystic fibrosis. *Pediatrics* 1968;41:723–732.

75. Boucher RGM, Kreuter J. Fundamentals of the ultrasonic atomization of medicated solutions. *Ann Allergy* 1968;26:59.

76. Lewis RA, Ellis CJ, Fleming JS, Balachandran W. Ultrasonic and jet nebulizers: Differences in the physical properties and fractional deposition on the airway responses to nebulized water and saline aerosols. *Thorax.* 1984;39:712. (Abstract)

77. Glick RV. Drug reconcentration in aerosol generators. *Inhal Ther* 1970;15:179.

78. Papo MC, Frank J, Thompson AE: A prospective, randomized study of continuous versus intermittent nebulized albuterol for severe status asthmaticus in children. *Crit Care Med.* 1993;21:1478–1486.

79. Moler FW, Johnson CE, Van Leanen C, et al. Continuous versus intermittent nebulized terbutaline: Plasma levels and effects. *Am J Respir Crit Care Med.* 1995;151:602–606.

80. Lin RY, Smith AJ, Hergenroeder. High serum albuterol levels and tachycardia in adult asthmatics treated with high-dose continuously aerosolized albuterol. *Chest.* 1993;103:221–225.

81. Levitt MA, Gambrioli EF, Fink JB. Comparative trial of continuous nebulization versus metered-dose inhaler in the treatment of acute bronchospasm. *Ann Emerg Med.* 1995;26(3):273–237.

82. Dahlback M, Wollmer P, Drefeldt B, Johnson B. Controlled aerosol delivery during mechanical ventilation. *J Aerosol Med.* 1989;4:339–347.

83. MacIntyre NR, Silver RM, Miller CW, et al. Aerosol delivery in intubated, mechanically ventilated patients. *Crit Care Med.* 1985; 13:81–84.

84. Fuller HD, Dolovich MB, Posmituck G, et al. Pressurized aerosol versus jet aerosol delivery to mechanically ventilated patients: Comparison of dose to the lungs. *Am Rev Respir Dis.* 1990; 141:440–444.

85. O'Riordan TG, Greco MJ, Perry RJ, Smaldone GC. Nebulizer function during mechanical ventilation. *Am Rev Respir Dis.* 1992; 145:1117–1122.

86. McPeck M, O'Riordan TG, Smaldone GC. Choice of mechanical ventilator: influence of nebulizer performance. *Respir Care.* 1993;38: 887–895.

87. Hughes JM, Saez J. Effects of nebulizer mode and position in a mechanical ventilator circuit on dose efficiency. *Respir Care.* 1987;32:1131–1135.

88. Fink JB, Cohen N, Covington J, Mahlmeister M. Titration for optimal dose response to bronchodilators using MDI and spacer in 120 ventilated adults. *Respir Care.* 1991;36–1321.

89. Fink JB, Dhand R, Duarte AG, Jenne JW, Tobin MJ. Aerosol delivery from a metered-dose inhaler during mechanical ventilation. *Am J Respir Crit Care Med.* 1996;154:382–387.

90. Dhand R, Jubran A, Tobin MJ. Bronchodilator delivery by metered-dose inhaler in ventilator supported patients. *Am J Respir Crit Care Med.* 1995;154:388–393.

91. Manthous CA, Hall JB, Schmidt Ga, Wood LDH. Metered-dose inhaler versus nebulized albuterol in mechanically ventilated patient. *Am Rev Respir Dis.* 1993;148:1567–1570.

92. Dhand R, Duarte AG, Jubran A, Jenne JW, Fink JB, Fahey PJ, Tobin MJ. Dose response to bronchodilator delivered by metered-dose inhaler in ventilator-supported patients. *Am J. Respir Crit Care Med.* 1996;154:388–393.

93. Duarte AG, Dhand, R, Reid R, Fink JB, Fahey PJ, Tobin MJ, Jenne JW. Serum albuterol levels in mechanically ventilated patients and healthy subjects after metered-dose inhaler administration. *Am J. Respir Crit Care Med.* 1996;154:1658–1663.

13

Bronchial Hygiene and Lung Expansion

James B. Fink

Key Terms

atelectasis
autogenic drainage
bronchial hygiene
continuous positive airway
 pressure (CPAP)
deep breathing
diaphragmatic breathing
directed cough
expiratory positive airway
 pressure (EPAP)
fixed orifice resistor
flow-oriented incentive
 device
hyperinflation therapy
incentive spirometry (IS)
intermittent positive-
 pressure breathing (IPPB)
positioning
positive airway pressure
 (PAP)
positive expiratory pressure
 (PEP)
postural drainage therapy
 (PDT)
sustained maximal
 inspiration (SMI)
threshold resistor
volume displacement

Objectives

- Identify mechanisms and risk factors for the development of atelectasis and retained secretions.

- Differentiate the therapeutic alternatives to prevent and treat atelectasis.

- Describe the role and rationale of each major technique of bronchial hygiene.

- Explain the use, indications, contraindications, and hazards associated with lung expansion and bronchial hygiene techniques.

- Compare and contrast clinical efficacy, comfort, and cost of each therapeutic option.

- Distinguish among different lung expansion devices in terms of their functional characteristics.

- Determine which option best meets a patient's needs.

- Modify the technique or frequency of application in light of the patient's response to therapy.

Bronchial hygiene comprises a variety of techniques that promote mobilization and clearance of secretions. Lung expansion is a subset of bronchial hygiene therapy, with the specific goal of assisting the patient to attain or maintain optimal lung volumes. Lung volumes are directly related to expiratory flows, cough effectiveness, and the ability to clear secretions from the airways. Lung expansion therapy incorporates bronchial hygiene techniques, such as **directed cough**, breathing exercises, and **postural drainage therapy** (PDT). The emphasis of lung expansion therapy is focused on the treatment and prevention of **atelectasis**. Treatments for atelectasis include **positioning** (turning and mobilization), **deep breathing,** directed cough, **incentive spirometry** (IS), **intermittent positive-pressure breathing** (IPPB), positive airway pressure (PAP), PDT, manipulation of the thorax, and bronchodilator therapy. Although each technique may prove to be effective under specific circumstances, no one treatment works all the time for all patients. In fact, most patients do not require therapy of any sort to avoid or resolve atelectasis. For most patients at risk of atelectasis, instruction and reminders to perform periodic deep breathing preoperatively and postoperatively are sufficient.[1,2] In the late 1970s, respiratory care was broadly criticized for the overuse of lung expansion therapies, with a special focus on IPPB. When IPPB fell into disfavor in the early 1980s, it was quickly replaced, in part, with IS, nebulizer treatments, and PDT, in some cases further escalating the cost of respiratory care.[3] The role of the respiratory care practitioner is to identify patients at risk, to recommend or initiate the level of intervention for each patient that provides the best care at the lowest cost, and to include a critical reevaluation of the care plan with each patient interaction or treatment throughout the course of care. To that end, this chapter examines briefly the need for lung expansion and bronchial hygiene therapies, including a detailed look at the available options in terms of efficacy, comfort, and cost.

ATELECTASIS

Atelectasis, or collapsed lung parenchyma, ranges in severity from microatelectasis (invisible on radiograph) to macroatelectasis. Although macroatelectasis is estimated to occur in less than 6% of patients undergoing surgery, estimates range as high as 60% of patients undergoing upper abdominal procedures.[4] Atelectasis leads to decreased alveolar size, which reduces compliance, leading to a further decrease in alveolar tidal volume. Microatelectasis may progress to involve subsegmental or larger areas, becoming visible on chest radiograph. The radiographic signs of atelectasis include localized increase in radiographic density, displacement of lobar fissures, elevation of the ipsilateral diaphragm, mediastinal shift, hilar displacement, regional approximation of ribs, and compensatory **hyperinflation** of the surrounding segments. Clinical features of atelectasis resolve after relief of the airway obstruction without treatment with antibiotics, hence distinguishing

atelectasis from a pulmonary infection. Atelectasis may cause pulmonary shunting and hypoxemia.[5] The presence of fever has been thought to be associated with atelectasis, but Engoren[6] reported no correlation between fever and the amount of atelectasis in 100 postoperative cardiac surgery patients. This contradicts common textbook dogma but agrees with previous human study and animal experiments.

The following factors are important in causing atelectasis:

Retained secretions: When an airway is obstructed with secretions and the alveoli distal to it collapse, lobar, segmental, or subsegmental atelectasis can occur. With the primary airway occluded, volume in the alveoli is reduced as gas is absorbed into the pulmonary capillaries, unless fresh gas enters by collateral channels.

Pain associated with surgery or trauma (especially upper abdominal and thoracic): Surgery and trauma to the abdomen and thorax may leave incisions or bruised areas that are sore and sensitive to stretching that occurs with deep breaths and coughing. This pain results in an altered breathing pattern characterized by shallow breaths, no sighing, and hesitation to cough effectively.

Altered patterns of breathing: After upper abdominal surgery, there is a 20% decrease in tidal volume, a 26% increase in respiratory rate, and a decrease in the frequency of sighing (taking deep breaths, at least three times normal tidal volume). This altered pattern of breathing is associated with decreased pulmonary compliance and increased closure of small airways.[7]

Alterations in small airway function: The postoperative state is associated with characteristic changes in small airway functions. Closing volume (CV), the lung volume at which small bronchioles close during exhalation, is usually less than expiratory reserve volume (ERV), so small airways remain patent throughout the normal respiratory cycle. Postoperatively, ERV may be reduced to less than CV, so airways are closed or occluded during tidal breathing. CV is increased in patients who smoke cigarettes, in those with chronic obstructive pulmonary disease (COPD), and in elderly patients. The greater the patient's CV, the greater is that patient's risk of developing atelectasis.

Prolonged supine position: Functional residual capacity (FRC) is reduced in normal subjects while in the supine position. In 1956, Miller and colleagues[8] demonstrated that changing from the supine to the lateral decubitus (right or left) position causes a small volume reduction in the dependent lung and a larger increase in the superior lung, producing an overall increase in FRC (Fig. 13–1). In critically ill patients, the prone position has been shown to improve FRC and oxygenation.[9,10] Torres and coworkers[11] demonstrated that the longer a ventilated patient remains in the supine position, the greater is the incidence of aspiration of gastric contents and associated pulmonary

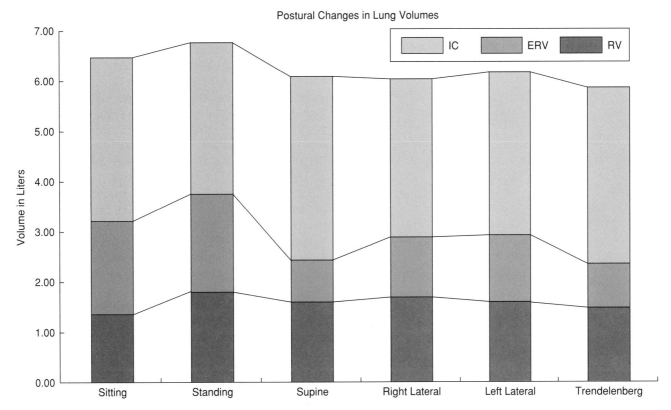

FIGURE 13−1 • Changes in lung volumes with position. Functional residual capacity (expiratory reserve volume [ERV] plus residual volume [RV]) is reduced in the supine position, with net increases in either lateral position. Note further reduction with patient in Trendelenburg's position. IC, inspiratory capacity.

complications, concluding that frequent position changes reduce risk.

Increased abdominal pressure after laparotomy: Increased general pressure in the abdomen translates to pressure against the diaphragm and reduced volumes in the lung.

Musculoskeletal or neurologic abnormalities: Abnormalities such as muscular dystrophy, spinal muscular atrophy, myasthenia, poliomyelitis, or cerebral palsy may be associated with compromised bellows function and reduced lung volumes.

Restrictive defects: These result in smaller vital capacities and reduced FRC.

Surgical procedures: Procedures such as open heart surgery, in which the left lung is deflated during the surgery, can result in postoperative atelectasis that typically requires several days to resolve, with or without therapy.

General Approach to the Prevention of Atelectasis

In patients with underlying pulmonary disease, aggressive preoperative preparation (eg, smoking cessation, bronchodilators, humidified air, and chest physical therapy) has been reported to result in a three-fold reduction in postoperative complications. Preoperatively, the patient is much more receptive to learning, practicing maneuvers, and consciously cooperating with the practitioner. Postoperatively, pain and medication taken to reduce pain may inhibit many factors, including cough, deep inspiration, early mobilization, attention span, and cooperation with respiratory care staff. Preoperative training is of particular importance in cigarette smokers, patients with COPD, the elderly, and obese (high-risk) patients.[12] Without preoperative instruction, the patient, on awaking from anesthesia, is instructed to take a deep breath and is rewarded with abdomen-splitting, gut-wrenching, and totally unexpected pain. Because patients tend to distrust people who surprise them with pain, they may be less than cooperative the next time some well-intentioned practitioner asks them to cough. In contrast, preoperative instruction allows the patient to be forewarned that coughing will hurt and that techniques such as splinting an abdominal incision with a pillow can minimize (not eliminate) the pain. The patient, who may be anxious before surgery, needs to understand that the consequences of *not* coughing include possible pulmonary complications, a slower recovery, and even more discomfort. Deep breathing and coughing provide patients with an active maneuver to perform that will help them speed their recovery. Forearmed with this knowledge, the patient awakens from anesthesia realizing that coughing will hurt but must be

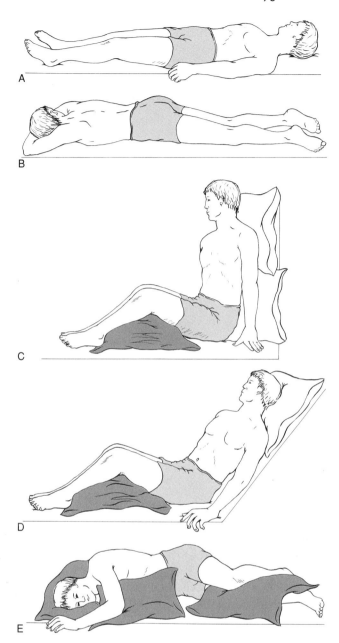

FIGURE 13–2 • Common positions: Supine (*A*), prone (*B*), Fowler's (*C*), semi-Fowler's (*D*), and side lying (*E*).

done, using the previously taught maneuvers. After preoperative instruction, when the practitioner coaches the patient to cough, the pain is not a surprise, and the trust relationship (and further cooperation) is not compromised.

PATIENT POSITIONING: KEEP IT MOVING

The primary technique for lung expansion is turning patients.[1,9] Patients should be encouraged to turn, or be turned, at least every 2 hours while awake. Even better than turning is sitting up and getting out of bed. Early mobilization of patients (who can safely get out of bed) pro-

vides a superb example of optimal lung expansion therapy, with minimal additional cost.[12]

In critical care and postoperative situations, where atelectasis is a major complication, factors such as pain and risk of dislodging tubes, monitor leads, and lines make it tempting to leave the patient in a supine position for a prolonged period. The longer a patient remains in the supine position, the greater is the chance that lung volumes will be reduced and that secretions, aspirated gastric contents, and third-space interstitial fluids will pool in gravity-dependent areas.[13,14]

Turning the patient from the supine to the lateral or prone position (Fig. 13–2) results in a net increase in lung volumes (FRC) and improved oxygenation.[8] As the patient is turned, the weight of the mediastinum, lung tissue, and abdominal contents tends to compress the gravity-dependent lung, whereas the superior lung is pulled open to a larger volume, resulting in a net increase in lung volume (see Fig. 13–1). Douglas and colleagues[9] demonstrated that the use of the supported prone position (supporting the patient at the hips and chest, allowing the abdominal contents to hang freely) results in larger lung volumes with similar increases in oxygen saturation as does the application of **continuous positive airway pressure** (CPAP) in COPD patients in acute respiratory failure.[9] Subsequently, use of the prone position, even without support, has been shown to offer significant benefits in oxygenation (Fig. 13–3).

Changing body position also affects distribution of both blood and lymphatic fluids because both pulmonary blood flow and lymphatic circulation are relatively low-pressure systems that are greatly affected by gravity. As the patient is turned, blood, lymphatic fluid, and third-space water preferentially redistribute to gravity-dependent areas of the lung (Fig. 13–4). In healthy lung tissue, ventilation also is increased in gravity-dependent areas, with smaller alveoli being more compliant than larger alveoli. When areas of atelectatic lung are moved to a superior position, the weight of the mediastinum and lung pulls on elastic tissue in the lung, expanding the airways and alveoli. Consequently, in the superior lung, there is reduced perfusion, increased forces expanding the airway, and reduced tidal ventilation secondary to the increased size of the airways. The strategy of placing the good lung down promotes good ventilation, matching areas of perfusion, whereas the superior lung is expanded and perfusion reduced.

Just as changes in body position can improve the matching of ventilation with perfusion in the dependent lung, turn-

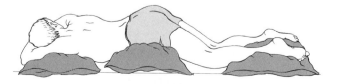

FIGURE 13–3 • Supported prone position.

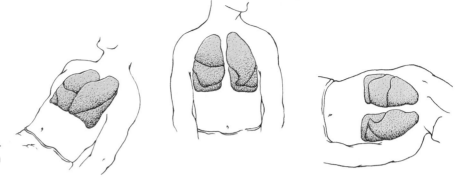

FIGURE 13-4 • Changes in perfusion and ventilation matching with position change.

ing may have deleterious effects, so that each change in position should be evaluated for patient tolerance.[15–17] When the bad lung is in the dependent position, decreased ventilation interfaces with increased perfusion, resulting in less effective oxygenation and possible hemodynamic instability. When turning unstable or critically ill patients, it is important to evaluate oxygen saturation, dyspnea, and changing blood pressures to determine patient response and tolerance.

In unilateral lung disease, it is tempting to place the good lung down for prolonged periods of time. The problem is that the gravity-dependent intercellular and lymphatic fluids and secretions migrate with gravity, transforming the good lung into the bad lung. In such cases, turning the patient so that the bad lung is down, even for short periods (eg, every 1 or 2 hours), helps to maintain the integrity of the good lung.

The use of rotating beds that continuously turn the patient from side to side (Fig. 13–5) has been advocated for critically ill patients, with reported reductions in pulmonary complications.[18–21] These beds are designed to shift position automatically, decreasing problems with pulled and disconnected lines from the patient, but are considerably more ex-

pensive than standard beds. Although preliminary study results have been encouraging, controlled studies are necessary to determine superiority of these expensive support devices over the standard practice of turning patients from side to side every 2 hours (Box 13–1).

Box • 13–1 PROCEDURE FOR POSITIONING (TURNING AND MOBILIZING) THE PATIENT

1. Explain to the patient that the reason for frequent position changes and mobility is to promote lung expansion and to improve oxygenation of the blood.
2. Encourage the patient to turn independently or assist the patient to change position as necessary. Optimal positions for lung expansion and secretion mobilization are the oblique side-lying position, with the bed at any degree of inclination tolerated by the patient, and prone. Sitting, dangling at the bedside, and ambulating also are effective in promoting lung expansion and secretion mobilization.
3. Repositioning frequency is determined in part by assessment of tissue tolerance. The reddened area marking the points of pressure should disappear within 30 minutes after the patient is repositioned. If the reddened area remains longer than 30 minutes, the turning frequency should be increased or the support surface changed.
4. Pillows and other positioning devices should be used to keep bony prominences from direct contact with one another, and to prop up or help support the patient in the desired position.
5. With each change in position, assess patient for increased dyspnea, decreased oxygen saturation, and discomfort.
6. Even when positions are poorly tolerated, position changes for as little as 5 minutes promote redistribution of ventilation, blood perfusion, and lymphatic flow.
7. Document patient response in the patient record.

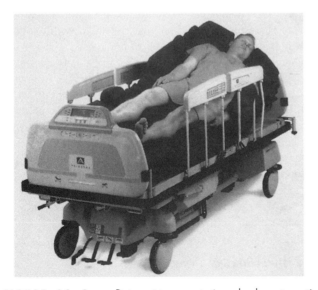

FIGURE 13-5 • Rotorest-type rotating bed automatically moves patient from side to side.

POSTURAL DRAINAGE THERAPY

Although turning is for everyone, a much smaller, select group of patients may benefit from additional assistance to help mobilize secretions and promote lung expansion with the help of gravity. PDT consists of positioning (posturing) the patient so that gravity helps to drain secretions from specific segments and lobes of the lung toward the central airways, where they can be more readily removed with cough or mechanical aspiration. This is accomplished by positioning the patient so that the affected segments of the lung are above the patient's carina, with each position maintained for at least 5 to 10 minutes. Twelve positions have been identified to drain all areas of the lungs (see later).

PDT was first described in the 1930s by a physical therapist in England to reduce postoperative complications for tuberculosis patients in that preantibiotic era, when bronchiectasis required removal of parts of the lungs of these patients. Bronchiectasis, with its large quantities of foul-smelling secretions, was thought to increase the risk of infection of the surgical site. PDT, or tipping the patient before surgery, helped to remove the secretions from the airway and reduce complications of surgery. From these humble beginnings, PDT became a commonly prescribed tool for prophylactic bronchial hygiene in a wide range of patients, from those with viral pneumonia to those with postoperative heart surgery, with negligible or questionable results.

There is evidence that PDT is effective in the treatment of acute and stable cystic fibrosis, bronchiectasis, and other conditions characterized by excessive sputum production that the patient has difficulty clearing.[22] PDT has been found to have little or no effect in conditions presenting with scant secretions. Consequently, the indications for PDT are limited largely to patients diagnosed with cystic fibrosis,[23–29] bronchiectasis,[24,30] or cavitating lung disease and to adult patients who produce at lease 30 mL/d of secretions and have difficulty clearing them.[31–42]

External Manipulation of the Thorax

Percussion

Percussion therapy involves rapidly striking the external thorax directly over the lung segment being drained, using either cupped hands or a mechanical device purported to assist secretion mobilization by shaking loose the secretions (Fig. 13–6). This procedure is also referred to as *cupping, clapping,* or *striking.*

There is little evidence that percussion improves mobilization of secretions during PDT and no evidence that percussion alone, without posturing, is of any value. There is no convincing research demonstrating superiority of manual or mechanical methods.[28,30,43–46]

Vibration

Vibrating the chest wall over the draining area with a fine tremorous action has also been advocated to assist mobilization of secretions during PDT. Vibration is performed manually by pressing in the direction that the ribs and soft tissue of the chest move during expiration. Mechanical vibrators also may be used (Fig. 13–7). Although some evidence suggests that vibration for 1 hour can increase movement of secretions, conclusive evidence has yet to be provided that supports the efficacy of this procedure, the superiority of manual methods over mechanical methods, or an optimal frequency.[22,26,30,32,33,37,47–52]

Patients should be evaluated for a variety of conditions that may be exacerbated by performing percussion or vibration to the thorax. It is important to inspect the thorax visually for irregularities of the skin, such as burns, open wounds, skin infections, and recent skin grafts. Review the patient's history, and palpate the tissue of the thorax to identify subcutaneous emphysema or a recently placed transvenous or subcutaneous pacemaker, particularly when using mechanical devices. Do not apply percussion if there has been recent epidural spinal infusion of anesthesia.

Whether or not vibration or percussion is effective for mobilization of secretions, the application of these procedures, especially with mechanical vibrators and percussors, may feel good to the patient. This may be the most convincing reason to consider applying these techniques during PDT sessions.

Contraindications

Positioning

Caution should be exercised when positioning any patient, especially in light of the conditions listed in Box 13–2.

Placing the patient in a head-down or Trendelenburg's position affects both hemodynamics and interaction of physical forces between the thorax and the abdomen. With the head down, there is increased blood flow to the head, and Trendelenburg's position should be avoided in patients who have increased intracranial pressure (ICP), for example, from neurosurgery, aneurysms, or eye surgery, of more than 20 mmHg;[53,54] uncontrolled hypertension; or gross hemoptysis (related to recent lung carcinoma treated surgically or with radiation therapy).[53] Shifting of abdominal and thoracic contents in Trendelenburg's position may be deleterious in patients at risk for aspiration because of an uncontrolled airway, distended abdomen, or recent esophageal surgery. Reverse Trendelenburg's position may be hazardous for patients with hypotension or for those on vasoactive medication.

Postural Drainage Therapy

The decision to use PDT requires assessment of potential benefits and risks. The specific modality and duration of

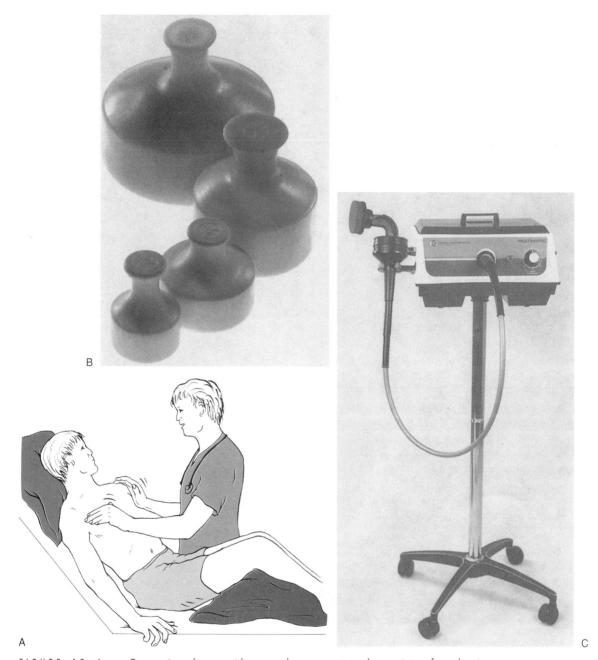

FIGURE 13–6 • Percussion shown with manual movement and a variety of mechanical devices. (*B*, Courtesy of DHD Medical Products, Canastota, NY; *C*, Courtesy of General Physiotherapy, St. Louis, MO.)

therapy should occur for no longer than is necessary to achieve the desired therapeutic results.[51]

During PDT, care should be taken to identify signs and symptoms of associated hazards and complications, including hypoxemia, bronchospasm, acute hypotension, increased ICP, pulmonary hemorrhage (blood in the sputum), pain or injury to the tissue, and vomiting with risk of aspiration.

If hypoxemia occurs or is likely to occur during positioning or PDT, administer additional oxygen during the procedure. If the patient becomes hypoxemic during treat-

ment, administer 100% oxygen, stop therapy immediately, return the patient to the original resting position, and consult the physician. Ensure adequate ventilation. Hypoxemia during PDT can be avoided in unilateral lung disease by placing the involved lung uppermost while the patient is in the side-lying position.[18,55–58]

With evidence suggesting increased ICP or acute hypotension, stop therapy, return the patient to the original resting position, and consult the physician. Consider the use of modified positions, such as a less severe angle of Trendelenburg's position, with future therapy. Moderate

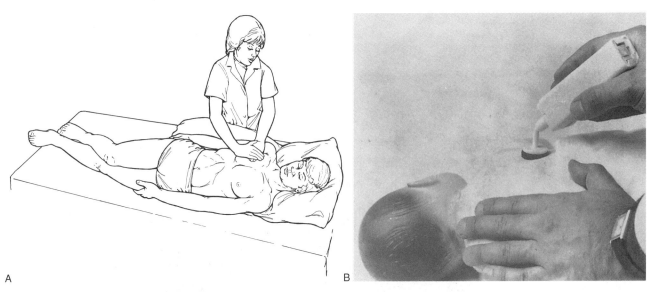

FIGURE 13-7 • Manual techniques and mechanical devices used for vibration. (*A*, Scanlon: *Egan's Fundamentals of Respiratory Care*. St. Louis: CV Mosby; 1995; *B*, Courtesy of General Physiotherapy, St. Louis, MO.)

changes in respiratory rate and pulse rate are expected. Bradycardia, tachycardia, increasingly irregular pulse, and a decrease or dramatic increase in blood pressure are indications for stopping therapy.

With signs of pulmonary hemorrhage or fresh blood in the sputum, stop therapy, return the patient to the original resting position, and call the physician immediately. Remain with the patient, administer oxygen, and ensure an open airway until the physician responds.

Box • 13-2   POSITIONING CONTRAINDICATIONS

- Intracranial pressure >20 mmHg[53,54]
- Head and neck injury until stabilized
- Active hemorrhage with hemodynamic instability
- Recent spinal surgery (eg, laminectomy)
- Acute spinal injury
- Active hemoptysis
- Empyema
- Bronchopleural fistula
- Pulmonary edema associated with congestive heart failure
- Large pleural effusions
- Pulmonary embolism
- Aged, confused, or nervous patient who does not tolerate position changes
- Rib fracture with or without flail chest

If the patient complains of pain or injury to muscles, ribs, or spine, stop the therapy that appears directly associated with the pain or problem and exercise care in moving the patient. Consult the physician or physical therapist.

To minimize the risk of vomiting and possible aspiration, perform therapy either before meals or more than 1 hour after meals. For patients receiving tube feedings, stop feeding 1 hour before and during therapy. If vomiting occurs, stop therapy, clear the patient's airway, suction as needed, administer oxygen, maintain the airway, return the patient to the previous resting position, and contact the physician immediately.

In patients with a history of bronchospasm, consider scheduling treatments to administer physician-ordered bronchodilators before PDT. A p.r.n. order for albuterol to treat increased wheezing or bronchospasm that occurs during therapy may be of some value. If more than mild bronchospasm occurs, stop therapy, return the patient to the previous resting position, and administer or increase oxygen delivery while contacting the physician.

With effective therapy, breath sounds may worsen as secretions move into the larger airways, increasing rhonchi. An increase of adventitious breath sounds often represents a marked improvement over absent or diminished breath sounds. Note any effect that coughing may have on breath sounds.

Sputum production of less than 25 mL/d with PDT is not enough to justify this procedure.[4,17,29,39,46,48,49,54] Some patients have productive coughs with sputum production from 15 to 30 mL/d (occasionally as high as 70 or 100 mL/d) without use of PDT. If PDT does not increase sputum clearance in a patient who produces more than 30 mL/d of sputum without PDT, the continued use of PDT is not indicated. Improved ease of clearing secretions during and after treatments supports continuation (Box 13–3).

Percussion

Percussion carries substantial additional risk, with little shown benefit. Because percussion is intended to shake loose secretions, it is contraindicated in patients with suspected pulmonary tuberculosis and resectable tumors of the thorax or neck, based on concern that it might shake loose or break up cysts and tumors, spreading bacteria or cancerous cells to other parts of the body (small lipomas and sebaceous cysts are not contraindications to percussion). Evaluate the presence of bronchospasm before and during therapy. Percussion has been associated with precipitating and increasing bronchospasm, resulting in increased wheezing, airway closure, and dyspnea. Potential damage to the thorax from percussion makes osteoporosis and osteomyelitis of the ribs, as well as complaints of chest pain, relative contraindica-

tions. Lung contusion and coagulopathies may be aggravated by percussion and vibration, resulting in increased bruising or bleeding within the chest wall or lung.

Clockwise Rotation for Complete Postural Drainage

A straightforward methodology for performing a complete PDT session with minimal movement of the patient might be viewed as a clockwise rotation of the patient, with each rotation draining a different segment of the lung. With modern hospital equipment, it is easier to modify the foot elevation of the bed than to make major position changes for the patient. Each position should be maintained for 5 to 10 minutes as tolerated, with the patient encouraged to deep breathe and cough during and between positions.

The following list starts with the patient flat on the back and proceeds through eight partial turns in a clockwise direction. The figures on the left indicate the body position and the position of the bed (Fig. 13–8).

(text continues on page 356)

Box • 13–3 PROCEDURE FOR POSTURAL DRAINAGE THERAPY

1. Assess whether PDT is indicated, and design a program to accomplish treatment objectives, identifying specific areas of the patient's lungs that might benefit from drainage.
2. Gather appropriate equipment, as follows:
   a. Bed or table that can assume range of positions, from Trendelenburg's to reverse Trendelenburg's position
   b. Pillows for supporting patient while in position
   c. Light towel for covering area of chest during percussion
   d. Tissues or basin for collecting expectorated sputum
   e. Suction equipment for patient unable to clear own secretions
   f. Gloves, goggles, gown, and mask
   g. Hand-held and mechanical percussor or vibrator (optional)
3. After initial patient treatment or training, communicate treatment plan to physician and nurse and provide instruction to nursing staff if required.
4. Explain to the patient that PD therapy is used to reexpand lung tissue and help mobilize secretions. Teach patient to perform active cycle of breathing and the huff-directed cough procedure.
5. Instruct the patient as follows:
   a. To assume each position with minimum of dis-

comfort and to maintain each position for 5 to 10 minutes
   b. To move from position to position with minimum of effort
   c. To take slow deep breaths
   d. To notify practitioner if feeling uncomfortable, short of breath, or dizzy
6. While draining a position, apply percussion or vibration over the affected area of the lung. Manual vibration often is performed on exhalation.
7. Encourage patient to take slow deep breaths and to cough between positions.
8. Modify positions to optimize patient tolerance and comfort (ie, reduce angle of head down tilt while draining posterior basal segments).
9. Assist patient in clearing and disposing of secretions. Note color, consistency, volume, and odor.
10. Evaluate the patient for their ability to self-administer. When appropriate, teach patient to self-administer. Observe patient self-administration on several occasions to ensure proper technique uncoached before allowing patient to self-administer without supervision.
11. Document procedures performed, positions drained, patient response to therapy, patient teaching provided, and patient ability to self-administer in the patient's medical record.

Start with bed flat.

1. Patient is in supine position with pillow under knees for comfort.

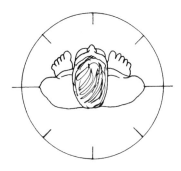

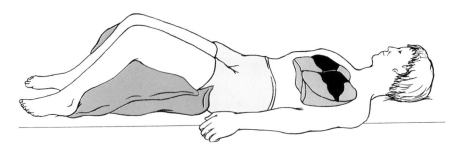

Area drained: anterior segment of both upper lobes.

Place the patient in a head-down position, with the foot of the bed elevated about 14 inches (or 20 degrees), as tolerated.

2. Patient rolls partially onto the right side, with pillow between the knees and left arm draped back over a pillow that is behind the back and shoulder.

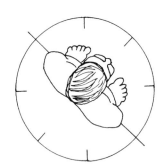

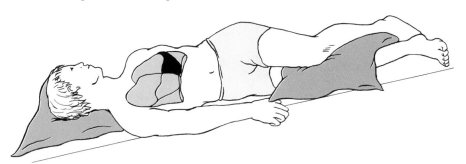

Area drained: lingular segment, left lower lobe.

Raise foot of bed an additional 4 inches (to 30 degrees), as tolerated.

3. Patient is on right side, not leaning forward or back. Foot of bed is raised another 4 inches as tolerated.

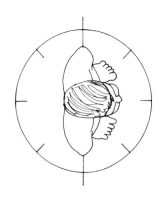

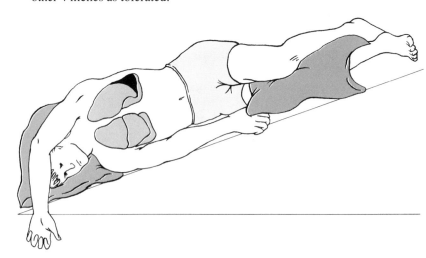

Area drained: anterior basal segment, left lower lobe.

FIGURE 13–8 • Twelve positions for postural drainage.

4. Patient lies with right side down and drapes arm forward, over the pillow in front of the thorax.

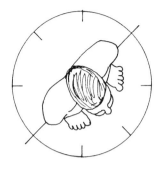

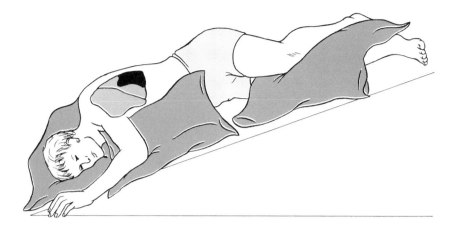

Area drained: lateral basal segment, left lower lobe.

Lower foot of bed to flat position.

5. Patient lies in prone position, with two pillows under hips and bed flat.

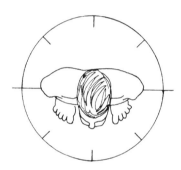

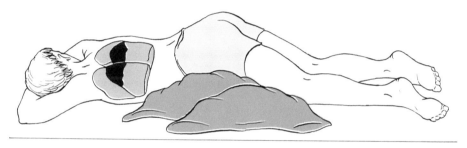

Area drained: Superior segment of both lower lobes.

Raise foot of bed an additional 4 inches (to 30 degrees), as tolerated.

6. Patient lies in prone position, with pillow under hips and foot of bed raised 18 inches (30 degrees), as tolerated.

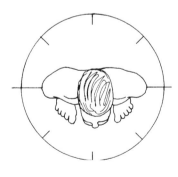

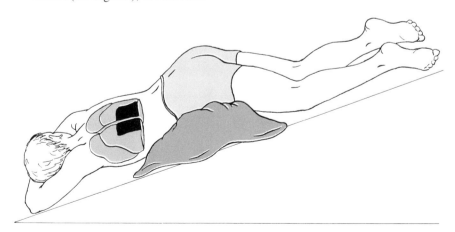

Area drained: posterior basal segments of both lower lobes.

FIGURE 13-8 • Continued.

7. Patient rolls onto left side, draping arm of pillow in front of chest and abdomen, with pillow between knees for comfort.

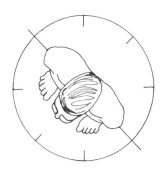

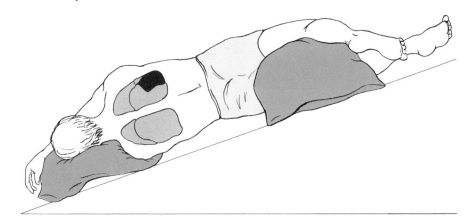

Area drained: lateral basal segment, right lower lobe.

8. Patient rolls directly onto right side, not leaning forward or back.

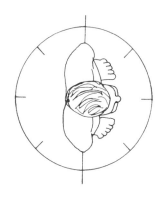

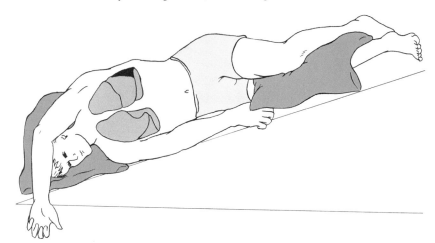

Area drained: anterior basal segment, right lower lobe.

Lower foot of bed by 4 inches to 20 degrees.

9. Patient lies on left side, drapes arm and shoulder back over pillow placed behind back and shoulders.

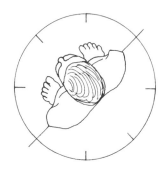

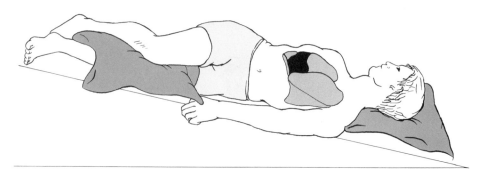

Area drained: right middle lobe.

FIGURE 13–8 • Continued.

Allow patient to roll over onto back and change bed position to Fowler's position.

10. Patient leans back in bed, with pillow under knees for comfort.

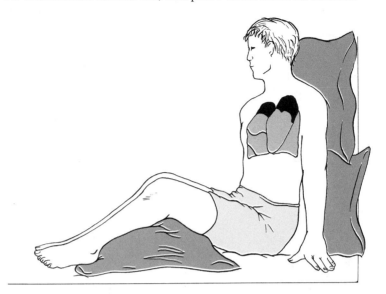

Area drained: apical segment of both upper lobes.

Place bed in semi-Fowler's position.

11. Patient in same position as in number 10.

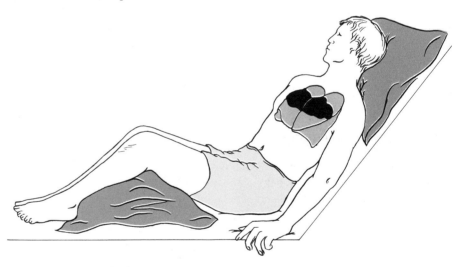

Area drained: anterior segment, left upper lobe.

12a. Patient rolls over to prone position with bed in semi-Fowler's position, pillow beneath head and chest, and pillows between knees for comfort, *or*
Area drained: posterior segment, left upper lobe.

FIGURE 13–8 • Continued.

12b. Patient sits up, dangling legs over side of bed, and leans forward over pillows on a bedside table, *or*

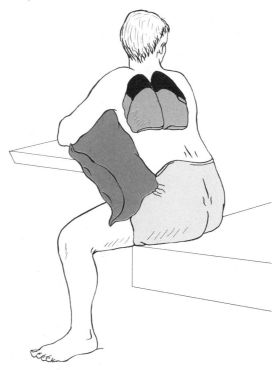

12c. Patient straddles chair, facing back rest and leaning forward against back rest.

FIGURE 13-8 • Continued.

Realistically, most patients spend a lot of time sitting up, or in semi-Fowler's position; thus, one may question the value of spending staff time in performing drainage for the upper lobes in most patients.

DEEP BREATHING AND COUGHING

The normal mechanism for lung expansion is spontaneous deep breathing (including yawn and sigh maneuvers) and an effective cough.[59] Instructing and encouraging the patient to take sustained deep breaths is among the safest, most effective, and least expensive strategies for keeping the lungs expanded.[60] The negative intrathoracic pressure generated during spontaneous deep breathing tends to inflate the less compliant, gravity-dependent areas of the lung better than do methods relying on lung inflation by application of PAP. A deep breath is a key component for a normal effective cough. Directed cough and active cycle of breathing (ACB; including the forced expiratory technique [FET] or huff-directed coughing) have been shown to be more effective in mobilizing secretions and increasing lung volumes than has PDT with percussion and vibration in patients with cystic fibrosis or chronic bronchitis.[61–66]

ACTIVE CYCLE OF BREATHING

The ACB techniques are a combination of three basic techniques:

• Breathing control
• Thoracic expansion control
• FET

Breathing control, commonly referred to with the misnomer of **diaphragmatic breathing,** has been described by Webber[66] as gentle breathing with the lower chest. While the upper chest and shoulders are relaxed, the patient breathes at normal tidal volume and rate. On inspiration, the patient should feel a swelling around the waist, which subsides while exhaling. Breathing control is basically the default maneuver between the more active techniques.

Thoracic expansion exercises are simply large breaths with active inspiration and relaxed expiration. Increasing lung volume increases air flow through small airways and collateral ventilation channels, increasing the volume of gas available to help mobilize secretions on expiration. This is limited to three or four deep breaths to avoid fatigue and hyperventilation.

The FET consists of one or two forced expirations or huffs, combined with a period of controlled breathing. A normal breath is taken in, and then the air is squeezed out by contracting the chest wall and abdominal muscles. The mouth and glottis are kept open. The huff should not be a violent or explosive exhalation. Some people find that physical compression of the chest wall helps during the huff.

> ### Box • 13–4   ACTIVE CYCLE OF BREATHING
>
> - Patient in a relaxed sitting or reclined position
> - Several minutes of relaxed diaphragmatic breathing (breathing control)
> - Three to four active deep inspirations with passive relaxed exhalation (thoracic expansion)
> - Relaxed diaphragmatic breathing
> - As the patient feels secretions entering the larger central airway, two to three huffs (forced expiratory techniques) followed by relaxed breathing control
> - Cycle repeated two to four times, as tolerated

The active cycle can be taught to parents with children from the age of about 2 years, with children working independently from about age 8 or 9 years. Exercise should be encouraged; patients often find increased exercise is associated with shorter requirements for ACB sessions (Box 13–4).

An effective cough is a vital component of lung expansion therapy. The normal cough (Fig. 13–9) involves taking a deep breath, closing the glottis, and compressing abdominal and thoracic muscles (generating pressures in excess of 80 mmHg), followed by an explosive release of gas as the glottis opens. In addition to mobilizing and expelling secretions, the high pressures generated during a cough may be an important factor in reexpanding lung tissue. Comparable pressures generated by positive pressure applied to the airway have been associated with barotrauma, which does not appear to be a problem with controlled cough maneuvers. The downside of the normal coughing maneuver is that it can be extremely painful for the patient (especially after upper abdominal surgery), and although coughing does not compromise coronary blood flow,[67] it has been reported to dislodge central venous catheters.[68] Paroxysms of uncontrolled coughing have been associated with neurologic symptoms[69] and gastroesophageal reflux.[70]

In patients with COPD and unstable airways, high pressures and flow combine in the dynamic compression of the airways, trapping gas and secretions. For these patients, ACB with the FET or huff appears to be the maneuver of choice.[71–74] Huff coughing is an FET that is performed by exhaling from high to middle lung volumes through an open glottis. The individual takes in a slow, deep breath, followed by a 1- to 3-second breath hold, and then performs short, quick, forced exhalations with the glottis open. The subject may be instructed to say the word huff during exhalation. Small children can be taught to flap their arms to their lateral chest as they perform the huff cough, a technique referred to as the *chicken (flapping wings) breath,* to focus on the expiratory maneuver, associating positive reinforcement and play with the huff technique[75] (Box 13–5; Figs. 13–10 and 13–11).

AUTOGENIC DRAINAGE

Autogenic drainage is a system of breathing exercises that has been shown to be as effective as PDT in mobilizing secretions in patients with cystic fibrosis and COPD. This technique depends on staged breathing at different lung volumes, starting with small tidal breaths from ERV, repeated until secretions are felt gathering in the airways. At that point, the cough is suppressed, and a larger tidal volume is taken for a series of 10 to 20 breaths, followed by a series of larger (approaching vital capacity) breaths, followed by several huff coughs (Fig. 13–12). Although this technique has been shown to be effective, it requires a great deal of patient cooperation and is recommended only in children older than 8 years and in patients who have a good sense of their own breathing.

INCENTIVE SPIROMETRY: ENCOURAGING SPONTANEOUS DEEP BREATHING

Incentive spirometry is an artifice developed to coax the patient to mimic natural sighing or yawning maneuvers by taking slow, deep breaths, also referred to as **sustained maximal inspiration** (SMI).[76,77] Because patients often

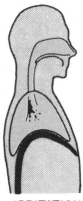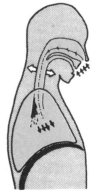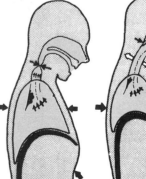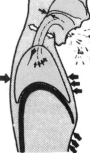

FIGURE 13–9 • Sequence of a normal cough. (Cherniak RH, Cherniak L. *Respiration in Health and Disease.* 3rd. ed. Philadelphia: WB Saunders; 1983.)

IRRITATION   INSPIRATION   COMPRESSION   EXPULSION

Box • 13–5   PROCEDURE FOR DIRECTED COUGH

1. Explain to the patient that deep breathing and coughing will help to keep the lungs expanded and clear of secretions.
2. Assist the patient to a sitting position or to a semi-Fowler's position if sitting position is not possible.
3. Begin standard directed cough procedure (see below for modifications).
   a. Instruct patient to take a deep breath, then hold the breath, using abdominal muscles to force air against a closed glottis, then cough with a single exhalation.
   b. The patient should take several relaxed breaths before the next cough effort.
   c. Document teaching accomplished, procedures performed, and patient response in the patient's medical record.
4. Begin alternate standard huff-directed cough procedure.
   a. Instruct patient to take three to five slow deep breaths, inhaling through the nose, exhaling through pursed lips, using diaphragmatic breathing. Have patient take a deep breath and hold the breath for 1 to 3 seconds.
   b. The patient should exhale from middle lung volumes to low lung volumes (to clear secretions from peripheral airways). The patient should take a normal breath and then squeeze the breath out by contracting the abdominal and chest wall mus-

cles, with the mouth (and glottis) open, while whispering the word huff (sounds like a forced sigh) during exhalation. This is repeated several times.
   c. As secretions enter the larger airways, the patient exhales from high to middle lung volumes to clear secretions from more proximal airways. This maneuver is repeated two or three times.
   d. Several relaxed diaphragmatic breaths should be taken before the next cough effort.
   e. Document teaching accomplished, procedures performed, and patient response in the patient record.
5. Use modified directed cough procedure in the following situations:
   a. Patients who have had abdominal or thoracic surgery: Instruct patient to place hand or a pillow over the incisional site and to apply gentle pressure while coughing (see Fig. 13-10). Personnel may assist with incisional support during coughing. Support chest tubes as necessary.
   b. Quadriplegic patients: Place your palms on the patient's abdomen, below the diaphragm, and instruct the patient to take three deep breaths (see Fig. 13-11). On exhalation of the third breath, push forcefully inward and upward as the patient coughs (similar to abdominal thrust maneuver performed on unconscious patient with an obstructed airway).

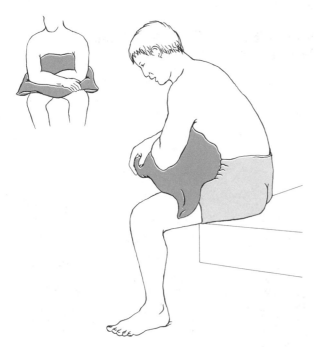

FIGURE 13–10 • Patient splinting abdomen with pillow while coughing.

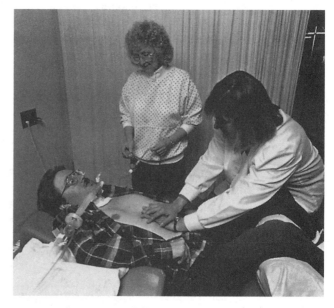

FIGURE 13–11 • RCP assisting a quadriplegic patient to cough.

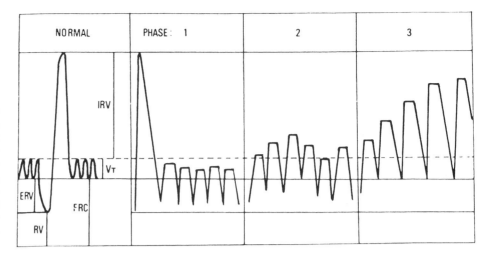

FIGURE 13-12 • Spirogram of autogenic drainage. ERV, expiratory reserve volume; FRC, functional residual capacity; IRV, inspiratory reserve volume; RV, residual volume; V$_T$, tidal volume. (Hardy KA. A review of airway clearance: New techniques, indications and recommendations. *Respir Care.* 1994; 39:446.)

stop sighing and adopt rapid, shallow breathing patterns after surgery, they should be encouraged to take 5 to 10 deep breaths every hour. Incisional pain and splinting may make those breaths painful after upper abdominal surgery, so IS devices provide patients with sensory feedback to quantify the deepness of their breaths. IS should provide patients with an objective comparison with the volumes (of flows) they were generating preoperatively, with the goal of attaining or returning to that preoperative volume despite the pain experienced. In addition, the IS device instruction should include how long the breaths should be held, how many times the breaths were attempted, and how many times the patient succeeded in meeting the volume goals.

Objectives of SMI are to increase transpulmonary pressure and inspiratory volumes to near preoperative or normal vital capacity, improve inspiratory muscle performance, and reestablish or simulate the normal pattern of pulmonary hyperinflation. When the SMI maneuver is repeated on a regular basis, airway patency may be maintained and lung atelectasis prevented and reversed.[78–80]

IS is indicated for use as prophylactic treatment of conditions predisposing to the development of pulmonary atelectasis, including upper abdominal surgery, and in thoracic patients with COPD, obesity, or advanced age. Although IS is valuable in the treatment of pulmonary atelectasis, it should not be used as the sole treatment for major lung collapse or consolidation, but rather as a part of a more comprehensive program of lung reexpansion.

Because SMI requires patient cooperation, as well as the ability to understand and demonstrate proper use of the device, IS is not a viable therapeutic option for the obtunded, confused, or uncooperative patient. IS is not the therapeutic option of choice for the patient who *cannot* spontaneously generate a vital capacity greater than 10 mL/kg or an inspiratory capacity more than one third of predicted value (generally considered the level of lung volume or capacity required for an effective cough).[81] For these patients, consider options such as IPPB or PAP.

As with many therapeutic modalities in respiratory care, IS is ineffective unless properly performed at ordered frequencies, making compliance a critical issue. If the patient experiences significant pain during deep inspiratory efforts, pain management or alternative options such as PAP should be considered.

When patient adherence appears to be a problem, the IS device used should record the number of breaths attempted and the number of times volume and breath-hold goals were accomplished. Although most IS devices are used with a mouthpiece, they may be adapted for use with an open tracheal stoma or artificial airway.

Evidence suggests that deep breathing alone, without mechanical aides, can be as beneficial as IS in preventing or reversing pulmonary complications, and controversy exists concerning overuse of the procedure.[1,2,5,60,82–85] If patients can take deep breaths without the IS device, encourage them to do so at regular intervals. Deep breathing, coughing, and IS work best as shared tasks among all the patient care personnel in the surgical units and wards, with each practitioner providing frequent reminders to the patients.

Need assessment for IS should focus on factors including surgical procedures involving the upper abdomen or thorax, conditions predisposing to development of atelectasis (eg, immobility, poor pain control, and abdominal binders), and the presence of neuromuscular disease involving respiratory musculature.[81] Outcome assessment should include absence of or improvement in signs of atelectasis (eg, decreased respiratory rate, improved breath sounds, normal chest radiograph, and improved P(A − a) O$_2$. For the surgical patient, increased vital capacity, peak expiratory flows, and return of FRC or vital capacity to preoperative values (in absence of lung resection) represent positive clinical outcomes. Improved inspiratory muscle performance and increased forced vital capacity (FVC) are desirable outcomes for patients with restrictive and neuromuscular problems.[81]

Equipment

The original Bartlett-Edwards incentive spirometer (McGraw) was a **volume displacement** device (Fig. 13–13). A piston-like plate rises as the patient inspires, and an indicator estimates the volume inspired while a battery-powered light flashes after a present volume goal is achieved. Other concepts in volume displacement include a cylindric bellows that is displaced upward as the patient inspires, with a scale on the side of the container with markers to indicate volume goals. These units do not record attempts or achieved goals and tend to be bulky, requiring a lot of space at the patient bedside and on the hospital supply shelves.

The volumetric incentive spirometer combines a quasi-volume displacement indicator (takes less space) and flow indicator (to encourage slow inspirations).

The other genre of IS device is the simple **flow-oriented incentive device**. Although the underlying premise of IS is taking deep breaths with an inspiratory hold, a large number of institutions have adopted IS flow-oriented devices to save space and costs. These devices usually direct the inspiratory flow through a tube to lift one or more light balls (or disks). The higher the patient's inspiratory flow rate, the higher or greater are the number of balls that are raised. The longer the flow is maintained, the larger is the volume, so the patient is encouraged to take slow deep breaths. Unfortunately, high flows can be generated (with low volumes) to raise the flow indicator to target levels, without the patient meeting therapeutic volume or breath-holding objectives. Although flow-oriented IS devices impose additional work of breathing, ranging from 0.33 to 0.66 J/L,[82]

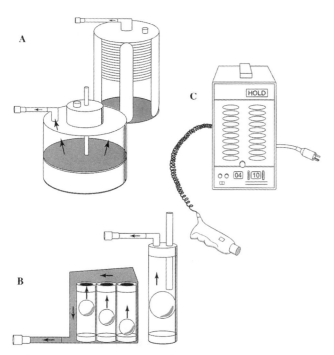

FIGURE 13–13 • Types of incentive spirometers.

it is unclear whether this additional work load is deleterious or part of the therapy. Successful use of these devices depends on effective patient education and compliance.

Another flow-based IS device uses a flow pneumotach to compute volumes based on flow and time. Increasing inhaled volumes results in lights on a scale ascending toward the level of a light on a parallel scale indicating the volume goal. When the goal is reached, a light goes on and stays on during the time that the patient should be holding the breath. Two digital counters indicate the number of attempts and number of times volume goal was achieved.

Lederer and colleagues[83] compared the Bartlett-Edwards Incentive Spirometer, the Triflo II, and the Spirocare in 79 patients divided into three groups. Patients were instructed preoperatively to take deep breaths (from resting volume, with 2- to 3-second hold) 10 times each hour while awake, with repeat instruction daily for five postoperative days. These investigators concluded that when left at the bedside with only one daily reinforcement of instructions, the three devices showed no clinically important differences. It is not known whether a clinical difference would exist with more frequent coaching. Certainly, a reduced frequency of use does not improve the relative efficacy of these devices.[84]

Independent of device, the inspiratory maneuver and the airway pressure pattern are the same (see Fig. 13–13). A number of researchers have demonstrated that IS is comparable in therapeutic effect to deep-breathing exercises,[85,86] coughing,[87] early mobilization,[88] and IPPB[85] in the postoperative patient. Hall and colleagues[89] demonstrated IS to be comparable to chest physical therapy after abdominal surgery, whereas mounting evidence suggests that IS may not have a viable role in thoracic surgery for patients with healthy lungs[86,87,90] (Box 13–6).

INTERMITTENT POSITIVE-PRESSURE BREATHING

Intermittent positive-pressure breathing is typically defined as short-term or episodic mechanical ventilation for the primary purpose of assisting ventilation and providing short-duration **hyperinflation therapy**.[91] Although IPPB historically has been administered with a variety of pneumatically driven, pressure-triggered, and pressure-limited ventilators (such as the Bird Mark 7 and Puritan Bennett AP-5 ventilators, which had significant inspiratory flow rate limitations), volume, pressure, time-limited, or flow-cycled ventilators may be used in the treatment of spontaneously breathing patients, with or without artificial airways.

IPPB originally was described in 1947; in the 1950s, the use of IPPB began to gain popularity as a method to treat and later prevent postoperative atelectasis and other lung problems. Its use corresponded with a perceived decrease in postoperative nosocomial pneumonia in surgical patients across the country, but support for IPPB was more anecdotal than empirically based. The use of IPPB expo-

---

Box • 13–6   PROCEDURE FOR INCENTIVE SPIROMETRY

1. Gather equipment.
2. Explain to the patient that taking deep breaths and coughing will keep the lungs expanded and that using the incentive spirometer will show how big a breath is being taken with the goal of returning to the normal volume before surgery. Warn patients that taking deep breaths and coughing may be painful after surgery but that deep breathing is essential for speedy recovery.
3. When possible, determine the patient's maximal lung volume achieved before surgery (or illness) and use that volume as the volume goal for incentive spirometry. If unable to assess preoperative volumes, set volume goal of 15 to 25 mL/kg of ideal body weight, as a minimum, with their predicted vital capacity as a maximum.
4. Assist the patient to a sitting position or to a semi-Fowler's position.
5. Instruct or assist the patient to splint incision when appropriate.
6. Introduce the patient to the incentive spirometer, describing how it works per manufacturer's instruction. Instruct the patient as follows:
    a. Place the spirometer on a flat surface or hold in an upright position.
    b. Place lips firmly around the mouthpiece.
    c. After a normal exhalation, inhale slowly through the mouthpiece, raising the volume indicator, and taking as deep a breath as possible.
    d. Hold breath for 3 to 5 seconds.
    e. Remove mouthpiece and exhale normally (or through pursed lips).
    f. Relax and breathe normally for several breaths.
    g. Repeat the maneuver to a total of 10 breaths each session (encourage the patient to take progressively deeper breaths up to the maximal goal).
    h. Repeat series of breaths once each hour while awake.
7. Observe the patient's color, heart rate, respiratory rate, and degree of dyspnea before, during, and after treatment. Care should be taken to avoid fatigue or dizziness.
8. Document procedures performed (including volume goals set, volume achieved, breaths per session, and frequency), patient response, and patient education in the patient medical record. Also document the ability of the patient to perform the maneuver without coaching.
9. Visit patient postoperatively to reinforce instruction and adjust volume goals as appropriate. Communicate with patient and nursing staff to determine compliance with self-administration; reassess or instruct as necessary.

---

nentially increased in the hospital, home, and beyond. The 1960s became the decade of the "puff parlor," typically a large room where a multitude of patients with COPD and other disorders would come, on an outpatient basis, to receive IPPB treatments with aerosol medications. In 1974, participants at the Sugarloaf Conference investigating the scientific basis for respiratory care concluded that there was little scientific basis for the use of IPPB. This was soon followed by members of the US Congress questioning the huge annual Medicare expenditure for IPPB therapy nationwide in light of the lack of evidence to support its use. IPPB soon became the treatment non grata of respiratory care departments, and its use was abolished in many institutions.[3]

IPPB has been advocated as a method for administration of aerosolized medication but has not been shown to provide any therapeutic advantage over the use of nebulizers or metered dose inhalers (MDIs) for spontaneously breathing patients.[91] In fact, Dolovich and coworkers[92] demonstrated that nebulized medication administered with IPPB results in 32% less drug deposited in the lung than does spontaneous breathing with the same type of nebulizer. Consequently, IPPB should not be used for lung expansion or aerosol administration in spontaneously breathing pa-

tients when less expensive and less invasive therapies can reliably meet clinical objectives.

Indications for IPPB therapy are included in Box 13–7.[84] All of the mechanical effects of IPPB are short lived, lasting 1 hour or less after the treatment. The efficacy of an IPPB device for ventilation and aerosol delivery is technique dependent (eg, coordination, breathing pattern, selection of appropriate inspiratory flow, peak pressure, inspiratory hold) and design dependent (eg, flow, volume, and pressure capability as well as aerosol output and particle size).[84]

Assessment of the need for IPPB should include evidence of atelectasis, reduced pulmonary function (eg, FEV_1 less than 65% predicted, FVC less than 70% predicted, maximum voluntary ventilation less than 50% predicted, vital capacity less than 10 mL/kg), preclusion of effective coughing, neuromuscular disorders, or kyphoscoliosis with associated decreases in lung volumes and capacities. IPPB may be applicable in situations of fatigue or muscle weakness with impending respiratory failure as well as in the presence of acute severe bronchospasm or exacerbated COPD that fails to respond to other therapy.

IPPB should be volume oriented, with tidal volume during IPPB adjusted to deliver breaths that are at least 25%

- The need to improve lung expansion, based on the presence of clinically important pulmonary atelectasis, when other forms of therapy have been unsuccessful (eg, incentive spirometry, chest physiotherapy, deep-breathing exercises, positive airway pressure) or when the patient cannot cooperate
- The inability to clear secretions adequately because of pathology that severely limits the ability to ventilate or cough effectively and failure to respond to other modes of treatment
- The need for short-term ventilatory support for patients who are hypoventilating as an alternative to tracheal intubation and continuous ventilatory support
- The need to deliver aerosol medication in the presence of severe bronchospasm (eg, acute asthma, unstable or status asthmaticus, exacerbated COPD) using a careful closely supervised trial of IPPB when treatment using other techniques (MDI or nebulizer) has been unsuccessful. IPPB may be used to deliver aerosol medications to patients with fatigue as a result of ventilatory muscle weakness (eg, failure to wean from mechanical ventilation, neuromuscular disease, kyphoscoliosis) or chronic conditions in which intermittent ventilatory support has been used for home care patients or nasal intermittent positive-pressure ventilation has been used for respiratory insufficiency.

larger than the patient's spontaneous volumes. It may well be argued that IPPB breaths should be targeted as high as 15 to 20 mL/kg, approximating a normal effective sigh volume. The effects of increased volume with IPPB can be assessed by determining if secretion clearance is enhanced as a consequence of deep breathing and coughing (cough more effective during treatment) as well as improvement in breath sounds, chest radiograph, and patient subjective response. FEV_1 or peak flow increase may be transiently improved with improved volume, secretion clearance, or response to aerosolized bronchodilators. IPPB may be provided with any device with assist-control or pressure-support mode; volume-, pressure-, or time-limited ventilator; or manual resuscitation device.

IPPB has not been shown to offer long- or short-term benefit greater than other lung-expansion therapeutic options in spontaneously breathing patients.[93–95] Like other lung-expansion therapies, IPPB has been associated with increased work of breathing.[96] Its use for lung expansion

should be considered only after all less invasive and expensive alternatives have been exhausted.[91] This should not be confused with the role of IPPB in the treatment of hypoventilating patients as a form of noninvasive mechanical ventilation[97–99] (Box 13–8).

POSITIVE AIRWAY PRESSURE

Positive airway pressure,[92] as defined by the American Association of Respiratory Care Clinical Practice Guideline,[100] includes the use of CPAP, **positive expiratory pressure** (PEP), and **expiratory positive airway pressure** (EPAP) to mobilize secretions and treat atelectasis. PAP bronchial hygiene techniques have proved to provide effective alternatives to chest physical therapy in expanding the lungs and mobilizing secretions. Evidence suggests that PAP therapy is more effective than IS and IPPB in the management of postoperative atelectasis[101,102] and as an adjunct to enhance the benefits of aerosol bronchodilator delivery.[103,104] Cough and other airway clearance techniques are essential components of PAP therapy.

Definitions

Continuous positive airway pressure is the application of a PAP to the spontaneously breathing patient during both inspiration and expiration.[100] The patient breathes from a pressurized circuit with a **threshold resistor** on the expiratory limb of the breathing. CPAP maintains a consistent airway pressure (5 to 20 cm H_2O) throughout the respiratory cycle. CPAP requires a relatively high gas flow available to the patient's airway that is sufficient to maintain the desired PAP.

EPAP applies positive pressure to the airway, much like CPAP, but only during expiration. Unlike CPAP, patients generate subatmospheric pressures on inspiration to take a breath. During EPAP therapy, the patient exhales against a threshold resistor, generating preset pressures of 5 to 20 cm H_2O.

PEP consists of positive pressure generated as the patient exhales through a **fixed orifice resistor**, generating pressures ranging from 10 to 20 cm H_2O (although pressures up to 60 cm H_2O have been reported). The fixed orifice resistor, which differentiates PEP from EPAP, generates pressure only when expired flows are high enough to generate back pressure through the small orifice. EPAP, using a threshold resistor, does not produce the same mechanical or physiologic effects that PEP produces with a fixed orifice. Further study is required to determine how these differences affect clinical outcome.

Threshold resistors, in theory, exert a predictable, quantifiable, and constant force at the expiratory limb of a circuit. When the force is applied over a unit area, a constant threshold pressure is established. Pressures exceeding threshold open the valve and allow expiration, whereas pressures below threshold close the valve, stopping the flow of gas. A

Box • 13–8 PROCEDURE FOR INTERMITTENT POSITIVE-PRESSURE BREATHING ADMINISTRATION

1. Assess whether IPPB therapy is indicated, and design a treatment program to accomplish treatment objectives.
   a. Bring equipment to bedside, and provide initial therapy to patient, adjusting pressure settings to meet patient need.
   b. After initial patient treatment and training, communicate treatment plan to physician and nurse, and provide instruction to nursing staff if required.
2. Explain that IPPB therapy is used to reexpand lung tissue, increase ventilation, deliver aerosol, and help mobilize secretions.
3. Instruct the patient as follows:
   a. Sit comfortably.
   b. If using a mask, apply it tightly but comfortably over the nose and mouth. If mouthpiece is used, place lips firmly around it and breathe through mouth.
   c. Begin breathing by turning on the respirator and then passively allowing the respirator to provide a breath that is larger than normal.
   d. Length of inhalation should be about one third of the total breathing cycle (inspiration/exhalation of 1 : 3). If inspiration is too long, instruct patient to stop leaks by ensuring a tight seal (mask or mouthpiece). Reduce pressure for cycling or manually cycle respirator off. Instruct patient to re-

move mouthpiece or forcibly exhale to stop the breath whenever uncomfortable.
   e. Perform 10 to 20 breaths.
   f. Remove the mask or mouthpiece and perform and encourage the patient to rest and cough as needed.
   g. Repeat above cycle four to eight times, not to exceed 20 minutes (as a periodic therapy).
4. Monitor volume exhaled before and after an IPPB breath. Adjust pressure to deliver a volume of at least 15 mL/kg. Monitor inspiratory time, and observe patient to avoid hyperventilation.
5. When patient is receiving bronchodilator aerosol administered in conjunction with IPPB therapy, monitor for changes in vital capacity and peak flow (as well as adverse responses). Rinse mouthpiece or mask and nebulizer manifold assembly device with sterile water and shake or air dry after each treatment; disinfect circuit every 24 hours.
6. When appropriate, teach patient to self-administer. Evaluate the patient for ability to self-administer. Observation on several occasions of proper technique uncoached should precede allowing the patient to self-administer without supervision.
7. Document in the medical record procedures performed (including device, settings used, pressure developed, volumes achieved, number of breaths per treatment, and frequency), patient response to therapy, patient teaching provided, and patient ability to self-administer.

true threshold resistor maintains constant pressure in the circuit, independent of changing flow rates. Relatively few CPAP devices are *true* threshold resistors, in that they offer flow-dependent resistance once the valve is open so that pressure varies secondary to changes in flow rates, resulting in increased resistance and work of breathing.

Types of Resistors

Underwater seal: The expiratory limb of the circuit is submerged under water.[105] The height of the water above the terminal end of the expiratory limb (cm H_2O) corresponds to the threshold pressure generated (Fig. 13–14). A variant of the underwater seal is the water column, in which the threshold pressure is generated from a column of water above a diaphragm directly above the expiratory limb of the circuit. Pressure in the circuit must be greater than the pressure of the water to raise the diaphragm, allowing gas to exit. In this device, threshold pressure is a product of the water-column height and the surface area of the diaphragm.

Weighted ball: A precision ground ball of a specific weight is set above a calibrated orifice immediately above the expiratory limb of the circuit in a housing with expiratory ports. If the diameter of the orifice is not the narrowest point in the expiratory limb of the circuit, the weight of the ball determines the threshold pressure. Weighted-ball systems require meticulous attention to vertical orientation to maintain consistent pressures (see Fig. 13–14).

Spring-loaded valve: A spring holds a disk or diaphragm down over the end of the expiratory limb of the circuit. The force of the spring must be overcome for gas to leave the circuit. The function of the spring-loaded valve is independent of position (see Fig. 13–14).

Magnetic valve: A bar magnet attracts a ferromagnetic disk to a seat on the outlet orifice. As pressure exceeds the attraction of the magnet, the disk is displaced, allowing gas to exit the circuit. The greater the distance between the magnet and the disk, the lower is the pressure required for gas to leave the circuit.

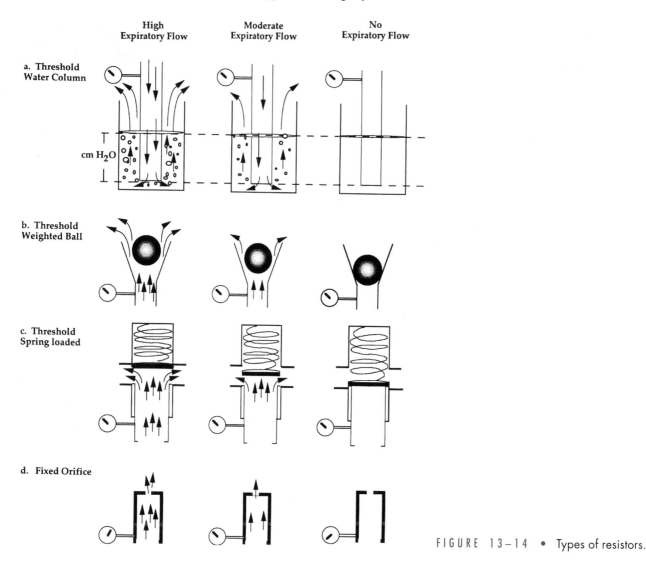

High
Expiratory Flow

Moderate
Expiratory Flow

No
Expiratory Flow

a. Threshold
Water Column

cm H₂O

b. Threshold
Weighted Ball

c. Threshold
Spring loaded

d. Fixed Orifice

FIGURE 13–14   •   Types of resistors.

Fixed orifice resistor: A restricted opening of a fixed size is placed at the end of the expiratory limb of a breathing circuit. As gas reaches the restricted orifice, turbulence and airway resistance result in increased pressure within the circuit. For any given gas flow, the smaller the orifice, the higher is the pressure generated. Expiratory pressure is flow dependent, so as flow decreases, pressure decreases. With this device, there is no threshold pressure to be overcome before gas can exit the system. In fact, there is no pressure generated until expiratory flow is high enough to create turbulence on exiting through the orifice (see Fig. 13–14). The fixed orifice resistor has long been a mainstay for producing CPAP (eg, the Gregory CPAP using a clamp to restrict the tail piece of a bag) in infants but was considered to be less than desirable in adults because of the high pressure that might be generated with changing flows (ie, coughing). In reality, it appears that the pressures generated with the fixed orifice resistor during a cough are of no greater consequence than those produced by the normal cough with the glottis closed.

Rationale

Pursed-lip breathing is a simple procedure that many patients with chronic obstructive lung disease have taught themselves to relieve air trapping caused by collapse of unstable airways during expiration[106] (Fig. 13–15). Resistance at the mouth during pursed-lip exhalation is believed to transmit back pressure to splint the airways open, preventing compression and premature closure (much like the fixed orifice resistor).[107,108] As an instinctive adaptation to disease, pursed-lip breathing represents a functional predecessor to many modern strategies of applying PEP to the airway.

In 1936, Poulton and Odon[109] described the use of the positive-pressure mask for the treatment of congestive heart failure and cardiogenic pulmonary edema. One year later, Barach and associates[110] reported the use of continuous positive-pressure breathing by mask in patients suffering from respiratory obstruction and pulmonary edema. At that time, the positive-pressure mask did not find application for the treatment or prophylaxis of postoperative pulmonary complications. Thirty years later, Cheney and colleagues[111] described improvements in PaO_2 after the ap-

A

B

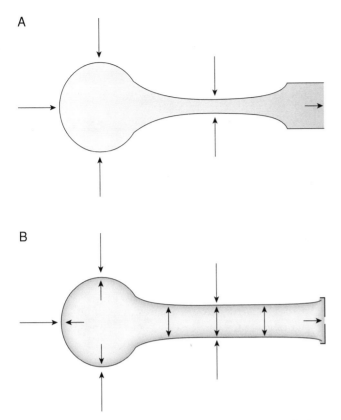

FIGURE 13-15 • (A) Forces that compress and close unstable airways during forced expiration. (B) The use of positive airway pressure to splint open the airway during expiration. (From Mahlmeister M. Pep Mask Therapy. *Respir Care.* 1991;36(11):1220–1221.)

plication of expiratory resistance in anesthetized patients on mechanical ventilation and speculated that this was caused by reversing alveolar collapse. In the late 1960s, articles by Ashbaugh and colleagues[112] established the concept of positive end-expiratory pressure (PEEP) as a technique to improve oxygenation in acute respiratory failure and adult respiratory distress syndrome. In 1971, Gregory and coworkers[113] reported a significant reduction in mortality when CPAP was used to treat respiratory distress syndrome of the neonate, leading to its widespread application in newborns.

Further research[114–116] established that PEEP and CPAP can be effective in reducing the alveolar-arterial oxygen difference $P(A - a)O_2$, and right-to-left intrapulmonary shunt, increasing FRC in the intubated patient with acute respiratory failure, with or without mechanical ventilation. In 1979, Andersen and colleagues[117] showed that reinflation of collapsed excised human lungs could be accomplished with CPAP by mechanisms involving collateral ventilation and noted that CPAP has a potential secretion-clearing effect in that pressure is built distal to an obstruction. The following year, Andersen and Jespersen[118] made castings of human lungs, identified communications between intersegmental respiratory bronchioles, and concluded that collateral ventilation might be of importance in normal lung function.

The prophylactic and therapeutic use of CPAP and PEEP in nonintubated patients did not receive much attention until the early 1980s.[119,120] In 1980, Andersen and associates[121] conducted a prospective, randomized, controlled clinical trial using a sequential analysis design to determine the effects of conventional therapy versus conventional therapy plus periodic mask CPAP in the treatment of 24 surgical patients with atelectasis. CPAP was given each hour for 25 to 35 breaths with a pressure averaging 15 cm H_2O. After 12 hours, patients in the CPAP group exhibited significantly greater improvement (PaO_2 and radiographic findings) than did those in the control group. This study prompted Pontoppidan[122] to consider periodic CPAP as a tool for treatment of postoperative pulmonary complications. Several studies during the early 1980s explored the application of PEEP and CPAP to nonintubated patients in different fashions with varying results,[2,123–128] including comparisons of mask CPAP to IS, deep breathing and coughing, and IPPB. As more effective strategies were developed, Stock and colleagues[127,128] concluded that intermittent mask CPAP was as effective as IS or deep breathing and coughing in the return of pulmonary function after thoracic or upper abdominal surgery. Additionally, these authors suggested that mask CPAP might be preferable because it represented a more effortless, painless type of postoperative respiratory care.

Ricksten and associates[102] performed a randomized comparative study of 43 upper abdominal surgery patients that looked at postoperative complications, $P(A - a)O_2$, peak expiratory flow, and FVC in patients using either CPAP or PEP against a control group using IS. All three groups took 30 breaths each hour while awake for 3 days postoperatively. Although peak flow did not change between groups, FVC was greater in the CPAP and PEP groups. $P(A - a)O_2$ increased uniformly in all groups for the first 24 hours, but then decreased in the CPAP and PEP groups (being insignificantly lower in the PEP group). Atelectasis was observed in 6 of 15 patients in the control group, 1 of 13 in the CPAP group, and 0 of 15 in the PEP group. The authors concluded that periodic PEP and CPAP are superior to deep-breathing exercises with respect to gas exchange, preservation of lung volumes, and prevention of postoperative atelectasis after upper abdominal surgery. They also concluded that the simple and commercially available mask PEP is as effective as the more complicated CPAP system. A simple PEP system as described earlier certainly represents a cost savings over the use of a more complex CPAP system, which requires a gas flow that will not change FIO_2 in response to back pressure, pressure monitor, and oxygen analyzer.

Lindner and colleagues,[129] in a randomized study of 34 upper abdominal surgery patients, compared postoperative physiotherapy with postoperative physiotherapy plus mask CPAP. Their findings indicated that the group treated with physiotherapy plus CPAP had a more rapid recovery of vital capacity and FRC with fewer pulmonary complications. Campbell and coworkers[130] randomized 71 abdominal surgery patients into group 1 (breathing exercises and huff coughing) and group 2 (same as group 1 plus PAP using a water-column threshold resistor adjusted to produce pressures of 5 to 15 cm H_2O with the patient exhaling through a mouthpiece). Differences in pulmonary function between the two groups, with a 31% incidence of respiratory complications in group 1 and a 22% incidence in group 2, were not statistically significant. The authors concluded that PEP could serve as an adjunct to routine chest physiotherapy, particularly with postoperative cigarette smokers, in that 43% of the smokers in their study developed respiratory complications, compared with none of the nonsmokers ($P < 0.01$).

By preventing expiratory collapse, PEP is thought to facilitate a more homogenous distribution of ventilation throughout the lung by way of these these collateral interbronchiolar channels.[131] Groth and colleagues[132] measured lung function from the expiratory port of the mask PEP in 12 patients with cystic fibrosis and found a significant increase in FRC ($P < 0.02$), decrease in volume of trapped gas ($P < 0.05$), and decrease of washout volume (p $<$ 0.05), as compared with pretreatment measurements. They concluded that the changes were attributed to an improvement in the distribution of ventilation (more evenly within the lung) and the opening up of airways otherwise closed during normal ventilation.

Because the patient must breathe down to subatmospheric pressures on inspiration, both EPAP and PEP are believed to require a higher work of breathing than CPAP.[133] Van der Schans and associates[134] examined the effect of EPAP with 5 cm H_2O using a threshold resistor (Vital Signs) in eight COPD patients. These investigators measured work of breathing and myoelectric activity of the scalene, parasternal, and abdominal muscles. During EPAP, work of breathing increased from 0.54 to 1.08 J/L. Expired minute volume decreased from 12.4 to 10.5 L/min, and dead space V_D/V_T decreased from 0.39 to 0.34. Increased phasic respiratory muscle activity was increased with EPAP. Dyspnea sensation during the exercise test was higher than during the test with undisturbed breathing.

Limitations of Method

Positive airway pressure therapy for bronchial hygiene requires spontaneously breathing patients. The level of cooperation depends on the device being used. CPAP and EPAP appear to require little or no patient coordination to be effective. In contrast, PEP works best when used by a conscious and cooperative patient (personal communications, Michael Mahlmeister, University of California, San Francisco). CPAP is an equipment-intensive procedure requiring an external gas source or compressor that will work in the face of back pressure as well as considerable training of personnel for proper set-up and maintenance. These factors make CPAP more expensive and less portable than other PAP treatments (Box 13–9).

Box • 13–9   VIABILITY OF POSITIVE AIRWAY PRESSURE THERAPY

Positive airway pressure appears to be a viable therapeutic option in the following situations[100]:

- Sputum retention that is not responsive to spontaneous or directed coughing
- History of pulmonary problems treated successfully with postural drainage therapy
- Decreased breath sounds or adventitious sounds suggesting secretions in the airway
- Change in vital signs with increase in breathing frequency, tachycardia
- Abnormal chest radiograph consistent with atelectasis, mucous plugging, or infiltrates
- Deterioration in arterial blood gas values or oxygen saturation
- Complaints of pain consistent with inability or unwillingness to take deep spontaneous breaths
- High closing volume

Positive Expiratory Pressure Administration Techniques

Positive expiratory pressure therapy is performed with the patient seated comfortably and the elbows resting on a table.[106] The equipment consists of a soft, transparent hand ventilation mask or mouthpiece, T assembly with a one-way valve, a variety of fixed orifice resistors (or adjustable expiratory resistor), and a manometer. The mask is applied tightly but comfortably over the mouth and nose. The patient is instructed to relax while performing diaphragmatic breathing, inspiring a volume of air larger than normal tidal volume but not to total lung capacity, through the one-way valve. Exhalation to FRC is active, but not forced, through the resistor chosen to achieve a peak airway pressure (PAP) between 10 and 20 cm H_2O (0.98 to 1.96 kPa) during exhalation.

A series of 10 to 20 breaths is performed with the mask or mouthpiece in place. The mask or mouthpiece is then removed, and the patient performs several coughs to raise secretions. This sequence of 10 to 20 PAP breaths followed by huff coughing is repeated four to six times per PEP therapy session. Each session for bronchial hygiene takes 10 to 20 minutes and may be performed one to four times a day, as needed. For lung expansion, patients should be encouraged to take 10 to 20 breaths every hour while awake and as needed.

Positive Expiratory Pressure Administration Considerations

Selection of a resistor with an appropriate orifice size is critical to proper technique. The therapeutic goal of exhalation is to achieve a PEP of 10 to 20 cm H_2O, with an inspiration/exhalation ratio of 1:3 to 1:4. When using a fixed orifice, most adults achieve this pressure range using a flow-restricting orifice between 2.5 and 4 mm in diameter. Selection of the proper resistor also produces the desired inspiration/exhalation ratio of 1:3 to 1:4. A manometer is placed in-line to measure the expiratory pressure while selecting the appropriate-sized orifice. Once the proper resistor orifice has been selected, the manometer may be removed from the system. Selection of a resistor with too large an orifice produces a short exhalation, with resulting failure to achieve the proper expiratory pressure. Too small an orifice prolongs the expiratory phase, elevates the pressure above 20 cm H_2O, and increases the work of breathing. Performing a PEP session for more than 20 minutes may lead to fatigue. During periods of exacerbation, patients are encouraged to increase the frequency with which PEP is performed, rather than extending the length of the session.

The equipment used to provide mask PEP therapy can be assembled easily from parts available in most respiratory care departments or may be purchased as a prefabricated system with variable orifice resistors. Figure 13–16 shows an example of a commercially available fixed orifice resistor, the Resistex (Mercury Medical, Clearwater, FL).

Aerosol Administration

Aerosol therapy may be instituted simultaneously with or just before a PEP session, either by hand-held nebulizer or MDI. Andersen and Klausen[103] applied face-mask PEEP while administering nebulized bronchodilators to eight patients with severe bronchospasm. A randomized crossover design was used, and each patient was subjected to two PEEP treatments and two control treatments with zero end-expiratory pressure at intervals of 3 hours between each treatment. FEV_1, FVC, and peak flow improved significantly after the PEEP treatments ($P < 0.05$). These investigators concluded that PEEP improved the efficacy of bronchodilator administration, probably mediated through a better distribution to the peripheral airways.

Frischknecht-Christensen and colleagues[104] examined the effect of mask PEP applied in conjunction with β_2-adrenergic receptor agonists administered by MDI with spacer. In a randomized crossover study, eight patients alternately received treatments of 2 puffs of terbutaline MDI without PEP, terbutaline MDI with PEP, and placebo MDI with PEP. Results showed statistically significant improvement ($P < 0.0001$) in peak expiratory flow rates when the terbutaline was taken in conjunction with face-mask PEP of 10 to 15 cm H_2O. We described the use of an MDI and chamber-style adapter with the Resistex system, which accepts a spacer device on the distal inspiratory limb of the PEP assembly[106] (Fig. 13–17).

Although no absolute contraindications to the use of PAP therapies have been reported, common sense dictates that patients with acute sinusitis, ear infection, epistaxis, or recent facial, oral, or skull injury or surgery be carefully

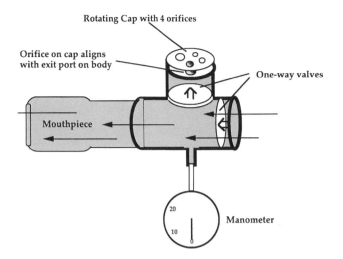

Inspiration

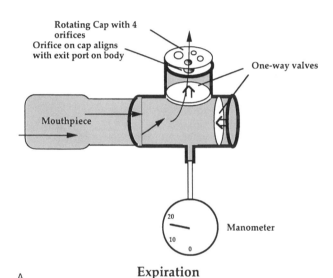

FIGURE 13–16 • Two commercially available positive expiratory pressure valves, Resistex (*A*) and DHD (*B*).

evaluated before a decision is made to initiate mask PEP therapy. Patients who are experiencing active hemoptysis and those with unresolved pneumothorax should avoid using PAP therapy until these acute pulmonary problems have resolved. Complications such as barotrauma or hemo-

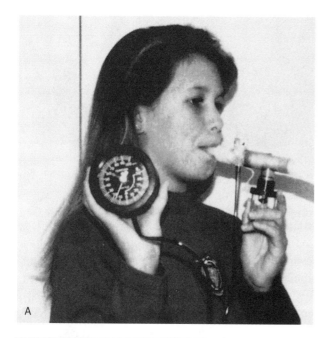

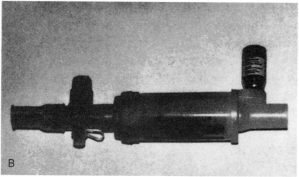

FIGURE 13–17 • Aerosol administration with positive expiratory pressure, small-volume nebulizer, and holding chamber. (From Mahlmeister M. Pep mask therapy. *Respir Care.* 1991;36(11):1220).

dynamic compromise are intuitive with the use of positive pressure; no complications have been reported when mask PEP therapy has been used for lung expansion or secretion clearance, in large part because of the techniques involved in the therapy and the patient population selected.

Because some authors have used different terms to describe PAP options, Figure 13–18 shows the different pressure patterns generated with CPAP, EPAP (threshold resistors), and PEP with fixed orifice resistor. Further studies are required to increase our understanding of the different effects of these three modalities (Box 13–10).

BLOW BOTTLE

Another procedure in vogue in the 1950s and 1960s was the blow bottle (Fig. 13–19). Two 1-L bottles were connected by a common conduit, with water filling one of the bottles. Tubing and a mouthpiece were attached to the top of each bottle. The patient is instructed to take a deep sustained breath and to blow into the tubing on the side of the full bottle, pushing water into the empty bottle.

Colgan and associates[135] studied the effects of the Valsalva maneuver, blow bottles, and sustained hyperinflation with an Elder Demand Valve Resuscitator. With the blow bottle, FRC increased significantly ($P = 0.04$) and shunt decreased slightly ($P = 0.07$). Inspiration resulted in airway pressures of -5 cm H_2O (-20 cm H_2O esophageal), with airway pressure rising to $+32$ cm H_2O ($+20$ cm H_2O esophageal) during aspiration. The authors concluded that the efficacy of blow bottles depends on an initial large and sustained deep breath, with prolonged gradual transfer of water from one bottle to another, and that a single sustained deep breath offers the same favorable transpulmonary gradient that occurs with blow bottles, but some patients may benefit from the challenge offered by transfer of water as evidence of progressing therapy. Iverson and

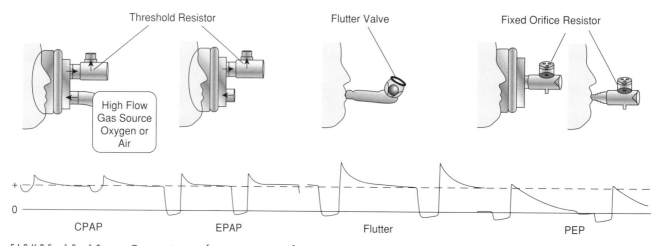

FIGURE 13–18 • Comparison of pressure waveforms, continuous positive airway pressure (CPAP), expiratory positive airway pressure (EPAP), positive expiratory pressure (PEP), and Flutter.

Box • 13–10   PROCEDURE FOR POSITIVE AIRWAY PRESSURE ADMINISTRATION

1. Assess whether PAP therapy is indicated, and design a treatment program to accomplish treatment objectives.
   a. Bring equipment to bedside, and provide initial therapy to patient, adjusting pressure settings to meet patient need.
   b. After initial patient treatment or training, communicate treatment plan to physician and nurse, and provide instruction to nursing staff if required.
2. Explain that PAP therapy is used to reexpand lung tissue and help mobilize secretions. Patients also should be taught to perform the huff-directed cough procedure.
3. Instruct the patient as follows:
   a. Sit comfortably.
   b. If using a mask, apply it tightly but comfortably over the nose and mouth. If mouthpiece is used, place lips firmly around it, and breathe through mouth.
   c. Take in a breath that is larger than normal, but do not fill lungs completely.
   d. Exhale actively, but not forcefully, creating a positive airway pressure of 10 to 20 cm H_2O during exhalation (determined with manometer during initial therapy sessions). Length of inhalation should be about one third of the total breathing cycle (inspiration/exhalation ratio of 1 : 3).

   e. Perform 10 to 20 breaths.
   f. Remove the mask or mouthpiece and perform two to three huff coughs, and rest as needed.
   g. Repeat above cycle four to eight times, not to exceed 20 minutes.
4. Evaluate the patient for ability to self-administer.
5. When appropriate, teach patient to self-administer. Observation on several occasions of proper technique uncoached should precede allowing the patient to self-administer without supervision.
6. When patient is also receiving bronchodilator aerosol, administer in conjunction with PAP therapy by placing an MDI with holding chamber or a nebulizer at the inspiratory port of the PAP device.
7. When visibly soiled, rinse PAP device with sterile water and shake or air dry; leave within reach at patient's bedside in a clear plastic bag.
8. Send the PAP device (if single patient use) home with the patient or discard it upon discharge. If nondisposable, send in-house for high-level disinfection.
9. Document in the medical record procedures performed (including device, settings used, pressure developed, number of breaths per treatment, and frequency), patient response to therapy, patient teaching provided, and patient ability to self-administer.

colleagues[136] compared IPPB, IS, and blow bottles in 145 post–cardiac surgery patients using 3 to 5 breaths every 3 hours. Pulmonary complications occurred in 30% of patients using IPPB, 15% of those using IS, and 8% of those using blow bottles ($P = 0.023$), with 20% of the IPPB patients complaining of gastrointestinal side effects.

Blow bottles have been criticized for emphasizing forced exhalation rather than SMI. The theory is that the overzealous patient, to achieve the goal of moving all of the water from one bottle to the next, may continue forced exhalation beyond CV, precipitating airway closure and possibly reducing FRC. Although intuitively attractive, this criticism of blow bottles has taken the form of textbook dogma that has not been substantiated with empiric observation.

In its defense, the blow bottle (see Fig. 13–19) acts as an expiratory threshold resistor that may stabilize the airway by splinting it open during a slow expiration (when dynamic compression tends to collapse airways), improve homogenous emptying of the lung, and improve distribution of ventilation. Blow bottles may be yet another valuable respiratory care technique driven to extinction before its time and could provide real benefit when applied to the appropriate patient population with the proper instructions (ie, "don't blow all the way out").

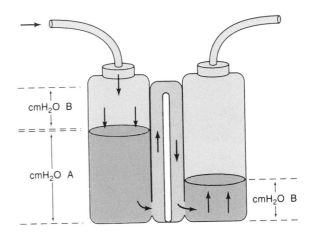

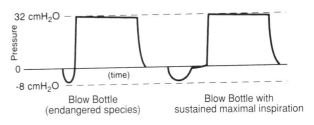

FIGURE 13–19 • Blow bottle.

HIGH FREQUENCY AIRWAY OSCILLATION

High frequency airway oscillation has been associated with improved mobilization of secretions. This was first identified during use of jet ventilation during laryngeal surgery. The principle has subsequently been applied to the devices discussed in the following two sections—the Flutter valve and the Percussionator used in intrapulmonary percussive ventilation.

FLUTTER VALVE

Developed in Switzerland, the Flutter mucus clearance device (VarioRaw SA, distributed by Scandipharm, Birmingham, AL) combines the techniques of PAP with high-frequency oscillations at the airway opening. A pipe-shaped device with a steel ball in the bowl is loosely covered by a perforated cap (Fig. 13–20). The weight of the ball serves as an EPAP device (at about 10 cm H$_2$O), and the internal shape of the bowl allows the ball to flutter, generating oscillations of about 15 Hz. In our laboratory, we found that the Flutter valve generated fluctuations in esophageal pressures similar to those generated during use of the ThAIRapy (described below).

Although the Flutter valve has been available in Europe for several years, little has been published on its efficacy.[137] In 1994, Konstan and coworkers[138] reported that the amount of sputum expectorated by 18 patients with cystic fibrosis was more than three times the amount ex-

pectorated with either voluntary cough (described as vigorous cough every 2 minutes for 15 minutes) or PDT (up to 10 positions in 15 minutes). It may be worthwhile to examine the study protocol from a more critical perspective than that taken by the Food and Drug Administration. Patients with cystic fibrosis or COPD tend to experience airway closure prematurely during vigorous coughing (rather than FET, huff, or ACB), resulting in trapped gas and secretions. National American Association of Respiratory Care guidelines suggest that effective PDT requires between 3 and 10 minutes per position,[14] so those 10 drainage positions would require between 30 and 100 minutes to provide effective results. It appears that neither the cough nor the PDT leg of the protocol was designed in light of available research to provide optimal results.

In 1994, Pryor and coworkers[139] studied 24 patients with cystic fibrosis who averaged more than 11.9 g/d of sputum using ACB as their standard bronchial hygiene. In this study, ACB alone resulted in significantly more sputum production than 10 minutes of Flutter use followed by ACB, and the authors expressed concern about the possibility of sputum retention when the Flutter was used.

To better understand how the Flutter device compares with other PAP devices, our laboratory[140] compared the Flutter valve with both threshold resistors and fixed orifice devices to determine the effects on the airway *in vitro.* Pressure patterns, peak expiratory flows, peak expiratory pressure, mean airway pressure, work of breathing, and changes in residual volume during passive exhalation were

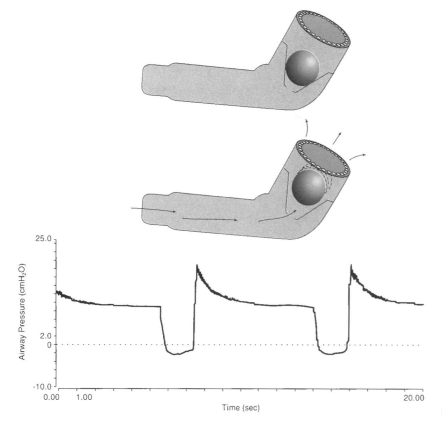

**FIGURE 13–20 • ** Flutter valve.

Table • 13–1 COMPARISON OF FLUTTER VALVE, THRESHOLD RESISTORS, AND FIXED ORIFICE DEVICES

Device	PEFR	P_{exp}	EPAP	W(pt)	MAP	RV
Flutter	27.1	18.8	8.4	1.406	7.5	450
TR 10 cm H_2O	39.0	15.5	7.5	1.255	6.6	450
TR 15 cm H_2O	40.0	20.6	12.5	1.694	9.9	700
FO 4.0 mm	23.7	9.5	0.3	0.738	0.8	0
FO 3.0 mm	13.4	10.2	0.3	0.714	1.6	0

PEFR, peak expiratory flow rate (L/min); P_{exp}, peak expiratory pressure (cm H_2O); EPAP, expiratory positive airway pressure; W(pt), work of breathing (J/L); MAP, mean airway pressure (cm H_2O); RV, changes in residual volume (milliliters above baseline during passive exhalation [V_T 500 mL, positive inspiratory force, 40 L/min]); TR, threshold resistor; FO, fixed orifice device.

measured using a test lung with a compliance of 0.02 cm H_2O/L. The results with the Flutter valve, two levels of threshold resistors, and two sizes of fixed orifice device are shown in Table 13–1.

The Flutter developed lower peak expiratory flow rates than did the threshold resistors but developed higher flow rates than the fixed orifice devices. In all other respects, the Flutter resembled the threshold resistors (see Fig. 13–18). The fixed orifice devices developed lower peak flows, peak and mean airway pressures, work of breathing, and residual volume than did the threshold resistors or the Flutter ($P < 0.001$).

EPAP requires greater work of breathing than does CPAP.[141] In this bench study, both the Flutter and threshold resistors produced a greater work of breathing than the fixed orifice devices. It is unclear what the effects may be of this increased patient work in severely obstructed COPD patients. Clearly, CPAP has a role in reducing dysp-

nea,[142,143] although EPAP may not (at least during exercise).[134] Further studies are required to determine whether the Flutter device (about $26) adds therapeutic benefit over other less expensive PAP devices ($6 to $20) or bronchial hygiene therapies (such as ACB, which is free; Box 13–11).

INTRAPULMONARY PERCUSSIVE VENTILATION

Intrapulmonary percussive ventilation (IPV) of the lungs is a therapeutic form of chest physical therapy advanced for the treatment of patients with COPD that consists of a pneumatic device called a Percussionator. IPV was designed to treat diffuse patchy atelectasis, enhance the mobilization and clearance of retained secretions, and deliver nebulized medications and wetting agents to the distal airways.[144]

With IPV, the patient breaths through a mouthpiece that delivers high-flow minibursts at rates of more than 200 cy-

Box • 13–11 PROCEDURE FOR FLUTTER ADMINISTRATION

1. Assess whether Flutter therapy is indicated, and design a treatment program to accomplish treatment objectives.
   a. Bring equipment to bedside, and provide initial therapy to patient, adjusting pressure settings to meet patient need.
   b. After initial patient treatment or training, communicate treatment plan to physician and nurse, and provide instruction to nursing staff if required.
2. Explain that Flutter therapy is used to reexpand lung tissue and help mobilize secretions. Patient also should be taught to perform the huff-directed cough procedure.
3. Instruct the patient as follows:
   a. Sit comfortably.
   b. Take in a breath that is larger than normal, but do not fill lungs completely.
   c. Place Flutter mouthpiece in mouth, lips sealed firmly, and exhale actively, but not forcefully, holding the Flutter valve at an angle that produces maximal oscillation.
   d. Perform 10 to 20 breaths.
   e. Remove the Flutter mouthpiece, and perform two or three huff-directed coughs, and rest as needed.
   f. Repeat above cycle four to eight times, not to exceed 20 minutes.
   g. Evaluate the patient for ability to self-administer.
4. When appropriate, teach patient to self-administer. Observation on several occasions of proper technique uncoached should precede allowing the patient to self-administer without supervision.
5. When patient also is receiving bronchodilator aerosol, administer in conjunction with Flutter by administering bronchodilator immediately preceding the flutter breaths.
6. When visibly soiled, rinse Flutter device with sterile water and shake or air dry; leave within reach at patient bedside.
7. Send the Flutter device home with the patient.
8. Document in the medical record procedures performed (including device, number of breaths per treatment, and frequency), patient response to therapy, patient teaching provided, and patient ability to self-administer.

cles/min (Fig. 13–21). During these percussive bursts of gas into the lungs, a continuous airway pressure is maintained while the pulsatile percussive intraairway pressure rises progressively. Each percussive cycle is programmed by the patient or clinician by holding down a thumb button for 5 to 10 seconds for percussive inspiratory cycle and then releasing the button for exhalation. Treatments lasting about 20 minutes are recommended by the manufacturer. Impaction pressures of 25 to 40 psig are delivered with a frequency of less than 100 to 225 percussive cycles/min at 40 psig. The IPV-2 includes nonoscillatory demand CPAP, oscillatory demand CPAP with intermittent mandatory ventilation, or both.

Natale and associates[145] reported that a single IPV treatment was as effective as standard chest physiotherapy in improving acute pulmonary function and enhancing sputum expectoration in nine patients with cystic fibrosis. (Note that huff-directed coughing, CPAP, PEP, and Flutter all have been shown to be *more* effective than standard chest physiotherapy in enhancing sputum expectoration.) Further studies would be valuable in determining the rela-tive merit of IPV in comparison to other lung-expansion and secretion-clearance techniques.

With so little published on the use of IPV,[146–148] one might assume that contraindications and hazards are similar to those associated with other forms of mechanical ventilation. The manufacturer lists potential side effects to include sore ribs, fatigue, stress, and irritation.

The role of airway oscillation or vibration on secretion clearance remains unclear. Van Henstum and coworkers[149] reported no effect of oral high-frequency oscillation combined with forced expiration maneuvers on tracheobronchial clearance in patients with chronic bronchitis. Further studies are warranted.

HIGH-FREQUENCY EXTERNAL CHEST WALL COMPRESSION

High-frequency chest wall compression has been shown to increase tracheal mucus clearance rates and to correlate with improved ventilation in both animal and clinical studies.[150,151]

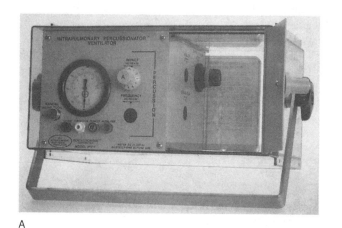

A

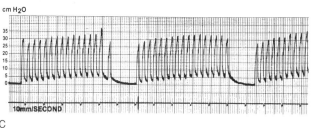

C

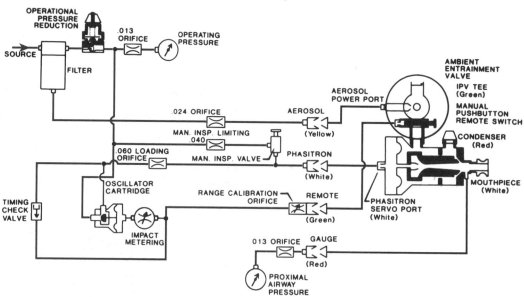

B

FIGURE 13–21 • Percussionator device (*A*) and waveform (*B*). IPV, intrapulmonary percussive ventilation. (Courtesy of Percussionator, Sandpoint, ID.)

ThAIRapy

ThAIRapy (American Biosystems Inc., St. Paul, MN) was designed for self-therapy and consists of a large-volume variable-frequency air-pulse delivery system attached to a nonstretchable inflatable vest that is worn by the patient and extends over the entire torso down to the iliac crest (Fig. 13–22). Pressure pulses that fill the vest and vibrate the chest wall are controlled by the patient (with a foot pedal) and applied during expiration. Pulse frequency is adjustable from 5 to 25 Hz, and pressure in the vest varies from 28 mmHg at 5 Hz to 39 mmHg at 25 Hz.

In theory, these vibrations to the chest wall cause transient increases in airflow in the lungs to improve gas–liquid interactions and the movement of mucus. Animal and clinical studies demonstrated that the frequency of oscillations (cycles/second) and flow bias (inspiratory versus expiratory) are important in determining effectiveness. Flow bias determines whether secretions move upstream or downstream.[151] Conjecture that this device may have a role in the lung expansion of patients other than those with cystic fibrosis in the acute care setting has not been empirically established.

In a limited study of patients with cystic fibrosis, ThAIRapy was shown to be more effective than PDT in secretion clearance,[152] but there has been no comparison in a controlled manner with ACB, PEP, or other bronchial hygiene measures. Such comparisons, however, would be important to justify a device that costs $500 a month (according to recent third-payor reimbursement rates).

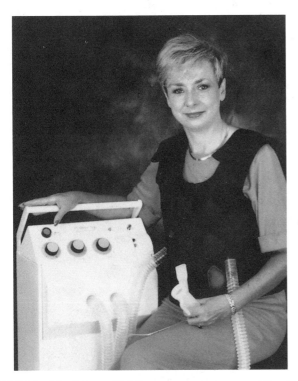

FIGURE 13–22 • ThAIRapy pneumatic vest. (Courtesy of American Biosystems, Inc., St. Paul, MN.)

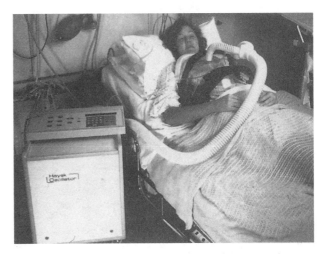

FIGURE 13–23 • Hayek oscillator. (Courtesy of Breasy Medical Equipment, Stamford, CT.)

HAYEK OSCILLATOR

The Hayek oscillator is an electrically powered, microprocessor-controlled, noninvasive oscillating ventilator that uses an external, flexible chest enclosure (cuirass) to apply negative and positive pressure to the chest wall to deliver noninvasive oscillation to the lungs (Fig. 13–23). The negative pressure generated in the cuirass causes the chest wall to expand for inspiration, while positive pressure compresses the chest to produce a forced expiration. Both inspiratory and expiratory phases may be active and not reliant on passive recoil of the chest. Expiratory pressure can be positive, atmospheric, or negative, allowing ventilation to occur above, at, or below the patient's normal FRC. Several groups have reported success in using this device as a method of ventilatory support.[153–155] Four adjustable parameters with the Hayek oscillator include frequency range (to 999 oscillations/min), inspiration/exhalation ratio (6:1 to 1:6), and inspiratory/expiratory pressure (-70 to $+70$ cm H_2O).

Clinicians' anecdotal observations of spontaneous expulsion of secretions[156,157] during high-frequency ventilation have led to development of several discrete secretion management program recommendations in which the chest is oscillated through two sets of cycles: several minutes at a high frequency of up to 999 (usually 600 to 720) cycles/min at an inspiration/exhalation ratio of 1:1, followed by 60 to 90 cycles/min at a ratio of 5:1. The setting can be changed according to the needs of the patient. Reports of efficacy of this or similar protocols for secretion management with the Hayek oscillator have yet to be published.

BRONCHODILATOR THERAPY

Salbutamol is thought to improve mucociliary clearance in addition to its bronchodilator functions. This has formed the foundation for the argument to use β_2-agonists such as albuterol or terbutaline perioperatively to reduce the incidence of pulmonary complications. Dilworth and col-

Table • 13–2 LUNG EXPANSION THERAPY

Therapy	Indications	Contraindications	Potential Complications	Frequency/Limitations/Costs
Turning/repositioning/mobility	Inability/reluctance of patient to change body position; Poor oxygenation associated with position; Potential for or development of atelectasis; Presence of artificial airway; Unprotected airway at risk for aspiration	All Positions; ICP > 20 mmHg; Head/neck injury; Active hemorrhage with hemodynamic instability; Recent spinal surgery or acute spinal injury; Reverse Trendelenburg; Hypotension; Vasoactive medication therapy	Hypoxemia; Increased ICP; Acute hypotension; Injury/discomfort of muscles, bones; Vomiting, aspiration; Bronchospasm; Arrhythmias	Turn supine to lateral q 2 h as tolerated; Pain management may be required; No additional costs beyond basic nursing care
Directed cough	Removal of retained secretions; Collection of sputum specimens; Atelectasis; Prophylactic use in surgical patients; Routine for patients with bronchiectasis and COPD	Elevated ICP or known intracranial aneurysm; Acute unstable head, neck, spinal injury; High risk for regurgitation/aspiration; Acute abdominal pathology; Flail chest	Reduced coronary artery perfusion; Reduced cerebral perfusion; Fatigue; Headache; Bronchospasm; Chest/incisional pain, evisceration; Rib or costochondral fracture; Gastroesophageal reflux	As needed to expel secretions and prophylactically for postoperative patients (q 2 h while awake); Limited value in paralyzed, obtunded, and uncooperative patient; No additional costs beyond basic nursing care
Incentive spirometry	Conditions predisposing to development of pulmonary atelectasis: Upper abdominal surgery; Thoracic surgery; Surgery on patients with COPD; Atelectasis; Restrictive lung deficit associated with quadriplegia and/or dysfunctional diaphragm	Patient cannot be instructed or supervised to ensure appropriate use of device; Patient cooperation is inconsistent; Patient cannot demonstrate proper use of device; Patient cannot deep breathe effectively with device	Hyperventilation; Discomfort secondary to inadequate pain control; Hypoxia; Exacerbation of bronchospasm; Fatigue	10 breaths per session every hour while awake; No evidence that IS is more effective than deep breathing alone; Concerns about overuse; Equipment <$5-$10 setup, minimum instruction and follow-up time
Positive airway pressure therapy (PAP)	To treat atelectasis; To aid in mobilization of retained secretions; To optimize delivery of bronchodilators in patients receiving bronchial hygiene therapy	Inability to tolerate increased work of breathing; ICP > 20 mmHg; Hemodynamic instability; Recent facial, oral, or skull surgery/trauma; Active hemoptysis	Discomfort; Hyperventilation, hypercarbia; Increased ICP; Skin breakdown/irritation; Cardiovascular compromise	Frequency 1–6 hours; Requires spontaneously breathing patient; CPAP setup may cost >$100, requiring high flow gas source. Flutter <$120, EPAP <$25, and PEP <$10; Flutter may be less effective than active cycle of breathing (directed cough) in mobilizing secretions
Intermittent positive pressure breathing (IPPB)	To improve lung expansion; Ineffective cough; Short-term ventilatory support for patients who are hypoventilating as an alternative to CMV; To deliver aerosol medication (when other less expensive, invasive, and complex options don't work)	Untreated pneumothorax; ICP > 15 mmHg; Hemodynamic instability; Recent facial, oral, or skull surgery; Uncontrolled hypertension; Active hemoptysis; Recent esophageal surgery; Tracheoesophageal fistula; Nausea or air swallowing; Active untreated tuberculosis; Singulation (hiccups)	Increased airway resistance; Barotrauma, pneumothorax; Nosocomial infection; Hypocarbia/hypoventilation; Hypoxemia/hyperoxia; Increased ICP; Gastric distension; Impaction of secretions; Psychological dependence; Impedance of venous return; Air trapping, auto-PEEP; Hypocarbia/hypoventilation	Frequency 1–6 hours; All mechanical effects last ≤ 1 hour; Less efficient for aerosol delivery than SVN or MDI; Efficacy is technique (coordination, selection of inspiratory flow, peak pressure) and device (flow, volume, pressure capabilities) dependent; Limited portability and convenience as aerosol delivery device; Equipment and labor intensive; Device costs >$500
Extrathoracic high frequency oscillation/vibration	To aid in mobilization of retained secretions (when other less expensive, invasive, and complex options don't work)	Untreated pneumothorax; ICP > 15 mmHg; Hemodynamic instability; Uncontrolled hypertension; Active hemoptysis; Tracheoesophageal fistula; Nausea or air swallowing; Active untreated tuberculosis; Singulation (hiccups)	Hypoxemia; Increased ICP; Impaction of secretions; Psychological dependence; Increased mismatch V̇/Q̇; Air trapping, auto-PEEP; Increased airway resistance	Frequency 1–6 hours; Not shown to be more effective than active cycle of breathing (FET) or PAP; Efficacy is technique (coordination, frequency, I:E ratio) and device dependent; Limited portability and convenience; Device costs >$10,000

leagues[158] performed a double-blind placebo-controlled study in which one group of patients received 5 mg of salbutamol and the other group received normal saline, every 6 hours for 2 days after abdominal surgery. These investigators found no useful reduction in the incidence of pulmonary infections with high-dose bronchodilator therapy in the perioperative period and no reduction of postoperative chest infection in high-risk patients.

ROLE OF THE PRACTITIONER IN LUNG EXPANSION AND BRONCHIAL HYGIENE THERAPY

With all these options available for lung-expansion therapy, and no one proved option superior for all patients, it is essential that the health care team consider which option best meets the needs of the individual patient. It is incumbent on the practitioner, or direct care provider, to assess the patient, no matter what the initial order may be, and to identify therapeutic alternatives that will reliably meet the therapeutic objectives. High among the considerations should be patient comfort and cost. Always start with the most comfortable, cost-effective option available; then, as you assess patient response to therapy, reevaluate the efficacy of the current order. Only with a balance of needs and outcomes assessment can the practitioner fine-tune a cost-effective program to meet the needs of the individual patient.

Table 13–2 lists a variety of techniques discussed in this chapter, starting with the least expensive and invasive procedures and culminating with the most expensive procedures. Also listed are indications, complications, hazards, recommended frequencies, and costs.

Now that you have the facts on bronchial hygiene tools and lung-expansion techniques, the next hurdle is selecting the appropriate tool or technique for a specific patient at a specific point in time (Fig. 13–24). We offer two decision-making trees that should help guide you through your initial assessments and evaluations.

The first algorithm (Fig. 13–25) guides you through some basic decision-making suggestions for evaluating the appropriate therapeutic interventions for a patient who has been ordered to receive lung-expansion therapy. Remember that boxes represent actions and diamonds represent decisions (decisions are like questions; an arrow indicates a yes, unless no is specified). For lung-expansion therapy, the first question is whether patient has or is at risk of developing atelectasis. If the patient is not at risk, expensive additional therapy is probably not warranted, and basic nursing care should be provided, including turning and mobilization. If the patient is at risk of developing atelectasis and is cooperative, the vital capacity should be determined. Remember that a vital capacity of less than 15 mL/kg is associated with lung volumes too low for an effective cough, and an effective cough is key to lung expansion and bronchial hygiene.

Figure 13–26 guides you through evaluation for an order for PDT. If the patient does not have a diagnosis of cystic fibrosis or bronchiectasis and does not produce more than 30 mL/d of sputum with difficulty, PDT is not indicated. In this situation, the algorithm guides you to the appropriate tool or technique to recommend or initiate.

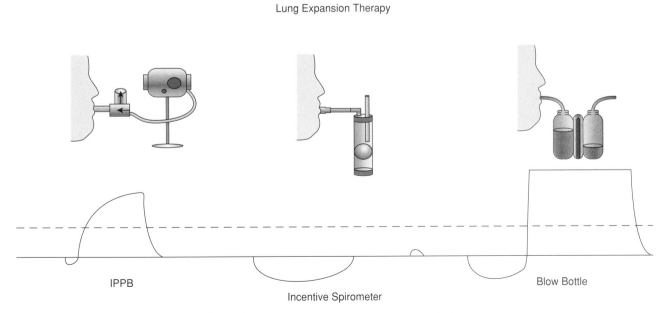

Lung Expansion Therapy

IPPB

Incentive Spirometer

Blow Bottle

FIGURE 13–24 • Comparison of waveforms for common lung expansion techniques. IPPB, intermittent positive-pressure breathing.

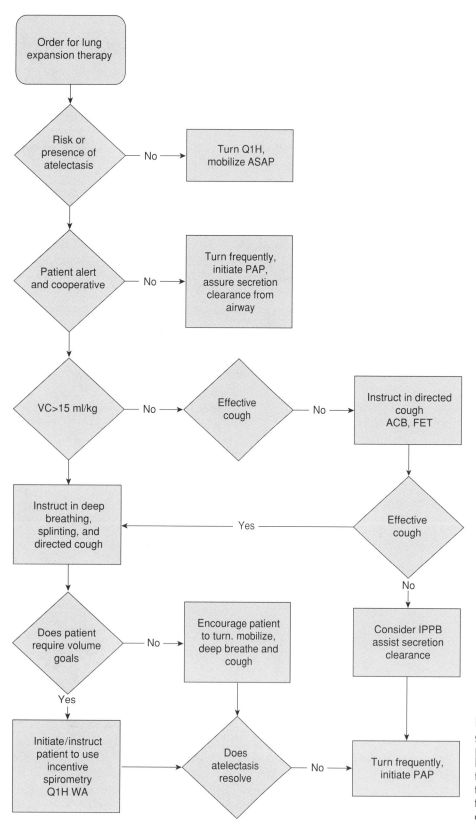

FIGURE 13–25 • Flow diagram for evaluation of lung expansion. ACB, active cycle of breathing; FET, forced expiratory technique, IPPB, intermittent positive-pressure breathing; PAP, positive airway pressure; VC, vital capacity.

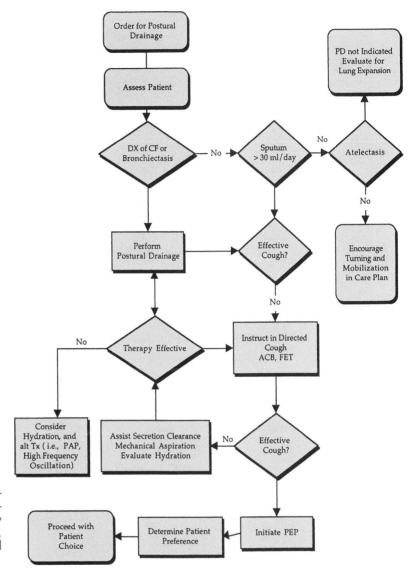

FIGURE 13–26 • Flow diagram for postural drainage. ACB, active cycle of breathing; CF, cystic fibrosis; FET, forced expiratory technique; PAP, positive airway pressure; PEP, positive expiratory pressure; PD, postural drainage.

CRITICAL THINKING CHALLENGES

Go Figure

Scenario one: A 64-year-old white woman with a 30-pack/year history of cigarette smoking and chronic cough is admitted for orthopedic surgery (hip replacement). Her vital capacity preoperatively is >20 mL/kg, and she does not have difficulty clearing secretions. You have been asked to do a preoperative evaluation. What would you recommend?

Scenario two: A 46-year-old, 200-lb, black man is admitted for an elective bunionectomy with no history of pulmonary complaints. The doctor orders IPPB q.i.d. with normal saline postoperatively. The patient has a pretreatment vital capacity of 5.4 L. What would you recommend?

Scenario three: A 38-year-old, 98-lb, Asian woman with a 10-pack/year history of cigarette smoking and a chronic

cough is admitted for a laparotomy. Her preoperative vital signs are normal, vital capacity is 2.6 L. What would you recommend preoperatively and postoperatively?

Scenario four: A 14-year-old, 95-lb, white boy with cystic fibrosis has been admitted for a "tune-up." The doctor has ordered postural drainage, and the patient has told you that he just does not have time to do postural drainage at home, is embarrassed to do it when he is away from home. What do you recommend?

Scenario five: A 63-year-old, 180-lb, white man had a triple coronary artery bypass graft 2 days ago and, despite being given an incentive spirometer, has increasing atelectasis on chest radiograph and a poor oxygen saturation (92%) of 40% oxygen. His vital capacity is 1.8 L. What do you recommend?

References

1. O'Donohue WJ Jr. Postoperative pulmonary complications: When are preventative and therapeutic measures necessary? *Postgrad Med.* 1992;91:167–175.

2. Pontoppidan H. Mechanical aids to lung expansion in non-intubated surgical patients. *Am Rev Respir Dis.* 1980;122(5 Pt 2): 109–119.

3. Agency for Health Care Policy and Research (AHCPR) Health Technology Reports. *Intermittent Positive Pressure Breathing (IPPB) Therapy.* 1991; No. 1.

4. O'Donohue WJ Jr. National survey of the usage of lung expansion modalities for the prevention and treatment of postoperative atelectasis following abdominal and thoracic surgery. *Chest.* 1985;87:76–80.

5. Tobin MJ. Perioperative problems. In: *Essentials of Critical Care Medicine.* New York: Churchill Livingstone; 1989:515–528.

6. Engoren N. Lack of association between atelectasis and fever. *Chest.* 1995;107:81–84.

7. Meyers JR, Lembeck L, OKane H, Baue AE. Changes in residual capacity of the lung after operation. *Arch Surg.* 1975;110: 567–583.

8. Miller RD, Fowler WS, Helmholz F. Changes of relative volume and ventilation of the two lungs with changes to the lateral decubitus position. *J Lab Clin Med.* 1956;47:297–304.

9. Douglas WW, Rehder K, Beynen FM, et al. Improved oxygenation in patients with acute respiratory failure: The prone position. *Am Rev Respir Dis.* 1977;115:559–566.

10. Brussel T, Hachenberg T, Roos N, et al. Mechanical ventilation in the prone position for acute respiratory failure after cardiac surgery. *J Cardiothorac Vasc Anesth.* 1993;7:541–546.

11. Torres A, Serra-Batlles J, Ros E, et al. Pulmonary aspiration of gastric contents inpatients receiving mechanical ventilation: The effect of body position. *Ann Intern Med.* 1992;116:540–543.

12. Stein M, Cassara EL. Preoperative pulmonary evaluation and therapy for surgery patients. *JAMA.* 1970;211(5):787–790.

13. Hilling L, Bakow E, Fink J, et al. AARC clinical practice guideline: Postural drainage therapy. *Respir Care.* 1993;36:1418–1426.

14. Zack MB, Pontoppidan H, Kazemi H. The effect of lateral positions on gas exchange in pulmonary disease: A prospective evaluation. *Am Rev Respir Dis.* 1974;110:49–55.

15. Chulary M, Brown J, Summer W. Effect of postoperative immobilization after coronary artery bypass surgery. *Crit Care Med.* 1982;10:176–179.

16. Piehl MA, Brown RS. Use of extreme position changes in acute respiratory failure. *Crit Care Med.* 1976;4:13–14.

17. Coonan TJ, Hope CE. Cardio-respiratory effects of change of body position. *Can Anaesth Soc J.* 1983;30:424–437.

18. Schimmel L, Civetta JM, Kirby RR. A new mechanical method to influence pulmonary perfusion in critically ill patients. *Crit Care Med.* 1977;5:277–279.

19. Gentilello L, Thompson DA, Ronnesen AS, et al. Effect of a rotating bed on the incidence of pulmonary complications in critically ill patients. *Crit Care Med.* 1988;16:783–786.

20. Summer WR, Curry P, Haponick EF, et al. Continuous mechanical turning of intensive care unit patients shortens length of stay in some diagnostic related groups. *J Crit Care.* 1989;4:45–53.

21. Fink MP, Helsmoortel CM, Stein KL, et al. The efficacy of an oscillating bed in the prevention of lower respiratory tract infection in critically ill victims of blunt trauma: A prospective study. *Chest.* 1990;97:132–137.

22. Lorin MP, Denning CR. Evaluation of postural drainage by measurement of sputum volume and consistency. *Am J Phys Med.* 1974;50:5:215–219.

23. Tecklin J, Holsclaw D. Evaluation of bronchial drainage in patients with cystic fibrosis. *Phys Ther.* 1975;55:1081–1084.

24. Cochrane GM, Webber BA, Clarke SW. Effects of sputum on pulmonary function. *Br Med J.* 1977;2:1181–1183.

25. Wong JW, Keens TG, Wannamaker EM, et al. Effects of gravity on tracheal mucus transport rates in normal subjects and in patients with cystic fibrosis. *Pediatrics.* 1977;60:2:146–152.

26. Pryor JA, Webber BA, Hodson ME, Batten JC. Evaluation of the forced expiration technique as an adjunct to postural drainage in treatment of cystic fibrosis. *Br Med J.* 1979;2:417–418.

27. Pryor JA, Webber BA. An evaluation of the forced expiration technique as an adjunct to postural drainage. *Physiotherapy.* 1979;65:10:305–307.

28. Murphy MB, Concannon D, Fitzgerald MX. Chest percussion: Help or hindrance to postural drainage? *Irish Med J.* 1983;76:4: 189–190.

29. DeBoeck C, Zinman R. Cough versus chest physiotherapy: A comparison of the acute effects on pulmonary function in patients with cystic fibrosis. *Am Rev Respir Dis.* 1984;129:182–184.

30. Bateman JRM, Newman SP, Daunt KM, et al. Is cough as effective as chest physiotherapy in the removal of excessive tracheobronchial secretions? *Thorax.* 1981;36:683–687.

31. Anthonisen P, Riis P, Sogaard-Anderson T. The value of lung physiotherapy in the treatment of acute exacerbations in chronic bronchitis. *Acta Med Scand.* 1964;175:6:715–719.

32. Campbell AH, O'Connell JM, Wilson F. The effect of chest physiotherapy upon the FEV1 in chronic bronchitis. *Med J Aust.* 1975;1:33–35.

33. Newton DAG, Stephenson A. The effect of physiotherapy on pulmonary function: A laboratory study. *Lancet.* 1978;312(29): 228–230.

34. Murray JF. The ketchup-bottle method. *N Engl J Med.* 1979;300: 20:1155–1157.

35. Oldenburg FA, Dolovich MB, Montgomery JM, Newhouse MT. Effects of postural drainage, exercise, and cough on mucus clearance in chronic bronchitis. *Am Rev Respir Dis.* 1979;120: 739–745.

36. Rochester DF, Goldberg SK. Techniques of respiratory physical therapy. *Am Rev Respir Dis.* 1980;122(2):133–146.

37. Connors AF, Hammon WE, Martin RJ, Rogers RM. Chest physical therapy: The immediate effect on oxygenation in acutely ill patients. *Chest.* 1980;78:4:559–564.

38. Hodgkin JE. The scientific status of chest physiotherapy. *Respir Care.* 1981;26:7:6657–6659.

39. Sutton PP, Pavia D, Bateman JRM, Clarke SW. Chest physiotherapy: A review. *Eur J Respir Dis.* 1982;63:188–201.

40. Wollmer P, Ursing K, Midgren B, Eriksson L. Inefficiency of chest percussion in the physical therapy of chronic bronchitis. *Eur J Respir Dis.* 1985;66:233–239.

41. Kirilloff LH, Owens GR, Rogers RM, Mazzocco MC: Does chest physical therapy work? *Chest.* 1985;88:3:436–444.

42. Faling LJ. Pulmonary rehabilitation physical modalities. *Clin Chest Med.* 1986;7:4:599–618.

43. Pavia D, Thomson ML, Phillipakos D. A preliminary study of the effect of a vibrating pad on bronchial clearance. *Am Rev Respir Dis.* 1976;113:92–96.

44. Maxwell M, Redmond A. Comparative trial of manual and mechanical percussion technique with gravity-assisted bronchial drainage in patients with cystic fibrosis. *Arch Dis Child.* 1979; 54:542–544.

45. Holody B, Goldberg HS. The effect of mechanical vibration physiotherapy in arterial oxygenation in acutely ill patients with atelectasis or pneumonia. *Am Rev Respir Dis.* 1981;124:372–375.

46. Radford R, Barutt J, Billingsley JG, et al. A rational basis for percussion augmented mucociliary clearance. *Respir Care.* 1982;27:5:556–563.

47. MacKenzie CF, Shin B, McAslan TC. Chest physiotherapy: The effect on arterial oxygenation. *Anesth Analg.* 1978;57:28–30.

48. Barrell SE, Abbas HM. Monitoring during physiotherapy after open heart surgery. *Physiotherapy.* 1978;64:9:272–273.

49. Bateman JRM, Newman SP, Daunt KM, et al. Regional lung clearance of excessive bronchial secretions during chest physiotherapy in patients with stable chronic airways obstruction. *Lancet.* 1979;Feb 10:294–297.

50. Feldman J, Traver GA, Taussig LM. Maximal expiratory flows after postural drainage. *Am Rev Respir Dis.* 1979;119:239–245.

51. Hammon WE, Martin RJ. Chest physical therapy for acute atelectasis. *Phys Ther.* 1981;61:2:217–220.

52. Stiller K, App B, Geake T, et al. Acute lobar atelectasis: A comparison of two chest physiotherapy regimens. *Chest.* 1990;98: 1336–1340.

53. Tyler ML. Complications of positioning and chest physiotherapy. *Respir Care.* 1982;27:4:458–466.

54. MacKenzie CF, Ciesla N, Imle PC, et al. In: *Chest Physiotherapy in the Intensive Care Unit.* Baltimore: Williams & Wilkins; 1990.

55. Zack MB, Pontoppidan H, Kazemi H. The effect of lateral posi-

tions on gas exchange in pulmonary disease: A prospective evaluation. *Am Rev Respir Dis.* 1974;110:49–55.

56. Sonnenblick M, Melzer E, Rosin AJ. Body position effect on gas exchange in unilateral pleural effusion. *Chest.* 1983;83:5:784–786.

57. Heaf DP, Helms P, Gordon I, Turner HM. Postural effects on gas exchange in infants. *N Engl J Med.* 1983;308:25:1505–1508.

58. Hasan FM, Beller TA, Sobonya RE, et al. Effect of positive and expiratory pressure and body position in unilateral lung injury. *J Appl Physiol.* 1982;52:1:147–154.

59. Hilling L, Bakow E, Fink J, et al: AARC clinical practice guideline: Directed cough. *Respir Care.* 1993;38:495–499.

60. Roukema JA, Carol EJ, Prins JG. The prevention of pulmonary complications after upper abdominal surgery in patients with noncompromised pulmonary status. *Arch Surg.* 1988;123:30–34.

61. Partridge C, Pryor J, Webber B. Characteristics of the forced expiratory technique. *Physiotherapy.* 1989;75(3):193–194.

62. Pryor JA, Webber BA. An evaluation of the forced expiration technique as an adjunct to postural drainage. *Physiotherapy.* 1979;65:304–307.

63. Pryor JA, Webber BA, Hodson ME, Batten JC. Evaluation of the forced expiration technique as an adjunct to postural drainage in the treatment of cystic fibrosis. *Br Med J.* 1979;2:417–418.

64. Bateman JRM, Newman SP, Daunt KM, et al. Is cough as effective as chest physiotherapy in the removal of excessive secretions? *Thorax.* 1981;36:683–687.

65. DeBoeck C, Zinman R. Cough versus chest physiotherapy: A comparison of the acute effects on pulmonary function in patients with cystic fibrosis. *Am Rev Respir Dis.* 1984;129:182.

66. Webber BA, Hofmeyer JL, Morgan MDL, Hodson ME. Effects of postural drainage, incorporating the forced expiration technique, on pulmonary function in cystic fibrosis. *Br J Dis Chest.* 1986;80:353–359.

67. Kern JM, Gadipati C, Tatineni S, et al. Effect of abruptly increased intrathoracic pressure on coronary blood flow velocity in patients. *Am Heart J.* 1990;119:863–870.

68. Jacobs WR, Zaroukian MH. Coughing and central venous catheter dislodgement. *JPEN.* 1991;15(4):491–493.

69. Stern RC, Horwitz SJ, Doerslock CF. Neurologic symptoms during coughing paroxysms in cystic fibrosis. *J Pediatr.* 1988;112:909–912.

70. Ing AJ, Ngu MC, Breslin AB. Chronic persistent cough and gastro-oesophageal reflux. *Thorax.* 1991;46(7):479–483.

71. Bain J, Bishop J, Olinsky A. Evaluation of directed coughing in cystic Fibrosis. *Br J Dis Chest.* 1988;82:138–148.

72. Hie T, Pas BG, Roth RD, Jensen WM. Huff coughing and airway patency. *Respir Care.* 1979;24:710–713.

73. Oldenburg FA, Dolovich MD, Montgomery JM, Newhouse MT. Effects of postural drainage, exercise and cough on mucus clearance in chronic bronchitis. *Am Rev Respir Dis.* 1979;120:739–745.

74. Sutton PP, Parker RA, et al. Assessment of the forced expiration technique, postural drainage and directed coughing in chest physiotherapy. *Eur J Respir Dis.* 1983;64:62–68.

75. Hardy KA. A review of airway clearance: new techniques, indications and recommendations. *Respir Care.* 1994;39:440–452.

76. Hilling L, Bakow E, Fink J, et al. AARC clinical practice guideline: Incentive spirometry. *Respir Care.* 1991;36:1402–1405.

77. Bartlett RH, Krop P, Hanson EL, Moore FD. Physiology of yawning and its application to postoperative care. *Surg Forum.* 1970;21:223–224.

78. Craven JL, Evans GA, Davenprot PJ, Wiolliam RHP. The evaluation of incentive spirometry in the management of postoperative pulmonary complications. *Br J Surg.* 1974;61:793–797.

79. Scuderi J, Olsen GN. Respiratory therapy in the management of postoperative complications. *Respir Care.* 1989;34:281–291.

80. Dohi S, Gold MI. Comparison of two methods of postoperative respiratory care. *Chest.* 1978;73:592–595.

81. Walter J, Cooney M, Norton S. Improved pulmonary function in chronic quadriplegics after pulmonary therapy and arm ergometry. *Paraplegia.* 1989;27:278–283.

82. Mang H, Obermayer A. Imposed work of breathing during sustained maximal inspiration: Comparison of six incentive spirometers. *Respir Care.* 1989;34:1122–1128.

83. Lederer DH, Vandewater JM, Indech RB. Which breathing device should the postoperative patient use? *Chest.* 1980;77:610–613.

84. Rau JL, Thomas L, Haynes RL. The effect of method of administering incentive spirometry on postoperative pulmonary complications in coronary bypass patients. *Respir Care.* 1988;33:771–778.

85. Celli BR, Rodriguez KS, Snider GL. A controlled trial of intermittent positive pressure breathing, incentive spirometry, and deep breathing exercises in preventing pulmonary complication after abdominal surgery. *Am Rev Respir Dis.* 1984;130:12–15.

86. Jenkins, SC, Soutar SA, Loukota JM, et al. Physiotherapy after coronary artery surgery: Are breathing exercises necessary? *Thorax.* 1989;44:634–639.

87. Stiller K, Montarello J, Wallace M, et al. Efficacy of breathing and coughing exercises in the prevention of pulmonary complications after coronary artery surgery. *Chest.* 1994;105:741–747.

88. Dull JL, Dull WL. Are maximal inspiratory breathing exercises better or incentive spirometry better than early mobilization after cardiopulmonary bypass. *Phys Ther.* 1983;63:655–659.

89. Hall JC, Tarala R, Harris J, et al. Incentive spirometry versus routine chest physiotherapy for prevention of pulmonary complications after abdominal surgery. *Lancet.* 1991;337:953–956.

90. Stiller K, Geake T, Taylor H, et al. Acute lobar atelectasis: A comparison of two chest physiotherapy regimens. *Chest.* 1990;98:1336–1340.

91. Nilsestuen J, Fink J, Stoller J, et al. AARC clinical practice guideline: Intermittent positive pressure breathing. *Respir Care.* 1993;38:1189–1195.

92. Dolovich MB, Killian D, Wolff RK, et al. Pulmonary aerosol deposition in chronic bronchitis: Intermittent positive pressure breathing versus quiet breathing. *Am Rev Respir Dis.* 1977;115:397–402.

93. The IPPB Trial Group. Intermittent positive pressure breathing therapy of chronic obstructive pulmonary disease: A clinical trial. *Ann Intern Med.* 1983;99;612–620.

94. Pedersen JZ, Bundgaard A. Comparative efficacy of different methods of nebulizing terbutaline. *Eur J Clin Pharmacol.* 1983;25:739–742.

95. Bartlett RH. Respiratory therapy to prevent pulmonary complications of surgery. *Respir Care.* 1984;29:667–669.

96. DeTroyer A, Deisser P. The effects of intermittent positive pressure breathing on patients with respiratory muscle weakness. *Am Rev Respir Dis.* 1981;124:132–137.

97. Moore RB, Cotton EK, Pinney MA. The effect of intermittent positive pressure breathing on airway resistance in normal and asthmatic children. *J Allergy Clin Immunol.* 1972;49:137–141.

98. Rodenstien DO, Stanescu DC, Delguste P, et al. Adaptation to intermittent positive pressure ventilation applied through the nose during day and night. *Eur Respir J.* 1989;2:473–478.

99. Bach JR, Alba A, Mosher R, Delaubier A. Intermittent positive pressure ventilation via nasal access in the management of respiratory insufficiency. *Chest.* 1987;92:168–170.

100. Hilling L, Bakow E, Fink J, et al. AARC clinical practice guideline: Use of positive airway pressure adjuncts to bronchial hygiene therapy. *Respir Care.* 1993;38:516–521.

101. Paul WL, Downs JB. Postoperative atelectasis: Intermittent positive pressure breathing, incentive spirometry, and face-mask positive end-expiratory pressure. *Arch Surg.* 1981;116:861–863.

102. Ricksten SE, Bengtsson A, Soderberg C, et al. Effects of periodic positive airway pressure by mask on postoperative pulmonary function. *Chest.* 1986;89:774–781.

103. Andersen JB, Klausen NO. A new mode of administration of nebulized bronchodilator in severe bronchospasm. *Eur J Respir Dis.* 1982;63(suppl 119):97–100.

104. Frischknecht-Christensen E, Norregaard O, Dahl R. Treatment of bronchial asthma with terbutaline inhaled by conespacer combined with positive expiratory pressure mask. *Chest.* 1991;100(2):317–321.

105. Kacmarek RM, Dimas S, Reynolds J, Shapiro B. Technical aspects of positive end expiratory pressure (PEEP). I. Physics of PEEP devices. *Respir Care.* 1982;27:1478–1489.

106. Mahlmeister MJ, Fink JB, Hoffman GL, Fifer LF. Positive-expiratory-pressure mask therapy: Theoretical and practical considerations and a review of the literature. *Respir Care.* 1991;36:1218–1230.

107. Thoman RL, Stoker GL, Ross JC. The efficacy of pursed-lips breathing in patients with chronic obstructive pulmonary disease. *Am Rev Respir Dis.* 1968;93:100–106.

108. Petty TL. Chronic obstructive pulmonary disease. New York: Marcel Dekker; 1978.

109. Poulton EP, Odon DM. Left-sided heart failure with pulmonary oedema: Its treatment with the "pulmonary plus pressure machine." *Lancet.* 1936;231:981–983.

110. Barach AL, Martin J, Eckman L. Positive pressure respiration and its application to the treatment of acute pulmonary edema and respiratory obstruction. *Proc Am Soc Clin Invest.* 1937;16:664–680.

111. Cheney FW, Hornbein TF, Crawford EW. The effect of expiratory resistance on the blood gas tensions of anesthetized patients. *Anesthesiology.* 1967;28(4):670–676.

112. Ashbaugh DG, Petty TL, Bigelow DB, Harris TM. Continuous positive pressure breathing (CPPB) in adult respiratory distress syndrome. *J Thorac Cardiovasc Surg.* 1969;57:31–41.

113. Gregory GA, Kitterman JA, Phibbs RH. Treatment of the idiopathic respiratory distress syndrome with continuous positive airway pressure. *N Engl J Med.* 1971;284:1333–1340.

114. Pontoppidan H, Wilson RS, Rie MA, Schneider RC. Respiratory intensive care. *Anesthesiology.* 1977;47:96–116.

115. Katz JA. PEEP and CPAP in perioperative respiratory care. *Respir Care.* 1984;29:6:614–623.

116. Garrard CS, Shah M. The effects of expiratory positive airway pressure on function residual capacity in normal subjects. *Crit Care Med.* 1978;6:320–332.

117. Andersen JB, Qvist H, Kann T. Recruiting collapsed lung through collateral channels with positive end-expiratory pressure. *Scand J Respir Dis.* 1979;60:260–266.

118. Andersen JB, Jespersen W. Demonstration of intersegmental respiratory bronchioles in normal lungs. *Eur J Respir Dis.* 1980;61:337–341.

119. Branson RD, Hurst JM, DeHaven CB. Mask CPAP: State of the art. *Respir Care.* 1985;30:846–857.

120. Branson RD. PEEP without endotracheal intubation. *Respir Care.* 1988;33:598–610.

121. Andersen JB, Olesen KP, Eikard E, et al. Periodic continuous positive airway pressure, CPAP, by mask in the treatment of atelectasis: A sequential analysis. *Eur J Respir Dis.* 1980;61:20–25.

122. Pontoppidan H. Mechanical aids to lung expansion in nonintubated surgical patients. *Am Rev Respir Dis.* 1980;122:109–119.

123. Carlsson C, Sonden B, Thylen U. Can postoperative continuous positive airway pressure (CPAP) prevent pulmonary complications after abdominal surgery? *Intensive Care Med.* 1981;7:225–229.

124. Martin JG, Shore S, Engel LA. Effect of continuous positive pressure on respiratory mechanics and pattern of breathing in induced asthma. *Am Rev Respir Dis.* 1982;126:812–817.

125. Stock MC, Downs JB. Administration of continuous positive airway pressure by mask. *Acute Care.* 1983/84;10:184–188.

126. Stock MC, Downs JB, Corkran ML. Pulmonary function before and after prolonged positive airway pressure by mask. *Crit Care Med.* 1984;12:973–974.

127. Stock MC, Downs JB, Cooper RB, et al. Comparison of continuous positive airway pressure, incentive spirometry, and conservative therapy after cardiac operations. *Crit Care Med.* 1984;12:969–972.

128. Stock MC, Downs JB, Gauer PK, et al. Prevention of postoperative pulmonary complication with CPAP, incentive spirometry and conservative therapy. *Chest.* 1985;87:151–157.

129. Lindner KH, Lotz P, Ahnefeld FW. Continuous positive airway pressure effect on functional residual capacity, vital capacity and its subdivisions. *Chest.* 1987;92:1:66–70.

130. Campbell T, Ferguson N, McKinlay RGC. The use of a simple self-administered method of positive expiratory pressure (PEP) in chest physiotherapy after abdominal surgery. *Physiotherapy.* 1986;72:498–500.

131. Frolund L, Madsen F. Self-administered prophylactic postoperative positive expiratory pressure in thoracic surgery. *Acta Anaesthesiol Scand.* 1986;30:381–385.

132. Groth S, Stafanger G, Dirksen H, et al. Positive expiratory pressure (PEP mask) physiotherapy improves ventilation and reduces volume of trapped gas in cystic fibrosis. *Bull Eur Physiopathol Respir.* 1985;21:339–343.

133. Branson RD, Hurst JM, DeHaven CB. Mask CPAP: State of the art. *Respir Care.* 1985;30:846–857.

134. van der Schans CP, de Jong W, de Vries G, et al. Effects of positive expiratory pressure breathing during exercise in patients with COPD. *Chest.* 1994;105:782–789.

135. Colgan FJ, Mahoney PD, Fanning GL. Resistance breathing (blow bottles) and sustained hyperinflations in the treatment of atelectasis. *Anesthesiology.* 1970;32:543–550.

136. Iverson LIG, Ecker RR, Fox HE, May IA. A comparative study of IPPB, the incentive spirometer, and blow bottles: The prevention of atelectasis following surgery. *Ann Thorac Surg.* 1978;35:197–200.

137. Lindemann H. The value of physical therapy with VRP 1—Desitin (Flutter). *Pneumologie.* 1992;46:626–630.

138. Konstan MW, Stern RC, Doershuk CF. Efficacy of the Flutter device for airway mucus clearance in patients with cystic fibrosis. *J Pediatr.* 1994;124:689–693.

139. Pryor JA, Webber BA, Hodson ME, Warner JO. The Flutter VRP1 as an adjunct to chest physiotherapy in cystic fibrosis. *Respir Med.* 1994;88:677–681.

140. Fink J. A comparison of Flutter to other airway clearance valves: A laboratory study. *Chest.* 1995;108(3):147S. (Abstract)

141. Schlobohm RM, Fallrick RT, Quan SF, Katz JA. Lung volumes, mechanics and oxygenation during spontaneous positive pressure ventilation: The advantage of CPAP over EPAP. *Anesthesiology.* 1981;55:426–422.

142. Petrof BJ, Calderini E, Gottfried SB. Effect of CPAP on respiratory effort and dyspnea during exercise in severe COPD. *J Appl Physiol.* 1990;69(1):179–188.

143. Petrof BJ, Legare M, Godberg P, et al. Continuous positive airway pressure reduces work of breathing and dyspnea during weaning from mechanical ventilation in severe chronic obstructive pulmonary disease. *Am Rev Respir Dis.* 1990;141:281–289.

144. McInturff SL, Shaw LI. Intrapulmonary percussive ventilation. *Respir Care.* 1985;30:884–885.

145. Natale JE, Pfeifle J, Homnick DN. Comparison of intrapulmonary percussive ventilation and chest physiotherapy. *Chest.* 1994;105:1789–1793.

146. Davis KJ, Hurst JM, Branson RD. High frequency percussive ventilation. *Respir Care.* 1989;34:39–47.

147. Hurst JM, Branson RD. High-frequency percussive ventilation in the management of elevated intracranial pressure. *J Trauma.* 1988;28:1363–1367.

148. Cioffi WG, Major MC. High frequency percussive ventilation in patients with inhalation injury. *J Trauma.* 1989;29:350–354.

149. van Henstum M, Festen J, Buerskens C, et al. No effect of oral high frequency oscillation combined with forced expiration manoeuvres on tracheobronchial clearance in chronic bronchitis. *Eur Respir J.* 1990;3:14–18.

150. King M, Phillips DM, Zidulka A, et al. Tracheal mucus clearance with high-frequency chest wall compression. *Am Rev Respir Dis.* 1983; 128:511–515.

151. King M, Zidulka A, Phillips DM, et al. Tracheal mucus clearance in high-frequency oscillation: Effect of peak flow rate bias. *Eur Respir J.* 1990;3:6–13.

152. Hansen L, Warwick W. High frequency chest compression system to aid in clearance of mucus from the lung. *Biomed Instrum Technol.* 1990;24:289–294.

153. Spitzer SA, Fink G, Mittelman M. External high-frequency ventilation in severe chronic obstructive pulmonary disease. *Chest.* 1993;104:1698–1701.

154. Soo Hoo GW, Ellison MJ, Zhang C, et al. Effects of external chest wall oscillation in stable COPD patients. *Am J Respir Crit Care Med.* 1994;149:A637.

155. Smithline HA, Rivers EP, Rady MY, et al. Biphasic extrathoracic pressure CPR: A human pilot study. *Chest.* 1994;105:842–846.

156. Segawa J, Nakashima Y, Kuroirwa A, et al. The efficacy of external high frequency oscillation: Experience in a quadriplegic patient with alveolar hypoventilation. *Kokyu To Junkan.* 1993;41:271–275.

157. Gaitini L, Krimerman S, Smorgik J, et al. External high frequency ventilation for weaning from the mechanical ventilation. *Recent Advances Anaesth, Pain, Int Care, Emerg.* 1990;5:137–138.

158. Dilworth JP, Warley RH, Dawe C, White RJ. The effect of nebulized salbutamol therapy on the incidence of postoperative chest infection in high risk patients. *Respir Med.* 1994;88:665–668.

14

Airway Care

Robert M. Lewis

Key Terms

bag-mask ventilation
cricothyrotomy
esophageal obturator
head-tilt
chin-lift maneuver
laryngeal airway mask
percutaneous dilation
   tracheostomy
tracheostomy
ventilator-associated
   pneumonia (VAP)

Objectives

- Discuss the anatomy and physiology of the upper and lower airway.

- Describe the emergency management of the airway without an endotracheal tube.

- Outline the procedures for emergency and elective endotracheal intubation.

- Discuss ongoing care of the intubated patient.

- Summarize the etiology and prevention of nosocomial pneumonia in the intubated patient.

Maintenance of the airway is essential for the preservation of human life and is the most important skill required of respiratory care practitioners and all those who work with the critically ill. Establishment of an airway under emergency conditions is successful only when the practitioner and the institution prepare for emergencies through training of personnel and appropriate deployment of equipment.

In addition to skillful placement of the artificial airway, the respiratory care practitioner should be knowledgeable in the proper selection and maintenance of airway equipment and in the care and prevention of complications in the intubated patient. This chapter briefly reviews the anatomy and physiology of the airway; techniques of management without intubation; the process of emergent and nonemergent intubation; care of the established airway; recognition and prevention of complications; the care of tracheostomized patients; and airway management in spontaneously breathing patients who are not candidates for intubation.

RELEVANT ANATOMY AND PHYSIOLOGY

The Nose

The principle functions of the nose are to warm, humidify, and filter the inspired air. To fulfill these functions, a rich vascular supply is required to provide water and heat. As such, the nose is prone to edema and bleeds easily when subjected to trauma. It is also equipped with a rich supply of mucous glands, which can produce copious amounts of secretions, obstructing the airway. In addition, the mucosa is highly enervated to detect the inspiration of harmful substances. Stimulation of some of these nerves produces sneezing.

To provide the greatest possible interface between air and the moist nasal mucosa, the inspiratory airstream into the nose is distributed into several smaller passages formed by the nasal turbinates (three on each side). The first of these passages lies parallel to the nasal floor and provides the easiest route for nontraumatic passage of suction and endotracheal tubes to the pharynx (Fig. 14–1).

Communicating with the nasal cavity are four paranasal sinuses, or cavities, which are lined with the same type of mucosa as are the nasal passages. The sinuses produce mucus, which drains into the nasal passage and aids in the removal of foreign debris. If the sinus openings are occluded (eg, by an endotracheal tube), mucus stagnates and becomes infected, producing sinusitis.

The Mouth

The mouth is designed primarily for intake of food and for speech and only secondarily for air passage. Normally, humans can breathe through the nasal passages even with complete mouth closure. In the event of partial or complete nasal obstruction or with increased ventilatory demands, the mouth may be the sole airway. Factors that may impair the ability to breathe through the mouth include lack of teeth (in infants

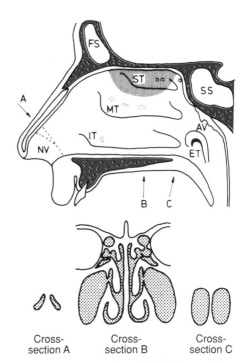

FIGURE 14–1 • Lateral wall of the nasal cavity and cross-sections of the internal ostium (*A*), the middle of the nasal cavity (*B*), and the choanae (*C*). IT, inferior turbinate; MT, middle turbinate; ST, superior turbinate. (Mygind)

and the elderly), an unusually large tongue (as in angioedema, certain congenital disorders, trauma, or tumors), and an unusually short or immobile mandible (which prevents full mouth opening), as occurs in certain congenital or acquired disorders, such as Pierre Robin syndrome.

The Pharynx

The pharynx is a cone-shaped structure lying behind the mouth and below the nasal cavity. It is the common passageway for food and air. Lining the lateral anterior walls of the pharynx are lymphoid structures called *tonsils*. These structures can increase significantly in size as a result of acute or chronic inflammation, leading to symptomatic airway obstruction. In some cases, infections can produce a tonsillar or retropharyngeal abscess, which can produce life-threatening airway obstruction.

The tissue of the pharynx is extremely soft and compliant, making it vulnerable to penetration during intubation attempts. The anterior pharynx leads into the larynx, whereas the posterior pharynx leads to the esophagus. The anterior location of the larynx, relative to the pharynx, accounts for much of the difficulties encountered in endotracheal intubation.

The Larynx

The larynx functions to conduct air to and from the lungs, to produce speech, and to protect the airway. It is funnel shaped, cartilaginous, and muscular. The opening of the larynx is called the *glottis.* Above the glottis is a structure called the *epiglottis,* which covers the glottis during swallowing to prevent food from entering the airway. The epiglottis is part of the defense system of the airway, with nerves that detect foreign-body intrusion, with reflex cough and laryngeospasm. The *vallecula* is an avascular, relatively insensitive area between the epiglottis and the base of the tongue, making it an important landmark for elective and emergency intubations. Painful swallowing is a possible indication of epiglottic swelling or injury.

The glottis is also closed during the compressive phase of a cough. Impairment of epiglottic mobility (as in epiglottitis) impairs the ability to cough.

The false vocal cords also assist in glottic closure during swallowing or coughing. These structures approximate and seal the laryngeal opening. They also partially close during normal exhalation, helping to maintain a normal functional residual capacity (FRC). This function is lost during endotracheal intubation, and, as a result, FRC may be reduced. Typically, 2 to 3 cm H_2O of positive end-expiratory pressure or continuous positive airway pressure is sufficient to restore the FRC to normal.

The anterior larynx is protected by the thyroid cartilage. The cricoid cartilage marks the lower border of the larynx. It is a complete ring, larger posteriorly than anteriorly (Fig. 14–2).

Trauma or disease can sometimes lead to paralysis of one or both cords. This results in failure of the cords to abduct (open) during inspiration and may result in significant airway obstruction. Trauma to the cords with resultant edema reduces vocal cord mobility and reduces the ability of the cords to adduct (come together) and close the airway. This reduces the efficacy of the cough and increases risk of aspiration during swallowing.

The Trachea

The trachea is supported by a series of C-shaped cartilaginous rings. The open parts of the rings face the esophagus. As such, there is the possibility of tracheal compression from foreign bodies in the esophagus. In contrast, the anterior tracheal wall is more rigid. Although this helps to resist collapse from external compression, it increases the risk of mucosal ischemia and ulceration from overinflated endotracheal tube cuffs.

EMERGENCY MANAGEMENT OF THE AIRWAY

Common Causes of Acute Airway Obstruction

The most common cause of airway obstruction encountered by the respiratory care practitioner is soft tissue obstruction secondary to loss of neural control of the airway. With loss of consciousness secondary to drug overdose, head injury, cardiac arrest, or other cause, the neural con-

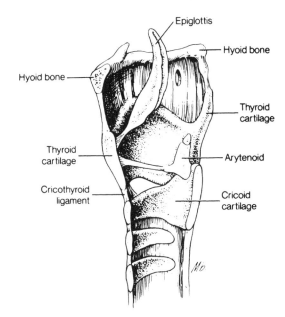

FIGURE 14–2 • Detailed view of the adult larynx. (BT Finucane, AH Santora (eds): Principles of Airway Management. Philadelphia, FA Davis, 1988, with permission.)

trol of the airway is depressed or lost. The patient therefore lacks the muscle tone needed to keep the pharyngeal structures open, and the tongue falls backward, causing obstruction. Along with posterior displacement of the tongue, the epiglottis is displaced downward over the glottic opening.

Manual Techniques

The first step in establishment of the airway is the **head-tilt, chin-lift maneuver.** This brings the tongue and epiglottis forward, reestablishing patency. In addition, this maneuver reduces the angle between the nasooropharynx and the larynx (Fig. 14–3). This maneuver is performed by placing the hand closest to the patient's head on the fore-

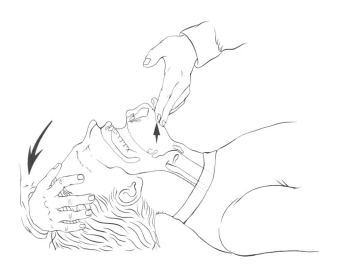

FIGURE 14–3 • Manual opening of the adult airway using the head-tilt chin-lift maneuver.

head, tilting the head back into the sniffing position. Next, two or three fingers are placed under the bony portion of the chin to lift the jaw. Care should be taken to avoid compression of the soft tissue posterior to the chin.

If the patient is approached from the rear, three fingers can be placed along the posterior rim of the mandible and the jaw thrust forward.

Oronasopharyngeal Airways

If an airway cannot be maintained easily with the manual methods and the resuscitation team is not yet ready for intubation, an oral airway may be inserted (Fig. 14–4). An oral airway of proper size holds the tongue in the anterior position, opening the posterior pharynx. In addition, it prevents complete mouth closure, decreasing resistance to airflow. This may be helpful in edentulous (toothless) patients. Use of too small an oral airway results in failure to hold the tongue in proper position. Too large an airway results in posterior displacement of the epiglottis. Improper insertion can result in extreme posterior displacement of the tongue. To prevent this, the airway is usually inserted upside-down, moved past the tongue, and rotated into correct position (Fig. 14–5). Alternately, a tongue blade can be used to depress the tongue during insertion. Finally, semiconscious patients may resist or gag during insertion attempts. Therefore, the oral airway is the only suitable method for severely obtunded patients.

Nasopharyngeal airways are usually soft and made of rubber. They are seldom used during emergency airway

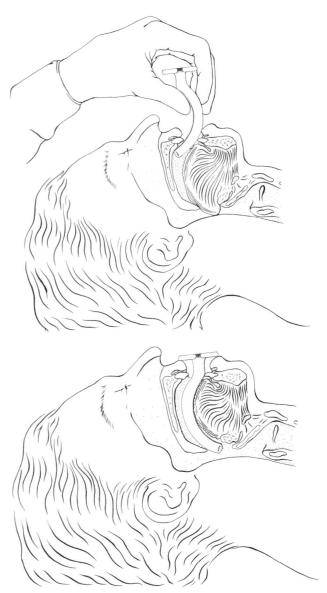

FIGURE 14–5 • (*A*) Insertion of an oropharyngeal airway should be initiated in the upside-down position. As the airway is advanced, it is rotated so the distal portion supports the posterior pharynx. (*B*) Airway shown in position.

management of the completely unconscious patient but may be useful in the semiconscious patient. They are especially helpful in patients who are able to breathe spontaneously but who need frequent nasotracheal suction (Fig. 14–6). Box 14–1 demonstrates the proper procedure for inserting a nasopharyngeal airway.

Bag-Mask Ventilation

After establishment of the airway, ventilation must be provided by means of **bag-mask ventilation**. A good fit is essential for proper ventilation. This may be difficult in patients without teeth, in obese patients, and in those with facial trauma. The ideal mask is transparent and has a soft, air-filled cuff to provide a good seal.

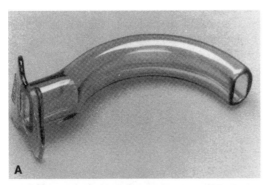

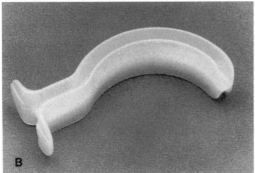

FIGURE 14–4 • Oropharyngeal airways. (*A*) Guedel-style. (*B*) Connel style.

CRITICAL THINKING CHALLENGES

Case Scenario

Taping in the Oral Airway

Mr. Fox is a 46-year-old, obese white man who is recovering from anesthesia postoperatively. After extubation, Mr. Fox exhibits signs of obstructed upper airway, and an oral airway is inserted. As Mr. Fox begins to awaken, he spits out the oral airway and resumes snoring, with episodes of obstructive apnea. The bedside attendant, after reinserting the airway three times, tapes the airway in position. As Mr. Fox awakens, he begins to gag on the airway, is unable to spit it out, vomits, and aspirates. Mr. Fox proceeds to develop aspiration pneumonitis, is taken to the ICU, and dies.

Never tape in an oral airway. If you need to secure the airway, consider the nasopharyngeal airway.

The mask must be held properly to ensure good seal and proper airway alignment. The technique is illustrated in Figure 14–7. Some operators prefer to use the dominant hand to hold the mask and the nondominant hand to squeeze the bag. Others prefer the opposite approach. When possible, two practitioners should be available to perform ventilation: one to use both hands to secure the airway and hold the mask (see Fig. 14–7); the second to squeeze the bag. Delivered tidal volumes can be increased by as much as 250 mL with this approach.[1,2]

Esophageal Obturators and Laryngeal Airway Masks

When intubation cannot be performed immediately, the airway may be maintained temporarily by the use of either

Box • 14–1 PROCEDURE FOR INSERTING THE NASOPHARYNGEAL AIRWAY

1. Estimate the length of airway to be inserted—the distance from the tip of the nose to the earlobe correlates to the distance from the nares to the base of the tongue. Select an airway of appropriate length or adjust the "stop" on the universal-size airway.
2. Determine which side of the nasal passage is less obstructed by feeling for best airflow through a naris when the other side is temporarily occluded (with your finger). If the patient is alert, ask him or her to sniff with each naris occluded. Proceed with insertion on side with best airflow.
3. Lubricate airway or nares.
4. Gently insert tip of airway with the bevel toward the nasal septum, diagonally up and back (to track above the medial turbinate) through the nasopharynx. Then rotate the airway to take advantage of the natural curve of the tube.
5. Insert gently; if obstruction is encountered, try the other side.
6. Insert to predetermined length, assess to ensure that the airway is not interfering with epiglottis or larynx function (cough or gag). Be sure that you have not intubated the patient's trachea.
7. Secure the airway. Place a safety pin through the side of the flare, distal to the nares. This will keep the tube from being aspirated into the nose beyond your reach with strong inspiratory maneuvers by the patient. These tubes are generally secured by nasal structures so that tape is not required.

---

an esophageal obturator or a laryngeal airway mask. These devices do not enter the trachea but rather separate the airway from the gastrointestinal tract, improving ventilation and reducing the risk of aspiration.

The **esophageal obturator** is used primarily in the management of the cardiac arrest victim in the prehospital setting. The device consists of a cuffed tube, with the distal end sealed, inserted into a mask. The proximal portion of the tube is patent and contains holes for air to enter the pharynx. The tube is inserted into the esophagus and the cuff inflated. This prevents air from entering the stomach and gastric contents from escaping into the airway (Fig. 14–8). A manual resuscitation device can be attached to the mask. With proper head position, the path of least resistance for gas flow is into the lungs, and ventilation can be accomplished with little difficulty. When the patient arrives in the emergency room, the trachea should be intubated before removal of the esophageal obturator to prevent aspiration.

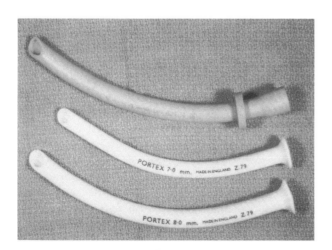

FIGURE 14–6 • Nasopharyngeal airways.

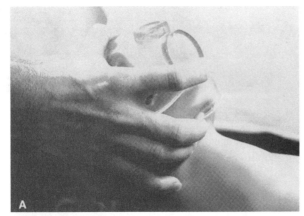

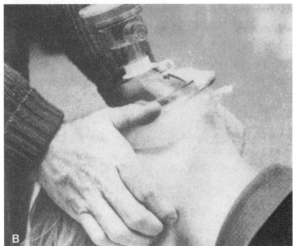

FIGURE 14–7 • (*A*) One-handed technique to apply a mask to the airway. Notice placement of the fingers under the mandible and maintenance of head extension. (*B*) Two-handed technique. (Hess D, Ness C, Oppel A, Rhoads K. Evaluation of mouth-to-mask ventilation devices. *Respir Care.* 1989;34:191.)

The **laryngeal airway mask** consists of a silicone rubber inflatable mask attached to the distal end of a short endotracheal tube (Fig. 14–9). The mask is designed to lie in the posterior pharynx, sealing off the esophagus but permitting ventilation of the larynx. It is useful in patients with depressed levels of consciousness.

ENDOTRACHEAL INTUBATION

Endotracheal intubation is indicated to achieve the following objectives:

• Maintain the airway
• Prevent aspiration
• Facilitate ventilation
• Improve pulmonary hygiene

Intubation of the patient in cardiac arrest does not require special patient preparation other than ventilation and preoxygenation. The conscious or semiconscious patient, however, usually requires pharmacologic preparation with muscle relaxants, topical anesthetics, and sedatives to pre-

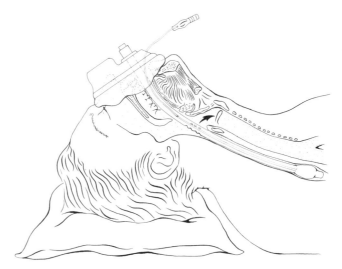

FIGURE 14–8 • Schematic drawing of the esophageal obturator airway in place in the esophagus.

vent untoward cardiovascular and intracranial reactions as well as to decrease patient resistance and improve comfort.

Equipment

Endotracheal Tubes

Endotracheal tubes are manufactured in accordance with standards developed by the F-29 subcommittee of the American Society for Testing and Materials. The basic design and features of a standard endotracheal tube are illustrated in Figure 14–10. Important elements of the tube include the following:

The patient connector. This device connects the proximal end of the endotracheal tube to respiratory support equipment, such as a manual or mechanical ventilator. The proximal end is always 15 mm in external diameter. The distal end is equal to the internal diameter of the endotracheal tube.

The tube body. The endotracheal tube is somewhat curved and is made of polyvinyl chloride or silicone. Materials used for endotracheal tube construction are tested in rabbit muscle (implantation tested) to ensure that they are nontoxic to tissues. The distal end of the tube is beveled and usually has an additional opening, or "Murphy's eye" in the wall of the tube to provide a means of ventilation if the distal end is occluded. Markings along the body of the tube include it size, length markings, brand name, and an indication that it meets American Society for Testing and Materials standards.

Inflatable cuff. An inflatable cuff is located just above the distal end of the tube. It is connected to a small-bore inflation tube that runs within the wall of the tube and exits several inches before the proximal end. The external portion of the inflating tube is usually several inches long and has a soft pilot balloon that

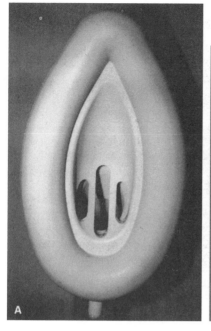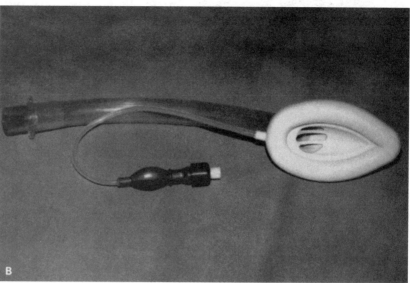

FIGURE 14–9 • (*A*) Laryngeal mask airway. (*B*) Detail of mask ventilating orifices at the junction of the tube and mask.

gives an indication of the pressure in the cuff. The tube ends with an inflation valve that opens when a syringe is inserted and seals when the syringe is withdrawn. The tube is inflated or deflated with a syringe placed into the inflation valve.

The purpose of the cuff is to prevent escape of inspired gases and to prevent or minimize the risk of aspiration. Most tubes intended for adult use are equipped with soft, low-pressure, high-volume cuffs. This type of cuff minimizes the pressure applied to the tracheal wall and reduces the risk of tracheal injury.

Laryngoscopes

The **laryngoscope** consists of two components: the handle and the blade. The handle is available in two sizes. The internal chamber of the blade contains a space for batteries, and the distal end contains a connector for the laryngoscope blade. Laryngoscope blades are either straight (Miller) or curved (McIntosh). Both types contain a small light bulb (Fig. 14–11).

The curved blade is designed to displace the tongue easily, and the tip of the blade is designed to insert into the vallecula (the space between the epiglottis and the base of the tongue). Elevation of the blade puts traction on the base of the epiglottis, lifting it away from the larynx (Fig. 14–12). The straight blade lifts the epiglottis directly, allowing greater exposure of the larynx (Fig. 14–13).

Additional Equipment

A stylet inserted into the endotracheal tube is sometimes helpful in facilitating intubation. Sterile, water-soluble lubricant may be helpful as well. A Magill forceps is especially helpful in nasal intubation. A list of supplies recommended for intubation is provided in Box 14–2.

Equipment Set-up and Patient Preparation

A properly functioning bag and mask connected to oxygen should be available. Suction equipment should be set up and tested for proper function. A rigid large-bore suction tube and soft suction catheters of various sizes should be on hand.

Selection and Preparation of the Endotracheal Tube

A tube of appropriate size should be selected according to the guidelines described in Table 14–1. A tube one-half

CRITICAL THINKING CHALLENGES

Challenging Assumptions

Although an indication of endotracheal intubation is to prevent aspiration, the placement of the tube virtually ensures microaspiration. The tube and the cuff keep out the peas and carrots but do not keep the soup from dripping past the cuff into the airway. The normal flora of the upper airway and gastric tube are the source of pathogens associated with VAP.

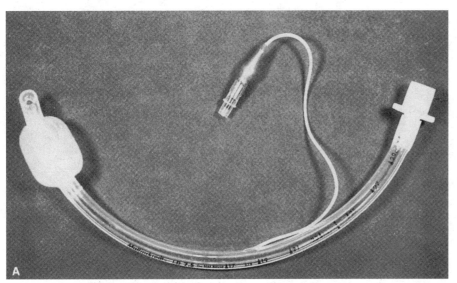

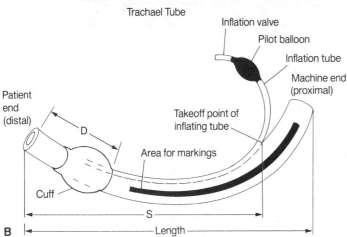

FIGURE 14–10 • (*A*) A cuffed endotracheal tube. (*B*) Diagram illustrating basic design features and dimensional zones. (American Society for Testing and Materials. Standards for cuffed and uncuffed tracheal tubes [F2290201]. Philadelphia: American Society for Testing and Materials; 1989.)

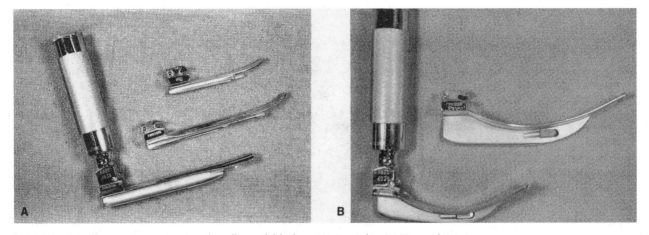

FIGURE 14–11 • Laryngoscope handle and blades. (*A*) Straight. (*B*) Curved (McIntosh) blades.

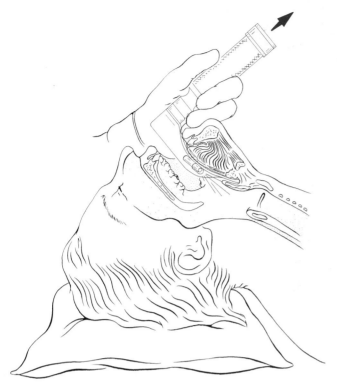

FIGURE 14–12 • Adult laryngoscopy with curved blade. Note that the wrist is straight.

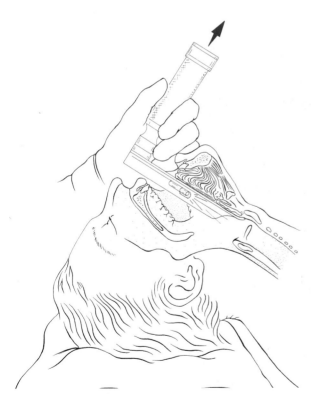

FIGURE 14–13 • Adult laryngoscopy with straight blade. (Barnes TA, Watson ME. Cardiopulmonary resuscitation and emergency cardiac care. In: Barnes TA, ed. *Core Textbook in Respiratory Care Practice*. 2nd ed. St. Louis: Mosby–Year Book; 1994:308.)

size smaller should be used for nasal intubation. The tube may be lubricated with sterile water-soluble lubricant. If desired, a stylet may be inserted to increase rigidity. This is especially useful with neonatal and pediatric intubation. The stylet should never be inserted beyond the level of the eye because tracheal perforation can result. The cuff should be inflated to detect leaks, then deflated.

A laryngoscope blade of the type and size preferred by the intubator should be attached to the laryngoscope handle. The bulb must be checked to ensure that it is securely attached and sufficiently bright. Additional sizes and types of blades should be immediately available.

Placement and Position of the Patient

The patient's bed should be placed so there is sufficient room at the head of the bed for the intubator and an assistant. The head of the bed is usually removed. The level of the bed is adjusted to allow the intubator to stand and maneuver comfortably. The patient is positioned in the sniffing position as shown in Figure 14–14.

Positive-pressure ventilation is continued, and the patient's SaO_2 and heart rate are continually monitored.

Box • 14–2 EQUIPMENT NEEDED FOR INTUBATION

- Ventilation devices
    Masks (variety of sizes)
    Manual resuscitation
- Airway management devices
    Oropharyngeal airways (variety of sizes)
    Nasopharyngeal airways (variety of sizes)
    Laryngeal mask airway
    Pharyngeotracheal lumen airway or esophageal
      tracheal combitude
    Intubation devices
        Laryngoscope handles (two), with variety of
          curved and straight blades
        Wire guide or stylet and introducer, changer,
          or bougie
        Forceps
- Supplies and miscellany
    Lubricant
    Syringe
    12- to 16-gauge intravenous catheter-over-the-
      needle device for transcatheter ventilation
    Tape, endotracheal tube ties, or other method for
      tube stabilization
    Endotracheal tubes (variety of sizes)
    Eye shields and gloves
    Source of suction and suction catheters

Table • 14–1   RECOMMENDED SIZES (ID) AND ESTIMATES FOR TRACHEAL TUBES

Uncuffed Tubes (Based on age or body weight)

Premature	2.5–3.0 mm	
<1 kg	2.5 mm	
2–3 kg	3.5 mm	*or* $\dfrac{\text{Gestational age (in weeks)}}{10} + 0.5 = \text{ID (mm)}$
1 to 6 months	3.0–4.0 mm	
>3 kg	4.0 mm	*or* $\dfrac{3.5 + \text{age}}{3} = \text{ID (mm)}$
6 months to 1 year	3.5–4.5 mm	*or* $\dfrac{4.5 + \text{age}}{4} = \text{ID (mm)}$

Uncuffed Tubes (Based on body dimension)
Choose a tube with an external diameter (OD) that is the same width as the distal portion of the patient's little finger.

Cuffed Tubes

8 year old	6 mm
12 year old	6.5 mm
16 year old	7.0 mm
Average adult female	7.0–7.5 mm
Average adult male	8.0–8.5 mm

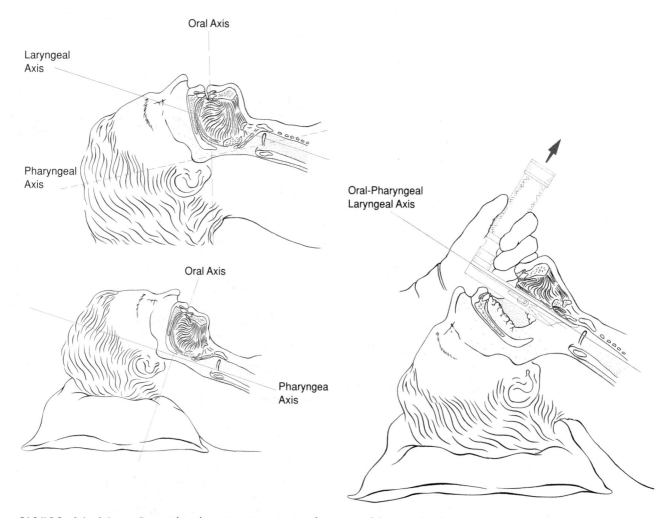

FIGURE 14–14 • Proper head position is important for successful orotracheal intubation. (*A*) The oral, pharyngeal, and laryngeal axes must be aligned for direct laryngoscopy. (*B*) Elevate the head 10 cm above the shoulders with a folded towel to align the pharyngeal and laryngeal axes. (*C*) Extend the atlanto-occipital joint to achieve the straightest possible line from the incisors to the glottis.

Direct Laryngoscopy and Intubation

If the patient is potentially combative or only semiconscious, a rapid sequence intubation is performed. This consists of administration of a rapidly acting sedative followed by administration of a rapidly acting muscle relaxant. Atropine may also be given to prevent bradycardia.

Once apnea is established, open the patient's mouth with the right hand. Grasp the laryngoscope with the left hand, and pass the blade through the oropharynx until the epiglottis is visualized. Gently put the tip of the blade under the epiglottis and lift upward. The glottis should now be visible. With the right hand, grasp the endotracheal tube, and insert it into the right side of the mouth. Try not to obstruct the view of the glottis. Advance the tube through the open glottis into the trachea. Usually, the tube needs to be advanced until the 21- (for women) or 23- (for men) cm mark reaches the teeth.[3] Advancement up to 30 cm may increase the risk of damage to the right mainstem bronchus. After advancing the tube, remove the laryngoscope blade, and while holding the tube firmly, assess for proper tube placement.

Alternate Techniques

For patients who are conscious and more cooperative, paralysis may not be required. Instead, sedation with a benzodiazepine and topical airway anesthesia with nebulized or sprayed lidocaine may suffice. Alternately, the patient may be asked to gargle viscous lidocaine.

When prolonged intubation is anticipated, nasotracheal intubation may be the technique of choice because nasotracheal tubes are usually better tolerated and more comfortable for the patient. Nasal tubes are often selected with a smaller diameter to ease passage, which may increase airway resistance and work of breathing. Nasotracheal intubation has also been associated with increased risk of sinus infection.

Process for Blind Nasal Intubation

Box 14–3 lists the proper steps for blind nasal intubation. To confirm tube placement, inflate the cuff, connect the endotracheal tube to a manual resuscitator, and give several breaths. Watch for even chest expansion, and listen for breath sounds over both sides of the chest. Next, listen over the left upper quadrant of the abdomen for air entry into the stomach. If placed correctly, breath sounds are heard in the chest bilaterally. Esophageal intubation produces harsh gurgling sounds over the stomach. If this occurs, the cuff should be deflated and the tube removed. The patient should be reoxygenated before an additional intubation attempt.

If breath sounds are heard over the right lung but not the left, a right mainstem bronchial intubation has occurred. The cuff should be deflated, the tube withdrawn several centimeters, and breath sounds reassessed.

Disposable end-tidal CO_2 detectors or capnographers can also be used to confirm proper placement. If the endotracheal tube is in the trachea, ventilation produces a positive reading for CO_2. With a capnogram, a plateau waveform is observed. With disposable colorimetric CO_2 detectors, the device changes from purple to yellow in the presence of normal levels of exhaled CO_2.

After tube placement has been confirmed, the tube should be secured in position. Commercially available tube holders (Fig. 14–16) or simple adhesive tape can be used. The face should be cleaned and coated with benzoin before the application of tape.

Intubation of the Difficult Airway

Some patients present special challenges in airway management. These include those with facial or airway burns (with resultant edema), cervical spine injury (head extension contraindicated), and disorders of the temporomandibular joint (with inability to open the mouth). If

---

CRITICAL THINKING CHALLENGES

Case Scenario

For the COPD patient who is awake and alert but in respiratory failure and requiring intubation, nasotracheal intubation can allow elective intubation without use of heavy sedation or paralysis, which could further aggravate the course of the respiratory failure.

To prepare the nose for intubation, a topical vasoconstrictor and anesthetic should be applied. This will minimize bleeding and increase the lumen of the nasal passage. A Magill forceps will be needed to facilitate passage of the tube from the posterior pharynx to the trachea (Fig. 14-15).

Some patients can be nasally intubated without the use of a conventional laryngoscope. Using a fiberoptic laryngoscope inserted into the lumen of the tube, the tube is directed through the nasopharynx into the larynx under direct vision. Blind nasal intubation may be performed by listening through the tube to determine when the tip of the tube is positioned above the glottis (on exhalation) so that the tube can be inserted on inspiration.

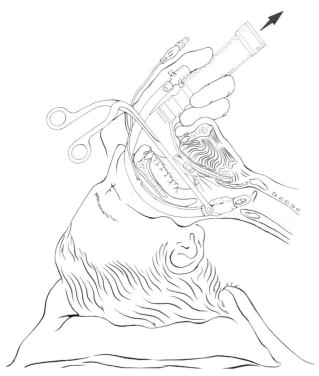

FIGURE 14–15 • Nasotracheal intubation using a McIntosh (curved) blade and a Magill forceps.

intubation is elective, provisions can be made for alternative techniques. Usually, awake intubation, perhaps with a fiberoptic laryngoscope, is performed. In more urgent intubations, it may not be possible to recognize difficult airways before attempted intubation. A list of conditions that can produce a difficult airway is included in Box 14–4.

Clinicians should be familiar with the American Society of Anesthesiologists' algorithm for management of the difficult airway[4] (Fig. 14–17). This algorithm outlines most of the decision-making steps needed to establish an airway in a difficult intubation. Most important, the clinician should call for help immediately if intubation proves difficult and bag-mask ventilation is difficult or impossible. Equipment for cricothyrotomy should be prepared and the anatomic landmarks located. In addition, a fiberoptic laryngoscope should be prepared and an individual trained in its use summoned.

A **cricothyrotomy** permits oxygenation of a patient, but ventilation is usually not feasible with this procedure. The procedure is performed by inserting a large-bore (14- or 16-gauge) needle into the trachea through the cricothyroid membrane. This membrane is located between the thyroid and cricoid cartilages. These are usually located easily because the thyroid cartilage (Adam's apple) is the largest cartilage in the trachea. The membrane is punctured easily and is relatively avascular. Once a needle cricothyrotomy is performed, supplemental oxygen should be delivered and additional attempts to establish a more stable airway continued.

Box • 14–3   PROCEDURE FOR BLIND NASAL INTUBATION

1. Determine distance that the tube should be inserted for placement immediately above the larynx (usually the distance from the tip of the nose to the earlobe).
2. Determine which side of the nasal passage is less obstructed by feeling for best airflow through a naris when the other side is temporarily occluded (with your finger). If the patient is alert, ask him or her to sniff with each naris occluded. Proceed with insertion on side with best airflow.
3. Lubricate airway or nares.
4. Gently insert tip of the tube with the bevel toward the nasal septum, diagonally up and back (to track above the medial turbinate) through the nasopharynx. Then rotate the tube to take advantage of the natural curve of the tube.
5. Insert gently; if obstruction is encountered, try the other side.
6. Insert to predetermined length, assess to ensure that the tip of the tube is above the glottis by placing your ear near the end of the tube and listening for gas flow on exhalation. If you do not hear gas flow on exhalation, the tip of the tube is either too low (in the esophagus) or too high (still in the nasopharynx).
7. With the tip of the tube above the glottis, insert on inspiration. Listen for cough and gas flow on expiration. If you do not hear gas flow on exhalation, withdraw tube to hear gas flow on exhalation, rotate tube one-quarter turn, and reinsert on patient inhalation. Repeat until tube enters trachea.
8. On insertion, inflate cuff, check breath sound, ensure proper position, secure tube, and call for chest film to confirm placement.

Tracheostomy

The patient who requires a long-term artificial airway usually receives a **tracheostomy**. Advantages of tracheostomy include improved patient comfort and reduced laryngeal, pharyngeal, oral, and nasal damage secondary to long-term endotracheal tube placement. Because tracheostomy tubes are much shorter than endotracheal tubes, airway resistance and dead space are less, and work of breathing should decrease. Many patients are able to swallow effectively with a tracheostomy tube in place, so eating and drinking without the use of nasogastric tubes is possible. In addition, management of oral secretions is improved. Many patients are able to speak with tracheostomy tubes, often with the use of adaptive devices such as the Passy-Muir valve.

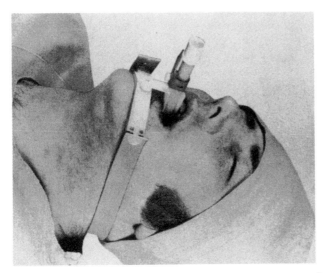

FIGURE 14–16 • Olympic Endolok. (Courtesy of Olympic Medical, Seattle, WA.)

The timing of and indications for tracheostomy vary among institutions. The National Association of Medical Directors of Respiratory Care suggests that tracheostomy is the airway of choice when intubation is required for more than 21 days.[5]

Technique

Tracheostomy has traditionally been performed in the operating room under general anesthesia. During the past decade, however, an alternative technique (**percutaneous dilation tracheostomy**) has become increasingly popular and has become the method of choice in many medical

---

Box • 14–4 CONDITIONS WITH POTENTIAL FOR DIFFICULT INTUBATION

- Limited access to the oropharynx
    Examples:
    Occluding nares
    Protruding teeth
    Large tongue (macroglossia)
    Temporomandibular joint immobility
- Poor visualization of the larynx
    Examples:
    Cervical spine immobility
    Soft tissue mass
    Upper airway hemorrhage
- Limited cross-sectional area of the larynx or trachea
    Examples:
    Laryngeal stenosis
    Tracheal stenosis
- Unexplained and unanticipated difficulties despite normal airway examination

---

centers. A needle is inserted in the first or second tracheal interspace, followed by a guidewire. A series of dilators is then used to enlarge the opening to allow placement of a standard tracheostomy tube. Complication rates with this technique are minimal and essentially the same as with standard, operating room tracheostomy.[6–11] The procedure usually takes less than 15 minutes and costs about half of the typical operating room tracheostomy charge.

CARE OF THE PATIENT WITH AN ARTIFICIAL AIRWAY

Physiologic Effects of Intubation

After establishment of an artificial airway, respiratory care and nursing personnel must be concerned with preventing complications, such as nosocomial pneumonia, and maximizing patient comfort. To plan effective care, an understanding of how endotracheal intubation affects normal physiology is important. Some important changes are as follows:

- The body's normal method of warming and humidifying inspired gas (the nose) is bypassed.
- The glottis is prevented from closing, which impairs the ability to cough, reduces end-expiratory lung volume, prevents swallowing, and prevents speech.
- The endotracheal tube is a foreign body, inducing inflammation. If sufficient pressure is applied to the tissues by the tube, ischemia can result.
- Airway resistance is often increased.
- A portion of the airway (ie, the tube) lacks a mucociliary clearance mechanism.
- The endotracheal tube promotes the development of a viscous biofilm, which promotes bacterial growth and adherence.

Patient care must be directed toward correcting or compensating for these changes as well as toward maintaining the endotracheal tube in place.

Care Techniques

Preventing Nosocomial Pneumonia in the Intubated Patient

Nosocomial pneumonia is a well-known and serious complication of intubation and mechanical ventilation, affecting as many as 25% of ventilated patients.[12]

Early studies on the cause and prevention of nosocomial pneumonia focused on the ventilator, ventilator tubing, and humidifier. Potential sources of infection were identified and systematically eliminated. For example, sterilization of ventilator circuits between patient use became universal. Eventually, disposable circuits became the norm. Use of sterile water in humidifiers was mandated. Control or elimination of ventilator condensate was achieved through use of water taps, and most experts strongly advised against the practice

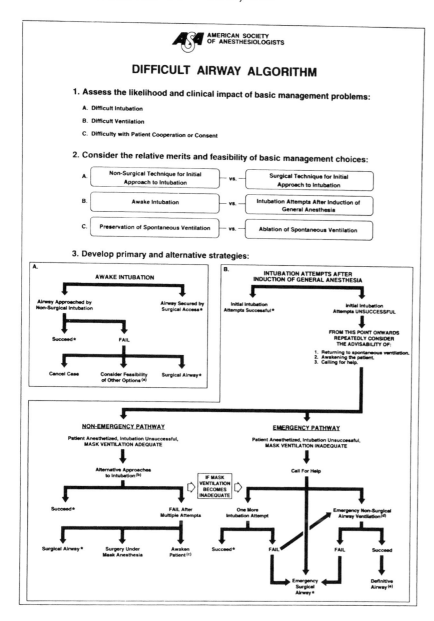

FIGURE 14-17 • Algorithm for management of the difficult airway. (American Society of Anesthesiologists. Practice guidelines for management of the difficult airway. *Anesthesiology.* 1993;78:597.)

of draining condensate back into the humidifier reservoir. Recognizing the importance of the ventilator and associated equipment in the pathogenesis of nosocomial pneumonia, most experts today prefer to use the term **ventilator-associated pneumonia (VAP) when discussing this problem.**

Some practices developed during the infancy of intensive respiratory care have since been found to be detrimental, or at least unnecessary. Studies have shown that daily changing of ventilator circuits does not reduce, and may increase, the risk of VAP.[12,13]

Technologic advances have also reduced some ventilator-associated factors in the development of VAP. The widespread use of metered dose inhalers has resulted in decreased use of nebulizers, with subsequent decreased risk of exposure to contaminated droplets. The use of heat–moisture exchangers and heated wire humidifiers has decreased patient exposure to contaminated condensate.

Despite these advances, VAP continues to be a substantial problem. During the past decade, attention has been focused on several new potential sources of infection in the intubated patient: the endotracheal tube and the feeding tubes and techniques required to nourish the intubated patient.

After a brief period of intubation, a thick, viscous biofilm is formed in the interior of the endotracheal tube, This film probably originates from upper-airway secretions[14] and is an excellent medium for bacterial growth. Bacteria can almost always be recovered from this film and grow unimpeded by the host's natural immune mechanisms or antibiotics, which do not penetrate the tube.[15]

The development of the biofilm is accelerated when there is any imperfection or irregularity in the tube wall. Increased concentrations of bacteria have been observed at

Murphy's eye and along the ridge created by the cuff-inflating tube.[14] Presumably, scratching the tube with a stylet or suction catheter would have the same effect.

The contaminated biofilm in the interior of the endotracheal tube almost certainly accounts for many cases of VAP. Portions of this biofilm can be dislodged with suctioning, normal saline instillation, condensation of moist inspired air, and high ventilator flow rates.[14] The development of endotracheal tubes that resist the formation of this biofilm would be a significant advance. In addition, a reexamination of suctioning techniques, with the aim of reducing the disruption of the biofilm, is needed. The endotracheal tube also contributes to VAP in other ways. First, as an irritating foreign body in the airway, it may increase the production of oral secretions. Next, because

the glottis is prevented from closing, swallowing is impossible. This results in accumulation of a large amount of secretions. These secretions eventually pool just above the cuff of the endotracheal tube in the trachea. Because they originate in the oropharynx, they are contaminated with normal oral flora in addition to other organisms easily acquired in the intensive care unit (ICU) setting.

Despite the use of cuffed endotracheal tubes, as many as 40% of patients routinely aspirate small amounts of secretions into the trachea.[16] Aspiration and subsequent VAP may be reduced by maintaining cuff pressures above 20 cm H_2O. Rello and colleagues[17] found that patients with cuff pressures less than 20 cm H_2O had a 2.5-fold increase in the rate of VAP. Continuous[17,18] or intermittent[12]

CRITICAL THINKING CHALLENGES

Shifting Care Plans

Preventing Unplanned Extubations

Unplanned extubations (UEs) are a common and serious event in the ICU. Formerly, these events were referred to as "accidental extubations." However, this terminology minimizes the responsibility of health care professionals to maintain a secure airway for the patient. The term "unplanned extubation" is also not altogether accurate because many of these events are indeed planned by the patient.

Several studies have been conducted in adult ICUs to determine the incidence, predictors, and consequences of UEs. Comparison between units is often difficult because investigators use different methods to express the rates of UEs. Some studies express the rate as simply the percentage of patients who experience at least one episode of UE. This method, however, fails to take into account the number of days a patient is intubated, and therefore underestimates or overestimates the total time the patient is at risk for a UE. Others have expressed the rates as the number of incidents per 100 days of mechanical ventilation. This method may be especially suitable for units with a large number of long-term patients. Ideally, investigators should report both indices to allow for more meaningful comparisons.

Reported rates vary considerably. Recent reports vary from 3[21] to 12%[22] of patients experiencing UEs. Furthermore, the search for modifiable or correctable risk factors has produced conflicting results. Tominaga and colleagues[23] were unable to demonstrate that the level of sedation affected the rate of UE, whereas Campbell and associates[24] cited poor sedation as a risk factor. Tominaga and colleagues[23] also found that failure to use hand restraints increased UE risk, whereas Campbell and associates[24] and Atkins and colleagues[25] noted that most UEs occurred in patients with hand restraints. Tominaga and colleagues[23] also noted a reduced risk when cloth tape or Velcro securing devices were replaced with waterproof

adhesive tape, whereas McAndrew and Brown[26] drew the opposite conclusion in a similar study.

Nasal intubation decreases the risk of UE.[27] Whether this is due to improved anchoring of the tube or to improved patient comfort is unclear. Up to 85% of UEs are a consequence of intentional action by the patient. Of the remaining cases, risk factors for UE include the use of rotary beds and transporting the patient.[28]

Among the studies reporting a mortality rate from 0% to 4%,[22] reintubation rates varied greatly, from 46%[21] to 78%.[22] Factors predicting a need for urgent reintubation include a high pre-UE FIO_2 and ventilator rate,[29] pre-UE tachycardia, altered mental status, and the presence of multisystem illness.[30]

The rate of UEs can be lowered by a multidisciplinary quality-assurance effort. By routinely monitoring the UE rate and identifying the presence of risk factors (eg, use of sedation, adequate restraints) and appropriate staff training, substantial and lasting reductions in the UE rate can be obtained.[26,27]

Adverse consequences of methods to prevent UE should be considered when planning care of the intubated patient. Heavy sedation and muscle paralysis can obviously reduce the risk of UE but may seriously delay weaning and have a detrimental impact on the patient's quality of life. Likewise, hand restraints impair the patient's ability to communicate and may cause panic and anxiety. The use of tight, circumferential adhesive tape may reduce the risk of UE but may be uncomfortable and damage skin integrity.

Patients' subjective experience of UEs has not been reported. Perhaps patients can inform caregivers about the most distressing aspects of intubation and assist in developing improved measures for patient comfort and communication.

aspiration of secretions from below the glottis may reduce VAP substantially.

Because the endotracheal tube interferes with swallowing, the patient is usually fed by means of orogastric or nasogastric tubes. These tubes may promote reflux of gastric secretions into the oropharynx and ultimately into the lung. Current feeding techniques and methods of stress ulcer prophylaxis may increase the risk that the aspirated fluids are contaminated.

Under normal circumstances, the acidic conditions in the stomach prevent significant bacterial growth. In critically ill patients, however, gastric pH is usually maintained at a higher than normal level. This is in part a result of the common practice of introducing liquid enteral feeding preparations in a continuous fashion. The presence of the formula increases pH and encourages bacterial growth.[12] Further increases in pH, with increased bacterial colonization and VAP, are seen when H_2-blocker therapy, with drugs such as ranitidine, is used to prevent stress ulcers.[19] VAP can be reduced by using sucralfate to prevent gastrointestinal bleeding.[19] This drug forms a protective barrier on the wall of the stomach but does not raise the pH of intragastric contents.

Other measures have been shown to decrease the risk of VAP in the enterally fed intubated patient. These include keeping the head of the bed elevated during and after feedings and removing residual formula after bolus feeding.[12,19,20]

Finally, nasotracheal intubation has been shown to increase the risk of VAP over oral intubation. This is presumably due to the development of sinusitis, which results in contamination of oral secretions and eventually of the lower airway.[12]

Preventing Extubation

Unplanned extubations are a common occurrence in the ICU. In patients who are unable to breathe spontaneously or whose airways are abnormal, the consequences can be disastrous. For less critical patients, unplanned extubations that require reintubation are uncomfortable, expose the patient to additional risks from repeat laryngoscopy and intubation, and may require the use of sedatives and muscle relaxants, which can increase the overall duration of intubation.

Unplanned extubations can be the result of patient action (deliberate self-extubation) or the result of action by ICU personnel. Judicious use of sedatives reduces the rate of extubation but may complicate weaning. Other causes of extubation can be minimized by ensuring proper taping of the tube at all times; minimizing traction on the endotracheal tube from ventilator circuits, resuscitation bags, and other equipment; and paying careful attention to tube stability during patient transport.

Provision of Humidification

Because the nose is bypassed, inspired air must be humidified to prevent inspissation of secretions and nosocomial pneumonia or tube obstruction. Humidification can be provided by heated humidifiers, with or without heated wire ventilator tubing or with the use of heat–moisture exchangers. Heat–moisture exchangers appear to be as effective, but less costly, than heated humidifiers; additionally, they may significantly reduce the risk of nosocomial pneumonia.[31,32] A detailed description of these devices appears elsewhere in this text.

Secretion Removal

Patients with artificial airways almost invariably require assistance with secretion removal by means of intermittent suctioning. The ideal frequency of suctioning has not been rigorously studied; however, suctioning in response to certain clinical signs seems more appropriate than suctioning according to a preset schedule. Some indications for suctioning include the following:

- Coarse or diminished breath sounds
- Unexplained increases in ventilator pressure
- Unexplained deterioration in blood gases

Many patients, especially those with tracheostomies, are capable of coughing secretions into, and occasionally out

CRITICAL THINKING CHALLENGES

Challenging Assumptions

Nasopharyngeal suctioning in nonmonitored patients, typically out of the ICU, is routinely done without benefit of procedures to hyperoxygenate and hyperinflate the patient, which are standard fare on ventilated ICU patients. Nasopharyngeal suctioning has been associated with arrhythmias secondary to vagal stimulation and hypoxemia. To minimize the hazards, and even occasionally eliminate the need to suction, the practitioner should consider instructing the patient to take a deep breath and cough or should provide manual hyperinflation before, during, and after suctioning. Effective coughs are volume dependent, so taking a large breath increases volumes. Manual stimulation of a cough, by pressing two fingers firmly on the trachea above the sternal notch, may also obviate the need for suctioning and is much less uncomfortable for the patient than is being suctioned. In many patients who are unable to cough and clear the airway on demand, providing a deep breath and mechanically stimulating a cough may help them to clear their airway.

of, the tube. Every effort should be made to encourage and assist patients in doing so. Patients with vigorous cough may be at increased risk of accidental extubation and must therefore have securely taped tubes.

Suctioning can cause hypoxemia as well as increase systemic arterial and intracranial pressure. Hypoxemia can be prevented or minimized by oxygenation with 100% oxygen for several minutes before suctioning; the suction catheter should not remain in the airway for more than 15 seconds. Most patients experience less hypoxemia and dyspnea if hyperinflation is performed between suctioning attempts. This can be performed using the ventilator or a manual resuscitation device. In addition, hyperinflation may improve secretion removal. Hyperinflation may be harmful in patients prone to air trapping and in those with elevated intracranial pressure or poor cardiac output.

When secretions are exceptionally thick and tenacious, several milliliters of sterile saline can be instilled, both to loosen secretions and promote coughing. The routine use of saline instillation has recently been challenged, however.

The American Association of Respiratory Care has issued clinical practice guidelines for suctioning of the ventilated patient. They are summarized in Box 14–5.

Suction catheters come in a variety of designs (Fig. 14–18 and Box 14–6); however, all are designed with one or more eyes near the tip. This prevents aspiration and injury to the airway mucosa. In-line catheters, which allow for suctioning without opening the ventilator circuit, are becoming increasingly popular. They permit some maintenance of ventilation and oxygenation during suctioning and are thought to reduce the risk of nosocomial pneumonia. Depending on the frequency of suctioning, they may be more expensive than single-use catheters. Until recently, it was common practice to change the in-line suction catheters every 24 hours. Changing the catheters on an as-needed basis only, however, significantly reduces costs and does not affect the incidence of nosocomial pneumonia.[34]

Suction techniques for the patient without an artificial airway are summarized in Box 14–7.

Management of the Cuff

The inflatable cuff of the endotracheal tube is designed to facilitate positive-pressure ventilation and to prevent aspiration. Low-pressure, high-volume cuffs seal the airway

---

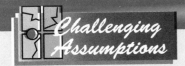

CRITICAL THINKING CHALLENGES

Challenging Assumptions

Normal Saline Instillation During Endotracheal Suction: Research Versus Ritual

Few practices are as universal as routine instillation of normal saline into the endotracheal tube during suctioning. The American Association of Respiratory Care Clinical Practice Guidelines for suctioning the ventilated patient recommends its use to loosen secretions. Many respiratory and critical care textbooks recommend the same.

Proponents of the routine use of normal saline instillation claim that it loosens secretions and promotes a cough. Critics have recently challenged these claims, however, and cast doubt on the overall clinical utility of this procedure. Reviewing the available research, Raymond[33] was unable to find any convincing evidence that routine saline instillation increased recovery of secretions from the lung. No improvement in blood gases could be attributed to this practice, and, in fact, a trend toward worsening oxygenation after saline instillation was noted.

Studies performed to date do not prove that saline instillation is useless or harmful, however. In part, this is because of research with inappropriate end points and inclusion of patients unlikely to benefit from the technique. Potential hazards of sputum retention include acute endotracheal tube obstruction, atelectasis, and nosocomial pneumonia. No studies have addressed the effects of saline instillation on these specific end points.

Patients with minimal sputum production and those who have loose secretions that are easily removed with con-

ventional suctioning would be unlikely to benefit from saline instillation. Yet most studies make no effort to exclude these patients. Future studies should focus on patients known to have excessively thick secretions, such as patients with COPD, pneumonia, or cystic fibrosis.

Even if a group of patients can be identified who have increased sputum removal after saline instillation, this would not justify the procedure. Despite increased secretion removal, the patients could be harmed by introduction of infectious material lining the endotracheal tube into the lower airway, resulting in lower respiratory tract infection.

Many clinical practices become "standards of care" without sufficient scientific evidence. Clinicians feel reluctant to abandon these procedures before the publication of well-controlled studies, however. Untoward events occurring after dropping such standard procedures may be construed as malpractice or negligence. Until the issue of normal saline instillation is resolved, the wisest approach may be to use saline instillation only when evidence of sputum retention is present after suctioning attempts without saline. Having a quality assurance program in place that monitors endotracheal tube occlusion, nosocomial pneumonia, and atelectasis will allow clinicians to monitor potential untoward events associated with any change in practice.

Box • 14–5 AARC CLINICAL PRACTICE GUIDELINE

ENDOTRACHEAL SUCTIONING OF MECHANICALLY VENTILATED ADULTS AND CHILDREN WITH ARTIFICIAL AIRWAYS

Indications: The need to remove accumulated pulmonary secretions as evidenced by one of the following: coarse breath sounds by auscultation or noisy breathing, increased peak inspiratory pressures during volume-controlled mechanical ventilation or decreased tidal volume during pressure-controlled ventilation, patient's inability to generate an effective spontaneous cough, visible secretions in the airway, changes in monitored flow and pressure graphics, suspected aspiration of gastric or upper airway secretions, clinically apparent increased work of breathing, deterioration of arterial blood gas values, radiologic changes consistent with retention of pulmonary secretions, the need to obtain a sputum specimen to rule out or identify pneumonia or other pulmonary infection or for sputum cytology, the need to maintain the patency and integrity of the artificial airway, the need to simulate a cough in patients unable to cough effectively secondary to changes in mental status or the influence of medication, presence of pulmonary atelectasis or consolidation presumed to be associated with secretion retention.

Contraindications: Endotracheal suctioning is a necessary procedure for patients with artificial airways. Most contraindications are relative to the patient's risk of developing adverse reactions or worsening clinical condition as a result of the procedure. When indicated, there is no absolute contraindication to endotracheal suctioning because the decision to abstain from suctioning to avoid a possible adverse reaction may, in fact, be lethal.

Assessment of Need: Qualified personnel should assess the need for endotracheal suctioning as a routine part of a patient or ventilator system check.

Assessment of Outcome: Improvement in breath sounds, decreased peak inspiratory pressure (Paw) with narrowing of inspiratory plateau pressure (PIP); decreased airway resistance or increased dynamic compliance; increased tidal volume delivery during pressure-limited ventilation, improvement in arterial blood gas values or saturation as reflected by pulse oximetry (SpO_2), removal of pulmonary secretions.

Monitoring: The following should be monitored before, during, and after the procedure: breath sounds, skin color, pulse oximeter (if available), respiratory rate and pattern, hemodynamic parameters, pulse rate, blood pressure (if indicated and available), ECG (if indicated and available), sputum characteristics (color, volume, consistency, odor), cough effort, intracranial pressure (if indicated and available), ventilator parameters (peak inspiratory pressure and plateau pressure, tidal volume), ventilator waveform graphics (if available), arterial blood gases (if indicated and available).

American Association of Respiratory Care. Clinical practice guideline: Endotracheal suctioning of mechanically ventilated adults and children with artificial airways. *Respir Care* 1993;38:500.

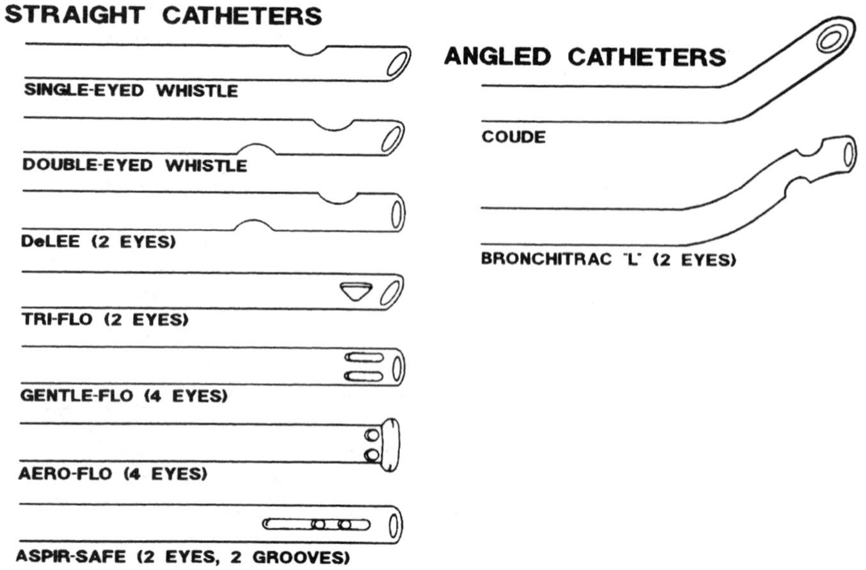

STRAIGHT CATHETERS

SINGLE-EYED WHISTLE

DOUBLE-EYED WHISTLE

DeLEE (2 EYES)

TRI-FLO (2 EYES)

GENTLE-FLO (4 EYES)

AERO-FLO (4 EYES)

ASPIR-SAFE (2 EYES, 2 GROOVES)

ANGLED CATHETERS

COUDE

BRONCHITRAC "L" (2 EYES)

FIGURE 14–18 • Straight-tip and curved-tip suction catheter designs.

Box • 14–6   SUCTIONING OF THE NONINTUBATED PATIENT

Patients without artificial airways often need assistance in removal of bronchial secretions. These may be recently extubated patients, postoperative patients whose cough ability is reduced by pain, or patients whose prognosis makes intubation inadvisable. Almost always, nasotracheal suction is safer and more comfortable than oropharyngeal suctioning.

The procedure should be explained to the patient. A lubricated catheter is introduced into the external naris and advanced along the floor of the nasopharynx. As the catheter advances into the posterior pharynx, breath sounds may be heard through the proximal opening of the catheter. Use a procedure similar to that used for blind insertion of a nasal endotracheal tube. Ask the patient to inhale slowly, and advance the catheter. This improves the chance of passing the catheter into the trachea rather than the esophagus. On entering the trachea, a cough usually is provoked. Apply suction, and gently remove the catheter into the oropharynx. In some cases, patient tolerance and comfort demand that the catheter

be removed completely after each pass into the trachea. It may be preferable, however, to leave the catheter in the nasopharynx (without suction applied) while the patient recovers and is reoxygenated. This spares the patient the trauma of repeated catheter insertion into the external nares. Repeat the above-mentioned procedure until breath sounds are satisfactorily improved.

Patients who require repeated nasotracheal suction may benefit from placement of a nasal airway. This reduces the trauma of repeated insertion.

Nasotracheal suction is less effective in the uncooperative patient. Many patients, however, respond to nasopharyngeal insertion of the catheter with a cough or sneeze, which effectively removes secretions without directly entering the trachea.

Topical anesthetics and decongestants are rarely needed for occasional nasotracheal suctioning, as is the case with intubation. When patient discomfort, bleeding, or nasal edema prevents effective suctioning, however, these options should be discussed with the patient's physician.

---

effectively, with only minor inflammation or trauma to the tracheal mucosa. In contrast, high-pressure, low-volume cuffs are associated with risk of severe tracheal ulceration and stenosis.

The pressure inside the cuff is measured easily (Box 14–8). A device that inflates the cuff and measures intracuff pressure is shown in Figure 14–19. Intracuff pressure should be maintained below 25 cm H_2O pressure to avoid disruption of perfusion of the mucosa. Prolonged

ischemia of the mucosa from cuff pressure is associated with stenosis and necrosis of the trachea.

Intracuff pressures may not equate to tracheal wall pressures, especially when the endotracheal tube is too small for the airway. This is a common occurrence with intubationists who think it is easier to hit the right hole with a smaller tube. Even 25 mmHg may be too much pressure in a hypotensive patient. An alternative to pressure monitoring is use of minimal occluding pressure. This technique uses empiric observation of the amount of air required in the cuff to seal the airway or to allow a small leak with peak inspiratory flow.

Facilitating Communication

Patients with oral or nasal endotracheal tubes obviously cannot speak, and alternate means of communication for alert patients should be available. Patients who have sufficient strength and coordination to write may find this the most convenient and practical method of communication. Others may prefer the use of a board with pictures or phrases to which the patient can point. For example, phrases such as "I am in pain" or "I cannot breath" can be written in large clear letters. When necessary, the patient points to the phrase or picture that best communicates his or her current needs.

Patients with tracheostomies can sometimes exhale a portion of their tidal volume around, rather than through, the tracheostomy tube. This permits some measure of speech.

A more reliable method is to use a commercially available tracheostomy speaking valve. These devices are one-

CRITICAL THINKING CHALLENGES

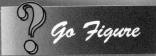
Go Figure

When to Use Closed-Suction Catheters

Practices at the bedside affect the costs of providing care. Such is the case with use of closed-suction catheters compared with individual catheters. Closed-suction catheters cost $8.50 each, whereas a single-use catheter with gloves costs $1.50.

How many times would a patient be suctioned before the closed-suction catheter becomes more cost-effective?

If a closed suction catheter could be used for 2 days between changes, what frequency of suctioning makes the closed-suction catheter a cost-effective option?

Box • 14–7 PROCEDURE FOR CLOSED-SUCTION AND STANDARD-SUCTION CATHETERS

USING A CLOSED-SUCTION CATHETER

1. Check suction regulator setting by occluding tubing (peak pressure between 80 and 120 mmHg for adults), and adjust. Explain procedure to patient.
2. Turn vent to allow suction to be applied to catheter and finger port.
3. Gently insert catheter into airway, as far as it will go.
4. Withdraw 1 to 2 cm, apply suction through finger port. Do not withdraw catheter while applying suction.
5. Take finger off port, withdraw catheter a few centimeters, and reapply suction. Repeat until catheter is removed from airway. Catheter should be in airway less than 15 seconds.
6. Withdraw catheter into sleeve, lavage catheter tip with saline while applying suction.
7. Turn off vent to suction regulator

USING A STANDARD-SUCTION CATHETER

1. Determine need to suction patient.
2. Wash hands.
3. Turn on regulator, check to ensure proper pressure (80 to 120 mmHg) with tubing occluded.
4. Explain procedure to patient.
5. Manually hyperinflate and oxygenate before procedure.
6. Don gloves, attach catheter to suction tubing, keeping suction catheter from touching any contaminated surfaces.
7. Gently insert catheter into airway as far as it will go, then withdraw 1 to 2 cm.
8. Apply suction for short periods of time, then withdraw catheter a few centimeters, and reapply suction. Repeat as needed, not to exceed a total of 15 seconds in the lower airway.
9. Remove catheter from airway.
10. Hyperinflate and oxygenate patient, resume previous therapy.
11. Flush suction tubing with water to clear.
12. Dispose of gloves and catheter.
13. Wash hands.

Box • 14–8 PROCEDURE FOR MINIMAL OCCLUSION AND MINIMAL LEAK

1. Inflate cuff.
2. Listen for air leakage around the cuff at the trachea as you mechanically ventilate patient (at setting they are currently on).
3. Withdraw air from cuff so that you just hear a small leak of air at the peak of inspiration (minimal leak).
4. Add just enough air so that you do not hear a leak (minimal occluding pressure).
5. Measure and record cuff pressure.

Note: Do not routinely deflate and inflate cuff totally to ascertain cuff volume. This practice allows secretions trapped above the cuff to lavage the lung, increasing the risk of infection.

way valves that are connected to the tracheostomy tube opening. The device opens during inspiration but closes during expiration, forcing exhalation to occur around the tube and past the vocal cords. Obviously, the tracheostomy tube cuff must remain deflated during use. Examples of this type of device are the Passy-Muir valve and the Olympic Trach-Talk (Fig. 14–20).

Because resistance to expiratory airflow may be greater when speaking valves are used, some patients may experience hyperinflation during their use. Careful monitoring of blood gases and patient comfort during an initial trial of the device is therefore essential.

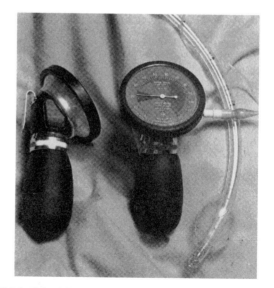

FIGURE 14–19 • Posey cuff pressure measurement system.

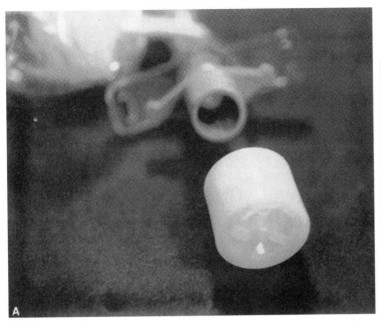
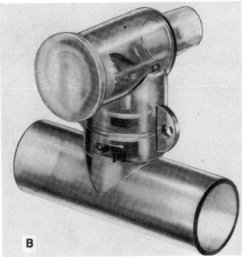

FIGURE 14–20 • Valves to facilitate speech with tracheostomy tubes. (A) Passy-Muir valve. (B) An Olympic Trach-Talk valve.

Additional benefits of tracheostomy speaking valves include a reduced risk of aspiration during feeding[35] and a reduction in the volume of secretions.[36]

Removal of the Artificial Airway

If the patient's airway was previously normal, extubation after return of adequate ventilatory function is usually uneventful. Just before removal of the tube, the oronasopharynx should be suctioned and the patency of the nares and oral airway assessed. The tube should be untapped and the cuff deflated. A large breath from a manual resuscitator is given, and the endotracheal tube is removed as the patient exhales. Humidified oxygen should be provided and the patient's respiratory status continuously assessed.

Some patients suffer from glottic edema, evidenced by respiratory distress and stridor developing shortly after extubation. This complication occurs most commonly in children but may occasionally be seen in adults as well. Patients who have no air leak around the endotracheal tube at 30 cm H_2O of pressure at the airway are at increased risk of postextubation stridor.[37]

A more common complication in the immediate postextubation period is laryngeal dysfunction. As a result of long-term disuse, edema, and inflammation, the glottis may not close properly during coughing and swallowing. Aspiration may occur in as many one third of patients during the first 24 hours after extubation,[37] As a result, patients are often kept NPO for 8 to 24 hours after extubation. Thereafter, fluids can be given under careful observation.

Removal of a tracheostomy tube is usually a more complicated process. First, the original reason for performing the tracheostomy (usually access to long-term mechanical ventilation) should be resolved. Progressively smaller tubes are used to enable the patient to breathe partially through the tube and partially through the natural airway. The smaller-sized tubes are intermittently capped to require the patient to breathe through the natural airway. This procedure allows the patient to reestablish laryngeal coordination gradually, preventing, for example, simultaneous inspiration and swallowing, which can result in aspiration when the tube is removed.

The use of a fenestrated tube is often helpful in decannulating the chronically intubated patient. Such a tube is shown in Figure 14–21. With the inner cannula removed and the external opening occluded, the patient can breathe through the natural airway. If the patient becomes fatigued or needs to return to positive-pressure ventilation temporarily, the inner cannula can be reinserted, closing the fenestration.

The tracheostomized patient has the ability to breathe and swallow simultaneously. Even with a properly inflated cuff, this may lead to microaspiration. After decannulation, some patients have difficulty reestablishing laryngeal coordination and may continue to inspire during swallowing, resulting in significant aspiration. Oral feedings should be monitored closely during the immediate decannulation period. Some patients may require the assistance of a speech therapist to retrain the larynx.

If it not certain that the patient will be able to maintain the airway after decannulation, the tracheal stoma can be kept open for a period of time with the use of tracheal "but-

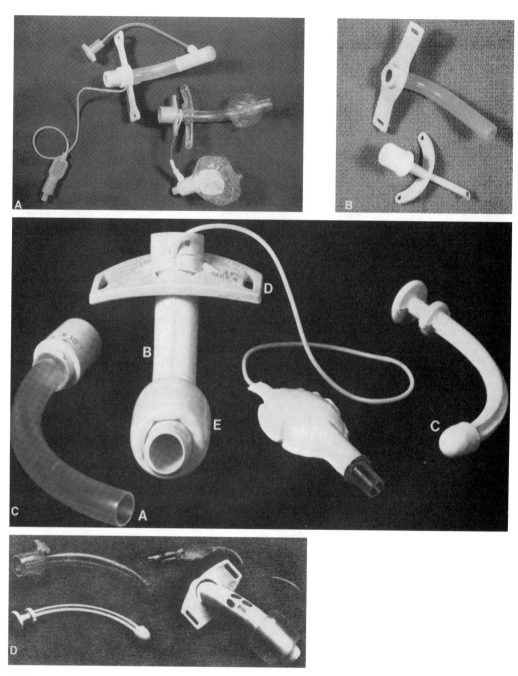

FIGURE 14-21 • Tracheostomy tubes. (*A*) Standard disposable cuffed tracheostomy tube. (*B*) Adult and pediatric uncuffed tracheostomy tubes. (*C*) Tracheostomy tube with removable inner cannula (*left*) and obdurator (*right*). (*D*) Fenestrated tracheostomy tube with inner cannula and obturator.

tons" that maintain the stoma without the presence of a tracheostomy tube.

References

1. Hess D, Goff G. The effects of two-handed versus one-handed ventilation on volumes delivered during bag-mask ventilation at various resistance and compliances. *Respir Care*. 1987;32:1025–1028.

2. Hess D, Goff G, Johnson K. The effect of hand size, resuscitator brand, and the use of two hands on volumes delivered during adult bag-valve ventilation. *Respir Care*. 1989;34:805–810.

3. Roberts JR, Spadafora M, Cone DC. Proper depth placement of oral endotracheal tubes in adults prior to radiographic confirmation. *Acad Emerg Med*. 1995;2:20–24.

4. American Society of Anesthesiologists. Practice guidelines for management of the difficult airway. *Anesthesiology*. 1993:78:597.

5. Plummer AL, Gracey DR. Consensus conference on artificial airways in patients receiving mechanical ventilation. *Chest*. 1989;96:178.

6. Graham JS, Mulloy RH, Sutherland FR, Rose S. Percutaneous versus open tracheostomy: A retrospective cohort outcome study. *J Trauma*. 1996;41:245–248.
7. Friedman Y, Mayer AD. Bedside percutaneous tracheostomy in critically ill patients. *Chest*. 1993;104:535.
8. Crofts SL, Alzeer A, McGuire GP, et al. A comparison of percutaneous and operative tracheostomies in intensive care patients. *Can J Anaesth*. 1995;42:775–779.
9. Cobean R, Beals M, Moss C, Bredenberg CE. Percutaneous dilatational tracheostomy: A safe, cost-effective bedside procedure. *Arch Surg*. 1996;131:265–271.
10. van Heurn LW, van Geffen GJ, Brink PR. Clinical experience with percutaneous dilatational tracheostomy: Report of 150 cases. *Eur J Surg*. 1996;162:531–535.
11. Hill BB, Zweng TN, Maley RH, et al. Percutaneous dilational tracheostomy: Report of 356 cases. *J Trauma*. 1996;41:238–243.
12. Craven DE, Steger KA. Nosocomial pneumonia in mechanically ventilated adult patients: Epidemiology and prevention in 1996. *Semin Respir Infect*. 1996;11:32–53.
13. Craven DE, Kunches LM, Kilinski V, et al. Risk factors for pneumonia and fatality in patients receiving continuous mechanical ventilation. *Am Rev Respir Dis*. 1986;133:792–796.
14. Koerner RJ. Contribution of endotracheal tubes to the pathogenesis of ventilator-associated pneumonia. *J Hosp Infect*. 1997;35:83–89.
15. Cassiere HA, Niederman MS. New etiopathogenic concepts of ventilator-associated pneumonia. *Semin Respir Infect*. 1996;11:13–23.
16. Stauffer JL. Complications of translaryngeal intubation. In: Tobin MJ, ed. *Principles and Practice of Mechanical Ventilation*. New York: McGraw-Hill; 19XX.
17. Rello J, Sonora R, Jubert P, et al. Pneumonia in intubated patients: Role of respiratory airway care. *Am J Respir Crit Care Med*. 1996;154(1):111–115.
18. Valles J, Artigas A, Rello J, et al. Continuous aspiration of subglottic secretions in preventing ventilator-associated pneumonia. *Ann Intern Med*. 1995;122:179–186.
19. Cook D. Prevention of stress ulcers and ventilator associated pneumonia: Examining the evidence. *Semin Respir Crit Care Med*. 1997;18:91–95.
20. Thompson R. Prevention of nosocomial pneumonia. *Med Clin North Am*. 1994;78:1185–1198.
21. Tindol GA, Di Benedetto RJ, Kosciuk L. Unplanned extubations. *Chest*. 1994;105:1804–1807.
22. Vassal T, Anh NG, Gabillet JM, et al. Prospective evaluation of self-extubations in a medical intensive care unit. *Intensive Care Med*. 1993;19:340–342.
23. Tominaga GT, Rudzwick H, Scannell G, Waxman K. Decreasing unplanned extubations in the surgical intensive care unit. *Am J Surg*. 1995;170:586–589.
24. Campbell R, Goldsberry DT, Michaela D, Hurst JM. Incidence, contributing factors, and outcomes of unplanned extubations in the intensive care unit. *Respir Care*. 1994;39:1111.
25. Atkins PM, Mion LC, Mendelson W, et al. Characteristics and outcomes of patients who self-extubate from ventilatory support: A case-control study. *Chest*. 19XX;112:1317–1323.
26. McAndrew J, Brown P. Reduction in self-extubation using comfit tracheal tube holder. *Respir Care*. 1994;39:1110.
27. Chiang AA, Lee KC, Lee JC, Wei CH. Effectiveness of a continuous quality improvement program aiming to reduce unplanned extubation: A prospective study. *Intensive Care Med*. 1996;22:1269–1271.
28. Christie JM, Dethlefsen M, Cane RD. Unplanned endotracheal extubation in the intensive care unit. *J Clin Anesth*. 1996;8:289–293.
29. Whelan J, Simpson SQ, Levy H. Unplanned extubation: Predictors of successful termination of mechanical ventilatory support. *Chest*. 1994;105:1808–1812.
30. Listello D, Sessler CN. Unplanned extubation: Clinical predictors for reintubation. *Chest*. 1994;105:1496–1503.
31. Kirton OC, DeHaven B, Morgan J, et al. A prospective, randomized comparison of an in-line heat moisture exchange filter and heated wire humidifiers rates of ventilator-associated early-onset (community-acquired) or late-onset (hospital-acquired) pneumonia and incidence of endotracheal tube occlusion. *Chest*. 1997;112:1055–1059.
32. Hurni JM, Feihl F, Lazor R, et al. Safety of combined heat and moisture exchanger filters in long-term mechanical ventilation. *Chest*. 1997;111:686–691.
33. Raymond SJ. Normal saline instillation before suctioning: Helpful or harmful? A review of the literature. *Am J Crit Care*. 1995;4:267–271.
34. Kollef MH, Prentice D, Shapiro SD, et al. Mechanical ventilation with or without daily changes of in-line suction catheters. *Am J Respir Crit Care Med*. 1997;156:466–472.
35. Dettelbach MA, Gross RD, Mahlmann J, Eibling DE. Effect of the Passy-Muir valve on aspiration in patients with tracheostomy. *Head Neck*. 1995;17:297–302.
36. Lichtman SW, Birnbaum IL, Sanfilippo MR, et al. Effect of a tracheostomy speaking valve on secretions, arterial oxygenation, and olfaction: A quantitative evaluation. *J Speech Hear Res*. 1995;38:549–555.
37. McCulloch TM, Bishop MJ. Complications of translaryngeal intubation. *Clin Chest Med*. 1991;12:507–521.

Mechanical Ventilation

15

Charles Vanderwarf

Key Terms

assist-control mode (AC)
auto–positive end-
  expiratory pressure (auto-
  PEEP)
external negative-pressure
  ventilation (ENVP)
mechanical ventilation
mode of ventilation
noninvasive positive-
  pressure ventilation
  (NPPV)
peak pressure
plateau pressure
pressure-support mode (PS)
rapid shallow breathing
  index (RSBI)
synchronized intermittent
  mandatory ventilation
  (SIMV)

Objectives

- Define mechanical ventilation, and discuss common clinical applications.

- Identify clinical objectives and indications for mechanical ventilation.

- List complications and hazards of mechanical ventilation.

- Describe the common modes of ventilation, and discuss their relative merits for different patient populations.

- Calculate compressible volume in a ventilator circuit.

- Describe the steps of mechanical ventilation.

- Evaluate strategies to adjust the ventilator for changes in $PaCO_2$, PaO_2, patient dysynchrony, and hemodynamic status.

- List criteria for readiness to wean.

- Identify two strength factors and endurance factors used to predict weaning success.

- Describe three strategies for weaning patients from controlled mechanical ventilation, and discuss the relative merits for each.

Part I
Overview of Modes

The fundamental importance of ventilation in the maintenance of life has been acknowledged for centuries. Biblical psalms describe how the withholding of breath ultimately results in death. Breathing originally was thought to cool the heart, which produced and circulated the vital "heat" of life. It was not until the Renaissance that Servetus proposed that air and blood somehow mixed in the lungs to cleanse the blood of waste products, a concept that ultimately resulted in his being burned at the stake for heresy. Vesalius, a contemporary of Servetus, was the first to describe the concept of artificial ventilation, which could be used to keep animals alive during dissection. He recommended tying a hollow reed into an opening in the trachea and blowing into it intermittently, so that the "motion of the heart and the arteries does not stop."[1] Vesalius had to take a trip to the Holy Land to avoid his turn at the stake; he died during the pilgrimage. The practice of artificial ventilation was limited to animals until the mid-1700s, when it was adapted in the form of mouth-to-mouth resuscitation as a treatment for drowning victims.[2] The technique was endorsed by the Paris Academy of Science, and over the years, many societies, including the Royal Humane Society in England, began to promote the practice. During the next 50 years, mechanical adjuncts were developed to assist in artificial ventilation, including devices to intubate the trachea and bellows compressors to provide positive-pressure breaths. In the early 1800s, however, experiments demonstrating pneumothorax as a complication of bellows ventilation resulted in abandonment of the technique of positive-pressure ventilation in humans for the next 100 years. As an alternative, negative-pressure ventilation techniques were investigated, but these were not widely used in patient care until the Drinker-Shaw iron lung was developed in the early 1920s. This was the classic cylindrically shaped iron lung, in which the patient's head protruded from a rubber collar at one end of the cylinder. A simplified version of the lung was built by Emerson in the 1930s and was used successfully well into the 1950s to treat polio patients with respiratory paralysis.[3] In the operating room, however, surgeons and anesthesiologists had rediscovered the benefits of positive-pressure ventilation just before the turn of the century. Trendelenburg added a cuff to an endotracheal tube in 1869, and the practice of positive-pressure ventilation grew in popularity. Surgeons appreciated the technique because it allowed them to operate in the thorax without creating a fatal pneumothorax. Anesthesiologists found this sealed tube an ideal way to deliver anesthetic gases, and the modern reintroduction of positive-pressure ventilation had begun.

MECHANICAL VENTILATION: WHY WE DO IT

Definition and Objectives

Mechanical ventilation may be defined as a life-support system designed to replace or support normal ventilatory function. The basic goals of instituting mechanical ventilation are to restore gas exchange and to correct work of breathing to normal levels. Common clinical objectives of mechanical ventilation are listed in Box 15–1. It is important to remember that mechanical ventilation is not in itself therapeutic; it *supports* the patient until the underlying condition can be corrected. The positive pressure can reinflate atelectatic or consolidated areas, improving the matching of ventilation to perfusion, and the elevated FIO_2 can improve oxygenation of poorly ventilated units. Positive-pressure breaths from the machine can also supplement or replace the inadequate efforts of the patient so that the extra oxygen consumed by the respiratory muscles can be "spent" by needier organs (eg, the brain or the heart). The "vent" can also be used to create abnormal states, which may be beneficial in some situations. For example, a patient with a dangerously elevated intracranial pressure can be hyperventilated to cause cerebral vasoconstriction, decreasing pressure in the skull and improving perfusion of the brain. Positive pressure can also be applied to stabilize the chest wall when severe flail chest prevents normal breathing.

Indications

The overriding indication for mechanical ventilation is respiratory failure or the clinical judgment that a patient is about to experience respiratory failure. Conditions that can

> **Box • 15–1 CLINICAL OBJECTIVES OF MECHANICAL VENTILATION**
>
> - Reverse hypoxemia
> - Reverse acute respiratory acidosis
> - Relieve respiratory distress
> - Prevent or reverse atelectasis
> - Reverse ventilatory muscle fatigue
> - Permit sedation or neuromuscular blockade
> - Decrease systemic or myocardial oxygen consumption
> - Reduce intracranial pressure
> - Stabilize the chest wall

lead to respiratory failure include refractory hypoxemia, acute hypercapnia, or a combination of both conditions. The most extreme example is respiratory arrest, during which gas exchange ceases and work of breathing drops to zero. Less dramatic examples are severe pneumonia in a patient who is hypoxic even on high concentrations of supplemental oxygen and exacerbation of chronic obstructive pulmonary disease (COPD) in a patient whose $PaCO_2$ rises suddenly, creating acidosis. Box 15–2 defines and lists the common causes of respiratory failure.

Patients who require mechanical support usually have obvious symptoms. If they are still able to speak, they usually tell you they need help. When they tell you that they feel like they are about to die, believe them. A comprehensive list of symptoms of respiratory failure is given in Figure 15–1. In general, symptoms of impending respiratory failure revolve around the body's attempts to either increase oxygenation or reduce work of breathing to prevent failure of the respiratory muscles. Hypoxemia can be improved somewhat by decreasing $PaCO_2$, and the initial response to hypoxemia is usually tachypnea. Tachypnea is also the initial response to an increased workload that threatens to fatigue the respiratory muscles. Rapid shallow breathing, although less effective at gas exchange, takes less energy to maintain than does a normal respiratory pattern. If the diaphragm begins to tire, a switch-over to the accessory muscles may occur, and you will see paradoxical movement of the abdomen during inspiration. Instead of the normal outward excursion of the abdomen during inspiration (as the abdominal contents are pushed out by the downward movement of the diaphragm), the abdomen moves inward. This change in pattern is due to negative pressure being developed in the chest by the accessory muscles, which pull up the resting diaphragm and the abdominal contents below. Another sign of impending failure is decreasing mental responsiveness. Acute increases in carbon dioxide can have sedative-like effects, but like other sedatives, if the patient is accustomed to an elevated carbon dioxide level, the sedative-like effect is not apparent. An end-stage COPD patient may have a chronic $PaCO_2$ of 80 mmHg and be perfectly alert, whereas an asthmatic patient whose $PaCO_2$ rises from 40 to 80 mmHg may become obtunded.

Hazards and Complications

The decision to begin mechanical ventilation is never easy. Seventy-five percent of patients who begin mechanical support need it for more than 48 hours.[4] If a patient is on mechanical ventilation for longer than 48 hours, the likelihood of being discharged alive from the hospital can be dismal. Statistically, chances of survival are directly related to the primary diagnosis, the patient's age, and the number of other organ systems in failure. Asthmatic patients have been reported to have a 90% or higher rate of survival to discharge, whereas a cancer patient's chances

---

Box • 15–2   COMMON CAUSES OF RESPIRATORY FAILURE

1. Hypoxic
   A. PaO_2 <60 mmHg or SpO_2 <90% on >50% FIO_2
   B. Shunt (eg, from atelectasis, pulmonary edema, pneumonia, pulmonary embolism)
   C. $\dot{V}/\dot{Q}$ mismatch or venous admixture (eg, asthma, COPD)
   D. Hypoventilation and high $PaCO_2$ (respiratory arrest, acute respiratory failure)
   E. Low FIO_2, low barometric pressure, and toxins (eg, fire, altitude, carbon monoxide poisoning)
   F. Inadequate diffusion equilibrium (eg, anemia, high cardiac output; typically a contributing factor rather than primary cause)
2. Hypercapnic ($PaCO_2$ >55 with acidosis or sudden rise in $PaCO_2$ from baseline with acidosis)
   A. Work capacity overwhelmed by increased workload from:
      i. Low compliance (eg, ARDS, chest burns, pleural effusion, obesity, pneumonia)
      ii. High resistance (eg, asthma, COPD, airway tumor or obstruction)
   B. Increased VCO_2 in the presence of limited capacity for work (eg, diet, COPD)
   C. Increased dead space requiring increased $\dot{V}E$ in the presence of limited capacity for work
   D. Work capacity decreased
      i. Reduced central drive (eg, drug overdose, central hypoventilation syndrome)
      ii. Neuromuscular disease (eg, myasthenia gravis, Guillain-Barré syndrome)
      iii. Mechanical disadvantage (eg, hyperinflation, auto-PEEP)
      iv. Atrophy (eg, malnutrition, long-term paralysis, corticosteroids)
      v. Metabolic disturbances (eg, acidosis, decreased O_2 delivery)
      vi. Exhaustion

---

of surviving can drop to less than 10%. Being older than 65 years decreases the patient's chance of survival to discharge to less than 50%.

Part of the reason for the poor outcomes in many ventilated patients can be directly related to the hazards that are associated with the process of mechanical ventilation (Box 15–3), especially positive pressure. Positive pressure does not belong in the chest, unless the patient is coughing. Outside of the occasional cough, however, the physiology inside the chest relies on negative pressure being created during breathing. Normal spontaneous ventilation depends on the respiratory muscles, primarily the diaphragm, to create a negative pressure in the thoracic cage. Gas transfer

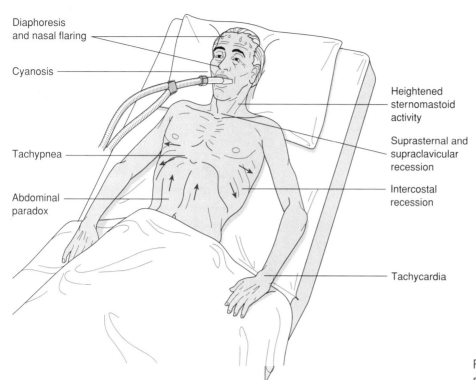

Diaphoresis
and nasal flaring

Cyanosis

Tachypnea

Abdominal
paradox

Heightened
sternomastoid
activity

Suprasternal and
supraclavicular
recession

Intercostal
recession

Tachycardia

FIGURE 15–1 • Signs and symptoms of respiratory failure.

Box • 15–3 COMPLICATIONS AND HAZARDS OF MECHANICAL VENTILATION

A. Barotrauma
B. Volutrauma
C. Hemodynamic effects
   1. Decreased CO
      a. Decreased venous return
      b. Increased pulmonary vascular resistance
D. Effects on ventilation–perfusion relationships
E. Effects on regional blood flow
   1. Kidney: PEEP and decreased urine output
   2. Brain: decreased cerebral perfusion pressure
F. Nosocomial pneumonia
G. Oxygen toxicity
H. Mechanical problems with the ventilator
   1. Increased loads
 I. Patient–ventilator synchrony problems
 J. Respiratory muscle fatigue and deconditioning
K. Intrinsic PEEP

into the chest is accomplished as air flows from a higher ambient pressure outside the chest toward the lower pressures at the alveolar space. Critical-care ventilators reverse this process by developing a positive ambient pressure in the airways to push gas down into the alveolar space. By inverting the normal process of ventilation, a series of complications can occur.

Changing the mean pressure in the thorax from slightly negative to positive can have an impact on blood flow into the chest and its distribution throughout the lungs. The extent of this disturbance is directly related to the amount of positive pressure applied and the fluid balance of the patient.

Ordinarily, the development of negative pressure in the chest during inspiration assists with venous return to the heart. As the pressure in the chest drops, it pulls in extra blood from the venous pool outside the chest. If positive pressure is applied during inspiration, this bonus flow is suspended. As positive pressure rises, blood flow into the thorax is obstructed; if it rises enough, so little blood returns to the heart that cardiac output decreases. This effect is exaggerated by dehydration, during which the impact on cardiac output occurs at respectively lower intrathoracic pressures.

Even if cardiac output is not decreased significantly by the positive pressure in the thorax, other organs can be negatively affected. For example, in a head injury, in which pressure has built up in the skull from edema, high mean airway pressures can decrease venous emptying into the chest, forcing the blood to back up in the skull and exacerbating the intracranial pressure problems. Changes in flow into the chest can also "trick" the body into perceiving it has too little fluid. To correct the perceived deficit, output of the hormone that promotes diuresis is reduced, and more fluid is retained.

Once blood finally enters the chest, its path through the lung is altered by positive-pressure ventilation. As the most compliant and well-ventilated areas of the lung pressurize, their associated capillary beds are compressed, reducing blood flow to that area. With enough pressure, blood flow is cut off entirely, turning the area into dead space, rerouting the blood to less well-ventilated spaces, and increasing shunt and $\dot{V}/\dot{Q}$ mismatch.

Positive pressure can also have severely damaging effects on the lung parenchyma. Present a high enough pressure to an alveolar space, and it will rupture. Gas then leaks into the pleural space and collapses the lung. Deliver enough pressure to distend the alveolus past its elastic limit but not to rupture it, and it will also be injured. Animals treated this way experimentally develop symptoms of severe lung injury (eg, acute respiratory distress syndrome [ARDS]) after less than 2 hours of hyperinflating ventilation.[5] In addition, the pressures required to induce injury are not all that high. It takes a mere 35 cm H_2O to inflate a normal lung (in a normal chest wall) to its elastic limit.[6] A ventilator can exceed that value easily if allowed. In fact, the ability to generate very high pressures was a selling point that manufacturers and users bragged about!

Another pressure-related complication of mechanical ventilation is gas trapping. If the ventilator is set at a high rate with a short expiratory time, the lung cannot empty completely before the next breath is delivered. This is easily detected because the circuit pressure does not fall to its expected level and can be corrected by decreasing the rate, increasing the expiratory time, or both. A more insidious version of gas trapping occurs in patients with COPD, asthma, or any disease that results in edema of the airways (eg, smoke inhalation, ARDS). Although the ventilator is successful at pushing the gas past the obstructed airways into the lung, the elastic recoil of the lung is not so successful at getting it all back out. This form of gas trapping is known as **auto–positive end-expiratory pressure** (auto-PEEP; also known as *intrinsic* or *occult* PEEP).[7] With auto-PEEP, the circuit pressure drops to the set level, but the alveolar pressures remain elevated because of the gas trapped behind the obstructed airways. This pressurized gas acts like, and has the same complications as, set PEEP. High enough auto-PEEP can reduce blood flow into the chest to insignificant levels, decreasing cardiac output to almost zero. A sure sign of severe auto-PEEP is seeing a patient's blood pressure decrease after being connected to the ventilator. An easy way to detect this is to disconnect the patient

and see if the blood pressure returns. Auto-PEEP can be measured accurately if the expiratory and inspiratory limbs are occluded at the end of expiration so that the pressure in the lung can equilibrate with the circuit, where it can be measured[8] (Fig. 15–2). Many machines have an automatic way to perform this maneuver. Manually, it can be performed by calculating the expiratory time, then turning the rate to zero after the delivery of a mechanical breath, waiting for the expiratory time to elapse, and then occluding the expiratory limb. If auto-PEEP is present, it will register within a few seconds. Your ability to measure auto-PEEP will depend on the patient's cooperation. If the patient makes respiratory efforts during the measurement, you will not be able to assess auto-PEEP accurately.

Lung injury can also result from high concentrations of oxygen that may be required to reverse hypoxemia. A lung ventilated with an FIO_2 of 100% will begin to show signs of oxidative injury in less than 24 hours.[9] Exactly what

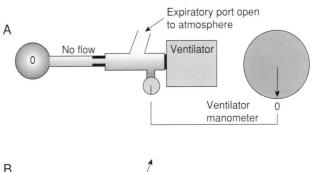

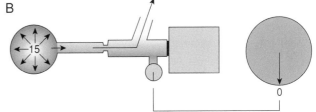

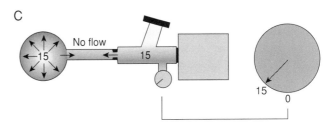

FIGURE 15–2 • Identifying auto–positive end-expiratory pressure (PEEP) during mechanical ventilation. When no auto-PEEP is present (*A*), alveolar and expiratory port pressures equilibrate. When airway resistance prevents complete alveolar emptying (*B*), positive pressure is trapped in the lung but is undetected by the ventilator as the postobstruction pressure drops to ambient. By occluding the expiratory port (*C*) at the end of expiration, the lung and ventilator circuit pressures equilibrate, and the trapped pressure can be identified.

FiO$_2$ above 21% is safe is controversial, but most clinicians strive to decrease the FiO$_2$ to 40% to 60% or less in an effort to avoid oxygen toxicity.

Intubating a patient to seal the airway so that positive pressure can be applied bypasses the normal protective mechanisms of the upper airway and increases the risk of nosocomial pneumonia. The mortality rate alone for such ventilator-associated pneumonia ranges from 40% to 80%![10]

As with the use of any device, there is always the risk of mechanical failure, and modern ventilators are typically stocked with an array of alarms to alert the user to problems. Regular maintenance and careful, frequent checks of the device are necessary to ensure it is operating as designed.

Even with careful maintenance, ventilators are less than perfect devices when it comes to replacing the spontaneous pump. Their ability to sense and respond to the patient's inspiratory efforts is limited by their design and technology, which can create significant problems. For example, an adult normally spends less than 5% of total oxygen consumption supporting spontaneous ventilation. In a study of mechanically ventilated patients in a coronary care unit, some patients were found to be spending in excess of 50% of their oxygen consumption on ventilation.[11] What is worse was that their ventilators were functioning as designed. It turned out that the patients wanted their breaths about twice as fast as the machine was set to deliver them. The resulting "fight" between the ventilator and the patient resulted in a doubling of the patients' oxygen consumption as they struggled to pull gas out of the machine to match their desired respiratory pattern. It is essential, therefore, to understand the function and limitations of the ventilator and to develop good patient assessment skills to ensure that patient tolerance and management are acceptable.

On the other end of the workload spectrum, too much unloading of ventilatory work can result in a loss of respiratory muscle strength, endurance, and eventually mass.[12] This complication appears to occur primarily at the extreme, that is, when the patient is completely controlled by the ventilator and makes no respiratory efforts whatsoever. It appears that as long as the patient is allowed to make respiratory efforts and trigger the ventilator, strength and endurance are relatively well preserved.[13]

MECHANICAL VENTILATION: WHAT WE DO IT WITH

The Machine

The full-featured intensive care unit (ICU) ventilator can be complex and intimidating in its operation, with more displays, alarms, menus, and flashing lights than the set of *Star Trek*. Often, you will wish that the Star Trek Science Officer were available to explain what the heck the machine is doing. The goal of this chapter is to demystify the ICU machine by simplifying it to its most important operations. With this basic understanding, you should be able to manage most of your patients competently regardless of the ventilator's design.

Modern ventilators are much more complex than they need to be for most operators and most patients. They are, in fact, potentially simple in their basic operation, but the mechanics and electronics are quite complex. For the purposes of this chapter, we will consider the internal mechanics of the ventilator to be a "black box" that will operate exactly as it is told.

The basic ICU ventilator is electronically powered and may or may not have a microprocessor to control its operations. Air and oxygen are fed into the machine at high pressure (about 50 psi), where they are blended to the desired FiO$_2$. Once mixed, the gas is available for delivery to the patient (some machines mix the gas as they deliver it to the patient). What happens next depends on the **mode of ventilation** that has been selected; the mode tells the machine what to do if the patient attempts to take a breath and, perhaps more importantly, what to do if the patient does not.

There are three conventional modes: **assist-control mode** (AC), **synchronized intermittent mandatory ventilation** (SIMV), and **pressure-support mode** (PS).[14] They were introduced chronologically, each being hailed as an advancement over its predecessor. Even AC mode, which we will begin with, was developed as an improvement over the original "control" mode. Before machines were developed for the early ICUs, most ventilators were designed to ventilate during anesthesia, when a patient was not expected to attempt spontaneous breathing. The operator could specify a tidal volume to be delivered and a rate at which to repeat the tidal breaths. The operator also needed to set the speed at which the breath was delivered, known as the inspiratory flow rate. The speed of the gas would fix the inspiratory time, and what time remained until the next breath was due became the expiratory time. With these parameters set, a minimum minute ventilation and the inspiratory pattern of the breath was established, or "fixed," because in control mode, rate was set regardless of the patient's actions. These early machines had no ability to detect a patient's efforts, so any effort by the patient was ignored. If, for example, you set a rate of 10 breaths/min and a tidal volume of 500 mL with an inspiratory flow of 30 L/min, every 6 seconds, the ventilator would begin to release gas at 30 L/min. The inspiratory flow would remain on for 1 second (500 mL is released) and then stop and open the expiratory valve. No other flow occurred until 5 seconds later, when the next breath was due. Patients who attempted to take bigger, smaller, or more frequent breaths were completely cut off. The word uncomfortable does not begin to describe the sensation that an alert patient experiences if ventilated in the control mode. Fortunately, there is no current indication for using this mode. It can be confusing, however, when clinicians refer to patients being in "controlled" ventilation; they are not referring to the original mode but are instead describing a situation in which the patient is not making any ef-

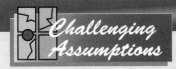

CRITICAL THINKING CHALLENGES

THE VENTILATOR CIRCUIT

The tubing that acts as a conduit for gas delivery has an impact on how much of that gas is supplied to the patient when fixed tidal volumes are set. As pressure in the circuit and the airways rises, the circuit expands, and the gas compresses. Gas that expands and compresses in the circuit is "lost" to the patient. How much gas is lost depends on the distensibility of the circuit used. The distensibility, or compliance, of the circuit can be measured by filling it with a small volume and measuring the pressure that results (off the patient, of course!). For example, if you cap the circuit at its Y connector, fill the circuit with 200 mL of gas, and see that the resulting peak pressure is 50 cm H_2O, the compliance of that circuit would be $200 \div 50 = 4$ mL/cm H_2O. You now know that your circuit will absorb about 4 mL of the patient's tidal volume for each cm H_2O of developed pressure. If you have set a tidal volume of 800 mL and have a peak pressure of 20, then 20×4, or 80 mL, of gas will stay in the circuit, and 720 mL will be delivered to the patient—a 10% loss, usually not a problem. However, if you have a 400-mL tidal volume and a peak pressure of 50 cm H_2O, then 50×4, or 200 mL, will be absorbed by the circuit, a 50% drop in the effective tidal volume! Tidal volume delivery can be improved in these situations by using stiffer tubing or shorter circuits, which absorb less gas.

Another common circuit modification can affect tidal volume: comfort tubing. Placed between the inspiratory and expiratory Y so that the weight of the heaviest part of the circuit is not directly attached to the artificial airway, this tubing effectively extends the patient's anatomic dead space. Five inches of typical wide-bore tubing holds roughly 50 mL of gas. Had we maintained comfort tubing on the above patient's circuit with pressures of 50 cm H_2O, effective tidal volume would have dropped by another 50 mL to only 150 of the 400 mL we had set! Under these circumstances (small volumes and higher pressures), comfort tubing should be eliminated.

---

forts and their ventilatory pattern is being controlled by the machine. As you will see, the primary difference between control, AC mode, and SIMV is what happens when the patient attempts to breathe spontaneously. If a patient makes no respiratory efforts, all three modes are essentially the same (Box 15–4).

Assist-Control Mode

As the need to ventilate patients outside of the operating room grew, new machines were developed and introduced in the 1950s. These early critical-care ventilators had a crucial advancement over their control mode–only counterparts: the ability to sense a patient's inspiratory effort. This was accomplished by installing a pressure sensor and connecting it to the breathing circuit. When the patient inspired and pulled gas out of the circuit, a pressure drop occurred. If enough of a pressure drop was created, the sensor triggered the machine to deliver an extra breath (see more on triggering on page 412. This extra, or "assisted," breath was identical in volume and flow to the mandatory or controlled breaths. This variation of the control mode was designated assist-control and prevailed as the only option to control mode until the 1970s (in adult ventilators; Fig. 15–3).

Advantages

Theoretically, the AC mode should reduce a patient's work of breathing significantly because each respiratory effort the patient attempts (that is also strong enough for the ventilator to sense) is supported by a mechanical breath.[15] Patients who have developed respiratory failure secondary to an in-

crease in work of breathing may receive the greatest benefit from this mode of support. There is also evidence that relieving even moderately elevated work of breathing in patients with severely limited cardiac reserves can be of value.

Disadvantages

Unfortunately, the theory behind AC mode assumes that the patient is planning on taking a breath that is identical in volume and flow to the pattern set on the ventilator. All

---

Box • 15–4 MODES OF POSITIVE-PRESSURE VENTILATION

- Control
- Assist-control (AC)
- Intermittent mandatory ventilation
- Synchronized intermittent mandatory ventilation (SIMV)
- Continuous positive-pressure ventilation
- Pressure support
- Assist-control pressure control
- SIMV pressure control
- Mandatory minute ventilation
- Pressure-regulated volume control
- Volume support
- Airway pressure release ventilation
- High-frequency jet ventilation
- High-frequency oscillation

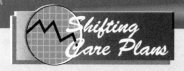

CRITICAL THINKING CHALLENGES

FLOW TRIGGERING

Pressure sensors were used for decades to trigger extra breaths from the ventilator and, because of their design limitations, created several problems, all of which conspired to increase the patient's work of breathing on the ventilator. By waiting for a pressure drop to occur, which in and of itself can be difficult for some patients to achieve, the ventilator is already behind in responding to the patient's effort and can be very slow to recover.

Enter flow triggering. With advances in technology, some ventilators now look for flow changes rather than

pressure drops. It works like this: the ventilator sends out a continuous flow of gas through the inspiratory circuit, constantly measuring how much is going out and comparing it with how much is coming back. When the patient inspires, some of the flow enters the airways, and this loss is sensed in the expiratory limb. The ventilator now triggers to this flow drop instead of waiting for a pressure change, which can reduce the work of breathing during spontaneous breaths by up to 50%.

---

too frequently, this assumption is false. If the ventilator is set to mimic the patient's respiratory pattern, AC mode significantly reduces the work of breathing. If not, the patient's oxygen consumption from the work of breathing in AC mode can increase 10-fold as the patient fights with the machine to achieve the desired respiratory pattern.[11] Symptoms include anxiety, tachypnea, accessory muscle use, and active exhalation maneuvers. Frequent monitoring of patients in AC mode for symptoms of distress associated with conflicting respiratory patterns is essential. Typically, the patient's distress is due to an inspiratory flow demand that is significantly greater than the preset flow rate on the ventilator. It is not unusual for ventilated patients to demand flow rates of 80 to 90 L/min or more

when their respiratory drive is increased by pulmonary disease. Although the ventilator can be adjusted to accommodate these high flow rates, you should also consider whether you want the patient to be working this intensely in the first place.

Mimicking the patient's respiratory pattern in AC mode can produce additional complications, especially if the patient is tachypneic. Anxious, air-hungry patients can easily hyperventilate in AC mode, resulting in a significant respiratory alkalosis. Tachypneic patients can also generate auto-PEEP, an insidious ventilator-induced gas trapping (reviewed later in the chapter). Patients who do not tolerate AC mode may tolerate other modes, but frequently, prescription of a sedative is necessary.

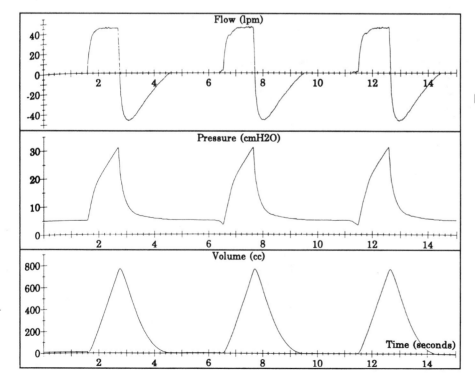

FIGURE 15–3 • Pressure, flow, and volume waveforms in assist-control mode (volume target). Inspiratory gas flow is delivered in a "square" wave pattern with a rapid rise to the set flow rate and maintenance of the flow rate throughout inspiration. Note that the last two breaths are patient triggered, indicated by the pressure drop just before the start of the breath. The first breath was delivered by the machine at the set rate because the patient failed to assist. (Kacmarek RM, Hess D. Basic principles of ventilator machinery. In: Tobin MJ. *Principles and Practice of Mechanical Ventilation.* New York: McGraw-Hill, 1994:77. Reproduced with permission of the McGraw-Hill Companies.)

Indications and Recommendations

Even though it provides nearly full support when set up properly, AC mode can be used through the entire course of ventilator support, assuming the patient tolerates it. In the past, it was thought that the respiratory muscles would not be stimulated enough in AC mode to prevent disuse atrophy, but there is no evidence to support this as long as the patient triggers some of the breaths.

Variations

The traditional AC mode delivers a fixed, preset tidal volume. Gas is delivered at the set flow rate until the prescribed volume is released. The peak airway pressure that results will depend on the obstacles that the ventilator has to push against. These obstacles include the resistance of the patient's airways (both anatomic and artificial) and the stiffness of their lungs, rib cage, and abdomen (static thoracic compliance). Peak pressure is also affected by the set flow rate and patient efforts. Higher flows generate higher resistance and higher pressures. If the patient inhales with the delivery of a breath, peak pressure is reduced; if the patient fights delivery of the gas, it is increased. To compensate for the hazards of high airway pressures, a pressure cutoff is built in so that delivery of the volume breath is halted when the upper pressure limit is reached.

A variation of AC mode, called **pressure-control mode**, was introduced in the late 1970s. Pressure-control mode replaces the volume limited breaths of AC mode with pressure-limited breaths. Instead of setting a tidal volume, a pressure target is set. Like with AC mode, a base rate is set, and extra efforts by the patient trigger extra pressure-limited breaths. Inspiratory flow is controlled by the ventilator and is adjusted so that the target pressure is achieved rapidly. The tidal volume that results depends on the obstacles listed previously. The duration of the breath is set directly with a control that fixes inspiratory time. Once the target pressure is achieved, it plateaus until the preset inspiratory time ends. An advantage of pressure-control mode is that airway pressure can be controlled more carefully to avoid the hazards associated with elevated airway pressures. The primary disadvantage is that volumes can vary and a minimum minute ventilation is no longer ensured (Fig. 15–4).

Troubleshooting

To evaluate if limited flow rate is the cause of or is contributing to a patient's distress, begin titrating up the flow rate. If you achieve 100 L/min without alleviating distress, flow rate limitations can be ruled out. If the ventilator has waveform display capabilities, this can assist you in evaluating flow limitations (Fig. 15–5). Another mechanical complication can occur with the pressure-trigger sensor. If malfunctioning or out of calibration, it can force the patient to make great efforts to initiate an assisted breath. At the other end of the spectrum, the trigger can be too sensitive, delivering extra mechanical breaths to the patient when none were requested. To assess pressure-triggering accuracy, observe the deflection in ventilator's pressure manometer during the patient's

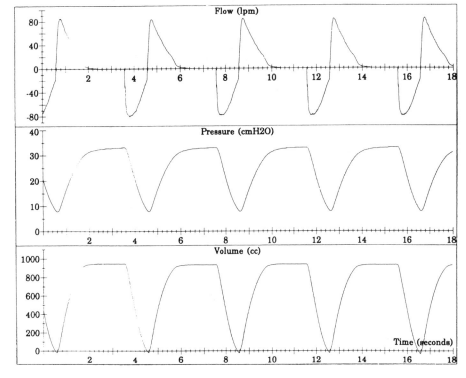

FIGURE 15–4 • Flow, pressure and volume waveforms during pressure-controlled ventilation. Note the rapid rise in flow and subsequent deceleration as the pressure target is achieved. In this example, the inspiration/exhalation ratio is inversed at 3:1. The short expiratory time does not allow for a complete exhalation, and airway pressures do not return to baseline, creating accidental positive end-expiratory pressure. (Kacmarek RM, Hess D. Basic principles of ventilator machinery. In: Tobin MJ. *Principles and Practice of Mechanical Ventilation.* New York: McGraw-Hill; 1994:82. Reproduced with permission of the McGraw-Hill Companies.)

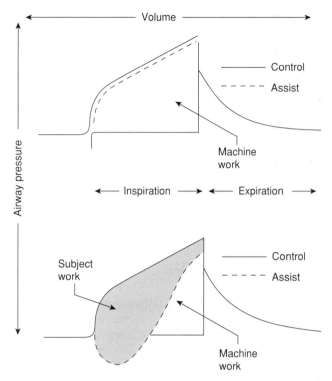

FIGURE 15–5 • Synchronized versus unsynchronized inspiratory pattern matching. (*A*) The patient's pressure volume curve follows the mechanically assisted breath, allowing the machine to assume the work of breathing. (*B*) The patient performs significant work, attempting to force the ventilator to match inspiratory pattern. (Marini JJ, Rodriguez M, Lamb V. The inspiratory workload of patient-initiated mechanical ventilation. *Am Rev Respir Dis*. 1986;134:902–909. Official Journal of the American Thoracic Society. © American Lung Association.)

inspiratory effort. When correctly set, a pressure drop of 2 cm H_2O or less should trigger an assisted breath. This assessment, however, can be confounded by the patient's inspiratory effort. If the effort is rapid and forced, the patient can outstrip the flow delivery capability of the machine, which will generate large pressure drops even with a properly functioning pressure sensor. If this is the case, you can remove the patient from the ventilator and manually ventilate. If this resolves the patient's distress, the triggering system may have been the culprit.

Intermittent Mandatory Ventilation

Another difficulty with the AC mode, clinicians discovered, is weaning. You cannot wean the patient in this mode, at least not while the patient is on the machine. Reducing the backup rate is ineffective because the patient will continue to receive mechanically supported breaths with each spontaneous inspiratory effort. Reductions in tidal volume will be countered by the patient with increases in respiratory rate to maintain the desired minute ventilation. The only true way to wean in AC mode is to remove the patient

from ventilatory support altogether. At the time, this meant placing the patient on an external supply of humidified oxygen (typically a heated aerosol delivered through large-bore corrugated tube attached to the airway with a T adapter). This "out of the frying pan and into the fire" method made for some nervous moments in the ICU for both patients and care providers. Monitoring was difficult and limited to perhaps an electrocardiogram monitor and visual observation of the patient's tolerance of the spontaneous work of breathing. Neither tidal volume nor minute ventilation could be easily monitored, and repeated blood gas analysis was necessary to evaluate adequacy of gas exchange. If the patient's strength and endurance were not up to the task, the patient was returned to mechanical support to rest and recover. These T-adapter trials would be repeated over a period of days, if necessary, with the duration of the trials extended to increase the patient's endurance until ventilatory support could be discontinued.

A breakthrough occurred in the early 1970s. What if the aerosol flow from the T-adapter system was plugged into the ventilator's circuit, and the pressure sensor to trigger extra breaths was turned off? This modification would allow the patient to breathe spontaneously from the continuous flow of gas through the circuit, but the patient's ability to initiate extra mechanical breaths would be eliminated. The clinician would now be able to limit the frequency of mechanically assisted breaths and could partition the work between the patient and the ventilator, as opposed to the all-or-nothing option in AC mode. Introduced for adults by Downs,[16] intermittent mandatory ventilation was proposed as a more efficient weaning tool than the T-adapter trial method. Because of the complexity of the circuit that was required to add continuous flow to the ventilator, the next generation of ICU ventilators came with a demand flow system.[17] This design tapped into the pressure sensor previously used to trigger extra volume breaths. In the new design, triggering the pressure sensor opened a valve that released fresh gas for spontaneous breathing, or, if it was time for one of the mandatory breaths, the ventilator would synchronize the mandatory breath with the inspiratory effort—hence the device was renamed synchronized intermittent mandatory ventilation (SIMV). A flow, pressure, and volume diagram representing ventilation in SIMV can be seen in Figure 15–5.

Advantages

VERSATILITY
With the ability to set the number of supportive breaths, SIMV can provide nearly full support if the rate is set at about the patient's spontaneous rate (Fig. 15–6). At lower rate settings, SIMV can provide partial support and allow the patient to assume more of the work of breathing. Determining how much work of breathing the patient can tolerate comfortably, however, can be difficult, and the risk of overworking the ventilatory pump is high.

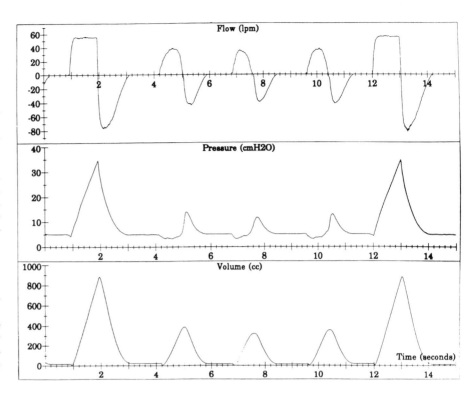

FIGURE 15–6 • Flow, pressure and volume waveforms during volume-targeted synchronized intermittent mandatory ventilation. The positive-pressure volume-targeted breath is identical to an assist-control supported breath. Note that the mechanical breaths are synchronized with an inspiratory effort (negative pressure deflection at start of breath) and are delivered with a square wave flow compared with the spontaneous breaths, which are sine wave in pattern. (Kacmarek RM, Hess D. Basic principles of ventilator machinery. In: Tobin MJ. *Principles and Practice of Mechanical Ventilation.* New York: McGraw-Hill, 1994:80. Reproduced with permission of the McGraw-Hill Companies.)

LOWER MEAN AIRWAY PRESSURES

By mixing positive-pressure mechanical breaths with negative-pressure spontaneous breaths, the mean pressures in the pleural space are lower than with AC mode, which may be advantageous if a patient cannot tolerate AC mode hemodynamically.[18] Again, the risk of increasing the work of breathing in a hemodynamically unstable patient when applying SIMV may outweigh the negative aspect of the increased positive pressure associated with AC mode.

Disadvantages

INCREASED WORK OF BREATHING

Triggering the machine for demand flow can increase the work of breathing to intolerable levels, fatiguing the respiratory muscles and potentially extending the time during which mechanical support is required. The lower the backup rate on the machine, the greater is the risk of overworking the respiratory muscles.[19]

Another factor in the increased workload involves the respiratory center's confusion with the support strategy of SIMV. The respiratory center in the brain determines how much work the respiratory muscles need to perform by taking a rolling average of the work required by previous breaths. If the previous breaths are spontaneous, then the respiratory center sets workload at the spontaneous level and turns on the respiratory muscles. If this triggers a mechanically supported breath, it is too late to back off. Once turned on, the respiratory muscles must complete their cycle before being reprogrammed by the respiratory center. Investigations into this phenomena have shown that, with

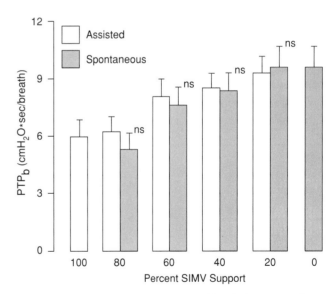

FIGURE 15–7 • Respiratory workload changes with increasing synchronized intermittent mandatory ventilation (SIMV) support. As the SIMV rate is decreased below 80% of the total rate, spontaneous workload, assessed by measuring the pressure-time product (PTP$_b$), increases significantly. At 20% of the total rate (SIMV set at 5 beats/min compared with total rate of 25 beats/min), spontaneous work is no different than if SIMV was set to 0 beats/min. Doubling the support to 40% only decreases spontaneous work by 13%. NS, not significant. (Marini JJ, Smith TC, Lamb VJ. External work output and force generation during synchronized intermittent mechanical ventilation: Effect of machine assistance breathing effort. *Am Rev Respir Dis.* 1988;138:1169–1179. Official Journal of the American Thoracic Society. © American Lung Association.)

SIMV rates at 20% to 40% of the total rate, the work of breathing during the mechanically supported breaths is the same as the work during spontaneous breaths[20] (Fig. 15–7).

DELAY OF WEANING

The traditional method of withdrawing rate to wean using SIMV has been demonstrated to prolong the weaning time in difficult-to-wean patients compared with other methods.[21,22] Weaning from mechanical ventilation is reviewed later in this chapter.

Indications and Recommendations

Because of its versatility, SIMV can be used in both acute and chronic ventilator support situations.[23] Caution must be exercised when applying SIMV in both circumstances to ensure that enough of the work of breathing has been unloaded to reduce stress on the hemodynamic system and to avoid overworking the respiratory muscles.[24]

Variations

A variation of traditional, volume-targeted SIMV is pressure-targeted SIMV. Similar to the pressure-control variation of AC mode, the mandatory breaths are pressure limited and are controlled just like the pressure-limited breaths of pressure-control mode. Between controlled breaths, the patient is allowed to breathe spontaneously. These spontaneous breaths may or may not be assisted. More information on assisting spontaneous efforts is provided in the Pressure-Support Mode section next.

Pressure-Support Mode

As it became apparent just how large the imposed workload was during spontaneous breaths in SIMV, an enhancement was developed. If we look at the problem from the patient's perspective, there appears to be a big resistance to gas flow in the circuit when the patient is breathing on a ventilator. Most of this resistance is created by the endotracheal tube, but the circuit and the demand system contribute to the problem. Even in the most technologically advanced ventilators, the patient has to generate an additional -5 to -10 cm H_2O of pleural pressure to pull gas for spontaneous breathing across these combined resistances. What if, the ventilator engineers said, we created a positive pressure during inspiration that would counter the negative pressure the patient had to generate? This positive "inspiratory-only" pressure is pressure support.[25] The pressure-support (PS) mode is a partial support mode that relies on the patient's innate respiratory drive; that is, there is no backup rate. If the patient does not breathe, neither does the ventilator. Attempting a respiratory effort, however, triggers the machine (PS mode does not reduce the work to trigger), and the machine begins delivering flow faster than the patient demands it until the dialed-in pressure gradient is achieved. Then, the machine maintains that pressure gradient, constantly monitoring inspiratory flow until the patient nears the end of the breath (different machines define this differently), at which point the pressure is allowed to return to baseline, and exhalation can begin (Fig. 15–8).

Think of PS mode as a turbocharger for spontaneous breaths or as the difference between drinking at a water fountain and drinking through a long straw. A long, skinny

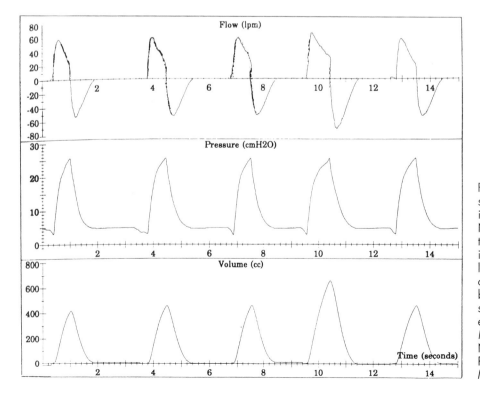

FIGURE 15–8 • Flow, pressure, and volume waveforms during pressure-support ventilation. Note that each breath is patient initiated (pressure drop from patient's inspiratory effort triggers the ventilator). In addition, inspiratory time and tidal volume vary with each breath. (Kacmarek RM, Hess D. Basic principles of ventilator machinery. In: Tobin MJ. *Principles and Practice of Mechanical Ventilation.* New York: McGraw-Hill; 1994:83. Reprinted with permission of the McGraw-Hill Companies.)

straw requires much more effort to obtain fluid than does a fountain, which pushes the water right up to your mouth. Figure 15–9 demonstrates the effects of differing levels of PS mode on flow and volume.[26]

Typically, PS mode can be combined with SIMV[27] so that the spontaneous breaths during SIMV are not completely unsupported. This reduces the confusion of the respiratory center by minimizing the all-or-nothing effect of SIMV alone and also reduces the risk of apnea occurring with PS mode alone because SIMV provides a backup rate. Low levels of pressure support, somewhere between 5 and 10 cm H_2O, overcome the resistance of the circuitry.[28] The higher end of the 5- to 10 cm H_2O range is reserved for patients with small endotracheal tubes relative to their size who need more help in overcoming the unusually high resistance of a small tube. Higher levels of pressure support begin to reduce the work of breathing secondary to the underlying disease, and eventually, as you titrate the level up, PS mode provides nearly full ventilatory support after the breath is triggered.[29]

Advantages

COMFORT

Ask a patient to compare AC, SIMV, and PS modes and they most likely will tell you (hopefully they are not actually talking) that they prefer PS mode.[25,30] The reason for this is simple: PS mode tries to follow the patient's breathing pattern instead of imposing a breathing pattern, as with AC mode or SIMV. If you want more flow, it will deliver more flow (up to a point). Want long inspiratory times or a large breath? No problem. This improvement in comfort usually translates to less need for sedation.[31] It also leads to improved ventilator–patient synchrony and improvement in the efficiency of a patients work, resulting in a decrease in the oxygen "cost" of breathing when compared with non–pressure-supported breaths in SIMV. Another reason that PS mode improves comfort may involve its regularity. As with AC mode, pressure-supported breaths receive the same amount of assistance with each breath, allowing the respiratory center to identify and set its workload more effectively.

POTENTIAL TO ASSESS A PATIENT'S ABILITY TO WEAN WITHOUT TAKING AWAY VENTILATORY SUPPORT

Placing the patient on a low level of pressure support as a trial may be a quick and efficient means of testing a patient's spontaneous breathing ability.[32] Whether this is as predictive as other weaning assessments remains to be tested.

Disadvantages

BACKUP VENTILATION

Used by itself, PS mode provides no backup support to patients should their respiratory drive or efforts decrease or stop altogether. Some ventilators switch modes if apnea occurs, as a corrective action to this problem. The use of PS mode alone in unstable, critically ill patients is not well

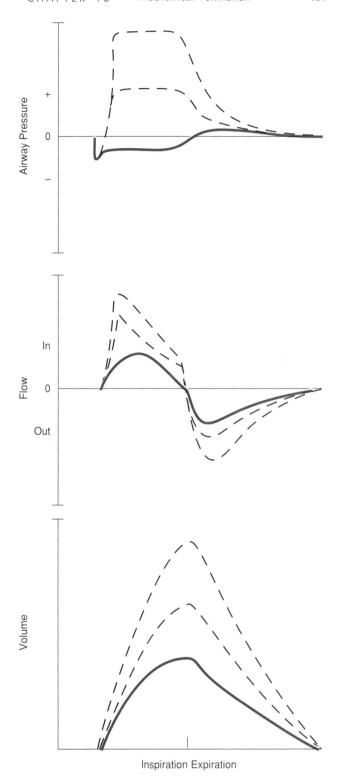

Inspiration Expiration

FIGURE 15–9 • Changes in airway pressure, flow, and volume with unassisted breaths (*solid line*) and with increasing levels of pressure support (*broken lines*). Note that the patient must maintain constant negative pressure to generate flow during unassisted breaths. Adding and increasing the pressure support levels results in increases in both flow rate and delivered volume during the spontaneous effort. (Brochard L, Pluskwa F, Lemaire F. Improved efficacy of spontaneous breathing with inspiratory pressure support. *Am Rev Respir Dis.* 1987;136:411–415. Official Journal of the American Thoracic Society. © American Lung Association.)

tested, although there is some evidence that it may work as well as AC mode in these patients.[33]

INABILITY TO IDENTIFY END OF EXPIRATION

Patients with leaks around their airway or with large bronchopleural fistulas can "fool" PS mode by keeping the inspired flow high through the leak, thus interfering with the machine's ability to sense the end of inspiration.[34] This complication reduces patient ventilator synchrony and increases work of breathing. Also, adding flow to the circuit of a pressure-triggered machine can interfere with its triggering abilities. Continuous nebulization of bronchodilators in a patient on PS mode was identified as the cause of hypoventilation in the patient, who could not over-breathe the flow from the nebulizer.[35]

Indications and Recommendations

Minimum levels of 5 to 10 cm H_2O of pressure support should always should be used to support spontaneous breathing when spontaneous breathing is allowed (SIMV or continuous positive airway pressure). Pressure support can also be titrated up from minimal levels to relieve pathologic increases in work of breathing, reducing the elevated workloads to tolerable levels.[31]

MECHANICAL VENTILATION: HOW WE DO IT

Strategies for Patient and Ventilator Management

Initiation of Mechanical Ventilation

When initiating mechanical ventilation, there are two primary goals: restoration of gas exchange and normalization of the work of breathing. It is usually possible to realize these goals with the ventilator. There will be occasions, however, when compromise will be necessary to avoid injury to the lung, requiring a switch to another approach. An algorithm for basic ventilator management is presented in Figure 15–10.

The first order of business after initiating the ventilator is to decide who is going to do the work of breathing. In respiratory arrest, the choice has already been made because the patient has essentially resigned from the competition, and the ventilator must take over all of the work of breathing. In a patient with less severe respiratory failure, you may want to allow the patient to perform some work of breathing, but not so much that you risk respiratory muscle fatigue or added stress on the hemodynamic system.

Controlling work of breathing can have several desirable effects. First, by reducing the oxygen expense incurred by the respiratory muscles to ventilate stiff lungs, the demand on the hemodynamic system to supply them with extra oxygen is minimized. Total oxygen transport can then be either reduced or rerouted to more critical organ systems. In patients with high shunt fractions, reducing oxygen con-

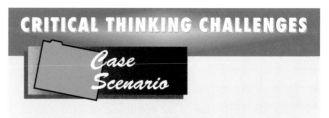

CRITICAL THINKING CHALLENGES

Case Scenario

OXYGEN CONSUMPTION AND HYPOXEMIA

If a patient has an oxygen delivery of 1000 mL/min and an oxygen consumption of 500 mL/min, then 50% of the total oxygen is consumed, and 50% remains in the venous blood. If this same patient has a 25% shunt fraction, one quarter of the blood passing through the lungs at a saturation of 50% will mix with the three quarters that has been saturated to 100%. The arterial saturation that will result from this 25–75 mix is 87%. If you were to reduce the work of breathing to normal, or even subnormal, levels and drop the oxygen consumption to 250 mL/min while our delivery remained at 1000 mL/min, the mixed venous saturation would rise to 75%. Now, mix the 75% saturated venous blood through the shunt, and you will have improved arterial saturation from 87% to 94%!

sumption can improve arterial oxygenation by raising the saturation of the venous blood that is being shunted. Taking over the work of breathing in patients who are failing from COPD can give the respiratory muscles time to recuperate from their exhausted state and allow them to improve in strength and endurance.

SELECTING A MODE

Deciding exactly how, or if, the ventilator will achieve the goal of normalizing the work of breathing depends primarily on the mode of support selected. As described earlier, there are three basic modes: AC, SIMV, and PS. In some ventilators, you can also choose volumes or pressures as a method of achieving tidal volume. In the presence of acute respiratory failure, this menu of three is reduced to two, because PS mode typically is not used when full support is required, although this approach is now being tested.[34] Much of the selection criteria for modes is based on personal preference and experience. If you have been trained with SIMV and PS mode, by all means, continue to use the modes you are comfortable with as long as you understand their limitations.

ASSIST-CONTROL MODE

It is entirely possible, and perhaps desirable, to ventilate a patient throughout the entire course of mechanical support using only AC mode. This mode has great potential for reducing work of breathing in a manner that is understood by the respiratory center; that is, the same level of support occurs with each breath. The real disadvantage to AC mode is the fixed respiratory pattern, which does not adjust to patient

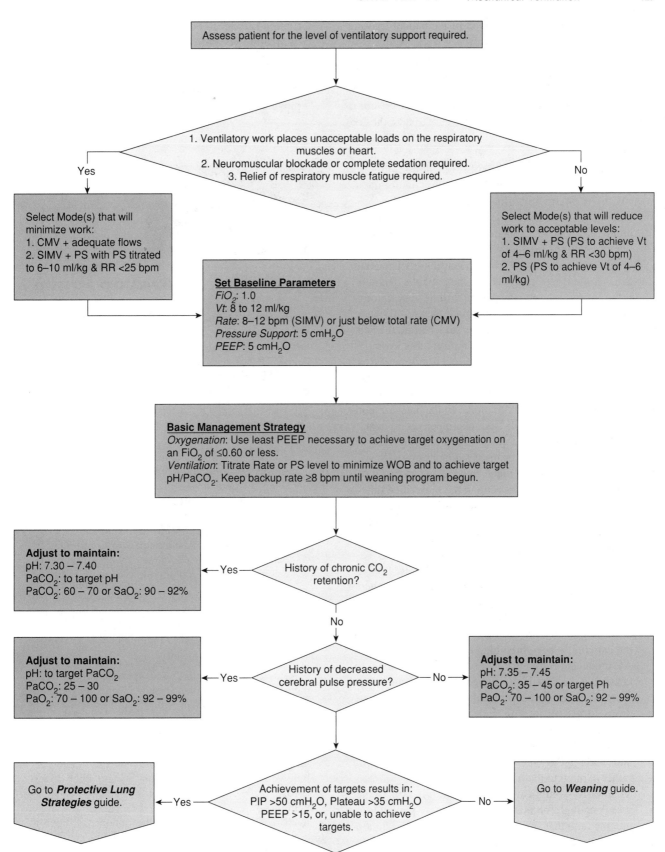

FIGURE 15-10 • Algorithm for basic ventilator management.

demand and increases the likelihood of the patient fighting the ventilator. When it works, however, it works well.

Recommendation: Use AC mode as the initial mode when ventilating patients with severe increases in work of breathing (eg, ARDS, thoracic burns, cardiogenic pulmonary edema), especially when the cardiovascular system is impaired by disease, injury, or age. Be sure to take the following steps:

- Set the peak flow high enough! A rate of 40 L/min is not good for everybody; in fact, it is too low for most situations. Start with a flow that will deliver the breath in at least 1 second. When using a volume breath, this can be calculated quickly by multiplying the tidal volume by 60. (When using a pressure breath, flow is controlled by the ventilator.) The goal is to set the flow slightly above the patient's demand. If the flow is too low, the patient will have symptoms of air hunger, and the pressure manometer will not show a crisp rise to the peak pressure. Titrate the peak flow up in increments of 5 L/min until these symptoms disappear. If you approach 100 L/min peak flow without achieving patient–ventilator synchrony, it is time for plan B. One option to consider is switching to the pressure version of AC mode. In the pressure-control mode, the ventilator attempts to deliver an overload of flow to achieve quickly the peak pressure goal that has been set. If the patient demands more flow, the ventilator accommodates the demand so that it can achieve the dialed-in pressure in the prescribed time frame. Another option to consider is increasing the dosage of sedation. Finally, chemical paralysis can be considered if all other methods fail to achieve adequate control of the work of breathing.
- Set the base rate near the patient's actual rate. It is slightly easier for the ventilator to synchronize when the machine's rate and the patient's rate are similar. Primarily, however, it is safer if the patient's rate decreases suddenly, for example, in a situation in which the patient has been breathing about 20 breaths/min in AC mode and is given a dose of sedation sufficient to knock out the ventilatory drive. If the base rate was set at 18 breaths/min, not much happens—the rate drops 2 to 18 breath/min, and the minute ventilation is essentially preserved. If the base rate was set at 10 breaths/min, the minute ventilation could decrease by half, and the $PaCO_2$ could double. Which would you rather explain to the judge?
- Monitor for complications of hyperventilation. Make it easy enough for an anxious, air-hungry patient to breathe (and that *is* your goal), and respiratory alkalosis can become a real problem. Most patients who drive themselves into respiratory alkalosis are sending a message that they need better sedation or pain control. Having a large tube in your trachea is not comfortable! This may also be an indication to test the patient in SIMV, in which the potential for hyperventilation is reduced but the potential for increased work of breathing is almost guaranteed.
- Check for auto-PEEP. This recommendation is true for all modes. As respiratory rates rise, especially in the presence of obstructive airway disease, gas trapping can be a problem (Fig. 15–11).

CRITICAL THINKING CHALLENGES

Case Scenario

AUTO–POSITIVE END-EXPIRATORY PRESSURE

As described earlier, auto-PEEP is a "hidden" pressure trapped in the lung because of inadequate expiratory time in combination with obstructive airways disease. Auto-PEEP has all the same complications as has applied PEEP, plus one. Eliminating auto-PEEP should be a priority. Outside of maximal bronchodilator therapy, strategies for eliminating auto-PEEP all center around the lengthening expiratory time. Start with 1; move down if 1 doesn't eliminate the auto-PEEP.

1. *Shorten inspiratory time.* In a volume mode, this is accomplished by increasing the peak flow setting. As peak flow is increased, however, the peak inspiratory pressure rises. Peak pressures over 60 cm H_2O may be risky. If you hit the peak pressure ceiling, consider shrinking the tidal volume. This will drop the peak pressure and shorten the inspiratory time as well. This may require allowing hypercapnia to develop to be successful.

2. *Lower the rate.* This allows more time between breaths and hence more expiratory time. This typically requires allowing hypercapnia to develop to be successful.

Auto-PEEP also interferes with ventilator triggering. If the alveolar pressure is +20 cm H_2O and the ventilator is set to trigger at −2 cm H_2O, the patient will have to generate an intrapleural pressure of at least −22 cm H_2O to trigger—enough to pull through all the positive alveolar pressure and past the trigger setting on the machine. When all attempts to eliminate auto-PEEP fail, you may want to consider adding PEEP to decrease work of breathing. For example, if the auto-PEEP is +12 cm H_2O and there is no PEEP in the circuit (with a −2 cm H_2O trigger), the patient will have to pull −14 cm H_2O to trigger. If we add +12 cm H_2O of PEEP to the circuit, the patient is able to trigger the ventilator with the normal −2 cm H_2O pressure change. Adding extrinsic PEEP usually has minimal effect on intrinsic or auto-PEEP because of the "waterfall" effect (see Fig. 15-11).

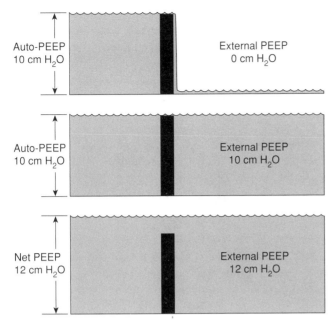

F I G U R E 1 5 – 1 1 • The waterfall effect. The gas trapped behind obstructive airways behaves like water trapped behind a dam. Increasing the water level (or the external positive end-expiratory pressure [PEEP]) does not increase the overall level of the water in the dam (or the pressure in the lung) until the external pressure exceeds the trapped pressure. Adding external PEEP to approximate auto-PEEP can improve patient triggering ability. (*Chest.* 1989;96:449.)

SYNCHRONIZED INTERMITTENT MANDATORY VENTILATION

As you will recall, SIMV was developed as a means of weaning patients who were being supported in AC mode. As it turns out, SIMV is not an effective weaning tool (more on weaning later) but can be used to support patients whose work of breathing is not critically elevated or patients who are not tolerating AC mode. SIMV should always be used in conjunction with PS mode if it is available. If PS mode is not available, it is preferable to stay in AC mode to avoid the work of breathing issues that SIMV presents when used alone. Also, if a patient is not breathing spontaneously, SIMV and AC mode are indistinguishable. Until the patient begins to breathe spontaneously, AC mode is a safer bet to guarantee that the patient's work of breathing does not become excessive.

The two-mode package of SIMV and PS mode allows you to set a minimum minute ventilation with the SIMV "rate X tidal volume" and to achieve an acceptable work of breathing during spontaneous ventilation by titrating appropriate pressure-support levels.

- Set the SIMV rate for a backup guarantee. This usually requires a rate of at least 10 or 12 breaths/min. Do not set rates lower than this. Remember, we are not weaning in SIMV. As with AC mode, ensure that the peak flow is set adequately to accommodate the patient's inspiratory demand for flow.
- Titrate pressure support. Start with 5 cm H_2O, and observe the spontaneous tidal volumes and the total res-

piratory rate that result. If the respiratory rate is more than 30 breaths/min, the patient's respiratory center is telling us that the workload is too high. Increase the pressure-support level in increments of 5 cm H_2O until the total respiratory rate is under 30 breaths/min and closer to 25 or 20 breaths/min. If it takes more than 20 cm H_2O in PS mode to achieve this respiratory rate goal, there could be additional problems.

The respiratory center may not be normal, a common issue in head injury and stroke patients. Institute a trial of AC mode. If the respiratory rate does not decrease in response to full support, the respiratory center is probably not functioning normally or the patient's pain and anxiety may not be adequately controlled. If the respiratory rate does decrease in AC mode, the respiratory center is telling you that the support in SIMV and PS modes was inadequate, even at 20 cm H_2O. Stay with AC mode, or with pressure-control mode if you need more aggressive initial flows, to control work of breathing.

If the patient does not respond to AC mode, reevaluate the respiratory center and potential pain and anxiety problems as the root cause of the tachypnea. In patients with head injury, stroke, and some pulmonary diseases like pulmonary fibrosis, a rapid shallow breathing pattern is the new base pattern. Determining whether to accept or treat this pattern can be difficult. Generally, if a more rapid shallow pattern is stable (ie, not worsening), gas exchange is stable, and the patient does not complain of or show signs of respiratory distress, it can be accepted as a new set point of the respiratory center. If the pattern or gas exchange does deteriorate, it should be treated with additional ventilatory support.

Restoring Gas Exchange

Once the appropriate mode has been selected to correct work of breathing, adequate gas exchange must be established without additional injury to the lung. From our previous discussions, we know that high oxygen concentrations and excessive alveolar volumes contribute to lung damage.

Oxygen concentrations of 100% are known to induce lung injury over time, although the exact FIO_2 below 100% that does not produce lung injury is not clearly established. Studies suggest that an FIO_2 at or below 60% does not contribute significantly to lung injury. It is also safe to say that 40% is probably less dangerous than 60%, so an FIO_2 strategy of "the lower the better" can be our guide.

There is also mounting evidence that even seemingly normal-sized tidal volumes, in combination with with a disease that shrinks the lung like ARDS, can exacerbate lung injury.[36-39] Because it is difficult, if not impossible, to determine the available volume of ventilated space in the lung, we must rely on the pressures that are associated with "excessive" to gauge hyperinflation of the lung. It requires about 35 cm H_2O of pressure applied to the alveolar space to bring a normal lung, in a normal chest, to its elastic limit.[40,41] Tidal volumes that result in alveolar pressures that exceed 35 cm H_2O can drive ventilated portions of lung past their elastic limits and injure them.

Alveolar pressures can be closely estimated by measuring plateau pressure. Plateau pressure is different from the peak pressure that accompanies the delivery of a tidal breath. **Peak pressure** is a result of the pressure necessary to overcome the resistance to airflow in combination with the pressure necessary to overcome the resistance of the lung to inflation. **Plateau pressure** is just the pressure necessary to overcome the resistance of the lung to inflation (compliance). To measure plateau pressure, have the ventilator delay exhalation for several seconds after the delivery of a mechanical breath. With the breath held, flow drops to zero, and the pressure generated to overcome the resistance of the airways drops out. The resulting plateau pressure closely approximates actual alveolar pressure generated from the delivery of the breath. Earlier recommendations for selecting tidal volume suggested a range of 10 to 15 mL/kg to ensure adequate inflation and to avoid atelectasis. Because of the risk of overdistention, current recommendations drop the lower end of this range to as little as 5 mL/kg to avoid lung injury. What is most important in selecting tidal volume, however, is not the whether you select 8 or 10 or 15 mL/kg, but that you avoid any volume that brings alveolar pressure above 35 cm H_2O.

There are some exceptions to this guideline that involve the complication of an abnormal chest wall. Problems such as thoracic burns, morbid obesity, and kyphoscoliosis alter the normal elasticity of the chest wall. Under these situations, it may take significantly more pressure than 35 cm H_2O to bring the lung to its elastic limit because of the increased pressure required to push the stiff chest wall out of the way. There is no simple way to delineate chest wall distending pressure from alveolar distending pressure at the bedside, which leaves you with a volume and pressure strategy similar to your FIO_2 strategy: the lower the pressure, the better.

With these oxygen and pressure thresholds in mind, you must now determine what are adequate gas exchange parameters for the patient. "Textbook" normal blood gas values for healthy adults are a pH of 7.35 to 7.45, a $PaCO_2$ of 35 to 45 mmHg, and a PaO_2 of 80 to 100 mmHg. If you happen to be ventilating a healthy adult, these goals are acceptable. For example, an otherwise healthy 35-year-old who requires ventilation after uncomplicated surgery to repair a prolapsed mitral valve should achieve these target blood gases easily without approaching any of the lung injury thresholds. When achieving textbook normal values means exceeding the thresholds or disturbing a patient's normal baseline values, your goals must be altered.

Permissive Hypercapnia: Patient Initiated

In a patient whose baseline pH and $PaCO_2$ are altered, your goal should be to return the gas exchange values to the patient's baseline, not to normalize them. A patient with a long history of COPD whose typical $PaCO_2$ is 65 mmHg

and pH is 7.34 should be ventilated back to these baseline values, not to normal values. If the exact preventilation blood gases are not known, ventilating to a low-normal pH, regardless of the $PaCO_2$, is a safe strategy. Attempting to ventilate a chronically hypercapneic patient down to a $PaCO_2$ of 40 mmHg will result in alkalosis from the extra buffer that has accumulated to compensate for the elevated CO_2. It would also be impossible to wean this patient using a normal CO_2 target because the patient was not able to achieve a normal CO_2 before ventilatory support.

Permissive Hypercapnia: Clinician Initiated

Protecting the lung from excessive pressures is another rationale for altering what is acceptable gas exchange. In ARDS, the lung can consolidate to only 25% of its normal size,[40] and regular-sized tidal volumes create tremendous alveolar pressures. Reducing the tidal volume so that the alveolar pressures are less than 35 cm H_2O typically creates small tidal volumes, resulting in hypoventilation, hypercapnia, and respiratory acidosis. A similar excessive elevation in alveolar pressures can occur when patients with severe obstructive lung disease are mechanically ventilated, resulting in significant intrinsic PEEP. In both of these disease processes, permitting hypercapnia and respiratory acidosis to occur while protecting the lung from hyperinflation results in better outcomes than does the conventional approach.[41,42] How to handle the acidosis is not well established. Some investigators have made no attempt to buffer the acidosis, allowing the kidneys to adjust the pH slowly.[43] Other investigators have suggested indirect interventions, such as reducing CO_2 production with paralysis, diet adjustment, and temperature regulation. Still another group of investigators advocate direct strike with bicarbonate administration,[41,44] tracheal gas insufflation,[45] or extracorporeal membrane oxygenation to decrease the CO_2 load, although the benefits of these approaches remains controversial. Your decision to intervene should probably center around the type of patient and the extent of the acidosis. In other words, what a previously healthy 20-year-old trauma patient will tolerate in acidosis is different than what an 80-year-old with congestive heart failure will tolerate. If buffering appears necessary, use the minimal amount necessary to return pH to the 7.20 range.

Correcting Hypoxemia

Most patients respond adequately to moderate increases in FIO_2. When potentially dangerous amounts of oxygen are required to correct hypoxemia, significant right to left shunting is occurring. The addition of PEEP can help restore lung volume lost to infiltrates and consolidation, reducing the shunt and allowing for a reduction in FIO_2 to safer levels. A simple strategy to use at the bedside in setting FIO_2 and PEEP is the "60–60 rule." That is, use the least amount of PEEP necessary to achieve a PaO_2 of greater than 60 mmHg on an FIO_2 of 0.60 or less. One ex-

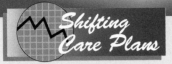

CRITICAL THINKING CHALLENGES

Shifting Care Plans

POSITIVE END-EXPIRATORY PRESSURE

Introduced in the late 1960s, PEEP was promoted as a way to prevent the lung from collapsing to an abnormally low end-expiratory volume. The original mechanics had the clinician place the expiratory line into a jug of water. If you wanted 10 cm H_2O of PEEP, you sunk the expiratory line 10 cm down into the jug. Current ventilators use various methods to maintain end-expiratory pressure.

PEEP has two positive side effects and several potential negative effects. On the positive side, the increase in lung volume improves ventilated alveolar space, decreasing shunt. In addition, the restoration of lung improves compliance by moving the tidal volume into a better pressure–volume curve, reducing work of breathing.

Being a positive pressure, however, PEEP has all the potential side effects of positive-pressure ventilation, most of which were discussed previously. One complication somewhat specific to PEEP is increased dead-space ventilation. Because of its continuous nature, PEEP that results in continuous alveolar pressures above pulmonary capillary pressures effectively shuts off blood flow to that unit, turning it into dead space. This problem, most common at higher levels of PEEP (above 10 cm H_2O), becomes evident when you are titrating PEEP up to correct hypoxemia, and suddenly the $PaCO_2$ rises even though you have not adjusted minute ventilation.

ception to this rule occurs in ARDS, in which the PEEP should be adjusted to help stent open the inflamed airways; this typically requires PEEP in the range of 8 to 12 cm H_2O. The titration of PEEP upward should also be halted if it results in excessive alveolar pressures, although you may want to consider decreasing the tidal volumes and allowing more PEEP if the FiO_2 is particularly high. Decreased cardiac output and hypotension are other stopping points in the titration of PEEP. The effects of PEEP on circulation are most pronounced in hypovolemic patients. Finally, if 15 cm H_2O of PEEP has not corrected the patient's hypoxemia adequately, more PEEP is not likely to help alveolar recruitment nor to increase functional lung volume. Functional residual capacity may increase, but it appears that most of that increase occurs from hyperinflation of already ventilated lung. As with permissive hypercapnia, your patient and your level of desperation can be your guide. A young, previously healthy patient with a strong heart and enough hemoglobin is more likely to tolerate moderate to severe hypoxemia and than is an elderly patient with limited cardiac function.

Hypoxemia Unresponsive to Positive End-Expiratory Pressure and FiO_2

Now what? Your patient is on 15 cm H_2O of PEEP and 100% oxygen, and the Sao_2 is only 85%. It is not clear at this time what the next step should be. One suggestion is to prolong the inspiratory time. This strategy is usually combined with the use of pressure-control mode. Instead of using only PEEP to increase mean airway pressure to recruit consolidated lung, somewhat less PEEP and long inspiratory times are combined to increase mean airway pressure. The higher pressures associated with inspiration may be more successful at recruitment than would be the lower background pressure of PEEP. Also, less PEEP is generally necessary, potentially reversing some of the dead space created with the higher PEEP level and allowing for a reduction in tidal volume or minute ventilation. Some advocate increasing the inspiratory time to the point that it is longer than the exhalation time. You can let your desperation and the circulation be your guide.

WEANING

Assessment of Readiness

Although potentially life-saving, the multitude of complications associated with mechanical ventilation suggest that support should be discontinued as soon as is reasonably possible. Most patients wean from the ventilator successfully with little effort regardless of the method used. The first step in weaning, or discontinuation of mechanical support, is deciding if the patient has recovered sufficiently to tolerate a return to spontaneous breathing. In general, this means that the patient should be better; the cause for ventilator support should be resolved or well controlled. Prematurely discontinuing ventilation in an unprepared patient is futile and potentially damaging. On the other hand, deciding when the patient is prepared is one of those issues in the management of mechanical ventilation for which practice is more of an art than a science. No exact criteria have been established to quantify when a patient is prepared for weaning, but a list of general assessment criteria is summarized in Box 15–5. None of these criteria is hard and fast; rather, they should be used as a group to develop a general sense of weaning readiness. Some of the criteria, however, are more sound than others. For example, if the patient meets all of the listed criteria but requires an FiO_2 of 0.60 to maintain an adequate SaO_2, weaning should be postponed on the basis of unresolved hypoxemia.

Predicting Weaning Success

Once weaning readiness has been established, the patient can be assessed for weaning potential. Over the years, an extensive list of assessment variables has been suggested to predict weaning success—some simple, and some outra-

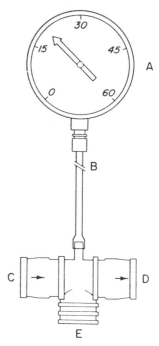

FIGURE 15–12 • Diagram of a circuit used to measure maximum inspiratory pressures (MIP). The manometer is attached to a T adapter with dual one-way valves at *C* and *D*. When *C* is occluded, the patient can exhale but cannot inhale. The negative pressure generated during each effort is displayed on the manometer (*A*).

geously complex. A list of criteria that are easy to measure at the bedside and have been demonstrated to be predictive of weaning success are listed in Box 15–6. Some of these criteria, such as vital capacity and negative inspiratory force, evaluate respiratory muscle strength. A minimum amount of strength is required to ensure that the patient can take a deep enough breath to generate an adequate cough to keep the airways clear. Strength is also an underlying component of endurance. Studies have shown that the respiratory muscles tolerate ongoing workloads that are less than 50% of a one-time maximum effort. The lower that one-time maximum effort, the lower is the respiratory workload that can be tolerated for extended periods.

A spirometer and pressure manometer are the basic equipment required to measure weaning parameters. The spirometer should meet recommended standards for volume and flow performance,[47] and the pressure manometer should be capable of measuring negative pressures down to −60 cm H_2O. A diagram of the circuit for the pressure manometer is given in Figure 15–12.

To calculate the **rapid shallow breathing index** (RSBI), measure the patient's respiratory rate and average tidal volume from the ventilator. Disconnect the patient from the ventilator, and attach the patient's airway to the spirometer. Count the frequency of respirations, and note the minute ventilation achieved on the spirometer in the first 60 seconds. Divide the minute ventilation by the respiratory frequency to calculate the average tidal volume achieved. Finally, divide the respiratory rate by the average tidal volume in liters. For example, a patient with a respiratory rate of 28 breaths/min and an average tidal volume of 0.24 L would have a RSBI of 117. An RSBI of less than 100 is predictive of weaning success. Return the patient to mechanical support briefly before measuring the remainder of the weaning variables.

To measure vital capacity, disconnect the patient from the ventilator, and reattach the spirometer circuit. Ask the patient to take as deep a breath as possible and then to exhale completely. Coach the patient through the maneuver to ensure a complete exhalation. Patients who cannot follow commands should be spared from this assessment because meaningful data cannot be collected.

To measure negative inspiratory force, connect the pressure manometer circuit to the airway, and ask the patient to breathe in with all of his or her strength. Have the patient repeat the maneuver several times. The circuit will allow the patient to exhale but not to inhale any fresh gas. This forces the patient to lower lung volumes during the measurement so that the respiratory muscles will have the greatest mechanical advantage. Measure for up to 20 seconds or until the patient becomes unstable. Use the highest value (most negative pressure) achieved in your assessment.

Patients should be assessed daily for weaning readiness so that you can ensure that the first possible opportunity is not missed to discontinue ventilatory support.

Methods of Discontinuation

Many methods of weaning have been proposed over the years. When AC mode was the only mode available, weaning could not be gradual. Decreasing the rate was futile because the patient could simply order up more mechanical breaths with each effort, and decreasing the tidal volume became counterproductive, leading only to a rapid shallow pattern. The only practical way to wean was to remove the patient from the ventilator altogether in a "trial-by-fire" type of setting. Because this could be overwhelming to both the patient and care provider, intermittent mandatory ventilation and then SIMV were developed so that weaning could be more gradual and comfortable. When it was discovered how difficult it was for a patient to breathe through an SIMV circuit, pressure support was introduced to ease the work of spontaneous breathing. Because pressure support could be used with SIMV or by itself, it too began to be used as a weaning tool. With four modes available to wean, untold numbers of strategies were developed as clinicians experimented to determine which was the best mode or combination of modes for weaning. Only recently have some of these been evaluated in a randomized and controlled fashion.

Before we discuss strategies, let us step back and look at patients on ventilatory support. Generally, we can divide them into two groups. In the first group are patients who require brief support for a few days or less and whose respiratory muscles retain their original strength and endurance. In the second group are all the other patients (Fig. 15–13). Patients in the first group are the easiest to wean, and once ready, it probably does not matter what method you use as long as it is quick so that you do not unnecessarily prolong the process. Patients in the second group typically fail the first attempt to wean once they appear to be ready; much of the controversy around the issue of weaning and most of the variations in weaning techniques relate to this group. Their failure to wean can also be divided into two general categories: respiratory failure and everything else. Respiratory failure indicates that the patient's current strength and endurance are not up to the task and the patient needs an exercise program to retrain the respiratory muscles. If the patient fails to wean for other reasons, your assessment of readiness was inaccurate and must be reevaluated before further weaning attempts are made.

Your strategies for weaning, therefore, must concentrate on "getting out of the way" for the short-term, uncomplicated group and on setting up an appropriate exercise program for the group of patients with weak muscles.

The most direct and simple way to wean the uncomplicated group is to simply stop or to minimize ventilatory support. This can be accomplished by removing the patient from the ventilator and placing the patient on a T adapter or by reducing mechanical support to about 5 cm H_2O of pressure support. The advantage of a T-adapter trial is its ability to mimic the work of breathing that the patient will be required to perform after extubation. T adapters also eliminate the potential problems associated with breathing spontaneously through the ventilator, like the work necessary to trigger demand flow. T adapters, however, eliminate the benefits of the ventilator, which allows you to monitor rate, tidal volume, and minute ventilation continuously during the trial. Whichever mode you choose, the patient should be observed regularly for signs of distress. It is also important to monitor the patient to ensure maintenance of a regular respiratory pattern. For example, postoperative patients who are still under the influence of anesthesia and patients receiving excessive sedatives or narcotics are prone to periodic breathing patterns and hypoventilation and may show no signs of distress.

After 30 to 60 minutes, the patient's vital signs and gas exchange should be assessed. Respiratory rates of less than 30 breath/min combined with stable hemodynamics are signs of a successful trial. In addition, assessment should be made of gas exchange, either from an arterial blood gas sample or from reliable pulse oximetry, and end-tidal CO_2 monitors. During the trial, the patient should continue to demonstrate adequate oxygenation and should be able to maintain baseline pH and $PaCO_2$ levels for about 30 minutes.

Once the trial is considered a success, and especially if the patient is intubated endotracheally, the need for maintenance of the artificial airway should be evaluated promptly. Do not confuse discontinuation of mechanical ventilation with extubation. Many patients do not require mechanical ventilation but do require an artificial airway for bronchial hygiene or to maintain a patent airway. Unnecessary endotracheal tubes, especially if they are narrow, should be removed quickly because they increase spontaneous work of breathing and may result in fatigue and respiratory failure if left in place while the patient is breathing spontaneously. If an endotracheally intubated patient requires a long-term artificial airway, a tracheostomy should be considered to avoid excessive work of breathing. Tracheostomy tubes of adequate diameter are shorter and less resistant to airflow than are endotracheal tubes and do not significantly impede work of breathing.

Patients who fail this first trial should be returned to full support and reassessed. Hypoventilation and periodic breathing are common reasons for failure in postoperative

Weaning Guide

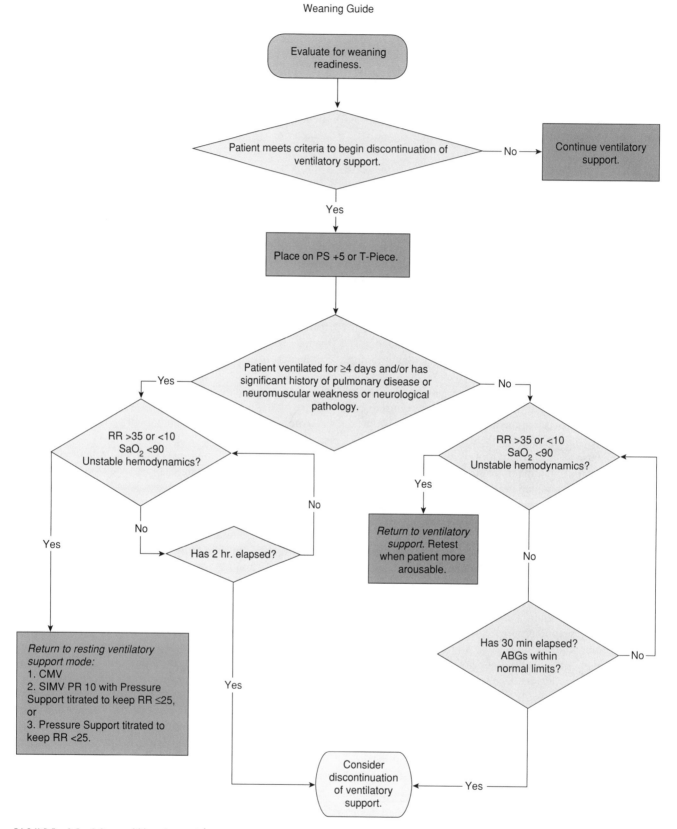

FIGURE 15–13 • Weaning guide.

patients and in patients taking sedatives. Both groups of patients can be retested in a similar fashion later in the day after the drug regimen has been changed or the anesthetics have cleared. Patients who fail the first trial because of respiratory distress or unstable hemodynamics may simply not be ready to assume the full work of breathing. If the failure was borderline, a second attempt can be considered after several hours of rest. If the failure was profound, a full night's rest is called for before another attempt is made. This delay may seem unnecessary, but it is tied to the physiology of the respiratory muscles. An exhausted respiratory muscle may require more than 24 hours to recover its baseline strength. Repeated trials only serve to push the muscle farther into metabolic debt, prolonging its recovery. These patients now advance to the complicated patient's weaning program.

Complicated patients who have had failed regular weaning may need more time for their underlying disease process to correct or may need improved respiratory muscle strength and endurance before they can assume all of the work of breathing. What constitutes a good exercise program for the respiratory muscles during mechanical ventilation is controversial. SIMV, the original mode developed to improve weaning time and comfort, has been shown to be the slowest weaning program for complicated patients. The fastest modes are AC mode with a T adapter and PS mode. The mode used may be less important than is the program employed.

Skeletal muscles should be exercised thoroughly to improve strength and endurance. Breathing spontaneously through a T adapter or on low levels of pressure support not only are good ways to test endurance but also provide thorough exercise in an undertrained muscle. From the exercise literature, we also know that the duration of exercise should be long enough to induce the **training effect.** In athletes, this is usually associated with achieving a target heart rate that is 70% of the maximum heart rate and maintaining that rate for at least 20 minutes. Such a target, however, is beyond the means of the ventilated patient. As the respiratory workload increases, the respiratory center switches over to a rapid shallow breathing pattern to forestall fatigue. Patients whose respiratory rates exceed 30 breaths/min during a weaning assessment are unlikely to succeed in the attempt. A respiratory rate in this range, then, appears to be a sign of significantly elevated work. A cutoff of 35 breaths/min as a signal that the patient has done enough work to achieve the training effect has been used in the studies cited previously. Remember that you want to exhaust the muscle only partially. Exhausting the muscle substantially may damage the muscle fiber structure, increasing recovery time from hours to days. If you have ever been a "weekend warrior" and have suffered through the intense muscle soreness that occurs after excessive exercise, you understand what we are trying to *avoid.*

Perhaps even more important in the exercise program is rest. The moderately exercised muscle needs about a day to recover adequately, and while rest does not mean "no work," it does mean avoiding the intensity of workload that exhausted the muscle in the first place. Again, a reliable indicator of work in most patients is the respiratory rate. Rates higher than 30 breaths/min are correlated with respiratory failure, so the mode and settings selected after a weaning trial should push the rate well below this number. How well below is not established, but targets that mimic normal resting respiratory rate (rates in the teens to low 20s) should do the trick.

The best mode for resting the muscle is also not well established, but SIMV by itself appears to be the loser in this regard. Remember that the respiratory center likes to see regular support when setting the work output of the next breath. Switching between supported and unsupported breaths, as in SIMV, fools the respiratory center into maintaining the higher work output; as a result, good rest is not achieved. Setting the SIMV rate at the patient's rate so that the respiratory center would see relatively consistent support is possible, but this is actually only a poor imitation of AC mode, and it is probably best to go with the real thing. AC mode is actually a good way to ensure rest, because every breath is assisted with the same support. If the patient's respiratory pattern is mimicked successfully (their demands should not be too excessive at this point), this mode is well tolerated. As long as the patient is working to trigger some of the breaths, disuse atrophy will not be a secondary complication.

Another option is PS mode. Titrated appropriately to reduce the respiratory rate to the target level, this mode also provides regular support with the advantage of a variable respiratory pattern that attempts to mimic the patient's demanded pattern. In the acute situation, the risk of no backup rate in pure pressure support is a concern, but at weaning, a stable respiratory drive should be well established before starting. If you must use SIMV, then ensure that the backup rate is set to achieve adequate minute ventilation in case the patient becomes apneic, and add pressure support titrated to achieve the target resting respiratory rate.

After developing your exercise and resting strategies, all you need is a schedule. After the exercise period, the patient will need a good day's rest to recover, so the trial is limited to once a day. Exercise once, rest until tomorrow. Do not become impatient, even if the insurance provider is pressuring! Each day before a trial is considered, the patient should be reevaluated to assess whether he or she still meets the weaning criteria. Is the patient febrile? Is the white blood cell count up? If the patient's condition deteriorates, do not add the extra stress of a spontaneous breathing trial to the mix. If the patient remains stable, go ahead and exercise. A patient who can tolerate 1 to 2 hours of exercise comfortably should be ready to sustain spontaneous breathing from then on. Use your judgment in this decision, however. If the patient has been ventilator dependent for 2 months, the first time they manage to achieve 2 hours of spontaneous breathing may not be predictive of readiness for weaning.

In summary, successful weaning involves waiting until the problem that put the patient on the ventilator is corrected or well controlled and the patient is otherwise stable. Then, the patient's spontaneous breathing ability must be tested during minimal support using the respiratory rate as a guide. Uncomplicated patients need only be tested for 30 minutes to predict success. Complicated patients may need to demonstrate up to 2 hours of spontaneous breathing on minimal support to predict success. Failure to achieve the target time goals successfully must be followed by a day's rest to allow adequate muscle recuperation.

AIRWAY ASSESSMENT

Once the patient successfully demonstrates an ability to breath spontaneously, it must be determined whether or not there is the need to maintain an artificial airway. This is not a small consideration because there is a 50% morbidity associated with extubation failure. There are three general reasons why you would maintain the airway after weaning: potential upper airway obstruction, inability to protect the airway, and inability to clear the airway.

Upper airway obstruction after extubation is uncommon but does occur. Patients with thermal injuries to their upper airways are at particular risk. One quick assessment technique involves deflating the cuff to the airway and seeing if gas will pass around it. No gas flow indicates an airway that remains edematous, and extubation in this situation would be high risk. Be sure to suction the secretions resting above the cuff before deflating it.

Obtunded patients are another group at risk because of their inability to protect their airways, increasing the risk of aspiration. Although not all obtunded patients aspirate, many do, and this potential should be considered carefully before extubation. Frequently, these patients are managed long-term with a tracheostomy.

Finally, inability to clear the airway is commonly associated with weaning and extubation failure. A weak cough combined with copious sputum production can be the "one-two punch" that pushes the patient back into respiratory failure. It may be safer to maintain the airway until this condition resolves.

References

1. Vesalius A. De humani corporis fabrica. Lib VII. Cap. XIX. *Devivorum sectione nonnulla.* Basle: Operinus; 1543:658.
2. Baker AB. Artificial respiration, the history of an idea. *Med Hist.* 1971;15:336–351.
3. Emerson JH. *The Evolution of Iron Lungs.* Cambridge: JH Emerson; 1978.
4. Nochomovitz ML, Montenegro HD, Parran S, Daly B. Placement alternatives for ventilator-dependent patients outside the intensive care units. *Respir Care.* 1991;36:199–205.
5. Hernandez LA, Peevy KJ, Moise AA, Parker JC. Chest wall restriction limits high airway pressure pulmonary edema: Respective effects of high airway pressure, high tidal volume, and positive end expiratory pressure. *Am Rev Respir Dis.* 1988;137:1159–1164.
6. West J. *Respiratory Physiology: The Essentials.* Baltimore: Williams & Wilkins; 1980.
7. Pepe PE, Marini JJ. Occult positive end-expiratory pressure in mechanically ventilated patients with airflow obstruction: The auto-PEEP effect. *Am Rev Respir Dis.* 1982;126:166–170.
8. Rossi A, Gottfried SB, Zocchi L, et al. Measurement of static compliance of the total respiratory system in patients with acute respiratory failure during mechanical ventilation: The effect of intrinsic positive end expiratory pressure. *Am Rev Respir Dis.* 1985;131:672–677.
9. Fife CE, Piantadosi CA. Oxygen toxicity. *Probl Respir Care.* 1991;4:150–171.
10. Kollef MH, Silver P. Ventilator-associated pneumonia: An update for clinicians. *Respir Care.* 1995;40:1130–1140.
11. Marini JJ, Rodriguez RM, Lamb B. The inspiratory workload of patient-initiated mechanical ventilation. *Am Rev Respir Dis.* 1986;134:902–909.
12. Anzueto A, Tobin MJ, Moore G, et al. Effect of prolonged mechanical ventilation on diaphragmatic function: A preliminary study of a baboon model. *Am Rev Respir Dis.* 1987;135:A201. (Abstract)
13. Muller DA. Influence of training and of inactivity on muscle strength. *Arch Phys Med Rehabil.* 1970;51:449–462.
14. Sassoon CSH, Mahutte CK, Light RW. Ventilator modes: Old and new. *Crit Care Clin.* 1990;6:605–634.
15. Ward ME, Corbeil C, Gibbons W, et al. Optimization of respiratory muscle relaxation during mechanical ventilation. *Anesthesiology.* 1988;69:29–35.
16. Downs JB, Klein EF, Desautels D, et al. Intermittent mandatory ventilation: A new approach to weaning patients from mechanical ventilators. *Chest.* 1973;64:331–335.
17. Shapiro BA, Harrison RA, Walton JR, Davison R. Intermittent demand ventilation (IDV): A new technique for support ventilation in critically ill patients. *Respir Care.* 1976;21:521–525.
18. Pinsky MR. The effects of mechanical ventilation on the cardiovascular system. *Crit Care Clin.* 1990;6:663–678.
19. Groeger JS, Levinson MR, Carlon GC. Assist control versus synchronized intermittent mandatory ventilation during acute respiratory failure. *Crit Care Med.* 1989;17:607–612.
20. Marini JJ, Smith TC, Lamb VJ. External work output and force generation during synchronized intermittent mechanical ventilation: Effect of machine assistance on breathing effort. *Am Rev Respir Dis.* 1988;138:1169–1179.
21. Esteban A, Frutos F, Tobin MJ, et al. *N Engl J Med.* 1995;332:345.
22. Brochard L, Rauss A, Benito S, et al. Comparison of three methods of gradual withdrawal from ventilator support during mechanical ventilation. *Am J Respir Crit Care Med.* 1993;104:1833–1859.
23. Downs JB, Stock MC, Tebeling B. Intermittent mandatory ventilation (IMV): A primary ventilatory support mode. *Ann Chir Gynaecol.* 1982;196(suppl):57–63.
24. Sassoon CSH, Mahutte CK, Te TT, et al. Work of breathing and airway occlusion pressure during assist-mode mechanical ventilation. *Chest.* 1988;93:571–576.
25. MacIntyre NR. Respiratory function during pressure support ventilation. *Chest.* 1986;89:677–683.
26. Brochard L, Pluskwa F, Lemaire F. Improved efficacy of spontaneous breathing with inspiratory pressure support. *Am Rev Respir Dis.* 1987;136:411–415.
27. Murphy DF, Dobb GD. Effect of pressure support on spontaneous ventilation during intermittent mandatory ventilation. *Crit Care Med.* 1987;15:612–613.
28. Marini JJ. Weaning from mechanical ventilation. *N Engl J Med.* 1991;324:1496–1497.
29. Brochard L, Harf A, Lorino H, Lemaire F. Inspiratory pressure support prevents diaphragmatic fatigue during weaning from mechanical ventilation. *Am Rev Respir Dis.* 1989;139:513–521.
30. Kanak R, Fahey PJ, Vanderwharf C. Oxygen cost of breathing changes dependent upon mode of mechanical ventilation. *Chest.* 1985;87:126–127.
31. Stewart KG. Clinical evaluation of pressure support ventilation. *Br J Anaesth.* 1989;63:362–364.
32. Brochard L. Pressure support ventilation. In: Marini JJ, Roussos C, eds. *Ventilatory Failure.* Berlin: Springer-Verlag; 1991:381–391.
33. Tejeda M, Boix JH, Alvarez F, et al. Comparison of pressure support ventilation and assist-control ventilation in the treatment of respiratory failure. *Chest.* 1997;111(5):1322.
34. Black JW, Brover GS. A hazard of pressure support ventilation. *Chest.* 1988;93:333–335.

35. Beaty CD, Ritz RM, Benson MS. Continuous in-line nebulizers complicate pressure support ventilation. *Chest.* 1989;96:1360–1363.

36. Jackson RM. Pulmonary oxygen toxicity. *Chest.* 1985;88:900–905.

37. Dreyfuss D, Soler P, Basset G, Saumon G. High inflation pressure pulmonary edema: Respective effects of high airway pressure, high tidal volume and positive end expiratory pressure. *Am Rev Respir Dis.* 1988;137:1159–1164.

38. Kolobow T, Moretti MP, Fumagalli R, et al. Severe impairment in lung function induced by high peak airway pressure during mechanical ventilation: An experimental study. *Am Rev Respir Dis.* 1987;135:312–315.

39. Hernandez LA, Coker PJ, May S, et al. Mechanical ventilation increases microvascular permeability in oleic acid-injured lungs. *J Appl Physiol.* 1990;69:2057–2061.

40. West J. *Respiratory Physiology: The Essentials.* Baltimore: Williams & Wilkins; 1980.

41. Gattinoni I, Pelosi P, Pesenti A, et al. CT scan in ARDS: Clinical and physiopathological insights. *Acta Anaesthesiol Scand.* 1991;35(suppl 95):87–96.

42. Tuxen D, Williams T, Scheinkestel C, et al. Limiting dynamic hyperinflation in mechanically ventilated patients with severe asthma reduces complications. *Anaesth Intensive Care.* 1993; 21(5):718.

43. Amato M, Barbas C, Medeiros D, et al. Improved lung mechanics and oxygenation achieved through a new approach to mechanical ventilation in ARDS: The importance of reducing the "mechanical stress" on the lung. *Am Rev Respir Dis.* 1993;147:A890.

44. Hickling K, Henderson S, Jackson R. Low mortality associated with low volume pressure limited ventilation with permissive hypercapnia in severe adult respiratory distress syndrome. *Intensive Care Med.* 1990;16:372–377.

45. Tuxen D, Williams T, Scheinkestel C, et al. Limiting dynamic hyperinflation in mechanically ventilated patients with severe asthma reduces complications. *Anaesth Intensive Care.* 1993; 21(5):718.

46. Nahum A, Burke W, Ravenscraft S, et al. Lung mechanics and gas exchange during pressure control ventilation in dogs: Augmentation of CO_2 elimination by an intratracheal catheter. *Am Rev Respir Dis.* 1992;146:965.

47. American Thoracic Society. Standardization of spirometry 1994 update. *Am J Respir Crit Care Med.* 1995;152(3):1107–1136.

Part II
Noninvasive Mechanical Ventilation

A remarkable number of complications are associated with artificial airways. Oral, pharyngeal, and tracheal damage can occur during insertion, use, and extubation, particularly when patients perform the extubation themselves. Intubated, mechanically ventilated patients have a higher risk of developing nosocomial pneumonia, which as an associated mortality rate of 55% to 71%.[1] See Box 15–7 for an *abbreviated* list of complications.

It would appear, then, that the ability to ventilate mechanically without an artificial airway would be preferable. In fact, one of the most widespread mechanical devices used to support ventilation during the first half of the 20th century was noninvasive: the **iron lung** (Box 15–8). An iron lung, or tank respiratory, was basically a large chamber that held a patient's entire body, with the head sticking out of one end. A vacuum pump was attached to the chamber to develop cyclical negative pressure around the thorax, simulating the negative pressure that the diaphragm would normally produce in the chest to drive breathing. A seal around the patient's neck kept the negative pressure localized around the lower end of the body, creating a pressure gradient between the patient's mouth, which remained at the higher atmospheric pressure, and the thorax. The amount of negative pressure applied controlled the tidal volume that developed. During the polio epidemics in the 1930s, iron lungs, especially the improved version created by Emerson, became the norm for ventilatory support of patients with respiratory paralysis.[2]

Although the complications of artificial airways are abolished with the iron lung, its use has several limitations (Fig. 15–14). First, the patient is trapped in an enormous cylinder with only the head exposed to the elements and with limited access to care providers. Opening the cylinder halts the machine's ability to ventilate, so one had to be very quick at changing the sheets. Even the positive-pressure ventilators developed later, which were adapted for

Box • 15–7 COMPLICATIONS OF INTUBATION
• Aspiration during and after intubation
• Obstruction of lumen by secretions
• Increased risk of nosocomial pneumonia
• Esophageal intubation
• Mainstem bronchus intubation
• Lip ulceration
• Glottic edema
• Laryngospasm during intubation
• Broken or dislocated tooth
• Tracheal edema and necrosis
• Tracheoarterial or tracheoesophageal fistula
• Tracheomalacia or dilation
• Reduced mucocilliary clearance
• Self-extubation
• Inability to verbalize
• Impaired cough
• Increased airway resistance from tube
• Tracheal narrowing from granuloma
• Vocal cord dysfunction, stridor

From Stauffer J. Complications of translaryngeal intubation. In Tobin MJ. *Principles and Practice of Mechanical Ventilation.* New York: McGraw-Hill; 1994.

Box • 15–8	TYPES OF EXTERNAL NEGATIVE-PRESSURE VENTILATION

Iron lung (tank respirator)
Chest cuirass
Rocking bed
Pneumobelt
Diaphragmatic pacing

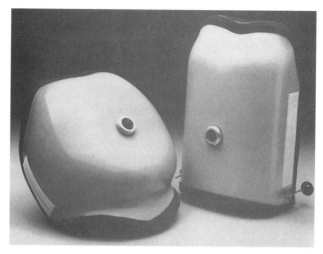

FIGURE 15–15 • Ready-made chest cuirass. (Courtesy of Respironics, Inc., Pittsburgh, PA.)

noninvasive use by the addition of a mouthpiece, were used only infrequently.

Another type of **external negative-pressure ventilator** (ENPV) introduced at the beginning of the 20th century is the chest cuirass ventilator (Fig. 15–15). A rigid, turtle-shell–shaped case, or cuirass, is sealed over the patient's thorax, and a negative-pressure pump is attached by a large-bore hose. Cycling the pump creates negative pressure, pulling out the patient's chest, and pulling air into the lungs. Because only half of the chest is exposed to negative pressure, the cuirass is less effective than the iron lung at ventilation, but it is a significant improvement when it comes to patient care and mobility. To fit the patient for the cuirass, a custom or semi-custom shell must be made, and even then, there are usually problems from the constant rubbing of the shell on the chest. Although not effective for critically ill patients, some stable, ventilation-dependent patients use a chest cuirass at home for support.

Also popular during the polio epidemics were the rocking bed and the pneumobelt, which were mechanical devices that used gravity to assist ventilation (Fig. 15–16). If you can imagine a wide, motorized see-saw with a mattress, you have visualized the rocking bed. Pivoting at the

patient's waist, the bed tilted up and down at a 45-degree angle. When the head moved down, gravity pulled the abdominal contents down against the diaphragm, assisting exhalation. When the head moved up, the abdominal contents fell away and pulled the diaphragm with them, assisting inspiration. Rocking beds were mostly used to assist weaning from iron lungs.[3]

The pneumobelt, another gravity-assist device, aided ventilation of a sitting patient (Fig. 15–17). A pneumobelt is a wide strap that wraps around the abdomen with an inflatable bladder in the front. The bladder was attached to a positive-pressure ventilator that would cyclically inflate the bladder. As the bladder inflated, the abdominal contents were compressed and pushed up against the diaphragm, assisting exhalation. When it deflated, the abdomen fell down, assisting inspiration. Pneumobelts were significantly less constraining than the iron lung and

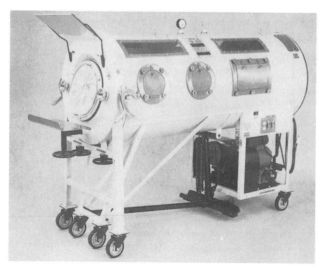

FIGURE 15–14 • The Emerson iron lung. (Courtesy of J.H. Emerson, Cambridge, MA.)

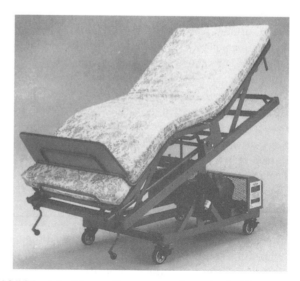

FIGURE 15–16 • Emerson rocking bed. (Courtesy of J.H. Emerson, Cambridge, MA.)

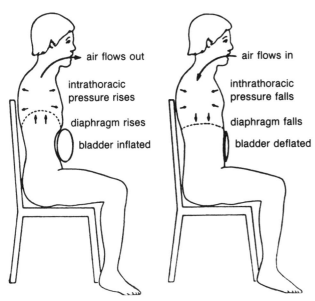

FIGURE 15-17 • A pneumobelt assists exhalation by compressing the abdomen and pushing up the diaphragm, and then deflating, allowing gravity to pull the diaphragm down, which assists inspiration. (From Hill NS, Clinical application of body ventilators. *Chest* 1986;90:897–905.)

rocking bed; patients could eat and use their arms while in a chair with the belt.

Advances in technology in the 1960s led to the development of a device that could electronically stimulate, or pace, the diaphragm when it has been cut off from the central nervous system. For **diaphragmatic pacing** to work, the patient must have relatively normal lungs and an intact phrenic nerve. This essentially limits the use of diaphragmatic pacing to two conditions: spinal cord injuries that paralyze the diaphragm and central hypoventilation syndrome, in which the respiratory center fails to maintain ventilation during sleep. Pacing must be initiated cautiously to prevent diaphragm fatigue and nerve trauma. A tracheostomy is required for most patients who have diaphragmatic pacing devices implanted, primarily to prevent upper airway obstruction and maintenance of bronchial hygiene.[4]

Positive-pressure devices have also been used to assist polio patients, typically using a tracheostomy, but in some cases using a mouthpiece. In 1987, Bach and colleagues[5] reported their experience in effectively ventilating 43 patients for a mean of 17.9 years using positive pressure and a mouthpiece, with relatively few complications in those patients who tolerated it.

Beginning in the 1960s, intermittent positive-pressure breathing (IPPB) therapy was evaluated for its effects on patients with chronic obstructive pulmonary disease (COPD). Although early studies demonstrated that IPPB was not beneficial,[6] widespread use of the therapy persisted. In 1983, the results of a large randomized controlled trial clearly demonstrated the ineffectiveness of IPPB in

patients with COPD.[7] These studies, however, focused more on the use of IPPB as a means of delivering aerosolized bronchodilators than as a ventilatory support device.

Improved positive-pressure ventilator technology, reduced cost, and better mask design have led to an increase in the use of **noninvasive positive-pressure ventilation** (NPPV). Beginning in the mid-1980s, a succession of (uncontrolled) studies demonstrated that NPPV is effective in reversing ventilatory failure in a number of diseases.

INDICATIONS

The goals of NPPV are identical to the goals of conventional ventilation: reduction in work of breathing and restoration of adequate gas exchange, just without placement of an artificial airway. This may be used to avoid the complications of an artificial airway, or when placement or maintenance of the artificial airway may be undesirable to the patient (Box 15–9). The most successful uses of NPPV identified are in patients with neuromuscular disorders, restrictive lung disease secondary to deformities of the spine or rib cage, and central hypoventilation syndrome[8–10] (Box 15–10). NPPV for the treatment of respiratory failure secondary to COPD is still controversial; some investigators have reported success, whereas others have found it less effective. NPPV has also been suggested as a strategy to prevent or postpone intubation and to assist in supporting patients who are failing after the withdrawal of conventional ventilatory support.[11] Other goals associated with the chronic aspects of NPPV are the prevention of the cardiovascular complications associated with chronic hypoxemia and hypercapnia, improved daytime alertness, and improved quality of life.

LIMITATIONS AND HAZARDS

The major limitations associated with NPPV involve the mask interface. The most often reported complaints are facial pain and discomfort, pressure sores, and difficulty sleeping secondary to the mask delivery system. Many of these problems can be avoided or minimized by ensuring

---

Box • 15–9 INDICATIONS FOR NONINVASIVE POSITIVE-PRESSURE VENTILATION

- Patient with respiratory failure, who refuses intubation but desires assistance
- To avoid intubation
- To assist failing patient after extubation
- Patient who requests decannulation
- To facilitate chronic home ventilation

Box • 15–10 PATIENTS IN WHOM NONINVASIVE POSITIVE-PRESSURE VENTILATION MAY BE EFFECTIVE

• Patients with progressive respiratory failure due to
    neuromuscular disease
    restrictive chest wall disease
    obesity hypoventilation syndrome
    central hypoventilation syndrome
    COPD

---

that the mask is fit carefully and that the patient is allowed sufficient time to acclimate to the mask and harness.

Leaks are a common problem with masks and lead to their own subset of complications. Oral leaks occur most commonly after the patient has fallen asleep and the mouth is open. Flow from the ventilator follows this open channel back out to the atmosphere, drying the oral and nasal cavities from the high flows of escaping gas. A chin strap can be added to the headgear to hold the mouth closed during sleep and may correct this problem. Mask leaks can also hinder the ventilator's ability to sense a patient's inspiratory effort, resulting in increased work of breathing from patient–ventilator dysynchrony.[12] Leaks can also interfere with a ventilator's ability to sense when to terminate pressure support. Some machines rely on the expiratory flow to fall to a threshold level before cycling off the pressure support. If a leak prevents the flow from falling to this level, inspiration can be extended beyond the patient's desired inspiratory time, again resulting in patient ventilator dysynchrony.

Gastric distention has also been reported but can be minimized if applied pressures are kept below 20 cm H_2O.[13] The patient must also be able to clear the secretions and maintain the airway. Finally, many patients, especially those with neuromuscular diseases, may require continuous assistance to use NPPV, although this would also be true of conventional invasive ventilation.

Generally, ENPV is less effective than NPPV at maintaining gas exchange, especially when airway resistance is high or lung compliance is low.[14] There is also an increased tendency for upper airway obstruction to occur during sleep secondary to the external negative pressure applied during ENPV. This obstruction results in cyclic arterial oxyhemoglobin desaturation similar to the desaturation that accompanies obstructive sleep apnea.[15]

NONINVASIVE POSITIVE-PRESSURE VENTILATION HARDWARE

Noninvasive positive-pressure ventilation has been attempted with just about every ventilator ever produced. The ideal NPPV ventilator would be easy to trigger, would adjust for leaks around the mask, and would be able to deliver large volumes quickly to minimize work of breathing. The ideal machine would also provide a variety of modes so that a good fit between the patient's condition and the level of support could be achieved.

It is possible to deliver NPPV with conventional pressure triggered, volume-cycled intensive care unit (ICU) ventilators. These ventilators typically have a variety of modes and are fully alarmed for safety. Their major limitation is in their pressure-triggering feature, which functions well with a sealed endotracheal tube but does not tolerate a leaky mask interface. In the presence of a leak, the circuit pressure can drop below the preset trigger sensitivity threshold, which cycles the ventilator on. This is fine if the patient was planning to take a breath but usually puts the ventilator and the patient "out of synch." Leaks in a pressure triggered system also "dilute" the patients inspiratory effort by allowing ambient gas to enter the circuit. This extra gas interferes with triggering sensitivity as the buildup of negative pressure in the circuit is delayed. Pressure triggered machines are best saved for patients with artificial airways.

Ventilators that are flow triggered can be adjusted to compensate for leaks function much more effectively during mask ventilation. An example of an ICU ventilator with adjustable flow triggering is the 7200 (Puritan Bennett, Carlsbad, CA) with the Flow-by 2.0 option. Flow-by mode activates a flow-triggering mechanism with parameters that can be set by the operator. A continuous flow in the circuit can be set from 5 to 20 L/min, and triggering can be adjusted to occur when that flow drops from 1 to 15 L/min below the continuous flow at the expiratory transducer. In a patient whose mask is regularly leaking 3 to 4 L/min, the continuous flow can be set at 20 L/min, and the trigger can be set 5 or 6 L/min under so that the leak of 3 to 4 L/min does not result in accidental triggering. A widely variable leak is more difficult because the trigger has to be set to compensate for the highest leak, but at the lowest leak, the patient is forced to generate a very high inspiratory flow to trigger a breath. The 7200 also has a short response time, can generate high pressures, and sets off an alarm and returns to timed ventilation if the patient becomes apneic. On the other hand, the 7200 is expensive, as are other full-featured ICU ventilators. If an institution is already using the device for conventional ventilation, then adapting it for occasional NPPV use is reasonable, but to purchase one only for NPPV use would not be cost-effective, especially in the home.

An example device to consider in the home or subacute care setting is the the BiPAP ventilator (Respironics, Pittsburgh, PA), which is flow triggered and adjusts its trigger automatically to compensate for leaks (Fig. 15–18). In fact, the BiPAP is designed to have a continuous leak from an adapter near the mask to flush exhaled CO_2 from the circuit (Fig. 15–19). Designed specifically for noninvasive use, the BiPAP evolved from earlier continuous positive airway pressure (CPAP) devices developed to administer CPAP by

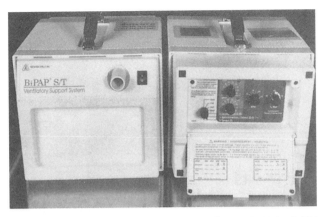

FIGURE 15-18 • The BiPAP ventilator (BiPAP S/T-D model pictured). (Courtesy of Respironics, Pittsburgh, PA.)

nasal mask for the treatment of obstructive sleep apnea. In addition to delivering CPAP (identified on the device as EPAP, for expiratory positive airway pressure), the BiPAP has an IPAP setting (for inspiratory positive airway pressure) that, if set higher than the EPAP level, causes the ventilator to deliver a pressure-support–type breath during inspiration when triggered by the patient. These two pres-

sure levels can be combined and controlled in four breathing modes: CPAP (EPAP only), spontaneous (IPAP and EPAP, like pressure support), spontaneous/timed (a backup rate and an inspiratory time percent can be set, and the mode operates like synchronized intermittent mandatory ventilation plus pressure control/pressure support), and timed (cycles between the pressures at the rate and inspiratory time percent set; the patient cannot trigger additional supported breaths). One major limitation of the BiPAP ventilator is its maximum generating pressure of 22 cm H_2O, which may not be able to ventilate patients effectively who have too low of a compliance or too high of an airway resistance. Another downside to the BiPAP is its lack of alarms. Without the addition of external alarms, only patients who can survive disconnection or mechanical failure should be considered for BiPAP ventilation.

The mask interface for NPPV comes in an assortment of applications, including full-face masks, nasal masks, and nasal pillows. A mouthpiece is available for patients who use ENPV at night and occasionally need NPPV during the day.[16]

Full-face masks are typically used in acute respiratory failure situations[13,17] (Fig. 15–20). Proper sizing and fit are essential for patient tolerance. The top of the mask should sit near the top of the bridge of the nose to prevent leaks into the eyes, and the bottom of the mask should sit just below the lower lip. The headgear should be adjusted so that a moderate but firm pressure is evenly distributed across the mask. The occasional leak is expected; the mask should not be on so tightly as to obliterate all leaks all the time. The complications of excessive mask pressure are a primary cause of patient intolerance.[18] Frequently, leaks are due to the mask being too tight at one point, tilting the mask off the face. Avoid the temptation to keep tightening the mask to seal a leak. It may be best to start over with a loose setting to ensure that the headgear is holding the mask evenly on the face. Other problems with full-face

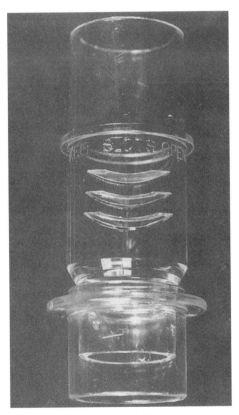

FIGURE 15-19 • "Whisper" swivel adapter for the Bi-PAP creates a continuous leak in the circuit. (From Kacmarek RM, Hess D. Equipment required for home mechanical ventilation. In: Tobin MJ, ed. *Principles and Practice of Mechanical Ventilation*. New York: McGraw-Hill, 1994. Reproduced with permission of the McGraw-Hill Companies.)

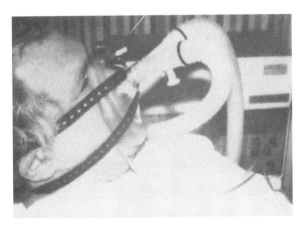

FIGURE 15-20 • Full-face mask and fastening headgear. (From Meduri GU, Conoscenti CC, Menashe PH, Nair S. Noninvasive face mask ventilation in patients with acute respiratory failure. *Chest* 1989;95:865–870.)

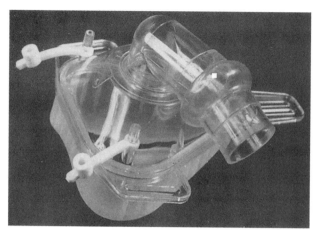

FIGURE 15–21 • Nasal mask with ports to bleed in O_2 or to monitor pressure. (From Kacmarek RM, Hess D. Equipment required for home mechanical ventilation. In: Tobin MJ, ed. *Principles and Practice of Mechanical Ventilation.* New York: McGraw-Hill, 1994. Reproduced with permission of the McGraw-Hill Companies.)

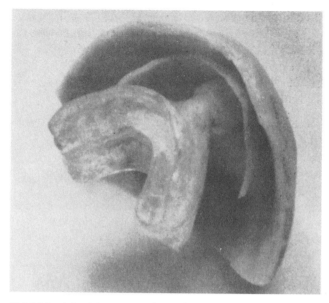

FIGURE 15–23 • Ready-made mouthpiece with flange. (From Back JR, Alba A, Saporito LR. Intermittent positive-pressure ventilation via the mouth as an alternative to tracheostomy for 257 ventilator users. *Chest* 1993;103:174–182.)

masks are the claustrophobia experienced by some patients and the large internal dead space that must be overcome.

Most NPPV applications are set up with a nasal mask (Fig. 15–21). A variety of mask sizes and shapes are being produced for nasal ventilation, and custom masks can be created. Again, mask fit is essential to success. A rule of thumb to consider when sizing is that the smaller the mask, the better is the fit.[18] The bottom of the fitted mask should ride close to the nares without occluding them, the sides should follow the contour of the sides of the nose, and the top should be near the top of the bridge of the nose. The least amount of pressure necessary to achieve a seal should be applied. Consider adding a chin strap to hold the mouth closed if oral leaks occur, although these straps are not always successful in preventing leaks.

A variation of the nasal mask is the nasal pillow (Fig. 15–22). Some patients find this interface more comfortable than a nasal mask. Nasal pillows can also be considered when pressure sores or irritation preclude ongoing use of the mask.

Mouthpieces have also been used successfully by some patients for up to 24 hours/d.[16] Ready-made mouthpieces are available, but patients tolerate custom-made mouthpieces better and for longer periods (Fig. 15–23). Nose clips may be necessary in some patients to prevent nasal leaks.

INITIATION AND MANAGEMENT OF NONINVASIVE POSITIVE-PRESSURE VENTILATION

For management of uncomplicated obstructive sleep apnea, a basic CPAP-generating device and a properly fitting nasal mask are generally effective. An applied pressure of between 5 and 10 cm H_2O is usually sufficient to keep the upper airway patent and prevent obstruction.[19] If apnea is not prevented by CPAP alone, consider testing the patient using a ventilator that can provide a backup rate like the BiPAP.

Patients with stable, chronic ventilator insufficiency from a variety of causes respond well to nasal pressure support. This has been tested using an ICU-type ventilator (Bird 6400 ST, Palm Springs, CA) in patients with stable

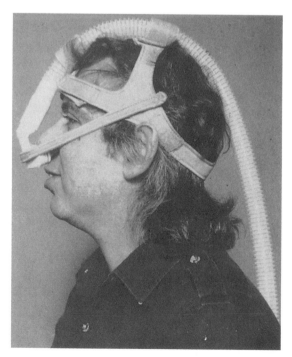

FIGURE 15–22 • Nasal pillows and fastening headgear. (Courtesy of Nellcor Puritan-Bennett Inc., Pleasanton, CA.)

but severe COPD.[20] Applying pressure-support values of 10 and 20 cm H_2O, patients demonstrated larger tidal volumes, lower respiratory frequencies, and reduced electromyogram activity of the diaphragm with nasal pressure support than with spontaneous breathing. Research using a BiPAP device demonstrated similar results in a group of patients with COPD and neuromuscular disease.[21] Both of these studies also applied 5 cm H_2O or more of positive end-expiratory pressure (PEEP) and found further improvements in respiratory parameters. PEEP levels of more than 5 cm H_2O were associated with a decreased CO_2 clearance, perhaps because of the higher PEEP-increased dead space/tidal volume ratios. Nasal pressure support can be applied and titrated with the same strategy as conventional pressure support. Titrate the pressure support up until respiratory work is reduced to a comfortable level based on the respiratory rate and other signs of respiratory muscle work. This may require higher pressure-support levels than typically used in conventional ventilation, particularly in patients with high impedance to gas flow.

In the acute rescue situation, in which NPPV is being used instead of or to avoid intubation, a full-face mask appears to be the interface of choice.[11] AC and PS modes have both undergone trial in acute situations, and there is some evidence that PS mode may be better tolerated than is assist-control mode.[22] As mentioned earlier, leaks may interfere with the effectiveness of pressure-support ventilation. Leaks also decrease the effectiveness of ventilation when assist-control mode is used because the ventilator does not increase the tidal volume in response to a leak. Frequently, this tidal volume loss is managed by increasing the tidal volume. Higher tidal volumes, however, can result in higher-peak pressures if the leak is variable and if a large volume combines with a small leak. This can lead to tightening of the mask to reduce the leak, which reduces patient tolerance of the mask and increases the risk of complications.

References

1. Meduri GU. Ventilator-associated pneumonia in patients with respiratory failure: A diagnostic approach. *Chest*. 1990;97:1208–1219.
2. Emerson JH. *The Evolution of Iron Lungs*. Cambridge: JH Emerson; 1978.
3. Lewis L, Hirschberg GG, Adamson JP. Respiratory rehabilitation in poliomyelitis. *Arch Phys Med Rehabil*. 1957;38:243–249.
4. Glenn WWL, Brouillette RT, Dentz B, et al. Fundamental considerations in pacing of the diaphragm for chronic ventilatory insufficiency: A multi-center study. *PACE*. 1988;11:2121–2127.
5. Bach JR, Alba AS, Bohatiuk G, et al. Mouth intermittent positive pressure ventilation in the management of post-polio respiratory insufficiency. *Chest*. 1987;91:859–864.
6. Thornton JA, Darke CS, Herbert P. Intermittent positive pressure breathing (IPPB) in chronic respiratory disease. *Anaesthesia*. 1974;29:44–49.
7. The Intermittent Positive Pressure Breathing Trial Group. Intermittent positive pressure breathing therapy of chronic obstructive pulmonary disease. *Ann Intern Med*. 1983;99:612–620.
8. Heckmatt JZ, Loh L, Dubowitz V. Night-time nasal ventilation in neuromuscular disease. *Lancet*. 1990;2:579–582.
9. Ellis ER, Grunstein RR, Chan S, et al. Noninvasive ventilatory support during sleep improves respiratory failure in kyphoscoliosis. *Chest*. 1988;94:811–815.
10. Caroll N, Branthwaite MA. Control of nocturnal hypoventilation by nasal intermittent positive pressure ventilation. *Thorax*. 1988;43:349–353.
11. Brochard L. Noninvasive ventilation in acute respiratory failure. *Respir Care*. 1996;41:456–465.
12. Carrey Z, Gottfried SB, Levy RD. Ventilatory muscle support in respiratory failure with nasal positive pressure ventilation. *Chest*. 1990;97(1):150–158.
13. Brochard L, Isabey D, Piquet J, et al. Reversal of acute exacerbations of chronic obstructive lung disease by inspiratory assistance with a face mask. *N Engl J Med*. 1990;323(22):1523–1530.
14. Ellis ER, Bye PTB, Bruderer JW, Sullivan CE. Treatment of respiratory failure during sleep in patients with neuromuscular disease. *Am Rev Respir Dis*. 1987;135:148–152.
15. Caroll N, Branthwaite MA. Control of nocturnal hypoventilation by nasal intermittent positive pressure ventilation. *Thorax*. 1988;43:349–353.
16. Back JR, Alba A, Saporito LR. Intermittent positive-pressure ventilation via the mouth as an alternative to tracheostomy for 257 ventilator users. *Chest*. 1993;103:174–182.
17. Meduri GU, Abou-Shala N, Fox RC, et al. Noninvasive face mask mechanical ventilation in patients with acute respiratory failure. *Chest*. 1991;100:445–454.
18. Kacmarek RM, Hess D. Equipment required for home mechanical ventilation. In: Tobin MJ, ed. *Principles and Practice of Mechanical Ventilation*. New York: McGraw-Hill; 1994.
19. Sullivan CE, Berthon Jones M, Issa FG. Reversal of obstructive sleep apnoea by continuous positive airway pressure applied through the nares. *Lancet*. 1983;1:862–865.
20. Nava S, Ambrosino N, Rubini F, et al. Effect of nasal pressure support ventilation and external PEEP on diaphragmatic activity in patients with severe stable COPD. *Chest*. 1993;103:143–150.
21. Elliot MW, Aquilina RA, Simonds AK. A comparison of the effects of nasal ventilation and CPAP on respiratory muscle function. *Eur Respir J*. 1992;5:482s. (Abstract)
22. Vitacca M, Rubini F, Foglio K, et al. Noninvasive modalities of positive pressure improve the outcome of acute exacerbations in COLD patients. *Intensive Care Med*. 1993;19(8):450–455.

Pediatric Considerations

16

Robert M. Lewis

Key Terms

bronchopulmonary
 dysplasia (BPD)
deceleration
intraventricular hemorrhage
 (IVH)
law of La Place
meconium
neutral thermal environment
newborn resuscitation
persistent pulmonary
 hypertension of the
 newborn (PPHN)
Poiseuille's law
retinopathy of prematurity
 (ROP)
time constant

Objectives

- Summarize the key patterns of the development of respiratory function and structure in the newborn, infant, and child.

- Discuss the etiology and prevention of respiratory care-related complications in the infant.

- List danger signs of impending deterioration in the newborn.

- Summarize controversies related to treatment of RSV infection in infants.

- Review the prevention and management of severe asthma.

- Discuss the similarities and differences in mechanical ventilation of the child and adult.

- Summarize the risks and benefits of chest physical therapy in the infant and child.

- Review the differentiation of upper and lower airway obstruction in the child.

Pulmonary structure and function in children differ from adult norms in a number of ways. A brief review will enable the practitioner to understand the differing presentations of respiratory disease and response to therapy in the premature and full-term newborn, the infant, and child.

GROWTH AND DEVELOPMENT OF LUNG STRUCTURES

The Airways

The most important function of the airways is to allow gas flow to and from the gas-exchanging portion of the lung. This is best accomplished when airway resistance is low. The factors influencing the ability of the airways to conduct air are best described by **Poiseuille's law,** which states the following:

$$Resistance = 8ln \div (\pi[r^4]),$$
where *l* refers to the length of the airway
and *n* is the viscosity of the inspired gas

Neither the length of the airway nor the viscosity of the inspired gas is likely to change in response to acute respiratory illness. Airway resistance, however, is exquisitely sensitive to changes in airway diameter. Small changes in airway diameter can have large effects on airway resistance.

In the healthy state, the infant's airway diameter ranges from one half (eg, the bronchioles) to one third (eg, the trachea) of the adult diameter.[1] Naturally, this results in a substantial increase in airway resistance. Because infants and children have lower minute ventilation, the impact on the overall work of breathing is minimized. The relatively small diameter of an infant's airway, however, does allow for clinically significant increases in the work of breathing after even small changes in airway diameter. As illustrated in Figure 16–1, 1 mm of edema produces a three-fold increase in resistance in adults but a 16-fold increase in infants.

The Upper Airways

For a number of reasons, upper airway obstruction is a common cause of respiratory distress in children. First, the newborn is considered an obligate nose breather for the first several months of life, partly because of the relatively large size of the tongue and the lack of teeth, which allows for complete mouth closure. In addition to being obviously smaller than an open mouth, the nasal airway is more easily affected by inflammatory processes, which cause mucus hypersecretion and obstruction. Assessing the patency of the nasal airway is essential to evaluating respiratory distress in an infant, and simple measures, such as frequent nasal suctioning with a bulb syringe, can relieve respiratory distress in many infants.

The larynx of an infant or child also differs from that of an adult in several important aspects. First, it is shaped more like a funnel, with the narrowest portion being at the cricoid cartilage at the beginning of the trachea.[2] Because the cricoid cartilage encircles the airway completely, edema developing at this point is at the expense of the internal diameter of the airway. This location is the most likely site of obstruction, for example, after removal of an endotracheal tube. The larynx is also prone to collapse because of the relative weakness of the supporting cartilage.

The Lower Airways

The most clinically relevant characteristic of the lower airway is the thinness of the airway wall, largely caused by the relative lack of cartilage and connective tissue. Airway stability is maintained, in part, by the resting tone of the bronchial smooth muscle. When this resting tone is abolished or decreased by the use of β_2-adrenergic receptor agents, the airway may be more prone to collapse, especially when high expiratory transmural pressures are generated, such as when crying or coughing.[1] Infants should

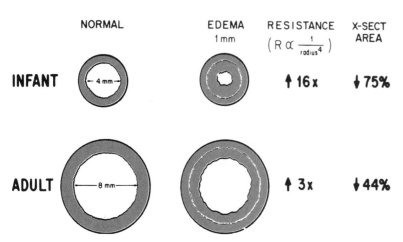

FIGURE 16–1 • Comparison of the effects of edema on airway resistance in infants and adults. Normal airways are represented on the left, edematous airways (with 1 mm of circumferential edema) on the right. Resistance to flow is inversely proportional to the fourth power of the lumen radius for laminar flow and to the fifth power for turbulent flow. The net result is a 75% decrease in cross-sectional area and a 16-fold increase in resistance in the infant versus 44% and three-fold in the adult during quiet breathing. Turbulent flow in the child (eg, crying) would increase the work of breathing 32-fold. (Cotes CJ, Todres ID. The pediatric airway. In: Cotes CJ, Ryan JF, Todres ID, Goudsouzian NH, eds. *A Practice of Anesthesia for Infants and Children.* Orlando: Grune & Stratton; 1986:39.)

be assessed for paradoxical airway collapse after β_2-agonist administration. Possible signs include increased respiratory rate, retractions, and blood gas deterioration.

The Alveoli

The lung of a newborn infant has about 20 million alveoli. The average diameter of each alveolus is substantially smaller than that of adult alveoli, and the structure is far less complex. Throughout the first 3 years of life, the number of alveoli multiplies rapidly, reaching the adult value of about 300 million. During this period, alveoli do not grow much in size.[3,4] After about 3 years of age, however, alveolar growth occurs chiefly in size, not number. That is, few if any new alveoli develop after this time.

The **law of La Place** states the following:

$$P = 2st \div r,$$

where P is intraalveolar pressure,
st is surface tension, and r is alveolar radius

This law suggests that the alveoli of infants and small children are inherently unstable because of their smaller diameter. This instability may make alveolar collapse more likely, especially when surfactant production is decreased.

The Chest Wall

The compliance of the chest wall in infants and children is much higher than that in adults.[1] This is primarily the result of the cartilaginous nature of the ribs. This proves to be advantageous during vaginal delivery because it allows the chest to pass more easily through the birth canal. This reduces trauma to the baby and mother, and the compression of the chest allows for expulsion of fetal lung fluid during birth. Furthermore, the elastic recoil after compression assists in the infant's first postnatal breath.

Beyond this, however, the highly compliant chest wall may actually predispose the pediatric patient to respiratory problems. In the intact chest, resting lung volume is maintained by a balance of the natural retractile forces of the lung and the natural expansive tendencies of the ribs. When the retractile forces of the lung increase, such as in surfactant deficiency states, the loss of lung volume is increased in the infant and child because the extremely flexible (ie, compliant) nature of the chest wall allows it to draw inward.

The lower lung volume, reflected in a lower functional residual capacity (FRC), increases the degree of hypoxemia seen when the retractile forces of the lung increase. Furthermore, the law of La Place suggests that the work required to inflate alveoli increases when inspiration begins at low alveolar diameter. When the infant attempts to inflate the low-volume alveoli, the resultant decrease in intrapleural pressure often results paradoxically in further inward motion of the chest wall, rather than alveolar inflation. Because the soft tissue between the ribs draws inward to a greater extent than the ribs themselves, this phenomenon manifests as retractions, a classic hallmark of respiratory distress in infants and children.

Ventilatory Muscles

Infants and children have less intercostal muscle mass than the adult. This contributes to the increased chest wall compliance and its consequences, already discussed. Furthermore, the diaphragm of the infant and child is also histologically different. That is, there are fewer high oxidative muscle fibers capable of prolonged activity without fatigue. In the preterm infant, these fibers make up 10% of the total; in the full-term infant, 25%, and in the adult, 40%.[5] This leaves the pediatric patient more prone to respiratory muscle fatigue.

The Developing Lung: Physiologic Considerations

Closing Volume

The closing volume is the lung volume at which airways begin to close during expiration. In healthy adults, the closing volume is usually below the FRC. This means that most airways remain patent throughout the ventilatory cycle, maximizing exchange of CO_2 and O_2.

In children, however, the closing volume is often above the FRC, meaning some portion of the airways close toward the end of exhalation, preventing normal alveolar emptying. Likewise, these airways may remain closed for part of the inspiratory phase, reducing alveolar ventilation. The closing volume may rise even higher, above the tidal volume range, when airway or alveolar disease is present.[4]

Oxygen Consumption and Oxygen Reserve

Oxygen consumption may be as much as 200% higher in infants and children than in adults.[1] This accounts, in part, for the relatively higher minute ventilation and cardiac output in children. If ventilation is interrupted for a period of time (eg, during muscle paralysis to facilitate intubation), the infant is dependent on oxygen reserve to meet the body's demands. The most important part of the oxygen reserve is the infant's FRC. The FRC of infants and children is about 30 mL/kg, about the same as the adult value. Furthermore, the alveolar surface area, which determines in part the rate at which oxygen in the alveoli is made available to the red blood cells, is also about equal to the adult value of 1 M^2/kg.[1] Therefore, the infant's ability to replace the oxygen rapidly consumed at the tissue level is not increased in proportion to the increased demands. These data support the common clinical observation that infants and children become hypoxemic more rapidly than adults during periods of hypoventilation and apnea.

Table • 16–1. COMPARISON OF NORMAL VALUES OF LUNG FUNCTION IN NEWBORNS AND ADULTS

	Newborn	Adult	Fold Change
Tidal volume (mL)	20 (5–7 mL/kg)	450 (6 mL/kg)	22
Alveolar ventilation (mL/min)	400	4200	10
(mL/m²/min)	2.3	2.3	1
Dead space, V_D/V_T ratio	0.3	0.33	1
Anatomic dead space (mL)	7.0	150	20
(mL/kg)	2.5	2	2
Respiratory quotient	0.8	0.8	1
Oxygen consumption (mL/min)	18	250	14
(mL/kg/min)	6.0–6.7	3.5	0.5
CO_2 output (mL/kg/min)	6	3	0.5
Body surface area (m²)	0.21	1.70	8
Body weight (kg)	3	70	23
Lung weight (g)	50	800	15
FRC (mL)	90	2400	24
(mL/kg)	30	34	1
Lung surface area (m²)	2.8	64–75	30
(m²/kg)	1	1	1
Respiratory rate	34–36	12–14	2–3

FRC, functional residual capacity.

Modified from Doershuk CF, Fisher BJ, Matthews LW. Pulmonary physiology of the young child. In: Scarpelli EM, ed. *Pulmonary Physiology of the Fetus, Newborn, and Child.* Philadelphia; Lea & Febiger; 1975:174.

Table 16–1 lists some important differences between newborn and adult respiratory anatomy and physiology. Table 16–2 highlights some factors that influence the development of respiratory failure in children.

Table • 16–2. ANATOMIC AND PHYSIOLOGIC FEATURES OF THE DEVELOPING RESPIRATORY SYSTEM

Physiologic or Anatomic Feature	Clinical Implications
Upper Airway	Prone to obstruction
Nose breather*	
Large tongue	
No teeth*	
Large tonsils and adenoids	
Teeth easily dislodged†	Trauma or aspiration with intubation
Airways	Prone to collapse, obstruction
Small, weak	
Little bronchial smooth muscle*	Poor response to bronchodilators
Alveoli	Increased closing capacity
Less elasticity	
Chest Wall	Prone to collapse, retractions
Less muscle mass	
Soft ribs and sternum	
Ventilatory Muscles	Prone to fatigue
Few high oxidation muscle fibers*	
Pulmonary Vasculature	Insufficient vasoconstriction
Less muscular†	
Increased Oxygen Consumption	Decreased oxygen reserves

*Primarily infants.
†Primarily children beyond infancy.

RESPIRATORY CARE OF THE NEWBORN

Prenatal Considerations

The transition from intrauterine to extrauterine life requires the newborn infant to inflate the lungs with air, begin regular respiration, and establish the normal adult pattern of circulation. In utero, the placenta is the organ of gas exchange and is perfused by the infant's circulatory system by the two umbilical arteries. Oxygenated blood (with a PaO_2 of about 35 mmHg) returning from the placenta by the umbilical vein enters the vena cava by the ductus venous and the portal circulation. It mixes with deoxygenated blood from both the inferior and superior vena cava, lowering the PO_2 somewhat.[6]

Because the lung is not the organ of gas exchange, the fetal circulation is designed to minimize pulmonary perfusion, shunting the blood entering the right side of the heart to the systemic circulation by the foramen ovale (located between the atria) and the ductus arteriosus (located between the pulmonary artery and the aortic arch). Right-to-left shunting is facilitated by the high pulmonary vascular resistance and low systemic vascular resistance maintained by the fetus in utero. Pulmonary vascular resistance is high for several reasons. First, the low tissue PO_2 present in the fetal lung prompts pulmonary vasoconstriction. Second, in the fluid-filled lung, alveolar geometry results in compression and kinking of pulmonary capillaries. Systemic vascular resistance is low, primarily because of the contribution of the placenta's low-resistance circulation.

At birth, the infant's transition to extrauterine life begins with expulsion of fetal lung fluid by means of thoracic compression in the birth canal. Next, the infant must inflate the lungs with air, overcoming considerable resistance to inflation because of the high surface tension present in the fetal lung. Inflation pressures of −80 mmHg are often required.[6]

Immediately on inflation of the lungs with air, pulmonary vascular resistance falls, owing to the increased PaO_2, with a subsequent increase in pulmonary blood flow. The ductus arteriosus constricts because of the increased PaO_2, further reducing the right-to-left shunt. Also, as pulmonary venous return increases, left atrial volume and pressure increase, and shunting by the foramen ovale ceases.

Recognition and Management of the High-Risk Newborn

Many infants have difficulty making the transition to extrauterine life successfully. **Newborn resuscitation** is the term used to describe all those techniques required to assist the distressed newborn in making this transition successfully. The task of practitioners in the delivery room is to identify infants likely to require resuscitation as soon as possible and to apply the resuscitative measures correctly.

A variety of fetal and maternal factors can be identified that increase the risk of perinatal distress. These are detailed in Box 16–1. Practitioners should be most concerned when life-threatening maternal conditions are present, such as uncontrolled hypertension or seizures (as seen in the preeclampsia and eclampsia syndromes), maternal hemorrhage, fever, hypotension, or drug intoxication.

During the immediate perinatal period, fetal heart monitoring is often used to assess fetal well-being and guide decisions concerning the management of labor and delivery.

Box • 16–1. RISK FACTORS AND WARNING SIGNS OF DISTRESSED NEWBORN

HISTORICAL FACTORS

Multiple gestation
Previous history of distressed newborn
Maternal drug abuse
Maternal diabetes
Advanced maternal age

PERINATAL FACTORS

Uncontrolled hypertension
Prolonged or difficult labor
Abnormal presentation (eg, breech)
Placental abruption
Late decelerations
Persistent fetal bradycardia
Persistent fetal tachycardia

Ideally, fetal heart rate should be maintained at 120 to 180 beats/min between contractions. When a uterine contraction occurs, the fetal head is compressed against the cervix, producing a brief reduction in the fetal heart rate, called a **deceleration**. Recovery should be prompt, with a normal fetal heart rate restored at the end of the contraction.[7]

When fetal oxygenation is compromised, another type of deceleration can be observed. Called *late* deceleration, the drop in heart rate begins later during the course of a contraction, and recovery is prolonged, lasting beyond the end of the contraction. These are thought to occur when the fetus is hypoxic, and the uterine contraction compromises blood flow even further, resulting in profound tissue ischemia.[7]

When late decelerations are evident, measures should be taken to improve fetal oxygenation in utero. Such measures depend on the exact cause of fetal compromise but may include maternal oxygen and fluid administration or altering maternal position to improve uterine blood flow. If unsuccessful, obstetricians may consider options to hasten delivery, including cesarean section. In any case, preparations for neonatal resuscitation should be made.

Additional measures are occasionally used to assess fetal well-being. For example, fetal scalp pH can be measured from intermittent sampling of scalp capillary blood. If the pH is less than 7.20, fetal distress is present.[7]

An additional warning sign of fetal distress that deserves special management is the presence of meconium-stained amniotic fluid. **Meconium** is the substance that lines the fetal bowel in utero. When the fetus is severely distressed, reflex colonic contraction and anal sphincter relaxation occur, expelling the meconium into the amniotic fluid. Because the distressed fetus also responds to severe asphyxia with deep, gasping respiration, aspiration of meconium into the airway may occur. Suctioning the oropharynx, larynx, and trachea under direct laryngoscopic visualization, as soon as the head is delivered (but before the chest is delivered), has proved effective in reducing pulmonary complications of meconium aspiration.[7]

Newborn Resuscitation: Initial Management

The delivery of a limp, cyanotic infant should prompt an immediate response by the delivery room team. A series of diagnostic and therapeutic measures must begin simultaneously. The infant should be placed on a radiant warmer and gently blotted dry to prevent heat loss. Failure to prevent heat loss dooms many resuscitative measures to failure. In the presence of a cool environment, the newborn, in an attempt to increase heat production and minimize heat loss, increases metabolism and oxygen consumption in the process of thermogenesis and undergoes diffuse peripheral vasoconstriction. Because the asphyxiated newborn obviously has limited oxygen delivery capacity, anaerobic metabolism and lactic acidosis develop, initiating a vicious cycle of events and resulting in death[8] (Fig. 16–2).

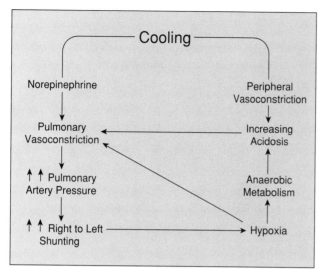

FIGURE 16-2 • The vicious cycle resulting from cooling in the neonate. (Klaus M, Fanaroff A. *Care of the High Risk Neonate.* 3rd ed. Philadelphia: WB Saunders, 1986:100.)

Next, the infant's respiratory efforts should be assessed. If absent or weak, positive-pressure ventilation with oxygen using a bag-and-mask assembly is begun. Heart rate should be determined by direct auscultation. In contrast to adult resuscitation, cardiac compressions may be instituted when a heart rate is present but below 60 beats/min. When a heart rate of 60 beats/min, but less than 100 beats/min, is present, positive-pressure ventilation is continued for 15 to 30 seconds, and the heart rate is reassessed. If the heart rate is not improving or is still below 80 beats/min, chest compression is begun. After 30 seconds to 1 minute of cardiopulmonary resuscitation, vascular access should be obtained (usually the umbilical vein) and intubation performed.

Epinephrine is the most important resuscitation drug, and doses are listed in Box 16-2. Epinephrine may also be given in a dilute solution by endotracheal tube if vascular access cannot be established. Naloxone may be given if a history of maternal narcotic administration is present. Volume expansion and glucose administration may be needed if evidence of hypovolemia and hypoglycemia are present. Sodium bicarbonate should be given only if severe metabolic acidosis is documented and adequate ventilation is established. An umbilical arterial line should be placed to provide for blood gas and blood pressure analysis. Arterial oxygenation should also be assessed by means of pulse oximetry.[7,8] The accompanying Figure 16-3 details more fully the sequence of events in newborn resuscitation.

Postresuscitation Care

After initial resuscitation and stabilization, the infant's ability to maintain adequate ventilation and oxygenation should be assessed and appropriate therapies and supportive care implemented. The differential diagnosis, treatment, and risk of complications of therapy differ greatly depending on the degree of maturity of the infant. Therefore, the postresuscitation care of the preterm and term infant are discussed separately.

Care of the Preterm Infant

If arterial oxygenation is not adequate when ventilated with 100% oxygen, practitioners should attempt to establish if cardiac or respiratory disease (or both) are present. Pulmonary disease is most often the cause of inadequate oxygenation in the preterm infant. Before 36 weeks' gestation, surfactant production is minimal and easily disrupted by an inhospitable biochemical environment. The presence of intercostal retractions, tachypnea, grunting, and nasal flaring, together with characteristic chest radiograph changes, helps to establish the diagnosis of respiratory distress syndrome (RDS) in such an infant. RDS is difficult to distinguish on clinical grounds from group B streptococcal pneumonia, which requires antibiotic therapy. Infants in whom RDS is suspected should be treated promptly with surfactant replacement therapy by endotracheal tube. A complete discussion of this therapy is beyond the scope of this text.

Certain congenital anomalies occur occasionally in preterm infants and should be considered in the differential diagnosis as well. Chief among these is esophageal atresia–tracheoesophageal fistula malformations. This condition should be suspected in pregnancies characterized by excessive amniotic fluid (polyhydramnios). The presence of esophageal atresia prevents the fetus from swallowing and absorbing amniotic fluid, a normal mechanism of maintaining normal intrauterine amniotic fluid volume. The increased quantity of amniotic fluid may be what causes most infants with this anomaly to be born prematurely. Further evidence of this anomaly includes the rapid accumulation and overflow of saliva in the oropharynx.[2]

Box • 16–2. NEONATAL RESUSCITATION DRUGS

Epinephrine: 0.01–0.03 mg/kg IV or per endotracheal tube every 3–5 min (0.1–0.3 mL/kg of a 1:10,000 solution). For endotracheal tube instillation, dilute with 3–5 mL normal saline.

Naloxone: 0.1 mg/kg IV or per endotracheal tube every 3–5 min (0.1 mL/kg of a 1-mg/mL concentration). For endotracheal tube instillation, dilute with 3–5 mL normal saline.

Source: American Heart Association.

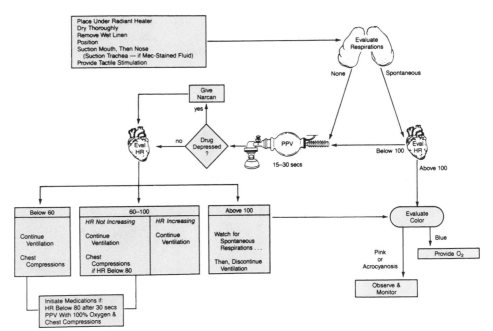

FIGURE 16-3 • Flow diagram for neonatal resuscitation. PPV, positive-pressure ventilation. (Reproduced with permission from Bloom RS, Cropley CS, Chameides L., Ed. *Textbook of Neonatal Resuscitation.* 1994. Dallas, TX: American Heart Association.)

Important Physiologic Considerations in the Care of the Preterm Infant

The Pulmonary Vascular Bed and the Ductus Arteriosus

Pulmonary vascular smooth muscle increases steadily throughout gestation. In the preterm infant, there is sufficient smooth muscle to accomplish the principal intrauterine task of this structure: to vasoconstrict sufficiently to promote right-to-left shunting through the ductus arteriosus and foramen ovale, for reasons already discussed. Likewise, the ductus arteriosus is much less muscular than in the full-term infant because it is normally not necessary for the ductus to constrict until birth, that is, after 38 to 40 weeks' gestation.[6]

Following birth, then, the preterm infant may not undergo the normal circulatory changes seen in the full-term infant. The ductus may remain open, for example. In the early course of RDS, hypoxemia usually causes some degree of pulmonary vasoconstriction, and some degree of right-to-left shunting through the ductus arteriosus may be present.

During recovery and after the establishment of PaO_2 values above the normal intrauterine levels, hypoxic pulmonary vasoconstriction is abolished. This results in a decrease in pulmonary artery pressure and resistance. The ductus arteriosus, meanwhile, remains patent because of the immaturity of its smooth muscle. Now that pulmonary artery pressure is lower than aortic pressure, blood flow through the ductus is left to right, and pulmonary blood flow increases substantially. This leads to pulmonary edema and heart failure. A patent ductus arteriosus should be suspected in any infant who has delayed recovery from RDS.

Control of Ventilation

Because of an immature central nervous system, the preterm infant often suffers from apnea and blunted respiratory drive. Apnea may be idiopathic or a reflection of a variety of systemic illnesses, such as acidosis and sepsis (Fig. 16-4). When confronted with an infant displaying periods of apnea, the practitioner should avoid the temptation to mask the problem by increasing the ventilator rate or instituting pharmacotherapy; rather, in addition to these measures, the infant should be assessed for signs and

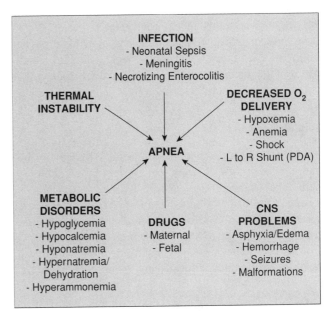

FIGURE 16-4 • Some of the causes of apnea. (Klaus M, Fanaroff A. *Care of the High Risk Neonate,* 3rd ed. Philadelphia: WB Saunders, 1986:193.)

symptoms of life-threatening conditions associated with apnea, such as sepsis and hypoglycemia.

Some causes of apnea in the nonintubated infant are iatrogenic and easily prevented or reversed. Forward flexion of the head causes the infant's flexible larynx to collapse. A small cloth rolled and placed under the shoulders can prevent obstructive apnea. Obstruction of the nares from tape (eg, for securing a nasogastric tube) or from eye shields used during phototherapy can be implicated as a cause of apnea.

Apnea is more likely to occur during periods of rapid-eye-movement sleep. This stage of sleep is associated with neurologic disorganization. In addition to apnea, control of the ventilatory muscles is reduced, with loss of muscle tone in the intercostal muscles. This reduces further the stability of the chest wall, reducing lung volume and decreasing oxygenation. Preterm infants spend most of their total sleep time in rapid-eye-movement sleep.[1]

Other Aspects of Care

Thermal Regulation

Perhaps the most important aspect of general care of the premature infant is the maintenance of an adequate thermal environment. A brief description of the importance of attention to thermoregulation during the resuscitation phase of care has already been presented and remains of prime importance throughout the premature infant's stay in the neonatal intensive care unit (NICU). The use of temperature support equipment is guided by the concept of the **neutral thermal environment**. This is defined as the ambient temperature at which oxygen consumption is minimal. Environmental temperatures above or below this level result in increased oxygen consumption as the infant attempts to maintain normal body temperature.[2]

Extreme variations in environmental temperature can have immediate disastrous consequences, including metabolic acidosis, hypoxemia, and shock (see Fig. 16–2). More subtle deviations from ideal thermal environment result in weight loss or decreased weight gain.

Infection Control

The preterm infant is extremely vulnerable to infection because of decreased efficiency of barriers to infection (eg, skin, mucous membranes) as well as an immature immune system. Careful attention to hand washing can help prevent disastrous nursery epidemics of infections such as respiratory syncytial virus (RSV). Furthermore, the possibility of infectious disease must be considered in any infant who has a deterioration in clinical status, no matter how subtle.

Neurologic Organization and Stimulation

During the past decade, much attention has been focused on creating an environment that minimizes noxious stimuli and enhances the preterm infant's ability to adjust. The infant's natural sleep–wake cycle should be noted and respected as much as possible. That is, routine procedures, assessments, linen changes, and so forth should be withheld if possible until the infant's awake periods. Furthermore, as many of these activities as possible should be clustered into limited time periods to permit more uninterrupted sleep periods. Environmental stimuli, such as noise and light, should be kept to a minimum. Caretakers should be familiar with methods for soothing irritable infants before and after painful procedures. Consistent use of these methods has been shown to reduce mortality and morbidity in the NICU.

Preventing Complications

The newborn infant is exquisitely sensitive to complications related to the application of respiratory care. This section reviews the causes and and prevention of complications to the central nervous system, eye, and lung.

Central Nervous System Complications

One of the most devastating complications of preterm birth is **intraventricular hemorrhage** (IVH), which is hemorrhage in one of the four reservoirs (or ventricles) of cerebrospinal fluid found in the infant's brain. During later fetal life, this area is highly vascular, containing many fragile capillaries, designed to nourish the rapidly growing brain. These blood vessels lack the capacity of autoregulation; that is, they do not effectively constrict to prevent rapid changes in blood flow when systemic venous or arterial blood pressures rise.

A number of risk factors have been identified that predispose to IVH. These include rapid volume administration (especially highly osmolar solutions, such as $NaHCO_3^-$), hypercarbia, and pneumothorax. For these reasons, most neonatologists administer fluid boluses slowly and carefully and avoid the liberal use of bicarbonate. Although moderate levels of hypercarbia may be allowed, severe and sudden hypercarbia (60 to 70 mmHg) should be avoided.

Positive airway pressure applied to the lung can also influence intracranial blood pressure and flow, especially during periods of rapid improvement in lung compliance, such as during the recovery phase of RDS.[9] When lung compliance is high, increased airway pressure results in a greater change in alveolar volume, compressing intrathoracic vessels and minimizing intracranial venous return. Cyclic changes in cerebral blood flow, corresponding to cyclic changes in airway pressure, have been documented in infants recovering from RDS.[9] Such detrimental changes can be avoided by adjusting peak airway pressures and inspiratory times frequently to the minimum level needed during recovery from RDS. In addition, the use of a low-compliance ventilator circuit, low ventilator flow rates, and short inspiratory times have been shown to minimize adverse changes in volume and pressure in a lung model study.[10]

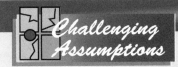

CRITICAL THINKING CHALLENGES

Developmental Care: What Is It?

The term *developmental care* is being used with increasing frequency in the NICU. This refers to a comprehensive approach to care of the sick preterm newborn, which attempts to minimize the effects of inappropriate stimulation on the infant's overall physiologic and neurologic development. Experienced clinicians in the NICU are familiar with the effects of painful or uncomfortable procedures on the infant's status. Deterioration of vital signs and oxygenation is a common result. Prolonged crying and thrashing often occur, making ventilation difficult, and undoubtedly increasing blood pressure. Increased FiO₂ and ventilator settings, as well as sedation, were often required. It was no wonder that so many of these infants suffered from IVH and BPD.

Heidelise Als,[72] a developmental psychologist, was the first to show that care providers can modify their interventions to reduce infant stress and its adverse consequences. The first step is training staff in recognition of the signs of infant stress. Some signs, such as crying and thrashing, are obvious. More subtle signs of infant stress include yawning, sneezing, and hiccuping; extreme flaccidity, excessive alertness, and uncoordinated eye movement. Finger extension or splaying is also a sign of stress, as is arching or hyperextension of the spine.[72,73]

When these or other signs of stress are present, the care provider should terminate the stressful intervention and help the infant to become calm. Surprisingly, some methods intuitively used by parents are counterproductive in the premature infant, including stroking or patting the infant, rocking, and talking in a soft voice. Effective comfort measures seem to imitate conditions in the womb. For example, the infant is held in a flexed position. The infant is not stroked or patted but rather held with a firm, gentle pressure with one or both hands. The infant is gently prevented from extending the arms or legs. Padding can be placed in the incubator to assist the infant in maintaining this position when a care provider cannot be present. This is called *nesting* or *bundling*. The padding also gives the infant a clear sense of boundaries, reinforcing the sense of being in the womb.

Additional measures to minimize stress and promote comfort include allowing the infant to grasp an object or an adult finger during painful procedures and providing a pacifier.[72,73] The methods of assessment and care needed to apply the concepts of developmental care are too complex to be taught in a book; direct contact with an expert is required. Some improvement in care, however, can be achieved by implementing the above procedures.

In addition to modification of individual care, the entire NICU environment can be modified to reduce sensory input. Such measures include systematic reduction of noise and bright lights.

The most recent evidence in a controlled trial demonstrates that adopting this approach to developmental care significantly reduces morbidity associated with premature birth. Specifically, the risks of BPD and IVH are reduced, and the length of time on mechanical ventilation is decreased. Developmental status at 9 months was significantly improved.[74,75]

Head-down positioning (eg, during chest physical therapy [CPT]) may also increase intracranial pressure. In fact, a significant increase in the rate of severe IVH was noted in one study of routine application of CPT in preterm infants with RDS.[11] Other factors may have contributed to the increased risk of IVH, such as chest percussion and suctioning.

Active expiration against the ventilator during the inspiratory phase also adversely affects intracranial hemodynamics and may predispose to IVH as well as pneumothorax. The incidence of both IVH and pneumothorax can be decreased by the use of muscle relaxants during mechanical ventilation.[12] Active expiration against the ventilator can also be minimized by the use of short inspiratory times or by the use of synchronized ventilation.[13]

Airway Complications

Among the most common complications of the application of modern ventilatory techniques to the newborn is damage to the airway secondary to prolonged endotracheal intubation. Most troublesome is the development of subglottic stenosis. This complication is seen most commonly in premature infants who have been intubated for prolonged periods. The size of the endotracheal tube appears to be the most important controllable etiologic factor. In a prospective study designed to decrease the rate of subglottic stenosis, it was found that selecting an endotracheal tube with an internal diameter that was one tenth the infant's gestational age virtually eliminated subglottic stenosis. Using this method, an infant of 31 weeks' gestation would require a 3.1-mm internal diameter endotracheal tube. Because this size is not commonly manufactured, the next *smaller* size (3.0-mm) would be used.[14] Another study documented a reduced risk of subglottic stenosis when an audible airway leak was heard when airway pressures were raised to 25 mmHg.[15]

Other complications of prolonged endotracheal intubation include impaired dentition and palatal abnormalities. The first complication results from prolonged resting of the endotracheal tube on the gums. The most common palatal abnormality seen is the formation of a groove in the palate. The may be the result of pressure from the tube or of the fact that the intubated infant cannot swallow, which normally serves to smooth out and flatten the palate. In any case, this abnormality can be prevented by the use of a specially designed oral prosthetic device.[16] Use of such devices does not appear to be widespread, however.

Complications can be seen in the lower airway as well. These are thought to be a result of vigorous suctioning of the airway with introduction of the suction catheter below the end of the endotracheal tube. Bronchial stenosis and granulomas may form, resulting in recurrent atelectasis and prolonged ventilator dependence.[17] These complications can be minimized by suctioning only when necessary rather than on a preset schedule. Indications for suctioning include coarse breath sounds, especially when accompanied by respiratory distress or blood gas abnormalities. Decreased frequency of suctioning does not appear to increase the risk of atelectasis or pneumonia.[18]

Additional measures to decrease airway trauma include limiting the depth of catheter insertion to no more than the length of the endotracheal tube. This ensures the catheter will not abut against the bronchial mucosa, and minimizes trauma.[19]

Lung Complications

Pulmonary dysfunction after recovery from acute RDS is one of the most common and dreaded complications of neonatal mechanical ventilation. This condition is known as **bronchopulmonary dysplasia** (BPD) and is characterized by diffuse airway obstruction, alveolar fibrosis, and hyperinflation, among other abnormalities. The diagnosis is usually made on clinical grounds, the chief criteria being oxygen dependence at 28 days of age in an infant with a history of RDS.

The cause of BPD is unclear and is probably multifactorial. When first described in the late 1960s, most investigators thought the disease was secondary to pulmonary oxygen toxicity. Indeed, the risk seemed proportional to the duration and magnitude of supplemental oxygen administration. The lung of the premature infant has less antioxidants, such as superoxide dismutase, than does the mature lung.[6] Antioxidants presumably protect the lung from oxygen-free radicals, which are oxygen molecules with an abnormal number of electrons. These molecules are formed in excessive quantities when a high oxygen concentration is present and are harmful to cell membranes. The addition of a naturally occurring antioxidant, vitamin A, has been shown to reduce the risk of BPD in some studies.[20]

Later, other investigators speculated that positive-pressure ventilation itself, and not high inspired oxygen concentrations, may be responsible for BPD. The occurrence of BPD in infants receiving high oxygen concentrations, but not mechanical ventilation, is rare. These observations led to various modifications in the style of positive-pressure ventilation used in the NICU. Peak airway pressure was limited to avoid alveolar and airway overdistention.

Higher respiratory rates were used to compensate for the decreased tidal volume. To date, however, no specific ventilatory strategy has been clearly shown to reduce the risk of BPD. Nonetheless, most neonatologists recommend limiting peak inspiratory pressures (PIPs) to the level necessary to maintain $PaCO_2$ at about 50 to 55 mmHg.[6] Attempts to achieve normal $PaCO_2$ levels (35 to 40 mmHg) necessitate higher airway pressures and increase trauma.

Ocular Complications

Retinopathy of prematurity (ROP) is characterized by widespread proliferation of blood vessels behind the infant's retina, leading to, in extreme cases, retinal detachment and blindness. The most commonly noted risk factors for ROP are prematurity and high arterial oxygen tension. ROP is rare in full-term infants, and clinically significant ROP is unusual in infants who weight more than 1600 g.[6] With increasing survival of very-low-birth-weight infants, the incidence of ROP is increasing, despite efforts to maintain oxygen saturation in the low-normal range (90% to 95%).

Care of the Term and Near-Term Infant

Differences From the Preterm Infant

The most notable difference in risk factors for pulmonary problems in the full-term infant is the maturity of the surfactant production system. Not only is the absolute quantity of surfactant increased, but the production of surfactant is less likely to be disturbed by negative biochemical influences, such as acidosis or hypoxemia. When present, surfactant deficiency is usually secondary to severe lung insult, such as meconium aspiration or pneumonia.

The supporting structures of the respiratory system, including airway cartilage and muscle mass, are more developed, providing more stability to the chest wall and airways. This is only a matter of degree, however; the stability of these structures is far less in infants than in adults.

Neurologic maturity results in a decreased frequency of REM sleep, and the frequency of apnea and arterial oxygen desaturation is reduced. Naturally occurring antioxidant systems are more developed, and the risk of pulmonary and retinal oxygen toxicity are reduced substantially. The greater muscle mass and subcutaneous fat work to insulate the full-term infant, so thermoregulation is less troublesome.

The differential diagnoses of impaired oxygenation and respiratory distress in term and near-term infants differ from those in preterm infants. Although RDS always remains a possibility, practitioners should maintain a higher index of suspicion that a congenital defect is responsible for cyanosis and respiratory distress. Many cardiac lesions present with cyanosis at birth, as does congenital diaphragmatic hernia. These lesions are rare in preterm infants. Meconium aspiration syndrome is also more common than in preterm infants. Physical examination, chest radiographs, and echocardiograms can assist in establishing the diagnosis.

While assessing and planning the treatment of term and near-term infants, it is essential to understand the role of the mature pulmonary circulation in the presentation and course of respiratory disease. At term, the pulmonary vascular smooth muscle of the infant is fully developed. This is the result of 9 months of development in a very-low-oxygen environment. In the presence of chronic fetal hypoxemia, the pulmonary vascular smooth muscle is even more hypertrophied.[2] As a result, the term infant is often exquisitely sensitive to even minor abnormalities in arterial oxygenation or pH. For example, an infant undergoing an extremely prolonged and difficult delivery is asphyxiated; that is, the infant is hypoxic and acidotic. This causes even more intense vasoconstriction. For reasons not entirely understood, pulmonary vasoconstriction may persist after birth even when normal arterial oxygenation and pH are restored. This condition is known as **persistent pulmonary hypertension of the newborn** (PPHN) or sometimes (less accurately) as *persistent fetal circulation.* An overview of the pathophysiology of PPHN is depicted in Figure 16–5.

In response to the elevated pulmonary artery pressures, the ductus arteriosus and foramen ovale remain patent, and right-to-left shunting persists, resulting in hypoxemia. In addition, the shunting of desaturated blood from the pulmonary artery to the aortic arch provides an important diagnostic clue to this disorder. Because the blood vessels supplying the right arm branch off the aorta before the intersection with the ductus arteriosus, arterial oxygen saturation is higher there than in the blood flowing after the

intersection. The PaO_2 of blood obtained from a right radial artery sample can be compared with that of blood obtained from the descending aorta (usually an umbilical arterial sample). If the umbilical (or postductal) sample shows a lower PaO_2 than that found in the preductal (right radial artery) sample, a right-to-left ductal shunt is almost certainly present. Continuous monitoring of oxygen saturation measured on the right hand and either of the feet can provide practitioners with a continuous indicator of the presence and magnitude of ductal shunting.

PPHN can also be a component of parenchymal lung disorders. It is nearly universal in congenital diaphragmatic hernia and meconium aspiration syndrome.

The mainstay of treatment of PPHN is mechanical ventilation with 100% oxygen and the maintenance of either respiratory or metabolic alkalosis. Some infants with profound vasoconstriction at normal PaO_2 levels (80 to 100 mmHg) have some vasodilation when PaO_2 is maintained well above normal (eg, 150 to 200 mmHg). Likewise, raising the pH to 7.55 or higher results in pulmonary vasodilation in some infants. Muscle relaxation and sedation are also employed, and handling of the infant is kept to a minimum.[6,21]

For infants who fail to respond to the above measures, extracorporeal membrane oxygenation has proved highly successful. More recently, many infants appear to have benefited from continuous inhalation of low-dose nitric oxide.[21,22]

Application of Respiratory Care Techniques in the Newborn

Monitoring

There is extensive experience with the application of noninvasive monitors in the NICU. Pulse oximetry is nearly universally employed and should be used on any infant undergoing mechanical ventilation. Compared with adults, pulse oximetry in infants is more prone to motion artifacts, and in some infants, the frequency of motion-induced artifacts makes monitoring extremely frustrating. The use of electrocardiogram-synchronized pulse oximetry can reduce this problem. Some pulse oximeters are subject to inaccuracy when exposed to intense ambient light (eg, phototherapy).[23] Covering the probe with a thick cloth may improve function.

Pulse oximeters are far superior to transcutaneous oxygen monitors for assessment of arterial oxygenation; however, transcutaneous measurement of carbon dioxide is accurate and clinically useful. Accuracy is improved when monitoring temperature is 44° to 44.5°C. This requires frequent changing of the monitoring site (every 2 to 3 hours) to prevent burns.[1,24,25]

End-tidal CO_2 monitoring represents an additional means of estimating the arterial $PaCO_2$. Practitioners should be careful to select a light-weight, low-dead-space

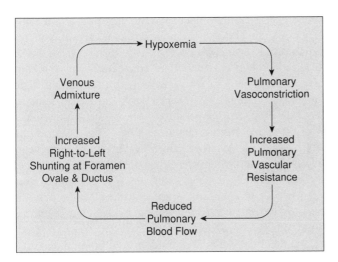

FIGURE 16–5 • Interrelationship between hypoxemia, pulmonary vascular resistance, and shunting. (Goldsmith J, Karotkin E. *Assisted Ventilation of the Neonate*, 2nd ed. Philadelphia: WB Saunders, 1988:56.)

adapter. In addition, a unit that permits display of the exhaled CO_2 waveform can assist the practitioner in determining the accuracy of the device. This form of monitoring is less accurate at high ventilator rates and in extremely small infants.[23]

Intermittent arterial puncture for blood gas analysis can be performed but is extremely difficult in small infants. Furthermore, it is painful and may cause changes in ventilation, making interpretation of results difficult.

Arterial cannulation is a more practical means of obtaining samples for blood gas analysis. Most commonly, the umbilical artery is cannulated. Blood gases measured here, however, may reflect right-to-left ductal shunting and may not reflect accurately the oxygen delivery to the brain. The radial artery is often cannulated as well.

Most arterial lines are continually flushed with saline solution to prevent occlusion. This solution must be removed from the catheter before obtaining a specimen for blood gas analysis. Failure to do so results in dilution of the sample and, most often, underestimation of both CO_2 and bicarbonate. Because blood samples obtained from newborn infants are small (0.2 mL or less), even a small amount of flush solution can have a dramatic effect on blood gas values. Dilution of the sample should be suspected when an unexplained decrease in hemoglobin, $PaCO_2$, and base excess are seen.[26]

After drawing a blood sample, umbilical arterial lines are usually flushed with a small amount of saline or heparinized saline. This should not be done when drawing blood from radial arterial lines, however, especially in premature infants. Cerebral air embolism has been reported as a complication of this technique.[27]

If arterial cannulation is not warranted, an arterialized capillary blood gas sample can be obtained from the infant's heel. Commercially available devices warm the foot to increase blood flow. Likewise, devices are available to facilitate skin puncture with minimal pain.[28] Capillary blood gas levels are inaccurate in conditions of shock and hyperoxia and should be interpreted with caution.[29]

Oxygen Therapy

In the acutely ill, nonintubated infant, oxygen therapy is usually provided by means of an oxygen hood. Oxygen delivered by hood should be warmed and humidified. Frequently, failure to warm the oxygen flowing into the hood results in hypothermia, despite the use of a radiant warmer or enclosed incubator. Practitioners should be careful to select equipment that is relatively quiet. Jet nebulizers, for example, may raise noise levels inside enclosed hoods and may damage the infant's hearing. Inexpensive sound meters are available at many hardware or electronic supply stores and can guide selection of equipment.[30]

Oxygen can also be delivered through infant nasal cannulas. These should be used with low-flow flowmeters, which allow precise control of flow at low-flow rates (eg,

less than 1 L/min). These are especially useful while feeding infants. Precise estimation of FIO_2 levels is difficult, and these levels may be higher than those typically delivered to adults by these devices. Oxygen masks are usually not well tolerated but may be used temporally while other equipment is being assembled.

Aerosol Therapy

Despite the relative lack of bronchial smooth muscle, many infants with BPD appear to benefit from aerosolized bronchodilators and steroids. Likewise, aerosolized vasoconstrictive agents are useful in treating subglottic edema. When using conventional nebulizers for aerosol delivery, the practitioner should operate the device in essentially the same fashion as when treating adults; that is, a flow rate should be selected to produce optimal particle size. Depending on the brand of nebulizer selected, this rate is between 6 and 8 L/min.[31] It is not necessary to reduce the flow rate to correspond to the infant's lower minute ventilation. Doing so will only increase particle size and reduce the efficacy of treatment.

Aerosol deposition is proportional to minute volume, and minute volume is proportional to weight. Consequently, the amount of drug placed in the nebulizer that is deposited in the lung is much less in infants than in older children and adults.[32,33] Most studies of aerosol deposition in infants cite deposition fractions of 1% or less,[34] whereas 10% to 15% is the typical figure for adult deposition. This suggests that the common practice of dosing aerosolized drugs by weight is misguided because the infant automatically adjusts the dose by having a lower minute ventilation. Fixed dose (ie, using the adult dose in children) has been shown in some studies to be safe and effective.[35]

Aerosolized medications can also be administered by mechanical ventilators. Usually, the nebulizer is inserted in the inspiratory limb, at a location that leaves about 15 to 30 cm of ventilator tubing between the nebulizer and the airway. This tubing serves as a reservoir for aerosol particles and improves drug delivery.[31,34]

The operation of a nebulizer connected to a ventilator may cause dangerous interactions with the ventilator and humidifier systems. First, when servo-controlled humidifiers are used, the temperature probe at the proximal airway is cooled by the nebulizer flow. This prompts the controller to increase humidifier heater output, superheating the water in the device. When nebulization is stopped, the temperature of the gas delivered to the infant rises sharply. For this reason, servo-controlled heated humidifiers should be inactivated during intermittent nebulization.

Nebulizer flow may also interfere with ventilator tidal volumes and pressures. This is more likely to occur with infant ventilators than with adult units. Infant ventilators operate on very-low-flow rates. The additional flow added by the nebulizer may cause total ventilator flow to double, with significant changes in peak and end-expiratory pressures.[31] Respiratory therapists should be alert for these changes, and temporarily adjust ventilator settings to accommodate them.

Metered dose inhalers (MDIs) may also be used in intubated and nonintubated infants. Holding chambers with masks are available commercially, and numerous studies have shown them to be at least as efficacious as nebulizers.[31,36–39] Adapters and spacer devices are also available for incorporation into neonatal ventilator circuits. Likewise, numerous studies have demonstrated that these devices are safe and effective in intubated patients.[31,40] Given the small tidal volumes of infants, reduction of the dose from the adult standard is not necessary.

Chest Physical Therapy

Although widely used, few studies document beneficial effects from routine CPT. The most commonly used indication for CPT in the newborn is the prevention of postextubation atelectasis of the right upper lobe.[41] This practice is based on a single study in 1979 that showed a reduction in right-upper-lobe atelectasis when CPT was applied to the right upper lobe every 2 hours for 24 hours.[42] This study did not control for suctioning, however. A recent attempt to verify the results of this study actually demonstrated an increase in atelectasis when routine CPT was employed.[43] This is consistent with other studies in children and animals showing that CPT (especially chest percussion) may increase the risk of atelectasis.[44,45] Given the high compliance of the infant's chest wall, it is not surprising that chest percussion is associated with a loss of lung volume.

As already noted, other studies demonstrated an increased risk of IVH when CPT was applied routinely to infants with RDS.

Despite the hazards associated with prophylactic CPT, when lobar atelectasis is present, a brief trial of CPT may be beneficial. Practitioners must be careful to maintain adequate lung volume during the procedure by use of manual ventilation. Gentle chest compression during exhalation only, rather than continuous chest percussion, may be more effective.[46] Head-down positioning should be avoided, especially in the preterm infant. If the infant does not respond to several treatments, prolonged therapy is usually not effective.

Mechanical Ventilation

General Considerations

The most common method of ventilation in the newborn is the use of pressure-limited, time-cycled continuous flow ventilators. Tidal volume is not set or measured directly but rather is primarily a function of the cycling pressure of the ventilator and the dynamic lung compliance of the infant. Inspiratory and expiratory times play an important but secondary role.

Cycling pressure is simply the difference between the end-expiratory pressure and the PIP. In most infant ventilators, these controls are not linked; that is, a change in the positive end-expiratory pressure (PEEP) does not result in an automatic corresponding change in PIP. For example, if the PIP is 20 cm H_2O and the PEEP is raised from 5 to 10 cm H_2O, the cycling pressure (the difference between PIP and PEEP) decreases from 15 to 10 cm H_2O, or by 33%. This results in a proportional decrease in tidal volume. If the practitioner wants to maintain the same tidal volume as before the change in PEEP, PIP must be increased accordingly. Those practitioners whose primary experience is with adult ventilators often fail to do so and mistakenly attribute the increased $PaCO_2$ to a PEEP-induced alteration in lung function.

When using pressure-limited ventilators, PIP does not vary, and changes in patient dynamic compliance (ie, change in airway resistance or lung compliance) lead to a proportional change in tidal volume. Again, practitioners accustomed to volume-preset ventilators often expect a change in PIP to signal events such as airway obstruction and pneumothorax. When ventilating infants, most ventilator alarm systems give no indication of a significant change in dynamic compliance. Usually, the only indication is a change in vital signs or oxygen saturation. Newer ventilators, however, often incorporate tidal volume monitors, which can indicate changes in compliance or resistance.

Inspiratory and Expiratory Times

To select an appropriate inspiratory and expiratory time for a ventilated infant, it is necessary to understand the concept of the **time constant**. The time constant is a number derived by multiplying the airway resistance by the lung compliance:

Time constant = airway resistance × lung compliance

This number can be used to predict how long it will take the lung to fill or empty. After three time constants have elapsed, the lung is virtually fully inflated (during inspiration) or deflated (during expiration).

It is seldom necessary to know the exact value of the time constant, but it is important to understand, in general, the conditions that may increase or decrease the time constant. For example, a 1000-g infant has much smaller lungs than a 4000-g infant, and lung compliance is about one fourth lower in the smaller infant. Assuming that there is little difference in the total airway resistance, the time constant of the smaller infant is much smaller than that of the larger infant. That is, at any given ventilator peak pressure, the lung of the smaller infant fills and empties faster, allowing for the use of shorter inspiratory and expiratory times (and higher rates).

In general, conditions that increase airway resistance increase the time constant and require longer inspiratory and expiratory times and lower rates. Common conditions that increase airway resistance in newborns include meconium aspiration syndrome and BPD. Conditions that lower lung compliance decrease the time constant, allowing for shorter inspiratory and expiratory times. Common conditions associated with lower time constants include pulmonary hypoplasia, RDS, and pneumonia, in addition to small size.

Failure to appreciate the role of the time constant can lead to significant errors in the selection of ventilator settings. For example, using an insufficient expiratory time when ventilating a large infant with meconium aspiration syndrome results in incomplete emptying of the lung, called *air-trapping*. This increased lung volume is reflected in an increase in the intrapulmonary end expiratory pressure (auto-PEEP). Because PIP is preset, as already discussed, the increased auto-PEEP results in reduced tidal volume and CO_2 retention.[10,47,48]

Commonly, practitioners respond to the rising $PaCO_2$ by increasing the ventilator rate, which further shortens the expiratory time and increases auto-PEEP and $PaCO_2$. Under these circumstances, the correct response would be to decrease the rate, permitting more complete alveolar emptying and reduction in auto-PEEP. Measurement of delivered tidal volume and analysis of lung mechanics may assist the practitioner in identifying such problems.

Inspiratory and Expiratory Timing: Clinical Trials

A number of studies have been conducted to assess the clinical results of various inspiratory times during mechanical ventilation of the newborn. Shorter inspiratory times have been shown to decrease the incidence of pneumothorax,[49,50] reduce patient–ventilator asynchrony,[13] and permit shorter weaning times.[51]

Ventilator Circuit Characteristics

Ventilator circuits used in infant ventilation must be light weight, have minimal dead space, and have as low a compliance as possible. Most commercially available infant ventilator circuits meet these criteria. It is possible, however, through modification or addition of elements to the circuit, to alter these characteristics unfavorably. For example, inserting a small segment of flexible tubing and a tracheostomy swivel adapter between the endotracheal tube and the patient Y of the ventilator circuit can add as much as 20 mL of mechanical dead space to the circuit. The amount of dead space present in these additions can be measured by determining how much water is required to fill them.

Likewise, using a large-volume, high-compliance humidifier increases total circuit compliance, which leads to increased auto-PEEP and lung overdistention.[10,52]

Newer Ventilators

Improvements in technology have resulted in the development of ventilators that allow for synchronization of the ventilator's output with the infant's spontaneous respiratory efforts. These devices are capable of sensing the infant's initial inspiratory efforts and rapidly delivering a positive-pressure breath. Some are also able to detect the end of the patient's active inspiratory efforts and terminate inspiration at that point. Usually, these devices incorporate sophisticated monitors, which allow for display of tidal volume and data concerning lung mechanics.

In some studies, use of synchronized ventilation (also known as *patient-triggered ventilation*) has resulted in shortened duration of mechanical ventilation and decreased morbidity.[53]

RESPIRATORY CARE OF THE INFANT AND CHILD

Common Respiratory Problems Beyond the Neonatal Period

After the first few months of life, the incidence of respiratory problems drops dramatically, and the nature of the problems change. The most common reason for hospital admission among children is asthma.[1] Other common respiratory conditions include RSV bronchiolitis, pneumonia, and croup. In specialized care centers, practitioners also see a substantial number of patients with cystic fibrosis as well as children suffering sequela of neonatal lung disease. In tertiary-care centers, children undergoing repair of congenital heart defects are seen, as are children with acute respiratory distress syndrome (ARDS) and systemic inflammatory response syndrome (SIRS) from a variety of causes.

Evaluation and Management of the Infant or Child with Respiratory Distress

Acute respiratory distress is a common presenting symptom in the pediatric emergency department. It may be the result of a primary pulmonary process or a manifestation of a multisystem illness, such as sepsis. For this reason, practitioners should avoid premature application of a pulmonary diagnosis in children with respiratory distress and should rapidly make a multisystem assessment to avoid missing other causes of life-threatening illness.

Warning Signs of Acute, Life-threatening Illness

One of the most reliable signs of an acute life-threatening process of any cause in infants and children is a change in the level of consciousness. Acutely ill infants are irritable, are difficult to console, are unable to focus attention on their parents or the examiner, and show no interest in their surroundings or in objects such as toys presented to them.

Additionally, they show no interest in bottle feeding or using a pacifier. A decrease in muscle tone may be present as well.[8,54]

The dehydration that accompanies many serious illnesses results in diminished or absent tears when crying and a dry or tacky oral mucosa. Skin turgor is poor; that is, when pinched, the skin does not readily return to its original shape. The skin over the knee cap is an excellent place to make this assessment. In addition, capillary refill is poor. This can be assessed by pinching the tip of a toe or finger, and counting the number of seconds until color returns. Ideally, this should be less than 2 seconds. If prolonged more than 4 seconds, serious circulatory impairment may be present. Light-skinned patients may manifest circulatory impairment by mottling, that is, a patchy alternation of pink and pale skin. Circulatory impairment may also be manifested by cool extremities.[8,54] Box 16–3 describes some "red flags" that should alert the practitioner to the possibility of a life-threatening illness. Table 16–3 summarizes essential features of pediatric assessment.

Specific signs of respiratory distress should also be noted and include tachypnea, grunting, nasal flaring, retractions, and cyanosis.

Infants and children displaying symptoms of shock or respiratory distress must be assessed and treated rapidly. The American Heart Association and the American Academy of Pediatrics[8] provide practical guidelines for this effort. In brief, they recommend rapid application of oxygen therapy, assisted ventilation if signs of respiratory distress

Table • 16–3. RAPID CARDIOPULMONARY ASSESSMENT

Respiratory Assessment	Cardiovascular Assessment
A. Airway patency	C. Circulation
• Able to maintain independently	Heart rate
• Requires adjuncts or assistance to maintain	Blood pressure
B. Breathing	Volume and strength of central pulses
Rate	Peripheral pulses
Mechanics	Present or absent
Retractions	Volume and strength
Grunting	Skin perfusion
Accessory muscles	Capillary refill time (consider ambient temperature)
Nasal flaring	Temperature
Air entry	Color
Chest expansion	Mottling
Breath sounds	CNS perfusion
Stridor	Responsiveness
Wheezing	Awake
Paradoxical chest movement	Responds to voice
Color	Responds to pain
	Unresponsive
	Recognizes parents
	Muscle tone
	Pupil size
	Posturing

Reproduced with permission. *Textbook of Pediatric Advanced Life Support*, 1994. Copyright, American Heart Association.

Box • 16–3. CONDITIONS REQUIRING RAPID CARDIOPULMONARY ASSESSMENT AND POTENTIAL CARDIOPULMONARY SUPPORT

Respiratory rate >60 beats/min

Heart rate

    Child ≤5 yr old: <80 or >180 beats/min

    Child >5 yr old: <60 or >160 beats/min

Increased work of breathing (retractions, nasal flaring, grunting)

Cyanosis or a decrease in oxyhemoglobin saturation

Altered level of consciousness (unusual irritability or lethargy or failure to respond to parents)

Seizures

Fever with petechiae

Trauma

Burns totaling >10% of body surface area

Reproduced with permission.
Textbook of Pediatric Advanced Life Support, 1994. Copyright, American Heart Association.

are present, and rapid establishment of vascular access. Shock is treated with the rapid delivery of a 20-mL/kg bolus of intravenous fluids. Intubation is considered in any patient who fails to show prompt improvement in signs of respiratory distress of shock. Note that the guidelines recommend rapid treatment *before* a definitive diagnosis is established and *before* objective measures of respiratory failure are obtained (eg, arterial blood gas values).

After initial assessment and therapy, the respiratory care practitioner focuses on determining the presence of specific respiratory disorders and their treatment. The assessment guidelines that follow can also be applied to the less acutely ill child.

Assessment begins by an observing the child's spontaneous respiratory pattern. In children of any age, but especially in infants, upper airway disorders are a common cause of respiratory distress. When upper airway obstruction is present, inspiration is usually prolonged and labored, whereas exhalation is effortless and brief. This is because the upper airway, when partially obstructed, tends to narrow or collapse further on inspiration (Fig. 16–6). Abnormal inspiratory sounds, such as stridor, wheeze, or rhonchi, are also more prominent on inspiration when upper airway obstruction is present. A summary of the diagnostic approach to stridor is presented in Figure 16–7.

The most common cause of symptomatic upper airway obstruction is laryngotracheobronchitis, or croup. This disorder is caused by a virus and rarely results in life-threaten-

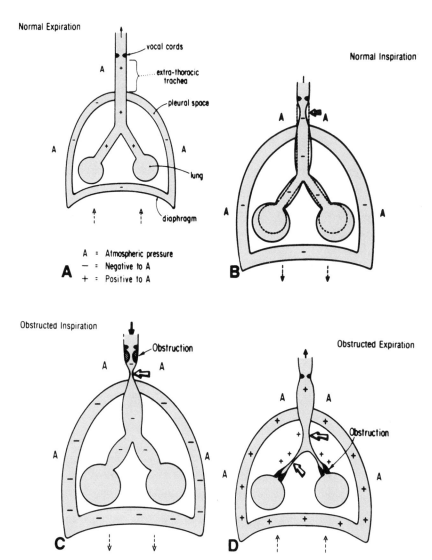

Normal Expiration

vocal cords

extra-thoracic trachea

pleural space

lung

diaphragm

A = Atmospheric pressure
− = Negative to A
+ = Positive to A

A

Normal Inspiration

B

Obstructed Inspiration

Obstruction

C

Obstructed Expiration

Obstruction

D

FIGURE 16–6 • (*A*) At end expiration, intrapleural pressure is less than atmospheric pressure, so it should maintain airway patency. In infants, the highly compliant chest does not provide the support required. Thus, airway closure occurs with each breath. Intraluminal pressures are slightly positive in relation to atmospheric pressure, so air is forced out of the lungs. Descent of the diaphragm and contraction of the intercostal muscles develop a greater negative intrathoracic pressure relative to intraluminal and atmospheric pressure.(*B*) The net result is a longitudinal stretching of the larynx and trachea, dilation of the intrathoracic trachea and bronchi, movement of air into the lungs, and some dynamic collapse of the extrathoracic trachea (*arrow*). The dynamic collapse is due to the increased compliance of the trachea and the negative intraluminal pressure in relation to atmospheric pressure. (*C*) Respiratory dynamics occurring with upper airway obstruction; note the severe dynamic collapse of the extrathoracic trachea below the level of obstruction. This collapse is greatest at the thoracic inlet, where the largest pressure gradient exists between negative intratracheal pressure and atmospheric pressure (*arrow*). (*D*) Respiratory dynamics occurring with lower airway obstruction. Breathing through a partially obstructed lower airway (such as occurs in bronchiolitis or asthma) results in greater positive intrathoracic pressures, with dynamic collapse of the intrathoracic airways (prolonged expiration or wheezing [*arrows*]). (Cotes CJ, Todres ID. The pediatric airway. In: Cotes CJ, Ryan JF, Todres ID, Goudsouzian, NH, eds. *A Practice of Anesthesia for Infants and Children.* Orlando: Grune & Stratton;1986:41.)

ing illness. Nonetheless, the stridor and barking cough may be dramatic at times. Treatment consists of inhalation of cool mist and oxygen if needed.[1] More severe cases may be treated with either systemic or inhaled steroids or with the inhaled vasoconstrictor racemic epinephrine.[55] When the latter is used, the infant should be observed for 3 to 4 hours before discharge to ensure that symptoms do not worsen as the effect of the drug decreases ("rebound phenomenon").

Some children with croup are at risk of respiratory failure and should be treated more aggressively. These include children with congenital or acquired lesions of the upper airway, such as subglottic stenosis, and those with preexisting lung disease, such as BPD.

Foreign body aspiration may also cause acute upper airway obstruction. Foreign body aspiration is more common in boys than girls and is most common between the ages of 1 and 3 years. Commonly aspirated objects include nuts, seeds, beads, and coins. Some tracheal foreign bodies can

be detected by a characteristic "slap" heard when the object hits the vocal cords on exhalation, and again when the object strikes the carina on inspiration. Laryngeal foreign bodies may cause hoarseness or drooling.[1]

If effective gas exchange and oxygenation can be maintained with oxygen therapy, the foreign body should be left in place until an experienced endoscopist can be present. If life-threatening hypoxemia is present, back blows and chest thrusts should be attempted in infants, and abdominal thrusts in children.[54] If unsuccessful, intubation should be attempted, and the foreign body pushed into one of the major bronchi, permitting ventilation of the other lung.[1]

Epiglottitis, a bacterial infection of the entire supraglottic area, is another cause of life-threatening airway obstruction. Since the recent introduction of a vaccine for *Haemophilus influenzae* type B infection, however, the incidence of this disease has fallen dramatically.[56] Occa-

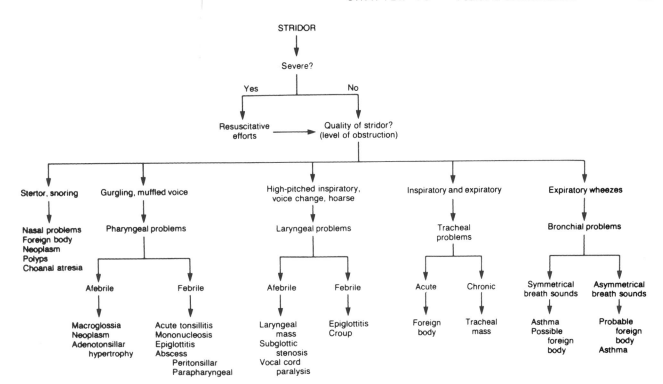

FIGURE 16–7 • Diagnostic approach to stridor. (Handler SD. Stridor. In: Fleisher GR, Ludwig S, eds. *Textbook of Pediatric Emergency Medicine.* Baltimore: Williams & Wilkins; 1988:301.)

sional cases are seen in children with immune deficiencies, however. History shows that compliance with immunizations waxes and wanes, so practitioners should be alert for the reemergence of this disease in the future.

Lower Airway Obstruction

Lower airway obstruction produces more prominent symptoms on expiration. Common signs and symptoms of lower airway obstruction include prolonged expiratory phase and pronounced expiratory wheeze. Occasionally, forced expiration with contraction of the abdominal muscles is present. Common causes of lower respiratory tract obstruction are discussed in this section, and a diagnostic approach to wheezing is presented in Figure 16–8.

Respiratory Syncytial Virus Infection

During the winter months in infants younger than 1 year, the most likely explanation for lower airway obstruction is bronchiolitis caused by RSV infection. This infection is usually accompanied by signs of upper respiratory infection. Most cases are benign and require no special intervention. Infants with coexisting medical problems, such as congenital heart disease, immune deficiency, and respiratory disorders, as well as infants younger than 6 weeks of age, are at higher risk for respiratory failure and death and require closer observation and more aggressive therapy.[1]

The treatment of these infants is controversial, and a review of the recent controversies is summarized in the following *Challenging Assumptions* display.

RSV is highly contagious. Therefore, infants admitted to the hospital with RSV infection should be placed in isolation. Caretakers of RSV-infected infants should not also be asked to care for premature infants, those with immune deficiencies, or other high-risk patients.

Asthma

By far, the most common explanation for acute lower airway obstruction is asthma. The incidence and severity of asthma appear to be increasing, especially in the inner cities. A comprehensive review of the management of asthma is beyond the scope of this chapter, but some recent trends are highlighted.

The mainstay of treatment of acute asthma is the delivery by aerosol of high doses of selective β_2-adrenergic agonists. Albuterol is the most commonly used drug. In mild cases, intermittent nebulizer treatments are effective, as is administration using MDIs. For children who fail to respond to three treatments or present with severe distress, continuous aerosolized administration of albuterol is warranted. Oral or intravenous steroids are also essential in these children if no immediate response is evident.[57] Recently, high-dose inhaled ipratropium bromide has been shown to speed recovery.[58]

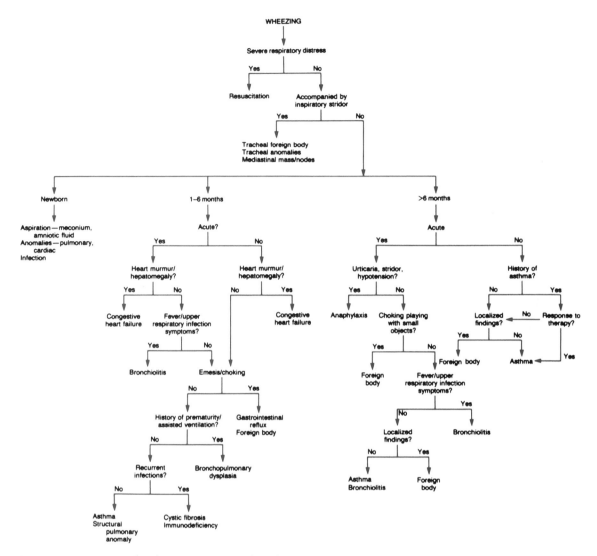

FIGURE 16–8 • The diagnostic approach to the wheezing infant or child. (Thompson AE. Wheezing. In: Fleisher GR, Ludwig S. eds. *Textbook of Pediatric Emergency Medicine.* Baltimore: Williams & Wilkins, 1988:273.)

Triggers of an acute exacerbation of asthma are variable. Pulmonary viral infections are a common trigger and should be considered in children who fail to respond to treatment.[1] Recognition and management of asthma triggers can reduce hospital admissions.

Also, children with a history of asthma are not immune to other causes of airway obstruction, such as foreign body aspiration.

When children fail to respond to inhaled therapy, and respiratory failure appears imminent, continuous intravenous administration of a selective β_2-adrenergic agonist is warranted.

Terbutaline is commonly used in the United States.[59] In Canada, intravenous salbutamol (known as albuterol in the United States) is available. Other therapies recently described for the treatment of severe asthma include intravenous magnesium sulfate[60] and use of helium–oxygen mixtures.[61]

Foreign Bodies

An overview of foreign bodies has already been presented. Those that lodge in the lower airway present different diagnostic challenges, however. In fact, it is not uncommon for the diagnosis to be delayed for weeks or months, in part because aspirated foreign bodies are often mobile, producing signs of obstruction in one location, then, as a result of a cough, moving to a location where symptoms are more benign.

If lodged in a large airway, the foreign body may produce symptoms similar to those of asthma. Theoretically, wheezing would be more prominent on the side where the foreign body is located. In practice, breath sounds are easily transmitted throughout the chest, and this may mislead the examiner.

The diagnosis of foreign body aspiration should be considered in any infant or child who presents with a history of

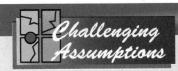

Controversies in Pediatric Respiratory Care: Treatment of Respiratory Syncytial Virus Infection

Respiratory syncytial virus infection, manifested clinically as bronchiolitis, pneumonia, or both, is a major cause of pediatric hospital and ICU admissions. In patients with co-existing medical problems, significant mortality and morbidity can result. Not surprisingly, the introduction of the antiviral agent ribavirin was greeted with much enthusiasm. Studies suggested that respiratory symptoms and blood gas abnormalities improved during ribavirin aerosol administration. Shortly after its introduction, aerosolized ribavirin use became widespread, being used in nearly every hospitalized infant with RSV infection. Because of its high cost, use eventually became limited to infants at high risk of death, that is, those with severe cardiac abnormalities, immune deficiencies, pre-existing lung disease, and other high-risk conditions.

Concern about the possible teratogenic effects of ribavirin on health care workers prompted most institutions to implement expensive and cumbersome methods to control environmental exposure. This, coupled with the apparent inability of ribavirin to produce significant improvements in outcome once in widespread use, prompted a critical reevaluation of its efficacy. Critics noted that the benefits reported in earlier studies were of limited clinical relevance; that is, researchers reported improvement in subjective symptom scores, duration of viral shedding, or slightly lower oxygen requirements in treated infants.[76,77] Newer studies looked at more clinically relevant outcome measures, such as overall mortality and duration of hospital or ICU stay.[76,78,79] Improvement in these variables would be of obvious value to patients and their families as well as to those responsible for health care costs.

A group of pediatricians and respiratory therapists from Ann Arbor, Michigan noted a significant flaw in most of the reported studies of ribavirin's efficacy. These studies used aerosolized distilled water as the placebo.[80] Far from being harmless, prolonged exposure to aerosolized water can lead to edema, bronchospasm, and hypoxemia. Later, other investigators conducted a trial of ribavirin therapy for intubated infants with RSV infection, using instead aerosolized normal saline in the placebo control group.[81] They were unable to demonstrate any significant difference between the two groups in terms of mortality, morbidity, length of stay, and other factors. A recent metaanalysis of all available studies on ribavirin failed to show any beneficial effect from therapy on mortality, morbidity, or length of hospitalization.[77]

In addition to antiviral therapy, investigators have focused attention on improving outcome and symptoms in bronchiolitis by the administration of various drugs to reduce airway obstruction and inflammation. Again, results are mixed. Studies evaluating the effects of albuterol are most confusing, with some studies showing a modest improvement in symptoms and oxygenation[82] and others showing no benefit or a worse outcome.[83-85] Some critics have suggested that the cause of airway obstruction may be variable in this disease, with only some patients suffering from bronchospasm. Airway edema may be a more important contributor to airway obstruction.

This view is supported by the results of several studies showing that racemic epinephrine, which has a significant α-adrenergic (vasoconstricting) effect, produces superior improvement in oxygenation, lung mechanics, and hospital admission rates.[86,87] Thus far, only studies of brief periods of treatment have been reported, and it is not clear if racemic epinephrine therapy should be continued for prolonged periods of time.

Several studies have examined the effects of inhaled or parenterally administered corticosteroids.[88,89] None has shown a clear benefit. Likewise, clinical trials of supplementation of vitamin A (a protector of epithelial cells and mucous membranes) have failed to show benefit.[90,91]

Preventing RSV-associated lung disease may be a more effective approach. In the hospital setting, this means protecting vulnerable infants from nosocomial spread of the virus. Identification and isolation of infected infants is key. For this reason, methods of rapidly detecting RSV antigens in infants with respiratory symptoms should be readily available in hospitals dealing with pediatric patients, especially during the Thanksgiving to Easter "RSV season."

Nosocomial spread occurs primarily as a result of infection of staff by autoinoculation of the virus from the hands to the mucous membranes of the eye or nose. For this reason, hand washing is essential, as is the use of masks with eye shields. Those who care for high-risk patients, such as premature infants or immune-suppressed children, should *not* also care for RSV infected infants.

A recently released RSV immune globulin has been shown to decrease the incidence of RSV infection in high-risk pediatric patients when administered before viral infection.[92] Administration after infection failed to produce benefit, however.[93]

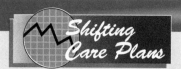

CRITICAL THINKING CHALLENGES

Preventing Hospitalizations in Asthmatic Children

Asthma is the leading pediatric respiratory disorder and one of the most common reasons for emergency room visits and hospitalizations among children. In theory, most exacerbations of asthma should be preventable. Key strategies in preventing acute exacerbations include prompt recognition of early warning signs through peak flow monitoring and early use of antiinflammatory agents, such as inhaled steroids.[57]

Just as important is recognition and elimination of triggers of asthmatic symptoms. One of the most common triggers of worsening asthma in children is environmental tobacco smoke (ETS). Asthmatic children living in homes where one or more smokers are present are nearly twice as likely to require an emergency room visit for treatment of symptoms.[94] On discharge, recovery from symptoms in these children is significantly delayed.[95]

Pediatric health professionals need to inform parents of the risk that ETS poses to their asthmatic children and encourage them to stop smoking. Smoking cessation is noto-

riously difficult, however, and clinicians should recognize that most parents will be unable to stop smoking immediately. Alternative strategies to minimize ETS include limiting smoking to an outdoor location or to a single, well-ventilated room of the house. Such measures, although not perfect, can reduce the frequency and severity of asthmatic symptoms.[96] One investigator estimated that, for every cigarette less smoked in the same room as the child per day, the FEV_1 increased 3%.[96]

Other children are highly sensitive to dust mites. Maintenance of a dust-free home would be ideal but is obviously difficult. Significant improvements in symptoms can be obtained by simple dust control measures applied to the child's bedroom. Covering the mattress and pillows (which can be infested with dust mites) with a polyurethane-coated cover has been shown to decrease the frequency and severity of symptoms.[97,98] Other indoor pollutants include mold from room humidifiers[99] and cockroaches.[100]

---

sudden, violent coughing spells, followed by signs of asthma. Expiratory chest radiographs assist in the diagnosis. The side with the foreign body remains hyperinflated during expiration.

Definitive therapy is removal of the foreign body with a bronchoscope. CPT should not be used to dislodge the object because this can lead to total obstruction and cardiac arrest.[1,62]

Parenchymal Disorders

Alveolar consolidation or collapse should be suspected in a child with respiratory distress who has diminished or absent breath sounds, or rales, over any area of the lung. Additional signs and symptoms include dullness to percussion and reduced movement over the affected area. Alveolar consolidation and collapse may coexist with signs and symptoms of airway obstruction. The diagnosis of asthma or bronchiolitis does not rule out coexistent pneumonia and should be suspected in infants or children who fail to respond to appropriate therapy. Premature or immune-deficient infants with RSV infection are more likely to have pneumonia along with RSV bronchiolitis. Asthmatic children with significant hypoxemia that worsens after administration of a β_2-adrenergic agonist are also likely to have alveolar consolidation.[63]

Most cases of pneumonia are associated with fever and an elevated white blood cell count. In general, both these values are higher in bacterial than in viral pneumonia, although no clear dividing line can be established. The chest

radiograph is useful for recognizing pneumonia. Infants younger than 2 months of age are more likely to have a life-threatening bacterial infection and are usually hospitalized.[2]

The practitioner should be alert for pediatric patients with recurrent pneumonia. These infants and children should be evaluated for immune deficiency, gastroesophageal reflux, cystic fibrosis, or foreign body aspiration, among other possible causes.

Application of Respiratory Care Techniques in Infants and Children

Most of the essential considerations in the application of respiratory care techniques in pediatric patients have already been discussed, but some additional considerations are considered here.

Monitoring

Pulse oximetry is an ideal monitoring tool for any child with respiratory distress. Transcutaneous oxygen monitoring is even less accurate in older children than it is in infants and is seldom useful. Transcutaneous CO_2 monitoring can be useful in infants and children.[24,25] Burning of the skin is less common, but routine changing of monitoring sites is still recommended. End-tidal CO_2 monitoring is generally more reliable in larger infants and children than in newborns because tidal volumes are larger and respiratory rates are lower in the former patient group. Capillary blood gas sampling is seldom reliable beyond the first few months of age.

Children beyond the age of 4 or 5 years can also usually cooperate with maneuvers required to obtain pulmonary function data, such as peak flows, flow–volume loops, and vital capacities.

Oxygen Therapy

Selecting appropriate oxygen therapy devices for toddlers can be extremely challenging. These children often are frightened of any device used to administer oxygen. Sometimes, placing an oxygen or aerosol mask in the infant's crib for a period, allowing the infant to play with it as a toy, helps the child to become familiar with the device before applying it to the face. Applying the device on a doll or teddy bear before placing it on the child may also be helpful.

Oxygen hoods are available to accommodate larger infants and are usually well tolerated. Toddlers may find them too confining. Oxygen tents are sometimes useful in toddlers but can often interfere with care.

Nasal cannulas are usually well tolerated once applied because the infant or toddler is unaware of their presence. The devices can be secured in place by applying Tegaderm or a similar adhesive over the portion of the cannula crossing the child's cheeks.

Aerosol Therapy

As with oxygen therapy devices, toddlers often resist application of treatment devices to the face. To minimize struggling and agitation, the treatment time should be as brief as possible. This can be accomplished by using high nebulizer flow rates and minimal dilution volumes. Parents may be better able to calm and restrain the patient than are professional care providers.

MDIs are available for most of the commonly used pediatric aerosolized medications and can be administered to a struggling pediatric patient in a fraction of the time needed for conventional nebulizer treatments. Of course, a spacer with mask is essential.

Older children can be taught to use MDIs in the same fashion as is recommended for adults, that is, with a slow inspiration and breath hold. Again, a holding chamber with mask or mouthpiece is desirable.

Chest Physical Therapy

The same problems relating to patient cooperation are a major factor in application of CPT. It is essential that the care provider spend some time gaining the child's confidence before beginning therapy. In this way, the child will consider therapy a play activity and be less resistant. Therapy sessions need not be prolonged because the child eventually will begin resisting therapy.

Current thinking regarding CPT suggests that procedures that use the patient's active expiratory air flow to mobilize and remove secretions are superior to passive techniques, such as chest percussion.[64,65] Getting toddlers and small children to exhale actively and forcibly is difficult. Some therapists have reported good results using soap-bubble kits. These devices require the child to produce a controlled, active exhalation to create bubbles. This is usually followed by a deep breath. Children can intuitively learn to perform this activity without detailed instruction by the therapist. A similar approach is described by Pryor,[66] who reported good results playing a game with small children that requires the child to move a crumpled piece of paper across a table by blowing at it through a cardboard paper towel roll. Alternately, a mouthpiece used for peak flow meters would suffice. Both of these devices require the child to keep the mouth wide open, which produces optimal flow rates for mucus mobilization. The practitioner may find that toy musical instruments, such as horns or flutes, encourage the patient to perform the desired expiratory maneuvers as well as to take deep breaths.

When possible, vigorous physical activity can be used to stimulate deep breathing and active expiration.[64] Of course, this may not be practical in the seriously ill child or in some crowded inpatient units. It should be considered as a form of bronchial hygiene therapy in, for example, the chronically ill patient with cystic fibrosis.

CHEST PHYSICAL THERAPY IN THE ACUTELY ILL CHILD

Recent reviews of CPT in the acutely ill patients suggest that there are few, if any, benefits to conventional CPT (percussion and postural drainage) in the treatment of acute respiratory conditions such as pneumonia, bronchiolitis, and asthma or in the treatment of postoperative patients.[64,65,67] In fact, routine application of CPT in postoperative pediatric heart patients has been shown to double the risk of postoperative atelectasis.[45] Other complications of routine CPT include hypoxemia and bronchospasm.[64]

One exception is the use of CPT for the treatment of acute lobar atelectasis. In a patient in whom a mucous plug is the likely cause of atelectasis, chest percussion or chest compression can produce resolution in one or two treatment sessions.[46,63] Methods to increase lung volume, such as deep breathing or manual hyperinflation of intubated patients, is essential as well. Prolonged therapy to prevent recurrence is probably not necessary, unless significant quantities of sputum are present. Also, practitioners should avoid prolonged therapy to reverse atelectasis that does not respond to a few CPT sessions. As noted, chest percussion can cause atelectasis when used prophylactically.

Newer CPT techniques, such as positive-expiratory pressure (PEP) therapy, may be useful in acute cases of atelectasis or sputum retention.[68] Successful application of PEP therapy requires some degree of patient cooperation, although some have reported successful application of PEP therapy in infants.[68] In addition, PEP therapy theoretically reduces air trapping in bronchospastic diseases.

CHEST PHYSICAL THERAPY IN THE CHRONICALLY ILL PATIENT

The most widely studied application of CPT in the chronically ill has been in patients with cystic fibrosis. For years, postural drainage and chest percussion were the mainstays of therapy. Studies supporting this form of therapy in cystic fibrosis patients were later criticized for failing to control for the effects of cough. Later, better designed studies showed that, in patients trained to cough properly and vigorously, the addition of chest percussion resulted in no additional sputum mobilization.[64,69,70]

These findings stimulated interest in techniques that use the patient's own expiratory airflow as a means of loosening and mobilizing secretions. Among the techniques developed and studied are PEP therapy, the forced expiratory technique (now known as the *active cycle of breathing*), and autogenic drainage. Our current level of knowledge about these techniques prevents a clear identification of the most effective technique. It is not clear whether there are fundamental differences between these techniques or whether they produce their results using similar or identical mechanisms.

All these techniques have as their primary advantage the fact that they can be performed independently. This is especially important for adolescents and young adults, who need to learn self-care skills. In younger children, some degree of therapist or parent supervision may be helpful.

Airway Management

The first step in endotracheal intubation is the selection of an appropriate-sized tube. This can be done with the following formula:

$$(\text{Age in years} + 16) \div 4$$

When the child's age is unknown, the width of the child's fifth fingernail can be used to approximate the required internal diameter.[69] Cuffed tubes should be used routinely in patients aged 8 years and older.[70] Younger children occasionally require cuffed tubes when high airway pressures are needed.

Mechanical Ventilation

It is difficult to compare and contrast ventilatory techniques used in the pediatric ICU with those used in the neonatal or adult ICU. Younger children are often ventilated with techniques borrowed from the NICU, whereas older children are managed with techniques adapted from the adult ICU.

In general, volume-controlled ventilation is the most commonly used technique. When using this technique in children, the practitioner must be aware of the importance of ventilator compliance. When appropriate-sized tubing and humidifiers are used (and ventilator circuit compliance is low), the ventilator accommodates changes in patient dynamic compliance by a corresponding change in airway pressure. In this way, reduction in ventilation is minimized when patient compliance decreases, and lung overdistention is avoided when patient compliance increases.[1] In addition, the change in ventilator pressure provides a useful signal to the care provider that compliance is changing.

When ventilator compliance is high, however, as when large-volume circuits and humidifiers are used, the ventilator pressure change is limited in response to patient dynamic compliance changes, and changes in lung volume are more dramatic. When small children are ventilated, this may be the case even when low-volume circuits are available. For this reason, practitioners must be alert for even small changes in airway pressure, which may reflect significant changes in patient compliance and volume.[1]

Knowledge of the ventilator's circuit compliance is important in calculating the delivered tidal volume. A portion of the preset tidal volume is compressed in the ventilator circuit during inspiration and does not participate in alveolar ventilation. Therefore, actual delivered volume is always less than preset volume. In adults, the difference is usually not clinically significant, and compensation is often not made. In children, however, the difference between the preset and delivered tidal volumes is usually clinically significant and must be known.

The first step is to determine the compliance of the ventilator circuit. Often, the ventilator's operating manual describes the procedure. Otherwise, it can be determined as follows: Before patient use, the circuit is occluded at the airway opening, and a tidal volume sufficient to generate 60 to 70 cm H_2O of pressure is selected. An inspiratory time similar to that used in the child's age group is selected. If this is unknown, an inspiratory time of 0.75 to 1 second should suffice. No PEEP is used. The preset volume is then divided by the observed PIP to obtain the circuit's compliance.

When adjusting the ventilator for patient use, a tidal volume slightly higher than the desired delivered tidal volume is selected. After connection to the patient, the cycling pressure (PIP − PEEP) is noted and is multiplied by the compliance of the ventilator circuit. Subtracting this volume from the preset volume yields the delivered tidal volume. If the delivered volume is thought to be inappropriate, the preset tidal volume can be increased and the calculations repeated. Further adjustments are made until an appropriate volume is obtained. Because this process is tedious and error prone, some practitioners prefer to use volume monitors that measure inspired and expired volumes at the airway.

The use of uncuffed tracheostomy and endotracheal tubes also complicates the application of volume-limited ventilation in children. A significant portion of the inspired tidal volume may be lost by leaking around the tube. This

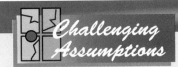

CRITICAL THINKING CHALLENGES

Reducing Sudden Infant Death Syndrome

The finding of an increased risk of sudden infant death syndrome (SIDS) in infants who sleep in the prone position was a major breakthrough in the understanding and prevention of this disorder.[101] The risks of prone positioning and the benefits of sleeping in the supine position were confirmed in recent studies. Deaths from SIDS dropped by as much as 50% when aggressive public education campaigns were launched to encourage parents to place their sleeping infants in the supine position.[102]

The message is not getting out to everyone, however. A recent study suggests that young, single mothers are more likely to continue placing infants in the prone position, even if aware of the risks.[103] This may reflect a lack of skill in assisting the infant to fall asleep. In any case, health care professionals should be sure to remind all parents of young infants of the hazards of the prone sleeping position. Furthermore, hospitalized infants should be treated according to these recommendations.

There are some legitimate exceptions to this general rule. Premature infants generally have improved oxygenation and less apnea when nursed in the prone position.[104-106] This can be done safely in the hospital setting, however, because of the common use of cardiac, apnea, and oxygen saturation monitors. Before discharge, however, it should be made clear to parents that prone positioning in the unmonitored home setting is risky.

---

loss of volume is not apparent when tidal volume delivery is calculated, or when it is measured at the ventilator's inspiratory port. Ideally, both inspiratory and expiratory volumes are measured at the airway, and appropriate adjustments are made more easily. When this is not possible, practitioners must rely on clinical assessment to gauge the adequacy of the tidal volume. There have been reports of serious hypoventilation in pediatric patients when using uncuffed tubes and volume ventilators, especially in the home setting and in patients with neuromuscular disease.[71] For these reasons, many practitioners prefer pressure-limited ventilation in all but the largest pediatric patients.

Certain developments in neonatal and adult ventilation have been applied to pediatric patients. These include the use of low-volume, high-frequency conventional ventilation in the treatment of ARDS and the use of inverse-ratio ventilation. Definitive answers regarding the ideal method of ventilation are lacking.

References

1. Lewis RM, Thompson SL, Goldberg AI. Respiratory care for the infant and child. In: Burton GG, ed. *Respiratory Care: A Guide to Clinical Practice*, 3rd ed. Philadelphia: JB Lippincott; 1991: 757–820.
2. Behrman RE, Kliegman RM. *Nelson's Essentials of Pediatrics*, 2nd ed. Philadelphia: WB Saunders; 1994.
3. Merkus PJFM, Ten Have-Oproek AAW, Quanjer PH. Human lung growth: A review. *Pediatr Pulmonol.* 1996;21:383.
4. Helfaer MA, Nichols DG, Rogers MC. Developmental physiology of the respiratory system. In: Rogers MC, ed. *Textbook of Pediatric Intensive Care*. Baltimore: Williams & Wilkins; 1992.
5. Keens TG, Bryan AC. Levison HG. Developmental pattern of muscle fiber types in human ventilator muscles. *J Appl Physiol.* 1978;44:909.
6. Lewis RM. Developmental considerations in the pulmonary care of the newborn. Educational Resources Consortium, Claremont CA, 1992.
7. DeCherney AH, Pernoll ML, eds. *Current Obstetric and Gynecologic Diagnosis and Treatment*, 8th ed. Norwalk CT: Appleton & Lange; 1994.
8. American Heart Association and The American Academy of Pediatrics. *Textbook of Pediatric Advanced Life Support*. Dallas: American Heart Association; 1994.
9. Cowan F, Thoresen M. The effects of intermittent positive pressure ventilation on cerebral arterial and venous blood velocities in the newborn infant. *Acta Paediatr Scand.* 1987; 76:239.
10. Lewis RM. Factors affecting lung overdistension during newborn mechanical ventilation: A bench study. *Respir Care.* 1992; 37:1153–1160.
11. Raval D, Cuevas D, Mora A, et al. Chest physiotherapy in preterm infants with RDS in the first 24 hours of life. *J Perinatol.* 1987;7:301–304.
12. Greenough A, Wood S, Morley CJ, Davis JD. Pancuronium prevents pneumothoraces in ventilated premature babies who actively expire against positive pressure ventilation. *Lancet.* 1984; 1:1–4.
13. Greenough A, Grenall F, Gamsu HR. Synchronous respiration: Which ventilator rate is best? *Acta Paediatr Scand.* 1987;76:713.
14. Sherman JM, Nelson H. Decreased incidence of subglottic stenosis using an appropriate sized endotracheal tube. *Pediatr Pulmonol.* 1989;6:183–185.
15. Connor GH, Bushey MJ, Maisels MJ. Prolonged endotracheal intubation in the newborn. *Ann Otol Rhinol Laryngol.* 1980;89: 459–461.
16. Angelos GM, Smith DR, Jorgenson R, et al. Oral complications associated with neonatal oral tracheal intubation: A critical review. *Pediatr Dent.* 1989;11:133–140.
17. Nagaraj HS, Shott R, Fellows R, Yacoub U. Recurrent lobar atelectasis due acquired bronchial stenosis in neonates. *J Pediatr Surg.* 1980;15:411.
18. Wilson G, Hughes G, Rennie J, Morley C. Evaluation of two endotracheal suction regimens in babies ventilated for respiratory distress syndrome. *Early Hum Dev.* 1991;25:87–90.
19. Bailey C, Kattwinkel J, Teja K, Buckley T. Shallow versus deep endotracheal suctioning in young rabbits: Pathologic effects on the tracheobronchial wall. *Pediatrics.* 1988;82:746–751.
20. Shenai JP, Kennedy KA, Chytil F, Stahlman MT. Clinical trial of vitamin A supplementation in infants with bronchopulmonary dysplasia. *J Pediatr.* 1987;111:269–277.
21. Avery GB, Fletcher MA, MacDonald MG. eds. *Neonatology: Pathophysiology and Management of the Newborn*, 4th ed. Philadelphia: JB Lippincott; 1993.
22. Goldsmith J, Karotkin E. *Assisted Ventilation of the Neonate*, 3rd ed. Philadelphia: WB Saunders; 1996.
23. Heyden WR, Greenberg RS, Nichols DG. Respiratory monitor-

ing. In: Rogers MC, ed. *Textbook of Pediatric Intensive Care.* Baltimore: Williams & Wilkins; 1992.

24. American Association for Respiratory Care. AARC clinical practice guideline: Transcutaneous blood gas monitoring for neonatal & pediatric patients. *Respir Care.* 1994;39:1176–1179.

25. Sivan Y, Eldadah MK, Cheah TE, Newth CJL. Estimation of arterial carbon dioxide by end-tidal and transcutaneous PCO_2 measurements in ventilated children. *Pediatr Pulmonol.* 1992;12: 153–157.

26. Lewis RM. Dilution of blood gas samples from radial and umbilical arterial lines. *Respir Care.* 1990;35:1120.

27. Butt WW, Gow R, Whyte H, et al. Complications resulting from use of arterial catheters: Retrograde flow and rapid elevation of blood pressure. *Pediatrics.* 1985;76:250–254.

28. Paes B, Janes M, Vegh P, et al. A comparative study of heel-stick devices for infant blood collection. *Am J Dis Child.* 1993;147: 346–348.

29. American Association for Respiratory Care. AARC clinical practice guideline: Capillary blood gas sampling for neonatal & pediatric patients. *Respir Care.* 1994;39:1180–1183.

30. American Association for Respiratory Care. AARC clinical practice guideline: Selection of an oxygen delivery device for neonatal and pediatric patients. *Respir Care.* 1996;41:637–646.

31. American Association for Respiratory Care. AARC clinical practice guideline: Selection of an aerosol delivery device for neonatal and pediatric patients *Respir Care.* 1995;40:1325–1335.

32. Pennea AC, Dawson KP, Manglick P, Tam J. Systemic absorption of salbutamol following nebulizer delivery in acute asthma. *Acta Paediatr.* 1993;82:963–966.

33. Chua HL, Collis GG, Newbury AM, et al. The influence of age on aerosol deposition in children with cystic fibrosis. *Eur Respir J.* 1994;7:2185–2191.

34. Cameron D, Caly M, Silverman M. Evaluation of nebulizers for use in neonatal ventilator circuits. *Crit Care Med.* 1990;18:866–870.

35. Oberklais F, Mellis CM, LeSouf PN, et al. A comparison of a bodyweight dose versus a fixed dose of nebulized salbutamol in acute asthma in children. *Med J Aust.* 1993;158:751–753.

36. Ba M, Spier S, Lapierie G, Lamarre A. Wet nebulizer versus spacer and metered dose inhaler via tidal breathing. *J Asthma* 1989;26:355–358.

37. Benton G, Thomas RC, Nickerson BG, et al. Experience with a metered dose inhaler with a spacer in the pediatric emergency room. *Am J Dis Child.* 1989;143:678–681.

38. Williams JR, Bothner JP, Swanton RD. Delivery of albuterol in a pediatric emergency department. *Pediatr Emerg Care.* 1996;12: 263–267.

39. Yung-Zen L, Hsieh KH. Metered dose inhaler and nebulizer in acute asthma. *Arch Dis Child.* 1995;72:214–218.

40. Grigg J, Arnon S, Jones T, et al. Delivery of therapeutic aerosols to intubated babies. *Arch Dis Child.* 1992;67(1 spec no):25–30.

41. Lewis R. Chest physical therapy in pediatrics: A national survey. *Respir Care.* 1991;36:1307–1309.

42. Finer NN, Moriartey RR, Boyd J, et al. Postextubation atelectasis: A retrospective review and a prospective controlled study. *J Pediatr.* 1979;94:110–113.

43. Al-Alaivan S, Dyer D. The role of chest physiotherapy in preventing post-extubation atelectasis in neonates. *Pediatr Res.* 1994;35:323A.

44. Zidulka A, Chrome JF, Wight DW, et al. Clapping or percussion causes atelectasis in dogs and influences gas exchange. *J Appl Physiol.* 1989;66:2833–2838.

45. Reines DH, Sade RM, Bradford BF, et al. Chest physiotherapy fails to prevent postoperative atelectasis in children after cardiac surgery. *Ann Surg.* 1982;195:451–455.

46. Galvis AG, Reyes G, Nelson WB. Bedside management of lung collapse in children on mechanical ventilation. *Pediatr Pulmonol.* 1994;17:326–330.

47. Simbruner G. Inadvertent positive end-expiratory pressure in mechanically ventilated infants: Detection and effect on lung mechanics and gas exchange. *J Pediatr.* 1986;108:589–595.

48. Hird M, Greenough A, Gamsu H. Gas trapping during high frequency positive pressure ventilation using conventional ventilators. *Early Hum Dev.* 1990;22:51–56.

49. Greenough A, Dixon AK, Robertson NRC. Pulmonary interstitial emphysema. *Arch Dis Child.* 1984;59:1046–1051.

50. Heicher DA, Kastling DS, Harrod JR. Prospective clinical trial of two methods for mechanical ventilation of neonates: Rapid rate and short inspiratory time versus slow rate and long inspiratory time. *J Pediatr.* 1981;98:957.

51. Greenough G, Grenall F, Gamsu HR. Inspiratory times when weaning from mechanical ventilation. *Arch Dis Child.* 1987;62: 1269.

52. Scott LA, Benson MS, Pierson DJ. Effect of inspiratory flowrate and circuit compressible volume on auto-PEEP during mechanical ventilation. *Respir Care.* 1986;31:1075–1079.

53. Bernstein G, Mannino FL, Heldt GP, et al. Randomized multicenter trial comparing synchronized and conventional intermittent mandatory ventilation in neonates. *J Pediatr.* 1996;128: 453–463.

54. Fleisher GR, Ludwig S, eds. Synopsis of pediatric emergency medicine. Baltimore: Williams & Wilkins; 1996.

55. Klassen TP. Recent advances in the treatment of bronchiolitis and laryngitis. *Pediatr Clin North Am.* 1997;44:249–261.

56. Hickerson SL, Kirby RS, Wheeler JG, Schutze GE. Epiglottitis: A 9-year case review. *South Med J.* 1996;89(5):487–490.

57. National Asthma Education Program. *Expert Panel Report II: Guidelines for the Diagnosis and Management of Asthma.* Washington: US Department of Health and Human Services; 1997.

58. Schuh S, Johnson DW, Callahan S, et al. Efficacy of frequent nebulized ipratropium bromide added to frequent high-dose albuterol therapy in severe childhood asthma. *J Pediatr.* 1995;126: 639–645.

59. Allen ED, McCoy KS. Airway disorders. In: Barnhart S, Czervinske M, eds. Perinatal and pediatric respiratory care. Philadelphia: WB Saunders; 1995.

60. Ciarallo L, Sauer AH, Shannon MW. Intravenous magnesium therapy for moderate to severe pediatric asthma: Results of a randomized, placebo-controlled trial. *J Pediatr.* 1996;129:809–814.

61. Kudukis TM, Manthous CA, Schmidt GA, et al. Inhaled helium oxygen revisited: Effect of inhaled helium-oxygen during treatment of status asthmaticus in children. *J Pediatr.* 1997;130: 217–224.

62. Kosloske A. Tracheobronchial foreign bodies in children: Back to the bronchoscope and a balloon. *Pediatrics.* 1980;66:321.

63. Connett G, Lenney W. Prolonged hypoxaemia after nebulized salbutamol. *Thorax.* 1993;48:574–575.

64. Lewis RM. Chest physical therapy. In: Barnhart S, Czervinske M, eds. *Perinatal and Pediatric Respiratory Care,* chap 14. Philadelphia: WB Saunders; 1995.

65 Selsby D, Jones JG. Chest physiotherapy: Physiological and clinical aspects. *Br J Anaesth.* 1990;64:621–631.

66. Pryor JA. The forced expiration technique. In: Pryor JA, ed. International perspectives in physical therapy. 7. Respiratory care. Edinburgh: Churchill Livingstone; 1991:79–100.

67. Eid N, Buchheit J, Neuling, et al. Chest physiotherapy in review. *Respir Care.* 1991; 36:270–282.

68. Mahlmeister MJ, Fink JB, Hoffman GL, et al. Positive-expiratory-pressure mask therapy: Theoretical and practical considerations and a review of the literature. *Respir Care.* 1991;XX:1218–1230.

69. King BR, Baker MD, Braitman LE, et al. Endotracheal tube selection in children: A comparison of four methods. *Ann Emerg Med.* 1993;22:530–34.

70. Bachofen JE, Rogers MC. Emergency management of the airway. In: Rogers MC, ed. *Textbook of Pediatric Intensive Care.* Baltimore: Williams & Wilkins; 1992.

71. Gilgoff IS, Peng R, Keens TG. Hypoventilation and apnea in children during mechanically assisted ventilation. *Chest.* 1992; 101:1500–1506.

72. Als H, Lawhon G, Brown E, et al. Individualized behavioral and environmental care for the very low birth weight preterm infant at high risk for bronchopulmonary dysplasia: Neonatal intensive care unit and developmental outcome. *Pediatrics.* 1986;78: 1123–1132.

73. Wong DL. *Whaley and Wong's Nursing Care of Infants and Children,* 5th ed. St. Louis: CV Mosby; 1995.

74. Als H, Lawhon G, Duffy FH, et al. Individualized developmental care for the very-low-birth-weight preterm infant: Medical and neurofunctional effects. *JAMA.* 1994;272:853–858.

75. Fleisher BE, VandenBerg K, Constantinou J, et al. Individualized developmental care for very-low-birth-weight premature infants. *Clin Pediatr.* 1995;34:523–529.

76. Law BJ, Wang EEL, MacDonald N, et al. Does ribavirin impact hospital course of children with respiratory syncytial virus infection? An analysis using the Pediatric Investigators Collaborative Network on Infections in Canada (PICNIC) RSV database. *Pediatrics.* 1997;99:7

77. Randolph AG, Wang EEL. Ribavirin for respiratory syncytial virus lower respiratory infection: A systematic overview. *Arch Pediatr Adolesc Med.* 1996;150:942–947.

78. Ohmit SE, Moler FW, Monto AS, Khan AS. Ribavirin utilization and clinical effectiveness in children hospitalized with respiratory syncytial virus infection. *J Clin Epidemiol.* 1996;49:963–967.

79. Moler FW, Steinhart CM, Ohmit SE, Stidham GL. Effectiveness of ribavirin in otherwise well infants with respiratory syncytial virus-associated respiratory failure. *J Pediatr.* 1996;128:422–428.

80. Moler FW, Bandy KP, Custer JR. Ribavirin for severe RSV infection. *N Engl J Med.* 1991;325:1884.

81. Meert KL, Sarnaik AP, Gelini MJ, Lieh-Lai MW. Aerosolized ribavirin in mechanically ventilated children with respiratory syncytial virus lower respiratory tract disease: A prospective, double-blind randomized trial. *Crit Care Med.* 1994;22:566–572.

82. Schuh S, Canny G, Reisman JJ, et al. Nebulized albuterol in acute bronchiolitis. *J Pediatr.* 1990;117:633–637.

83. Wang, EEL, Milner R, Allen U, Maj H. Bronchodilators for treatment of mild bronchiolitis: A factorial randomized trial. *Arch Dis Child.* 1992;67:289–293.

84. Hughes DM, LeSouef PN, Landau LI. Effect of salbutamol on respiratory mechanics in bronchiolitis. *Pediatr Res.* 1987;22:83–86.

85. Kisson N. Bronchodilator therapy in wheezy infants: A commentary. *Pediatr Emerg Care.* 1993;9:121–122.

86. Menon K, Sutcliffe T, Klassen TP. A randomized trial comparing the efficacy of epinephrine with salbutamol in the treatment of acute bronchiolitis. *J Pediatr.* 1995;126:1004–1007.

87. Reijonen T, Korppi M, Pitkakangas S, et al. The clinical efficacy of nebulized racemic epinephrine and albuterol in acute bronchiolitis. *Arch Pediatr Adolesc Med.* 1995;149:686–692.

88. Roosevelt G, Sheehan K, Grupp-Phelan J, et al. Dexamethasone in bronchiolitis: A randomised controlled trial. *Lancet.* 1996;348 (9023):292–295.

89. Klassen TP, Sutcliffe T, Watters LK, et al. Dexamethasone in salbutamol-treated inpatients with acute bronchiolitis: A randomized, controlled trial. *J Pediatr.* 1997;130:191–196.

90. Kyran P, Quinlan, MD, Karen C, Hayani MD. Vitamin A and respiratory syncytial virus infection serum levels and supplementation trial *Arch Pediatr Adolesc Med.* 1996;150:25–30.

91. Bresee JS, Fischer M, Dowell SF, et al. Vitamin A therapy for children with respiratory syncytial virus infection: A multicenter trial in the United States. *Pediatr Infect Dis J.* 1996;15:777–782.

92. The PREVENT Study Group. Reduction of respiratory syncytial virus hospitalization among premature infants and infants with bronchopulmonary dysplasia using respiratory syncytial virus immune globulin prophylaxis. *Pediatrics.* 1997;99:93–99.

93. Rodriguez WJ, Gruber WC, Welliver RC. Respiratory syncytial virus (RSV) immune globulin intravenous therapy for RSV lower respiratory tract infection in infants and young children at high risk for severe RSV infections. *Pediatrics.* 1997;99:454–461.

94. Cunningham J, O'Connor GT, Dockery DW, Speizer FE. Environmental tobacco smoke, wheezing, and asthma in children in 24 communities. *Am J Respir Crit Care Med.* 1996;153:218–224.

95. Abulhosn RS, Morray BH, Llewellyn CE, Redding GJ. Passive smoke exposure impairs recovery after hospitalization for acute asthma. *Arch Pediatr Adolesc Med.* 1997;151:135–139.

96. Murray AB, Morrison BJ. The decrease in severity of asthma in children of parents who smoke since the parents have been exposing them to less cigarette smoke. *J Allergy Clin Immunol.* 1993;91:102–110.

97. Etzel RA. Indoor air pollution and childhood asthma: Effective environmental interventions. *Environ Health Perspect.* 1995; 103(suppl 6):55–58.

98. Huss K, Rand CS, Butz AM. Home environmental risk factors in urban minority asthmatic children. *Ann Allergy.* 1994;72:173–177.

99. Dekker C, Dales R, Bartlett S, et al. Childhood asthma and the indoor environment. *Chest.* 1991;100:922–926.

100. Rosenstreich DL, Eggleston P, Kattan M, et al. The role of cockroach allergy and exposure to cockroach allergen in causing morbidity among inner-city children with asthma. *N Engl J Med.* 1997;336:1356–1363.

101. Beal SM, Finch CF. An overview of retrospective case-control studies investigating the relationship between prone sleeping position and SIDS. *J Paediatr Child Health.* 1991;27:334–339.

102. Spiers PS, Guntheroth WG. Recommendations to avoid the prone sleeping position and recent statistics for sudden infant death syndrome in the United States. *Arch Pediatr Adolesc Med.* 1994;148:141–146.

103. Taylor JA, Davis RL. Risk factors for the infant prone sleep position. *Arch Pediatr Adolesc Med.* 1996;150:834–837.

104. McEvoy C, Mendoza ME, Bowling S, et al. Prone positioning decreases episodes of hypoxemia in extremely low birth weight infants (1000 grams or less) with chronic lung disease. *J Pediatr.* 1997;130:305–309.

105. Dimaguila MA, Fiore JM, Martin RJ, Miller MJ. Characteristics of hypoxemic episodes in very low birth weight infants on ventilatory support. *J Pediatr.* 1997;130:577–583.

106. Kurlak LO, Ruggins NR, Stephenson TJ. Effect of nursing position on incidence, type, and duration of apnoea in preterm infants. *Arch Dis Child Fetal Neonatal Ed.* 1994;71:F16–F19.

17

Subacute Care

Robert Heidegger • John Walton

Key Terms

care plan
interdisciplinary team
    approach
point-of-care testing
routine cost limit (RCL)
scope of services
skilled nursing facility
    (SNF)

Objectives

• Define subacute care, and identify differences in types of patient service.

• Compare and contrast patient needs in the subacute care and home settings.

• List three settings in which subacute care is rendered.

• Discuss the economic incentives for providing subacute care.

• List advantages and disadvantages of the subacute care setting.

• Describe the roles of the team members and level of coordination of care required in subacute care, contrasted to the acute care setting.

• Contrast equipment needs and support requirements for subacute and acute services.

• Describe the role of the respiratory care practitioner in the subacute setting.

• Identify the typical scope of diagnostic services available in the subacute setting.

Although there is no universally accepted definition of subacute care, it can most simply be described as a level of inpatient care between the short-term acute hospital stay and the typical services rendered in a nursing home.[1]

Professional groups, such as the National Subacute Care Association, and accreditation agencies, such as the Joint Commission on Accreditation of Healthcare Organizations and the Committee on Accreditation of Rehabilitation Facilities, have adopted more lengthy definitions of subacute care. An interesting history of the term and its varying definitions is also available in a study commissioned by the Agency for Health Policy and Research of the Health Care Financing Administration published in December 1994 by the Lewin Group.[2] Adding confusion to the these distinctive definitions is a recent study implicating that subacute care patients in some settings may be sicker than the general acute care population as measured by both hospital and nursing home acuity scales.[3]

From a pragmatic standpoint, the respiratory care practitioner (RCP) should view the subacute care setting as appropriate for a patient who no longer needs the daily interventions offered only at acute care hospitals (eg, major surgery, high-level diagnostics, urgent care services). Although discharge home is possible for hospitalized respiratory patients who are capable of assisting in most of their activities of daily living, many patients do not meet these criteria and require further inpatient care. Patients whose needs fall in between those addressed by the hospital and home care settings are often best discharged to subacute sites.

SITES

Subacute care is rendered in three settings in the following order of prevalence: (1) free-standing **skilled nursing facilities** (SNFs), (2) hospital-based skilled nursing units, and (3) rehabilitation or other longer stay, acute care hospitals. The term SNF is restricted to an identified number of beds certified by the Health Care Financing Administration (HCFA) to participate in the Medicare program for servicing its long-term care benefits. Because there are Medicare reimbursement incentives to establishing such units over and above the traditional intermediate level of nursing homes, it is rare that a subacute facility is not Medicare certified as skilled or in an acute hospital. In 1996, there were 11,922 free-standing facilities with Medicare-certified SNF beds and 2055 hospitals with skilled nursing units in the United States.

For a hospital to be considered a longer-stay site and therefore exempt from the provisions of the HCFA's Prospective Payment System (PPS) for Medicare recipients (also known as *diagnostic-related grouping* [DRG] system), the hospital must demonstrate that its average length of stay exceeds 25 days. In 1996, there were about 100 hospitals meeting this definition of long-term stay (eg, Vencor hospitals, American Transitional Hospitals, Transitional Hospitals Corporation) in the United States. In the case of rehabilitation hospitals or units within short-term acute care hospitals, PPS exemption also requires that most diagnoses fit certain disease classifications.

ECONOMICS

From an economic perspective, development of subacute centers makes sense. Why should the patient, government, or insurance agency pay for services at the most expensive site (ie, short-term acute care hospital) when appropriate care can be rendered in a less costly subacute setting? Subacute care has often been described in such economic terms, and the birth of this type of care setting was associated with cost-containment initiatives from third-party payers and providers alike. Table 17–1 offers a comparison (albeit limited) of how direct bedside care in subacute care centers differs from that in acute hospitals and traditional nursing homes. Acute care hospitals are also burdened with high fixed-cost equipment and services that are not associated with subacute care facilities.[4]

Medicare Incentives

Becoming a new provider of Medicare SNF benefits provides an economic advantage. New providers are exempt from a geographically defined daily reimbursement ceiling called the **routine cost limit** (RCL) for a 3- to 4-year period. The RCL was designed to reimburse providers for nursing, administrative, supply, and capital costs in an up-and-running SNF. New providers are reimbursed under a cost-based system limited by the Tax Equity and Financial Responsibility Act (TEFRA), which recognizes both the direct and indirect (overhead) expenses of care during the start-up phase.

For existing providers of Medicare SNF benefits, HCFA has established a process to grant an exception to the RCL for a facility that can demonstrate that it has either atypical costs or services beyond those of regional SNFs. Because many subacute services entail nursing, social services, medical records, and other operating expenses that readily exceed the RCL ceiling, and because ventilator services per se are considered atypical, SNFs often file such RCL exception requests.

The number of new-provider exemption requests and filings for exceptions to the RCL has increased dramatically in the late 1990s. Short-term acute care hospitals can receive their full PPS reimbursement for a Medicare patient and then transfer that patient to their own SNF after 3 days, whereby they receive from Medicare either the TEFRA-limited cost-based reimbursement (as a new exempt provider) or an expense-related payment (as a provider meeting the exception to RCL). Nursing homes can also raise their overall level of reimbursement (which traditionally is state Medicaid-related or private pay) if they accept

Table • 17–1 DISTINGUISHING SUBACUTE CARE FROM SKILLED NURSING AND ACUTE HOSPITAL CARE*

Service	Acute Care Hospital	Subacute Care Unit	Skilled Nursing Facility
Nursing hours PPD	8–12 (ICU)	6–8 (ventilator)	2–3
	4–8 (general)	5–7 (other)	
Physician visits	Daily+	Weekly+	Monthly+
Professional staffing			
Dietitians	On admission	Weekly	Monthly
Occupational therapists	As needed	Daily	As needed
Physical therapists	Daily	Daily	As needed
Recreational therapists	As needed	Daily	Daily
Registered nurses	24 hours	24 hours	Daily
RCPs	24 hours	24 hours (ventilator)	As needed
		Daily (other)	
Social workers	As needed	As needed	Monthly
Speech therapists	As needed	Daily	As needed
Average costs PPD	$300–$800 (general)	$600–$700	$100–$150
(excluding physician)	$800–$2000 (ICU)		
Average length of stay	3–9 days	10–60 days	60+ days

*Actual figures will vary depending on specific treatment, facility location, and many other factors.
This table should be used as a general guide only.
  PPD, per patient day; ICU, intensive care unit; ventilator, ventilator in subacute care unit.

higher-acuity Medicare SNF patients because the RCL is usual greater than the typical non-Medicare payments. This reimbursement can be raised even beyond the RCL if the Medicare patients meet exception criteria. The growth of subacute care has logically been associated with these modifications to Medicare reimbursement policy.[5]

The growth of subacute care has also been linked to the implementation of Medicare PPS in hospitals between 1982 and 1986. Hospitals were given powerful financial incentives to reduce operating costs in the face of the set reimbursement under DRGs. For example, a hospital caring for a Medicare patient on a mechanical ventilator with no pre-existing respiratory disease (classified under DRG 475) would receive a set payment based on the weight of the DRG multiplied by the typical length of stay multiplied by the hospital-specific expense factor. This would typically be $10,000 to $20,000 during 1997 for most hospitals (excluding a modest provision for outlier cases). If the patient can be discharged to a subacute site before the hospital spent this fixed amount within DRG 475, the hospital keeps the profit under the current regulations. This same incentive system for all other diagnoses has led most hospitals with Medicare populations to discharge their patients "quicker and sicker" to alternative sites, such as subacute care.

Subacute care facilities that can safely manage ventilator and other patients requiring significant respiratory interventions present an outlet for hospitals to prevent their costs from exceeding the DRG reimbursement limit. Because the subacute center is often reimbursed by Medicare for its costs (either through the exemption or exception process), both the hospital and subacute facility gain economically by the transfer of respiratory patients.

Managed Care Influence

The proliferation of managed care (eg, health maintenance organizations, preferred provider organizations, provider-sponsored organizations) has also propelled the discharge of hospital patients to subacute care units. In an effort to reduce the length of hospital stay, the managed care plan sets strict utilization review criteria required to continue hospitalization. Once the managed care plan determines that the patient can be transferred safely to an alternate site, financial coverage of the stay at the hospital stops, further encouraging the hospital to work with the managed care plan to identify appropriate alternate care providers capable of serving this patient.

Managed care companies also view a distinction between a hospital-based SNF and a free-standing SNF. In 1994, the Prospective Payment Advisory Commission estimated that the average cost per day to care for hospital-based SNF patients is $443 versus $235 per day in a free-standing SNF.[6] Although part of this expense differential could be explained in terms of patient acuity, much of the higher cost in the hospital unit is related to the higher overhead allocated to the unit. If the care is comparable between the two SNFs, a managed care plan could offer a per diem payment rate of $300 to cover the patient. Although the average hospital-based SNF would lose $143 per patient per day (PPD) at this contracted price ($443 − $300), the free-standing SNF could gain $65 PPD over its costs ($300 − $235). Thus, it is common for a hospital-based SNF to restrict its admissions to Medicare patients, whereas the free-standing SNF is an outlet for both managed care and Medicare patients.

Referral Sources

For those contemplating building a subacute care unit in either a free-standing or hospital-based setting, maintaining a substantial volume of patients who meet this profile is essential. Box 17–1 describes the referral sources and typical diagnoses for subacute care admissions. The success of a subacute program lies in convincing these referral sources that the provider can deliver both safe and efficient care.

Unlike a hospital, where a person could literally walk in the front door to seek treatment, patients admitted to the subacute care unit are evaluated by a team both clinically (medical stability) and financially (reimbursement for subacute services). If the team determines that a patient would be appropriate for placement in the subacute care unit, the patient's attending physician must then write an order for the transfer.

Set-up

When a subacute ventilator unit is located within an SNF, significant investment is often made in upgrading the physical plant to include piped oxygen and vacuum. The facility must also purchase or rent high-technology equipment such as ventilators and monitoring devices. The facility also needs to acquire the necessary professional and support staff. Although this increases the operating costs over those of an SNF, those costs remain lower than the costs of running an acute care hospital.

The layout of the subacute unit includes areas for equipment and supply storage, office areas for the unit management, and an area for the respiratory care department. Patient rooms are generally private or semiprivate and are usually located in an area segregated from the rest of the SNF, with a separate dining area within the unit.

THE SUBACUTE CARE UNIT

Advantages and Disadvantages

The scope of services offered by various subacute providers differs just as hospitals differ in their expertise. Box 17–2 contains a summary of the relative advantages and disadvantages of such referrals.

Advantages of the subacute care environment include its ability to offer respiratory technologic support similar to that of an acute care hospital but in a less institutional atmosphere. Another significant advantage to this setting is the continuity of care. Caregivers and patients become familiar with each other because there is usually a staff of nursing personnel and RCPs dedicated to the unit. Additionally, many subacute respiratory care departments use protocols to expedite the ventilator weaning process. Respiratory care services may also be available outside of the subacute unit, in other areas of the SNF, although the highest-acuity respiratory patients are generally within the subacute unit, and the greatest portion of the RCP's time is spent there. Also, because patients must be assessed by the subacute care center staff before admission, the patient's medical and psychosocial conditions are generally known before the patient comes through the facility doors. With this initial information, clinical pathways and discharge planning can begin before admittance.

The subacute care setting also has some disadvantages. The subacute unit may not be capable of providing certain interventions in the event of an acute situation, such as the need for endotracheal intubation or advanced cardiac life support services. Because patients admitted to the subacute care setting are by definition more medically stable, the need for emergency intervention is rare. Still, if a patient should need invasive therapeutic or diagnostic services, such as bronchoscopy or videofluoroscopy, he or she would

---

Box • 17–1   COMMON REFERRALS

COMMON REFERRAL SOURCES TO SUBACUTE CARE

> Hospitals (including ICUs and emergency departments)
> Specialty rehabilitation hospitals
> Other subacute units
> Skilled nursing facilities
> Home care patients

THE MOST COMMON PATIENT REFERRAL TYPES TO SUBACUTE CARE

> Physical, occupational, and speech therapy
> Intravenous medication therapy
> Pulmonary rehabilitation
> Enterostomal therapy
> Chemotherapy

Box • 17–2   COMMON ADVANTAGES AND DISADVANTAGES OF SUBACUTE CARE

ADVANTAGES

- Lower cost than acute care
- Technologic capabilities similar to acute care
- Dedicated staff
- Less institution-like environment

DISADVANTAGES

- Need for certain services may require transfer to hospital.

have to be transferred to the hospital to receive these services.

The Subacute Care Team

Perhaps the greatest distinction between the subacute unit staff and their acute care counterparts is in the coordination of services provided. Rehabilitative services, such as those offered by physical, occupational, and speech therapists, are used extensively in the subacute care environment. In the acute care setting, where focus is generally targeted at resolving an immediate crisis, the subacute focus is geared toward the highest level of premorbid function that the patient can achieve. In the subacute care setting, daily physician intervention is rarely required. The nursing, respiratory care, and other professional staff need to use their clinical assessment skills constantly to follow clinical pathways and to keep the physician informed of the patient's condition.

Figure 17–1 shows a typical unit organization for a subacute ventilator unit in a free-standing or hospital-based SNF. State laws require the SNF to employ a director of nursing and a facility medical director. The SNF must also have a licensed nursing home administrator to manage the operations of the facility. The subacute unit may also have its own medical director, and if the subacute unit specializes in the treatment of respiratory impaired patients, a pulmonologist may serve as the medical director of the unit and possibly as the attending physician for patients admitted to the unit in cases in which the patient's previous physician chooses not to follow. Physician rounds are usually conducted at least weekly in the subacute care unit.

A director of nursing manages the overall nursing operation of the facility, although the unit probably has hired a clinical coordinator, who is a registered nurse, to oversee the management of the unit nursing and RCP staff. A respiratory care manager is sometimes used, depending on the size and volume of respiratory care services present in the facility.

The subacute care unit staff must also interact with the other SNF professional staff (physical, occupational, and speech therapists; social services; dietitians; and care plan coordinators) when determining the best approach for the care of the patient. This team approach is referred to as an **interdisciplinary team approach**. Meetings are scheduled regularly, and team members discuss the interventions they are providing and their ongoing **care plan** for the patient. Often, progress made in one area can influence the care plan in another. For example, if a patient is undergoing aggressive ventilator weaning by the RCP, he or she may not be able to tolerate extensive sessions in physical therapy. If the weaning trials were not communicated by the RCP to the physical therapist, the therapist may believe the patient had experienced a setback. By communicating important information such as this on a regular basis, the team can adjust the plan of care and the expectations associated with the treatment plan.

Respiratory Services

The RCP's role in the subacute care environment is dependent on the type of subacute services offered by the facility. Other factors, such as acuity and volume of respiratory patients, can affect the RCP's role. Subacute respiratory services are offered in two general categories: ventilator-related services and complex care services. Complex care respiratory services include oxygen and humidity administration, respiratory treatments, bilevel positive airway pressure (BiPAP), and tracheostomy care. The most significant differences between ventilator-related and complex

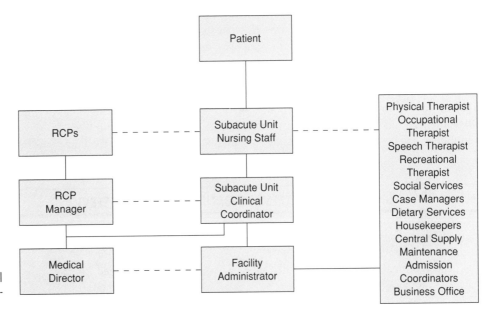

FIGURE 17–1 • Typical organization for a subacute respiratory unit.

care respiratory services are in the areas of RCP staffing and the physical plant. Table 17–2 describes these key differences.

Physical Plant and Equipment Considerations

In a subacute unit that is designed to care for ventilator-dependent patients, the use of piped medical gas, including oxygen and air, is desirable. If piped gases are unavailable, the facility must use electric air compressors and oxygen concentrators to provide the appropriate gas flow to the patient. Also, the addition of a piped vacuum eliminates the need for electronic suction machines, which can be limited in their power. Technologic advances in respiratory care equipment are beginning to address issues of equipment size, portability, and operation without the need for high-pressure gas sources. If the subacute unit is designed to provide respiratory services to complex care patients, the use of piped medical gases or vacuum is generally not required. With both types of subacute services, however, the facility must provide a backup source of electrical power capable of supporting the type of respiratory equipment used. This is usually a gas- or diesel-powered electric generator upgraded to handle the power requirements.

Most subacute units that are based outside of the hospital choose to rent rather than own most of the complex medical equipment. The main reasons are cost and maintenance of the equipment. Also, an SNF with Medicare as a predominant payer source is reimbursed for the direct costs associated with rented equipment. A facility would have to expend a considerable amount of capital to purchase enough ventilators to provide this service to patients. Additionally, the facility would then need to hire or contract a qualified biomedical technician to provide maintenance for the equipment, or the facility would have to purchase a service contract with the equipment vendor. The maintenance cost is factored into the rental price of the equipment. The facility also needs to maintain an appropriate amount of reserve equipment, such as ventilators and oxygen (concentrators and cylinders), in the event of disaster or equipment failure.

Staffing

Staffing levels for RCPs vary depending on the type of subacute care service. In a unit that provides mechanical ventilatory support, including ventilator weaning, RCP would typically be on site 24 hours per day, 7 days per week, at a level of about 3 to 4 hours PPD. The following Critical Thinking Challenge shows an example of RCP staffing using hours PPD. In a subacute unit that provides mechanical ventilatory support but in which the patients have been determined to be chronically ventilator dependent, RCP staffing levels are generally reduced because the level of the RCP intervention is reduced overall.

In a subacute unit that provides complex care respiratory services, RCP staffing levels are determined by the frequency with which the patients receive treatment. For instance, if patients are receiving respiratory care treatment four times daily, RCP staffing would need to include coverage for all four treatments, or about 12 hours per day. The use of 24-hour on-site RCP coverage in a complex care subacute unit is rarely required, unless the patient's condition or frequency of treatment administration warrants the additional hours of RCP service. Generally, around-the-clock respiratory care treatments in a complex care subacute unit are not required.

Technology

The technology available in subacute facilities has undergone significant advances during the past few years. When subacute services initially became available, the respiratory technology available to the subacute RCP was limited to the type of equipment found in the acute care setting or that used in home care. Although acute care hospital respiratory equipment could be applied in the subacute setting with the presence of piped oxygen and vacuum, there were some drawbacks. One of the largest expenditures for respiratory equipment in the subacute setting is allocated to ventilators. Because most hospital ventilators are capable of providing all modes of ventilatory support, their cost is usually high. Also, hospital ventilators are traditionally large in size and often require an external source of high-pressure gas (oxygen, medical air, or both). Because storage space in the subacute unit is often limited and the larger size of the hospital ventilator may be obtrusive in the patient room, this type of ventilator may not be appropriate for use in this setting. Additionally, because the subacute patient may not use the full capabilities of the hospital ventilator, the rental or purchase cost of such equipment may be prohibitive. On the other hand, the type of ventilator used in the home care setting, although modest in size and

Table • 17–2 DIFFERENTIATING TYPES OF SUBACUTE RESPIRATORY SERVICES

	Ventilator (Weaning)	Ventilator (Nonweaning)	Complex Care
Physical plant	Piped oxygen, air, and vacuum Backup electrical power Reserve respiratory equipment	Piped oxygen and air Backup electrical power Reserve respiratory equipment	Backup electrical power Reserve respiratory equipment
RCP staffing	24 hour/7 days per week 3 to 4 hours PPD	Up to 24 hours/7 days per week 2 to 3 hours PPD	As needed

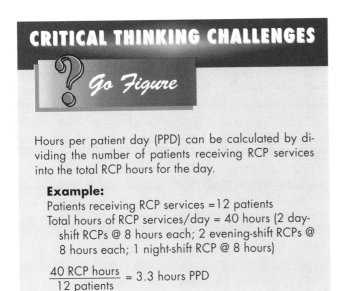

CRITICAL THINKING CHALLENGES

Go Figure

Hours per patient day (PPD) can be calculated by dividing the number of patients receiving RCP services into the total RCP hours for the day.

Example:
Patients receiving RCP services = 12 patients
Total hours of RCP services/day = 40 hours (2 day-shift RCPs @ 8 hours each; 2 evening-shift RCPs @ 8 hours each; 1 night-shift RCP @ 8 hours)

$$\frac{40 \text{ RCP hours}}{12 \text{ patients}} = 3.3 \text{ hours PPD}$$

cost, may not offer some of the capabilities required for ventilator weaning.

Of all the requirements respiratory care equipment in the subacute setting must meet, portability with advanced features stand out as the most important attributes. With mechanical ventilators, the ability to combine the features of a hospital ventilator with the size and portability of a home care ventilator would be ideal. Because patients in the subacute unit often spend a great deal of time outside of their rooms, whether receiving rehabilitation therapy services or eating a meal in the unit dining area, the mobility of the patient cannot be restricted by lack of appropriate equipment. The most frequently used diagnostic tool in the subacute unit is the pulse oximeter. Although arterial blood gas (ABG) measurements are vital during the weaning process, the use of routine ABG measurement in the subacute care setting is rare. Most subacute units use an outside contractor to provide ABG measurements because the cost associated with maintaining a laboratory within the facility can be excessive, especially if a limited number of ABG measurements are to be expected. With the advent of **point-of-care testing,** however, portable ABG measurement is making this a moot point. In point-of-care testing, pulse oximetry and capnometry measurements serve as an adjunct to ABG measurement, thus reducing the discomfort to the patient, reducing the overall cost to the facility and the patient, and providing accurate and timely data on which clinical decisions can be made.

ROLE OF THE RESPIRATORY CARE PRACTITIONER

In the subacute setting, the role of the RCP is not limited to providing respiratory therapy to the patient. The RCP's involvement in the care of a patient ideally begins before the patient's admission to the facility. For ventilator patients, a preadmission evaluation is conducted by a team from the subacute unit, which includes, at minimum, a nurse and an RCP. This preadmission evaluation is conducted at the referring facility to gather clinical information to determine if the subacute unit can provide the care necessary for the patient. The hospital or other site that desires to transfer a patient to the subacute unit notifies the facility social services department that it has received discharge orders from the patient's physician. After verification of appropriate financial resources, a clinical evaluation is conducted. Each subacute unit determines its own admission criteria. For example, patients with endotracheal tubes are generally not appropriate candidates for admission to subacute care units because these sites do not usually have the ability to reintubate and verify proper placement of endotracheal tubes.

Assessment Skills

The assessment skills of the RCP are used in a variety of ways in the subacute care unit. Generally, within 48 hours of admission, the patient is evaluated by a physician, whether by the patient's physician from the discharge origin or the subacute unit's medical director. At this point, the physician usually requests the RCP to conduct an evaluation of the patient and provide respiratory therapy recommendations. This initial evaluation of the patient gathers baseline information from the medical record and from direct assessment of the patient, such as breath sounds and pulse oximetry. Recommendations for treatment are then communicated to the physician.

If the subacute unit has developed and obtained appropriate written approval for protocols, the physician may order treatment or weaning based on the RCP following these protocols. Because a patient's continued treatment in a subacute unit is often limited in time by the payer, the use of protocols can result in a decreased length of stay. After a physician-prescribed respiratory treatment regimen, the RCP determines the appropriateness of the treatment based on measured progress (eg, improved breath sounds, decrease in shortness of breath), patient tolerance of the therapy, clinical observations, and the use of established criteria for continuation of therapy. These assessments are performed and documented with each treatment and are usually summarized in writing every 7 days. Any recommended change in the patient's respiratory plan of care is then immediately communicated to the physician for consideration.

The RCP must also communicate patient progress to other members of the interdisciplinary team. This is usually accomplished at predetermined intervals when the team meets to discuss the plan of care for all patients. A representative from the respiratory care department is selected to attend this meeting. Any significant changes in the respiratory plan of care are communicated to the patient's nurse and are documented in the patient's care plan, located in the medical record. Assessments of the patient are conducted at regular intervals, usually every 2 to 4 hours for ventilator and other tracheostomy patients. Complex care patients are generally assessed by the RCP with each treatment and at least once per shift.

Diagnostic Services

Diagnostic services play a key role in the patient's respiratory care plan. If a patient is receiving supplemental oxygen therapy, pulse oximetry measurements are performed routinely to assist in determining the continued need for the oxygen. Many payers require that patients meet certain criteria for the use of supplemental oxygen (eg, Blue Cross/Blue Shield Medical Necessity Guidelines). Other diagnostic services, such as chest radiograph or sputum culture and sensitivity, are provided mainly by an outside contractor and are performed only when clinically indicated. Table 17–3 shows some common respiratory diagnostic tools used in the subacute setting.

When performing diagnostic or therapeutic procedures, the RCP follows an established set of guidelines, which are usually found in the respiratory care department policy and procedure manual. These guidelines must be approved in writing by facility administration and by the facility or subacute unit medical director and reviewed or updated at least annually. The manner in which RCPs perform procedures is similar to that of their acute care counterparts. Most differences are found in the documentation of the procedure performed. Payers of subacute services often require evidence of necessity for therapeutic procedures to be documented each time a procedure is performed. The RCP must be aware of the clinical impact of each therapeutic procedure provided while administering the therapy and also must be aware of how it relates to therapy previously administered because clinical changes may manifest more subtly or over a longer period of time in a chronically ill patient. The documentation of the RCP must reflect the ap-

proaches to achieving the expected patient goals outlined in the overall plan of care. For instance, if a patient in the subacute unit is receiving hand-held nebulizer therapy to treat a pulmonary infiltrate but has demonstrated no progress toward meeting the defined patient goals for breath sounds, degree of dyspnea, or production of sputum, a review of this documentation should trigger the RCP to recommend to the physician an alternate approach, such as chest physical therapy. Box 17–3 describes some of the key elements relating to RCP documentation.

Documentation also plays a role in justifying the need for the RCP to provide respiratory care services to the patient. Documentation of respiratory procedures must include evidence that the skill level of the RCP is required, whether for the administration of the therapy or for the monitoring of its effects. Because the nursing staff in the subacute unit generally has minimal experience in treating the pulmonary impaired patient, the responsibility for providing respiratory services is often shared between the RCP and the unit nursing staff. For example, if the RCP determines that a patient is no longer making progress and that an alternate therapy is not indicated but the patient still requires the services to maintain a stable pulmonary status, the RCP would begin the transition of the patient's respiratory care to the subacute unit nursing staff. This is usually accomplished by in-servicing the nursing staff and by requiring return demonstration of proper therapy administration technique. It is rare for the RCP and the subacute unit nursing staff to share the provision of respiratory services to the same patient. Because third-party payers often require documented evidence to justify the expense of the RCP, sharing of the same respiratory services for the same patient may raise questions about the need for the RCP.

Another important aspect of the RCP's documentation is to assist in determining the appropriateness of the respiratory care services provided. For example, if a patient is receiving supplemental oxygen therapy at 4 L/min by nasal cannula, and documented pulse oximetry measurements show SpO_2 levels consistently above 96%, both at rest and during exertion, the appropriateness of this level of oxygen therapy may be questioned. Likewise, if a patient receiving aerosolized bronchodilator therapy for wheezing demonstrates clear breath sounds and absence of sputum produc-

Table • 17–3   COMMON DIAGNOSTIC TOOLS USED IN THE SUBACUTE SETTING

Diagnostic Tool	Frequency of Use
Arterial blood gas (ABG) measurement	When changes in ventilator rate, mode, or pressure support levels are made
	Within 2 hours after discontinuation of mechanical ventilatory support
	Within 2 hours after tracheal decannulation
Pulse oximetry	Every shift when receiving mechanical ventilatory support or supplemental oxygen therapy
	Within 2 hours after an adjustment or discontinuation in supplemental oxygen therapy
	Continuous use for monitoring and trending
Capnometry	As an adjunct to ABG measurement
	Continuous use for monitoring and recording trends

Box • 17–3   KEY POINTS OF RCP DOCUMENTATION

- Often used to justify RCP-level intervention
- Must demonstrate therapy appropriateness
- Documented procedural duration used to determine productivity
- All patient-related activities, direct or indirect, must be documented.

tion after a few days of treatment, the RCP needs to reevaluate the necessity of this type of treatment and contact the patient's physician to suggest a change in the treatment plan. Patient education also plays a key role when considering the RCP's documentation. Education can include breathing and coughing techniques, energy conservation, or the self-administration of respiratory procedures, such as metered dose inhalers and suctioning. Patient education is especially useful when the patient will be discharged home because the RCP is able to provide the instruction and observe the patient's progress in performing the procedures that have been instructed.

Another role for the RCP in the subacute setting involves participation with facility committees, including continuous quality improvement, infection control, safety, and interdisciplinary team meetings. The participation of the RCP in these activities is often required by regulatory agencies such as the Joint Commission for the Accreditation of Healthcare Organizations. In the acute care hospital setting, the respiratory care department director usually participates in the hospital quality assurance, infection control, and safety committee meetings. The RCP's involvement with these activities in acute care would be remote or nonexistent. In the subacute unit, however, the involvement of the entire respiratory care department is essential, especially with continuous quality improvement activities, because the RCP is responsible the collection of data relating to patient care. Interdisciplinary team meetings provide the RCP the opportunity to discuss the progress of the patient and the future plan of care. Each discipline providing care to the patient is represented at this meeting, allowing the RCP to get a complete picture of the patient's clinical condition and progress toward the discharge plan.

Respiratory Care Procedures

Although many of the procedures performed by RCPs in the subacute unit are similar to those performed by their acute care counterparts, there are some notable differences. In the subacute setting, RCPs generally provide most of the airway care, including suctioning and tracheostomy care. By providing this consistency with the patient's airway care, the RCP can be immediately alerted to changes in secretions or appearance of the stoma. Also, the subacute care RCP relies more on pulse oximetry and capnometry and less on ABG measurements mainly because many subacute units do not have the capability of providing ABG measurements on site. Another difference between services offered by the subacute respiratory care department and those generally available in the acute care hospital is the use of protocols in the subacute setting. In subacute care units, physician intervention is less intense and less frequent than that found in the acute care setting. The subacute respiratory care department often develops protocols for ventilator weaning, tracheostomy tube decannulation,

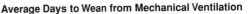

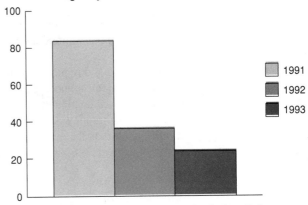

Note: Protocols for weaning from mechanical ventilation were implemented in this subacute unit at the end of 1990.

FIGURE 17-2 • The impact of protocol use at one subacute unit. (*Source: Integrated Health Services of Chicago at Brentwood, Burbank, IL*)

and supplemental oxygen therapy weaning. Once approved for use, a physician may order weaning to be conducted per protocol. This permits RCPs to use their assessment and decision-making skills and can often assist in expediting the weaning process (Fig. 17–2), although it should be noted that several factors can influence the ability to wean a patient from mechanical ventilation.

Each subacute respiratory care department develops a list of services available through the department. This list is usually maintained as a part of the respiratory care department policy and procedure manuals. These services are

Table • 17–4   SAMPLE SCOPE OF SUBACUTE RESPIRATORY SERVICES*

Therapeutic
Aerosolized medication nebulizer
Chest physical therapy
Postural drainage
Incentive spirometry
Breathing retraining
Oxygen therapy
Ventilator management and weaning
Tracheostomy care
Suctioning
Diagnostic
Arterial blood gas measurement
Pulse oximetry
Capnometry
Bedside spirometry
Sputum collection for analysis
Electrocardiogram
Respiratory assessment
Emergency
Basic life support

*This sample Scope of Services is not meant to be inclusive. Respiratory care services will vary among subacute units.

generally referred to as the **scope of services**. Table 17–4 shows what such a list may contain, although the scope of services for each subacute respiratory care department varies depending on the type of patients admitted and the capabilities of the facility.

As health care costs continue to rise and reimbursement for these services becomes more limited, the need for the services offered by the subacute unit will continue to grow. Concurrently, the need for the high-technology skills of the RCP in the subacute unit will increase as the acuity level and respiratory requirements of patients admitted to the subacute environment escalate.

References

1. Walton J, Heidegger R. Subacute care: A new opportunity for RCP's. *AARC Times*. 1993;17(5):49.
2. Lewin Group. *Subacute Care: Review of the Literature*. Fairfax, VA: Lewin Group; 1994.
3. McCormick W. Severity of illness: Comparisons between subacute care, acute care, and nursing facilities. *Nursing Home Medicine*. 1997;5(2):56–59.
4. Walton J. Understanding the costs of healthcare with specific attention to respiratory care. *Respiratory Care*. 1975; January.
5. Lewin Group. *Subacute Care: Policy Synthesis and Market Area Analysis*. Fairfax, VA: Lewin Group; 1995.
6. Lellis M, ed. Industry looks to case-mix demonstration for answers on new SNF PPS. *National Report on Subacute Care*. 1997;5(4).

18

Home Respiratory Care

Robert M. Lewis • Eileen M. Hagarty • Brian Lawlor

Key Terms

bilevel positive airway
    pressure (BiPAP)
clinical practice guidelines
concentrator
cylinders
liquid oxygen systems
quality of life

Objectives

- Describe the overall goals of home care.

- Discuss the process of patient assessment for home care.

- Outline problems with adherence to home care prescriptions.

- Describe the use of different types of oxygen delivery systems in the home.

- Review the assessment and planning required for successful discharge of the home ventilator-dependent patient.

- Discuss the application of noninvasive positive-pressure ventilation in the home.

Home respiratory care has undergone tremendous growth in the past two decades. This growth has been quantitative and qualitative; more patients are receiving care in the home, and the complexity of that care has increased steadily. In addition, outcome expectations have risen. Along with these changes, the roles of the home care agency, the home care provider, and the respiratory care practitioner (RCP) have evolved.

Several key trends in the evolution of home respiratory care have been identified,[1] including the following:

- A shift in focus from equipment set-up and maintenance to patient and caregiver education and consultation
- A recognition of the importance of the in-home caregiver
- A preference for a collaborative management approach
- An appreciation of the cultural context of home health care
- A recognition of quality of life as the most important outcome measure
- A desire for favorable cost/benefit ratios in all aspects of home care

This chapter begins with an overview of the home care process, including overall goals of home care; a generic overview of the assessment and care planning process; and an overview of patient education. This is followed by a discussion of the practical aspects of home respiratory care and an outline of some important aspects of the management of a home care agency.

HOME HEALTH CARE: AN OVERVIEW

The rapidly changing health care environment necessitates much more than a shift in the location of care delivery from the hospital to the home. Rather, health care providers must recognize that the ultimate responsibility for health maintenance is shifting from the health care provider to the patient. The shift in focus also recognizes that restoring or promoting patient independence and autonomy, rather than dependence, is an important health care goal.

Because of major advances in health care technology, people are living longer than ever before. Dramatic improvement in physiologic parameters or mere survival are no longer the exclusive measure of treatment success. Treatment outcomes must incorporate the functional, psychological, and social aspects of a person's life.[2–4] All care delivery strategies should be focused on attainment of realistic outcomes that foster wellness and an improved quality of life. **Quality of life** is a dynamic concept that is ever-changing and time-dependent[5] and that encompasses physical, psychological, and social domains[2–4] (Table 18–1).

Table • 18–1 QUALITY OF LIFE DOMAINS

Physical
Physical function
Ambulation and mobility
Self-care ability
Ability to work
Energy and stamina
Adequate sleep and rest
Nutritional balance
Absence of pain
Control of symptoms
Somatic comfort
Physical independence
Required lifestyle change
Sexual activity
Toxicity of treatment
Ability to take care of responsibilities
Ability to participate in recreational activities

Psychological
Level of stress
Coping ability
Control over life
Meaning of life
Healthy body image
Self-acceptance
Self-esteem and worth
Absence of negative mood
Psychological well-being
Achievement of life goals
Intellectual functioning
Perceived health status
Seriousness of illness
Illness worries and concerns
Illness prognosis
Confidence in treatment
Acceptability of treatment
Satisfaction with treatment
Satisfaction with health care
Adjustment to illness
Affect
Spiritual aspects
Depression
Creative expression
Hope
Enthusiasm for life and fortitude
Sense of security

Social
Ability to communicate
Role function
Usefulness to others
Recreational participation
Social interaction
Satisfaction with sexual life
Marital and family relationships
Family health and happiness
Financial independence
Socioeconomic status
Standard of living
Neighborhood
Employment status
Education
Friendships
Social life
Satisfaction with city, nation

THE DISCHARGE PLANNING PROCESS

Patients with chronic disease of any kind may experience problems in everyday living that can adversely affect their wellness and quality of life if adequate problem-solving strategies are not employed. Home health care providers should develop a plan of care and provide services that focus on assisting their patients to develop coping abilities in a number of areas.[6,7]

The discharge planning process includes a comprehensive patient assessment, development of a patient problem list, identification of services to meet the identified needs, development and implementation of a patient and caregiver training program, and evaluation of outcome. Depending on patient need, the discharge planning team may include a physician, professional nurse, respiratory care practitioner, dietitian, pharmacist, social worker, and/or physical, occupational, and speech therapists.

Patient Assessment

The performance of an in-depth, quality assessment of the patient, family, and environment assists the health care provider in identifying realistic and appropriate treatment outcomes and strategies. This assessment must examine the patient and family's ability to complete the training and lifestyle changes required for successful home care.

This process begins by assessing the patient and family's comfort with self-disclosure. Topics such as income, psychiatric histories, interfamily personal conflicts, and substance abuse are uncomfortable areas for many but must be explored to develop a comprehensive plan of care. Therefore, the assessment process must be carefully tailored to the patient's level of comfort.[8] A good introductory statement often puts the patient at ease. For example, the interview may begin with the statement, "To work with you thoroughly, I need to ask you some questions that may seem personal in nature. Would you be comfortable with that? If I ask you any questions that you do not want to answer or that you feel are too personal, please let me know. I do not want you to feel uncomfortable."

To understand even simple instructions for home care procedures, patients should be able to read at least at the fifth grade level. Sometimes, an estimate of the patient's reading ability can be ascertained informally through conversation, patient history, and observation. If any doubt exists, the patient's literacy level can be formally determined by use of diagnostic tests, such as the Wide Range Achievement Test or the Rapid Estimate of Literacy in Medicine.

Patients should be assessed for the presence of any form of mental illness, such as anxiety or depression, because these conditions can impair the patient's ability to participate in the training and self-care process. In addition, mental illness should be treated to improve the patient's quality of life.

In the assessment process, the patient and family's expectations and preferences regarding treatment and outcomes must be identified. Any discrepancy between the discharge team's expectations and those of the family should be resolved before discharge.

Baseline patient assessment can be accomplished by any member of the health care team as long as it incorporates investigative questions designed to identify problem areas that require more in-depth assessment. The collected data should be reviewed by the various disciplines involved in the patient's care. Team consensus with patient and family concurrence is essential for the success of a plan of care. Figure 18–1 provides examples of important data to obtain from an initial patient assessment.

Patient Care Plan

After assessment of the patient, a plan of care must be developed. The plan should include a listing of desired patient goals and outcomes related to the identified problem areas, such as the following:

- Fewer somatic complaints
- Increased exercise tolerance and energy level
- Correct medication administration
- Ability to function appropriately in crisis situation
- Decreased anxiety
- Prevention or delay of complications

CRITICAL THINKING CHALLENGES

Shifting Care Plans

Targeted Problem Areas of a Home Health Care Plan

☐ Symptom control
☐ Implementation of specific treatment regimens
☐ Prevention of or management of medical crises situations
☐ Adjustment to changes in the course of the disease
☐ Prevention of or delayed onset of chronic complications
☐ Prevention of or living with social isolation caused by lessened contact with others
☐ Implementation of healthy changes in lifestyle
☐ Finding ways to pay for the required medical care and to survive despite partial or complete loss of employment

Patient Assessment Parameters

Name _____ Height _____ Weight _____ Marital Status _____

Social Security Number _____ Occupation _____

Current Job Status _____ Are you experiencing any financial problems? _____

Do you have adequate health care coverage? _____

Primary Care Physician _____

Medical Diagnoses _____
_____

Past Medical History _____
_____

Present Symptoms _____
_____

Previous Hospitalizations _____
_____
_____

Known Allergies _____

Family Support systems _____

Literacy Level _____

Description of Home Environment _____

Comfort Level for Self-disclosure _____

Current Medications (name, dose, administration route, frequency, reason for taking) _____
_____

Home Medical Equipment _____

Do you use oxygen at home? _____ If yes, how much? _____

How many times have you had an infection this past year? _____

Do you have problems with your appetite? _____

Are you currently following a diet plan? _____ If yes, what type of diet are you following? _____

How many glasses of liquid do you drink every day? _____

Do you need assistance with bathing, dressing, walking, bathroom or eating? _____

Describe any physical activity that you do on a regular basis (type of activity, times per week) _____

Do you follow any type of exercise program at home? _____ If yes, how often do you exercise? _____

Do you have difficulty sleeping? _____

How many hours per day do you sleep? _____

Are you a nervous person? _____

Do you ever get depressed? _____

Do you experience mood swings? _____

Are you experiencing any tension in your relationship with your spouse, family members and/or significant others?
_____

Are you experiencing any difficulty with your sexual functioning? _____

Are you a spiritual person? _____

Do you currently smoke? _____ If yes, what do you smoke? _____

If yes, how many packs per day _____ If you quit smoking, when did you quit? _____

How many years have you smoked? _____

Are you currently exposed to second hand smoke? _____

Do you drink alcoholic beverages? _____ If so, what is your pattern of alcohol use? _____

Do you use any other recreational substances such as marijuana, cocaine, heroin, acid or prescription tranquilizers or pain killers? _____

If so, how much? _____

FIGURE 18–1 • Sample form incorporating patient assessment parameters.

- Decreased hospital use
- Increase in recreational activities

It is important that treatment goals be simple and easily measured. An example of a patient care plan is illustrated in the following Critical Thinking Challenge. The effectiveness of care and justification for continued services should be based on evaluation of achievement of the stated goals. The Joint Commission 1997-1998 Accreditation Manual for Home Care recommends that all of the goals and services for respiratory patients be evaluated every 30 days.[9]

Patient and Caregiver Training

Not all patients or their caregivers grasp the meaning behind health care instructions when they are provided. Certain conditions must be present to enhance memory and learning. Many factors, such as logic, experience, and language, must interact effectively for comprehension to take place.[10]

Patients and caregivers are not inclined to accept or learn new information unless this information is matched to their own logic, language, and experience. Cultural suitability must always be a consideration when written, audiotaped, or audiovisual material is used for instructional purposes. The use of audiotaped or videotaped instructions can increase teaching effectiveness and enhance patients' and caregivers' ability to learn new material. The problem with one-to-one oral instruction is that it takes a lot of time. Patients and caregivers tend to forget most of what they are told minutes after the educational intervention is provided. Easy-to-read educational materials produce a higher rate of patient and caregiver adherence.[10]

An overview of the patient and caregiver education process is given in the American Association of Respiratory Care (AARC) Clinical Practice Guideline on providing patient and caregiver training (Box 18–1).

CLINICAL APPLICATION OF RESPIRATORY CARE

Respiratory care is provided in the home to meet several broad categories of patient needs, including the following:

- Maintenance of arterial oxygenation
- Maintenance of alveolar ventilation
- Assurance of airway patency
- Delivery of medication to the respiratory tract

All of these treatment goals may require the use of sophisticated equipment. In addition, various forms of physical therapy can be used to improve mucociliary clearance. Often, several types of equipment or therapies are required to meet the patient's needs.

The role of the RCP, however, goes well beyond the correct set-up, maintenance, and operation of machines. Rather, the RCP's role is to use equipment and therapeutic

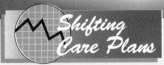

CRITICAL THINKING CHALLENGES
Shifting Care Plans

Home Oxygen Patient: Plan of Care

Goals and desired outcomes:

1. The patient and family will understand the following:
   - ☐ Reason why home oxygen therapy has been prescribed
   - ☐ Required oxygen flow (L/min)
   - ☐ Required hours per day of usage
   - ☐ Dangers of overusing oxygen from prescription
   - ☐ Dangers of underusing oxygen from prescription
   - ☐ Equipment operation requirements and problem solving
   - ☐ Who to contact when problems arise

2. The patient and family will not receive a burn or electrical injury as a result of having oxygen equipment in their home.

3. The patient or caregiver will adhere to the patient's home oxygen prescription.

Interventions:

1. Instruct the patient and the family or significant others on the following:
   - ☐ Reason why home oxygen therapy has been prescribed
   - ☐ Required oxygen flow (L/min)
   - ☐ Required hours per day of usage
   - ☐ Dangers of overusing oxygen from prescription
   - ☐ Dangers of underusing oxygen from prescription
   - ☐ Equipment operation requirements and problem solving
   - ☐ Who to contact when problems arise

2. Each patient or caregiver will be required to demonstrate proper equipment set-up and maintenance requirements.

3. Monitor patient compliance to prescription and safety requirements with every visit, as follows:
   - ☐ Document oxygen therapy device, flow, and duration of use.
   - ☐ Document the hour meter reading on the oxygen concentrator machine.
   - ☐ Monitor monthly portable tank usage.
   - ☐ Observe for any signs of smoking or other violations of safety rules.

Box • 18–1 AARC CLINICAL PRACTICE GUIDELINE

PROVIDING PATIENT AND CAREGIVER TRAINING

Description and definition: Patient and caregiver education provides the patient and family with the means of participating in the patient's health care management to the extent feasible, depending on physical condition and awareness. (The term *family* encompasses the persons who play a significant role in the patient's life and may include persons who are not legally related to the patient.) The training process should occur with every encounter between the health care provider (HCP) and the patient. The goal of the HCP should be to elicit a positive change in the patient's behavior through the use of verbal, written, and visual communication in the affective, cognitive, and psychomotor domains. Coordinated efforts by HCPs should provide the patient with an improved understanding of health care needs, therapy, and the importance of adherence to medical regimen and candid communication with caregivers. This should enable the patient to manage the disease better through cooperation with the caregiver and HCP in an active partnership. All members of the team need to be aware of these goals as an aspect of the patient's total care. A final goal of the HCP is to provide the patient and family with the means to reap the economic benefits of improved use of the health care system.

Limitations of method:

Patient limitations: lack of motivation or interest in acquiring knowledge or skills (this may include denial); impairment (eg, in hearing or vision, decreased energy or stamina, age-specific, pain, or medication side effects); inability to comprehend owing to factors such as anxiety, depression, hypoxemia, substance abuse; negative response to past educational experiences or encounters; illiteracy despite level of education completed, which may include functional illiteracy dealing with the health care process; a mind-set that leads to misapplication, misinterpretation, or rejection of instruction as irrelevant; language barriers; conflict of religious beliefs or cultural practices with material presented.

HCP limitations: lack of positive attitude or adaptability; limited understanding of knowledge or skill to be taught; inadequate assessment of patient's need or readiness to learn and inability to individualize the instructional approach to the patient, including age-specific needs; multiple patient needs to be met in the allotted time; inappropriate or inadequate communication skills (eg, unnecessary use of medical terminology, lack of listening skills); lack of documentation or discussion with other team members; inconsistency in information presented; inadequate knowledge of cultural or religious practice that may affect education process.

System limitations: hospital stay too brief; absence of interdisciplinary cooperation and communication; inconsistency in information provided; failure to provide interpreters.

Social limitations: absence of support system; reimbursement issues.

Environmental limitations: inadequate lighting, poor temperature control, uncomfortable seating, inadequate space for demonstrations; interruptions, distractions, and noise; poorly chosen resources, including inappropriate reading level and vocabulary.

Assessment of need: Determine the gap between what the patient already knows and what he or she needs to know. Interview the patient regarding past experience with topic being taught. A published self-generated guide may be used. Discuss what the patient perceives as knowledge relevant to his or her care. Observe the patient's performance of therapy and determine whether skills are adequate for self-care. (If psychomotor skills are markedly impaired, an occupational or physical therapy assessment may be indicated.) Determine whether the patient's attitude and outlook appear to be conducive to participation in his or her health care. By observation and questioning, determine whether the patient perceives himself or herself as able to cope with health care. By questioning patient and family, determine whether denial persists. (A psychological consult may be helpful.) Assess the patient's motivation or emotional readiness to learn and change behavior as it relates to his or her health care. Consider using quality-of-life profiles to determine the patient's general outlook and attitude or to determine the presence of low self-efficacy.

Assessment of outcome:

Assessment of knowledge gained: in a nonthreatening manner, question patient about specific aspects of information presented and note questions asked; request patient to repeat information given, in his or her own words.

Assessment of skills mastered: observe patient performing skill without prompting or assistance; observe patient's ability to adapt new skill to novel or unfamiliar situations; determine skill adaptability in home environment by telephone calls and home visits.

Assessment of patient outlook and attitude: observe patient and quantitate appropriate variables for evidence of life style changes (eg, weight change, smoking cessation, increased physical activity); determine through discussion with patient and family whether patient feels more in control of condition and care; use quality of life inventories.

American Association of Respiratory Care. Clinical practice guideline: Providing patient and caregiver training. *Respir Care* 1996;41(7):658–663.

techniques to improve or maintain the patient's health and well-being. Ideally, this is accomplished by meeting well-defined and measurable outcomes established by an interdisciplinary team of health care professionals.

ASSESSMENT OF THE PATIENT, FAMILY, AND ENVIRONMENT

The Patient

When selecting appropriate equipment and therapies to deliver respiratory care in the home, the RCP must consider not only the pathophysiology of the patient's disease but also the context in which the equipment or therapies will be used.

The first factor to be assessed is the patient. The RCP must consider to what extent patient cooperation is required to meet therapeutic goals. For all but the most dependent patients, cooperation with the therapeutic plan is important in achieving the desired outcome.

Determinants of patient compliance with therapy are complex and include the following:

- Patient motivation
- Patient education and skill level
- Patient expectations of benefits
- Patient values

Patients with severe chronic obstructive pulmonary disease (COPD), for example, often suffer from clinical depression. These patients may see no hope of recovery or improvement in their condition and may be unlikely to conform to complex and demanding treatment regimens. Likewise, patients who have had little success with other treatments in the past often do not believe the proposed treatments are likely to work. Cognitive impairment secondary to disease may render many patients incapable of operating sophisticated equipment or complying with demanding treatment schedules. Some patients may even view reliance on ventilators, oxygen therapy, or simple nebulizers as a sign of dependency and weakness and refuse to cooperate with treatment plans.

Finally, the RCP must consider the length of time that the patient is likely to require care. Patients with end-stage lung cancer, for example, may not require elaborate systems for oxygen delivery, whereas an active infant with

---

CRITICAL THINKING CHALLENGES

Case Scenario

Compliance With Home Respiratory Care

Successful outcomes in home respiratory care are dependent on patient cooperation. But securing the patient's cooperation is often difficult. Furthermore, the actual extent of patient compliance with therapy may be unknown to the health care provider. Actuarially measuring and ensuring patient compliance has been a common topic in recent commentaries and studies.

Pepin and colleagues[11] studied patient compliance with home oxygen therapy in France. Instead of relying on patient estimates of the actual number of hours of use, they installed utilization meters on the oxygen delivery devices. They noted that only 45% of patients actually used oxygen for 15 or more hours a day. (Fifteen hours was chosen as the minimum number of hours of daily oxygen therapy needed to improve mortality rates. Some authorities state that the actual number of hours of required therapy is much higher.) Improper therapy prescription and lack of patient education may be at fault, they suggest. Few patients are explicitly instructed to use their oxygen for a specific number of hours. Patients are often unaware that benefits beyond short-term symptom relief are obtainable through consistent use of oxygen. Likewise, patients are seldom explicitly instructed to use oxygen while in the bathroom or while eating. Compliance was further limited by failure to provide portable oxygen devices. Continuing education of the patient in the home by health care professionals improved compliance rates.

Given that compliance (and presumably, outcome) is improved with the use of liquid oxygen systems (with portable or ambulatory accessory devices), it would seem self-evident that these units should be used for most patients needing long-term oxygen therapy. However, in a review of home oxygen therapy in Medicare beneficiaries, Silverman and associates[12] found that only 19% of patients were using liquid systems. They speculated that failure to use liquid systems may be related to the lower costs associated with concentrator use. More explicit prescriptions for liquid systems by physicians may result in more appropriate use of portable, liquid systems.

Corden and coworkers[13] used similar methods to assess compliance with home nebulizer therapy. They found compliance rates were much lower than was stated by patients. Only 44% of patients complied with the frequency and duration of prescribed therapy. Poorly compliant patients tended to have an overall lower quality of life.

Improving compliance with therapy is a multifaceted problem. Patient education appears key. This begins when therapy is prescribed but must continue in the home. Proper matching of equipment and therapy to the patient is also helpful. Most important, health care providers should encourage an open and honest relationship with their patients. A nonjudgmental approach should be used to allow patients to feel comfortable discussing their actual use and concerns with the prescribed therapy.

bronchopulmonary dysplasia requires equipment that facilitates mobility.

The Family

Many patients requiring home respiratory care need the assistance of family members in the delivery of treatment. Family members must therefore be evaluated along the lines described previously. Usually one individual assumes the role of the primary in-home caregiver. In the case of the elderly, this often is a spouse, son, or daughter. Infants and children requiring home care usually are cared for by the mother. In addition to the demands of caring for the patient, the in-home care provider usually has additional demands, such as caring for other family members or working. Particularly among the elderly, the family member assuming responsibility for the patient's care may also be ill.

The interdisciplinary care team should attempt to identify and train care providers in addition to the principal caregiver. Because the principal provider may be reluctant to ask for help, members of the professional team may be better able to recruit others to assist.

The Home

Electricity

Before discharge, the RCP should inspect the home to ensure that respiratory care equipment can be used safely and reliably. Electrical outlets should be in good repair and well grounded. The RCP should estimate the amount of amperage that the proposed equipment will require and inspect the fuse box or circuit breaker to make sure such power is available. The RCP should also attempt to identify other electrical equipment operating on the same circuit. When possible, vital medical equipment should not be connected to the same circuit as air conditioners, microwave ovens, clothes dryers, or hair dryers. The RCP should assess the accessibility of the circuit breaker or fuse box. In some rental apartments, these devices are not accessible to tenants. The RCP or the family should discuss the patient's need to have access with the property manager and ensure that immediate access is provided. If the patient and caregiver are not sufficiently mobile, the RCP should seek to identify a neighbor who can assist in restoring

---

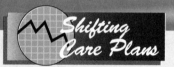

CRITICAL THINKING CHALLENGES

Shifting Care Plans

Evaluation of the Respiratory Home Care Patient's Quality of Life

Evaluation of the home respiratory care patient begins with the physical assessment skills applied in the inpatient setting, which are described elsewhere in this text. The unique circumstances of the home-bound respiratory patient, however, require a broader scope of assessment. The health care professional must assess not only the adequacy of respiratory function with a thorough physical examination but also the impact of the disease and therapy on the patient's overall functioning in the home, at work, and in the family. In addition, the effects of the disease and therapy on the patient's mental well-being must be considered.

Tu and colleagues[14] have devised a questionnaire (the Seattle Obstructive Lung Disease Questionnaire), which is designed to assess the severity of symptoms and their impact on the quality of life of home-bound (COPD) patients. Although designed as a formal research tool, the basic ideas contained in the survey can be adapted easily for home care professionals to use in their assessment of the home care patient.

The questionnaire covers several aspects of the patient's life, such as work and leisure activities and interpersonal relationships. The questions ask the patient to assess the impact of their disease on their ability to perform activities of everyday life, such as carrying grocery bags, walking a short distance, washing, and bathing.

In addition, the questionnaire attempts to assess the patient's interpersonal and psychological response to COPD. For example, patients are asked if they feel they are a burden to their family or are afraid to get angry for fear of acute breathlessness.

The scope of the questionnaire emphasizes that pulmonary disease is not simply an isolated physiologic derangement, but affects every aspect of the patient's life. When assessing the patient receiving home respiratory care, the health care professional can use the ideas contained in the questionnaire to form a more complete picture of the patient's physiologic functioning and quality of life.

Kiely and McNicholas[15] have demonstrated an additional dimension of assessment of the efficacy of home respiratory care: the impact of therapy on the patient's spouse or bed partner. They point out that many patients with obstructive sleep apnea are initially prompted to seek treatment because of complaints related to their snoring. Effective treatment of sleep apnea–related snoring should improve not only the patient's symptoms and quality of life but also the quality of life of the bed partner. In a study of 91 patients treated with nasal CPAP for sleep apnea, significant improvements were noted in the bed partner's sleep quality, daytime alertness, mood, and overall quality of life. The relationship between the patient and the patient's partner was also significantly improved

power if needed. In addition, the RCP should assist the patient and family in identifying an alternate outlet should the primary one fail.

Sources of Ignition

The practitioner should identify the source of heat for the home. Gas or propane space heaters pose an obvious hazard in the presence of oxygen, as can a gas stove. Their presence does not contraindicate the use of oxygen but does require additional safety measures and training and influences the location of oxygen reservoirs.

Characteristics of the Home Environment

Accessibility. Certain types of equipment may be impossible to deliver to some walk-up flats or high-rise apartments with small elevators. When houses or apartments are difficult to access, providers may wish to have replacement or back-up equipment in place before failure of the original equipment.

Space and layout. Large or bilevel homes may require several sources of oxygen or more than one ventilator, eliminating the need for the patient or family to carry heavy equipment throughout the house.

Box • 18–2   AARC CLINICAL PRACTICE GUIDELINE

OXYGEN THERAPY IN THE HOME OR EXTENDED CARE FACILITY

Indications: In adults, children and infants older than 28 days: $PaO_2 \leq 55$ mmHg (or $SaO_2 \leq 88\%$ in subjects breathing room air) or PaO_2 of 56 to 59 (or SaO_2 or $SpO_2 \leq 89\%$) in association with specific clinical conditions (eg, cor pulmonale, congestive heart failure, or erythrocythemia with hematocrit >56). Some patients may not qualify for oxygen therapy at rest but qualify for oxygen during ambulation, sleep, or exercise. Oxygen therapy is indicated during these specific activities when SaO_2 is demonstrated to fall to $\leq 88\%$.

Contraindications: No absolute contraindications to oxygen therapy exist when indications are present.

Assessment of need:

Initial assessment: Need is determined by the presence of clinical indicators as previously described and the presence of inadequate oxygen tension or saturation, or both, as demonstrated by the analysis of arterial blood. Concurrent pulse oximetry values must be documented and reconciled with the results of the baseline blood gas analysis if future assessment is to involve pulse oximetry.

Ongoing evaluation or reassessment: Additional arterial blood gas analysis is indicated whenever there is a major change in clinical status that may be cardiopulmonary related. Arterial blood gas measurements should be repeated in 1 to 3 months when oxygen therapy is begun in the hospital in a clinically unstable patient to determine the need for long-term oxygen therapy. Once the need for long-term oxygen therapy has been documented, repeated arterial blood gas analysis or oxygen saturation measurements are unnecessary other than to follow the course of the disease, to assess changes in clinical status, or to facilitate changes in the oxygen prescription.

Assessment of outcome: Outcome is determined by clinical and physiologic assessment to establish adequacy of patient response to therapy.

Monitoring: Clinical assessment should routinely be performed by the patient or the caregiver to determine changes in clinical status. Patients should be visited and monitored at least once a month by credentialed personnel unless conditions warrant more frequent visits. Measurement of baseline oxygen tension and saturation is essential before oxygen therapy is begun. These measurements should be repeated when clinically indicated or to follow the course of the disease. Measurements of SaO_2 also may be made to determine appropriate oxygen flow for ambulation, exercise, or sleep.

Equipment maintenance and supervision: All oxygen delivery equipment should be checked at least once daily by the patient or caregiver. Facets to be assessed include proper function of the equipment, prescribed flow rates, FDO_2, remaining liquid or compressed gas content, and backup supply. A respiratory care practitioner or equivalent should, during monthly visits, reinforce appropriate practices and performance by the patient and caregivers and ensure that the oxygen equipment is being maintained in accordance with manufacturers' recommendations. Liquid systems need to be checked to ensure adequate delivery. Oxygen concentrators should be checked regularly to ensure that they are delivering $\geq 85\%$ O_2 at 4 L/min.

American Association of Respiratory Care. Clinical practice guideline: Oxygen therapy in the home or extended care facility. *Respir Care* 1992;37:918.

Sanitation. Sources of clean water for equipment cleaning should be available as well clean areas for storage and assembly of equipment.

Miscellaneous hazards. Pets and small children may attempt to play with and disturb ventilators, oxygen tanks, and other equipment. Provisions to control these risks should be incorporated into the home care plan.

OXYGEN THERAPY IN THE HOME

Home oxygen therapy is indicated to correct arterial hypoxemia secondary to a variety of conditions. Specific criteria from the AARC Clinical Practice guidelines are reproduced Box 18–2. In addition, a summation of Medicare criteria for home oxygen therapy is provided in Table 18–2. Patients whose care is funded by private insurance may be governed by less stringent criteria.

In selecting an appropriate home oxygen delivery system, the RCP should consider the following:

1. How much oxygen (liters) will be required?
2. Where will the oxygen be used?
3. When will the oxygen be used?

When low-flow oxygen and/or an oxygen-conserving device is used for less than 24 hours a day, one or more large tanks may be sufficient. Likewise, patients who require oxygen only at night or are unable to move a significant distance from the bedroom seldom need more than a single stationary tank.

In contrast, patients who are on oxygen 24 hours a day and who are mobile benefit from more portable systems, such as liquid oxygen with a portable, refillable reservoir.

Petty and O'Donohue[16] recommend that oxygen therapy systems be classified as stationary, portable, and ambulatory. Depending on patient need, one or more types from these categories will be chosen. Stationary systems (such as large cylinders) are not easily moved from place to place but can, because of their size, contain large amounts of oxygen. A stationary system can be located, for example, in the patient's bedroom. Portable systems can be easily moved from place to place within the home and can be used in the car when the patient needs to travel. The assistance of a second person or a cart may be required for moving the devices. Ambulatory systems can be easily carried by the patient without assistance. A review of the most commonly used devices follows, and a summary is provided in Table 18–3.

Cylinders

Cylinders are available in large sizes as stationary systems and in smaller portable or ambulatory units. An H cylinder is the most commonly used stationary system in the home. This device can store 244 cubic feet of oxygen, which permits, at a rate of 2 L/min, about 3 days of oxygen therapy. However, the H cylinder is of limited utility for the patient requiring continuous oxygen therapy. It may be appropriate for bed-bound patients who require therapy only for acute breathlessness, or for infants and small children who require extremely low flows of oxygen. Likewise, they are suitable as an emergency backup system for more versatile

---

Table • 18–2 INDICATIONS AND REQUIREMENTS FOR HOME OXYGEN THERAPY FOR MEDICARE PATIENTS

A. Continuous long-term oxygen therapy when:
 1. $PaO_2 \leq 55$ mmHg or $SaO_2 \leq 88\%$, or
 2. PaO_2 56–59 mmHg or SaO_2 of 89%, with
  a. Edema due to heart failure, or
  b. Evidence of cor pulmonale, or
  c. Elevated hematocrit ≥56
 3. ABGs or arterial oxygen saturation by pulse oximetry obtained following optimum medical management
 4. Repeat ABGs or pulse oximetry 3 months after initial certification when
  a. Initial $PO_2 \geq 56$ mmHg or $SaO_2 \geq 89\%$, or
  b. The physician's initial estimated length of need was 1–3 months
 5. Certification of medical necessity and a prescription for therapy completed by the physician
 6. Revised certification when there is a change in O_2 prescription
B. Oxygen with exercise when:
 1. $SaO_2 \leq 88\%$ or $PaO_2 \leq 55$ mmHg during exercise, while resting $PaO_2 \geq 56$ mmHg or $SaO_2 \geq 89\%$, and
 2. Demonstration of improvement in hypoxemia that was evidenced when the patient exercised breathing room air
C. Nocturnal oxygen when:
 1. $SaO_2 \leq 88\%$ or $PaO_2 \leq 55$ mmHg evidenced during sleep, with $PaO_2 \geq 56$ mmHg or $SaO_2 \geq 89\%$ during day, or
 2. A decrease in arterial PO_2 more than 10 mmHg or saturation more than 5% associated with nocturnal restlessness, insomnia, or other physical or mental impairment attributable to nocturnal hypoxemia

---

Table • 18–3 CRITERIA FOR SELECTING THE APPROPRIATE OXYGEN SYSTEM

• Stationary oxygen delivery system, alone
  Patient is bed bound or unable to ambulate beyond the limits of a 50-ft length of tubing
  Patient requires nocturnal oxygen only
  Patient requires oxygen source for ventilator, CPAP, and so on
• Stationary and portable oxygen delivery system (eg, concentrator with E tank or liquid O_2 system)
  Continuous oxygen therapy is needed for a patient who only occasionally travels beyond the limits of a 50-ft length of tubing (eg, occasional visits to the physician)
• Stationary and ambulatory oxygen delivery system (eg, concentrator with lightweight cylinders <10 lb)
  Continuous oxygen therapy is needed for a patient who frequently travels beyond the limits of a 50-ft length of tubing (eg, frequent visits outside the home)
• Oxygen conserving device
  Continuous oxygen therapy is needed
   a. With portable or ambulatory system to reduce weight, extend functional time, and reduce need for refills
   b. With refractory hypoxemia and increased O_2 requirement
  Nasal cannula or transtracheal oxygen catheter requires the decision of physician and patient

systems. In any case, lightweight aluminum cylinders are preferable to heavier steel units.

Smaller cylinders, such as E (with 22 cubic feet) or D (with 13 cubic feet) cylinders, are suitable as portable or ambulatory systems. Because E cylinders and their carts are somewhat heavy, patients relying on them often require assistance with transport. At 2 L/min, an E cylinder allows for about 5 hours of therapy; a D cylinder permits about 3 hours.

Liquid Oxygen Systems

Liquid oxygen systems are the most versatile and popular of the methods available for home therapy. Steel containers, called *dewars,* contain oxygen in liquid form at a temperature of −170°C. Liquid oxygen passes through a warming coil, is converted into a gas, and is made available for patient delivery. Weighing about 100 lb when full, these systems can supply a patient with 2 L/min of continuous oxygen for about 7 days. Thus, among the stationary systems, they are capable of storing and delivering the largest volume of oxygen without occupying excessive space.

Perhaps most important, stationary liquid oxygen systems can be used to support portable and ambulatory systems. Small reservoirs can be filled easily and repeatedly with liquid oxygen from the main container. These small reservoirs weigh about 8 lb when filled and can provide 8 hours of therapy (at 2 L/min). Examples of both stationary and ambulatory liquid oxygen devices are depicted in Figure 18–2.

Some patients, however, are uncomfortable with liquid oxygen systems because of the loud noises they make when small reservoirs are transfilled or when the small reservoirs are placed flat. In addition, the connection between the large and small containers can become frozen if filling is not conducted properly. Finally, there is a continual small leakage of oxygen from the reservoir, which proves costly to patients who require only occasional oxygen administration.

Concentrators

Oxygen **concentrators** are electrically powered devices that extract oxygen from room air by means of a molecular filter or sieve. Obviously, these devices require a stable source of electricity and can add substantially to the patient's electric bill. They are easy to move from room to room, and, of course, can deliver oxygen without relying on deliveries from the medical supplier. An example is depicted in Figure 18–3.

Some drawbacks of oxygen concentrators are their need for periodic maintenance and the possibility of unexpected breakdown. They are not portable in the sense that they cannot be used away from a source of electricity. Finally, they may be noisy and can produce excess heat.

Oxygen concentrators may be ideal for patients who are not highly mobile and require oxygen in only one or two locations in a small house or apartment. With sufficient length of oxygen tubing (up to 50 feet), one concentrator may be able to supply oxygen to the patient in both the living room and bedroom, for example.

When selecting a concentrator for home oxygen therapy, special attention needs to be paid to the adequacy and reliability of the home's electrical supply. An alternate supply of oxygen needs to be available in case of an electrical or concentrator failure. Usually, an H cylinder suffices. Smaller

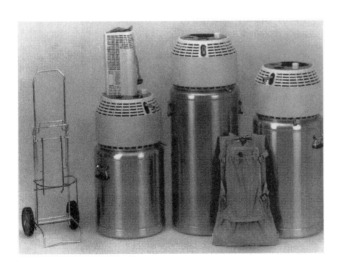

FIGURE 18–2 • Stationary and portable liquid oxygen systems. (Courtesy of Nellcor Puritan Bennett Inc., Pleasanton, CA.)

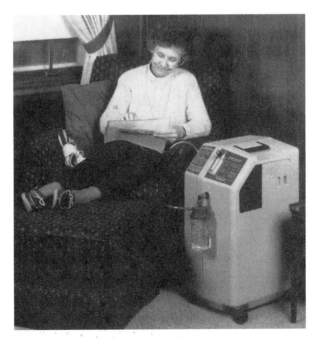

FIGURE 18–3 • Oxygen concentrator. (Courtesy of Nellcor Puritan Bennett Inc., Pleasanton, CA.)

tanks may be needed if the patient makes occasional trips outside the house.

Older oxygen concentrators may not have warning systems to alert the patient if the oxygen concentration produced by the device is falling. Suppliers should ensure that only devices with oxygen concentration indicators are used.

Monitoring and Assessment of the Patient on Home Oxygen Therapy

Patients on home oxygen therapy should be periodically evaluated to determine if the current oxygen prescription suits the patient's needs. In-home pulse oximetry can be used periodically to ensure that arterial oxygen saturation is within acceptable levels. In addition, using physiologic measurements, the patient's symptoms and quality of life should be evaluated. Providers should inquire about changes in the patient's level of activity, sleep duration and quality, appetite, and subjective assessment of breathlessness. Unfavorable changes in any of these indicators suggest that the patient's disease may be advancing, and a reevaluation of therapy is in order.

NONINVASIVE POSITIVE-PRESSURE SYSTEMS

Patients with a variety of disorders require or benefit from various modes of noninvasive ventilatory support.[17] Examples range from patients with advanced COPD who are awaiting transplants, patients with obstructive sleep apnea, and patients with neuromuscular disorders. Noninvasive ventilatory support is indicated when ventilatory muscle weakness or inadequate airway control mechanisms result in significant hypoventilation or apnea. Typically, patients require support only at night. Patients who lack adequate respiratory drive or who are completely dependent on mechanical ventilation are not candidates for noninvasive ventilation.

Noninvasive ventilatory support is usually provided by an electrically powered compressor that can provide a high flow rate at moderate levels of pressure. Pressure can be provided at a continuous level (continuous positive airway pressure, or CPAP) or at different inspiratory and expiratory levels. An example of a home CPAP system is illustrated in Figure 18–4. The term **bilevel positive airway pressure** (BiPAP) is usually used to describe the latter but is actually a registered trademark of the Respironics Corporation, not a generic term. A BiPAP device is shown in Figure 18–5.

Continuous Positive Airway Pressure

Noninvasive CPAP is indicated in patients who have adequate respiratory drive and respiratory muscle strength but who experience upper airway collapse during sleep. CPAP is usually delivered by means of a nasal mask, nasal prongs, or pillows, as illustrated in Figure 18–6. The RCP must often make several visits to the patient's home to ensure that the device is fitted properly. In addition to obtaining a good

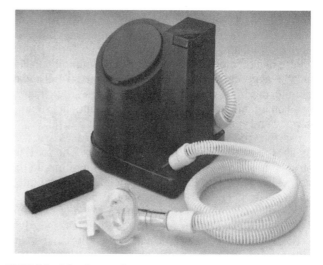

FIGURE 18–4 • Continuous positive airway pressure device for home therapy. (Courtesy of Respironics, Inc., Pittsburgh, PA.)

seal, it is important to ensure that skin integrity is not compromised by an overly tight mask or strapping device.

Patients treated with nasal CPAP for obstructive sleep apnea often initiate therapy as outpatients and do not have the benefit of a period of inpatient training and adjustment of therapy. The patient may not understand the rationale for therapy, or the expected benefits. Frequent visits by a nurse or RCP to ensure compliance during the initial phase of therapy are essential.

Some difficulties encountered by patients in the initial phase of therapy are an inability to tolerate the high flow rates required to attain the prescribed pressures. Ensuring a secure fit of the mask or nasal pillows minimizes the required flow. In addition, some units come equipped with a feature that gradually increases the level of CPAP (and hence, the level of flow) over a period of time, allowing the patient to fall asleep before full pressure is applied.

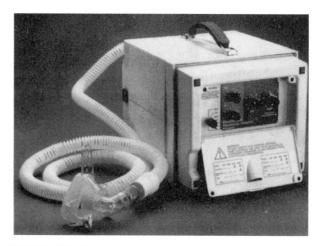

FIGURE 18–5 • Bilevel positive airway pressure (BiPAP) machine for bilevel pressure therapy. (Courtesy of Respironics, Inc., Pittsburgh, PA.)

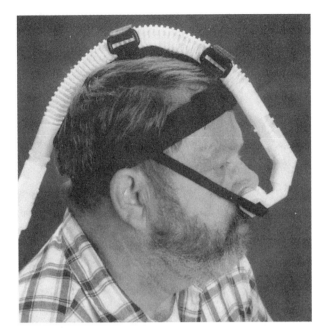

FIGURE 18–6 • Nasal pillows for continuous positive airway pressure. (Courtesy of Nellcor Puritan Bennett Inc., Pleasanton, CA.)

Noninvasive Positive-Pressure Ventilation

For patients with chronic lung disease and associated respiratory muscle weakness, noninvasive positive-pressure ventilation may provide symptomatic and physiologic improvement. Patients with chest wall or neuromuscular disorders may benefit as well.

The most commonly used device is the Respironics Bi-PAP device. This device uses a compressor-blower to generate flow. Independent levels of inspiratory and expiratory pressure can be set and can be used in the assist, assist-control, or control mode. Potential indications and contraindications to nocturnal noninvasive positive-pressure ventilation are summarized in Box 18–3.

Treatment with noninvasive positive-pressure ventilation can cause complications, either with the patient interface or

---

Box • 18–3 POTENTIAL INDICATIONS AND CONTRAINDICATIONS FOR A TRIAL OF NOCTURNAL NONINVASIVE VENTILATORY ASSISTANCE

Indications

Progressive respiratory failure due to neuromuscular or chest wall disease with excessive sleepiness, with or without* daytime hypercapnia

Obesity hypoventilation in the setting of obstructive sleep apnea that has not responded to CPAP

Disorders of ventilatory control associated with daytime hypercapnia or sleepiness

Progressive COPD despite maximal therapy accompanied by excessive sleepiness*

Documented elevations of carbon dioxide observed during polysomnography (eg, $PaCO_2 > 50$, or $P_{et}CO_2 > 55$, or $P_{pt}CO_2 > 60$)

Progressive respiratory failure due to COPD (eg, $PaCO_2 > 50$)*

Patients with existing tracheotomy who desire decannulation (see contraindications below)

Patients awaiting pulmonary transplantation

Contraindications

Absolute

　Bulbar dysfunction with inability to clear secretions

Relative

　Inability to tolerate noninvasive interfaces

　Inadequate caregiver in the home environment

---

*Efficacy not established.

Table • 18–4 ADVERSE EFFECTS OF INTERFACES AND POSSIBLE REMEDIES

Interface	Adverse Effect	Remedy
Nasal and oronasal masks	Discomfort	Proper fit, adjust strap tension, change mask type
	Nasal bridge redness, pressure sores	Reduce strap tension, use forehead spacer, try nasal pillows, use artificial skin
	Acneiform rash	Cortisone cream, alternative mask
Oronasal masks	Impeded speech and eating	Permit periodic removal if tolerated by the patient
	Claustrophobia	Choose clear masks with minimal bulk
	Aspiration	Exclude patients unable to protect airway; nasogastric tubes for patients with nausea and abdominal distention
Mouthpieces and lip seals	Interference with swallowing, salivary retention	Coaching, adaptation
	Pressure on lips, cheeks	Proper fit, strap adjustment
	Dental deformity	Orthodontic consultation
	Aerophagia	Simethicone, coaching
	Allergic reactions	Change prosthetic materials
	Nasal air leaking	Nose clips, pledgets
	Accidental disconnection	Appropriate alarms in ventilator-dependent patients

Table • 18–5   ADVERSE EFFECTS ASSOCIATED WITH AIR PRESSURE AND FLOW AND THEIR POSSIBLE REMEDIES

Adverse Effect	Remedy
Noise	Obtain muffler, alternative ventilator
Nasal, sinus, or ear pain	Reduce pressure
Nasal dryness, coldness, burning, or epistaxis	Nasal saline or emollient, heated humidifier
Nasal congestion	Topical nasal steroids, anticholinergics, oral decongestants and antihistamines, topical decongestants (temporary)
Oral dryness	Chin straps, humidifier
Gastric insufflation	Reassurance, pressure reduction, simethicone
Eye irritation	Proper mask fit, alternative mask
Barotrauma, pneumothorax	Inflation pressure reduction, pleurodesis
Poor synchrony, autocycling	Consider ventilator with adjustable sensitivity and rise time

with ventilation itself. Hill[18] has reviewed these complications and their remedies, which are summarized in Tables 18–4 and 18–5. Care givers should be especially vigilant for skin breakdown over the site of the patient interface (mask or nasal pillows). Patients at risk include those with impaired blood flow, such as patients with heart failure, diabetes, or extreme malnourishment. The bridge of the nose is especially vulnerable, as Figure 18–7 illustrates.

INVASIVE MECHANICAL VENTILATION

Patient Selection

Patients who cannot be weaned from mechanical ventilation in the hospital setting, but who are otherwise medically stable, can be ventilated successfully in the home. A

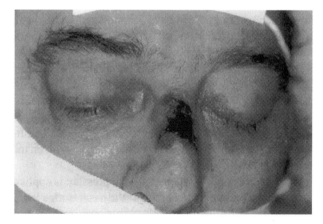

FIGURE 18–7 • Nasal ulceration induced by excessive pressure from a nasal continuous positive airway pressure mask used to deliver noninvasive ventilation. The patient was elderly, had congestive heart failure, and used the mask continuously for several days. All factors may have contributed to ulceration. (Hill NS. Complication of noninvasive positive pressure ventilation. *Respir Care.* 1997;42[4]:434.)

summary of some general medical criteria is given in Table 18–6. Typical candidates for prolonged mechanical ventilation in the home include patients with high spinal cord lesions, neuromuscular disorders, COPD, and bronchopulmonary dysplasia. Overall, patients with neuromuscular diseases survive longer and require fewer medical interventions and hospital admissions than do patients with COPD and cardiac disease (Box 18–4).

Discharge Planning and Patient Assessment

Planning and providing care for patients requiring long-term ventilation in the home is the most challenging and complex task confronting the home care professional. A complex assessment of the patient and family is required, including the patient's finances, the physical condition of the home, the family's means of transportation, and the strengths and weaknesses in the family's or other caregiver's ability to provide skilled care. Often, patients require other complex forms of therapy in the home as well, such as tube feedings, and may need wheelchairs or other devices to improve mobility.

Table • 18–6   CONDITIONS THAT MAY NECESSITATE LONG-TERM MECHANICAL VENTILATION

Neuromuscular Disorders
Central nervous system
   Central hypoventilation syndromes
   Ondine's curse
   Arnold-Chiari malformation
Spinal cord
   Traumatic injuries
   Thoracic myelomeningocele
   Syringomyelia
Anterior horn cell (lower motor neuron)
   Poliomyelitis
   Spinal muscle atrophy (Werdnig-Hoffman)
   Amyotrophic lateral sclerosis*
Muscle
   Muscular dystrophy (Duchenne's, limb girdle, myotonic dystrophy)
   Congenital myopathies
Peripheral nerve
   Phrenic neuropathies
   Diaphragmatic paralysis
      Idiopathic
      Postsurgical
   Guillain-Barré syndrome

Chest Wall and Diaphragmatic Defects
Kyphoscoliosis
Postsurgical (thoracoplasty)
Diaphragmatic hernia

Primary Pulmonary Disorders
Tracheomalacia
Bronchiectasis
Bronchopulmonary dysplasia
Chronic aspiration
Chronic bronchitis, emphysema*
Cystic fibrosis*
Interstitial lung disease (multiple causes)*
Adult respiratory distress syndrome

*Less appropriate disorders for home mechanical ventilation.

Box • 18–4 AARC CLINICAL PRACTICE GUIDELINE

LONG-TERM INVASIVE MECHANICAL VENTILATION IN THE HOME

Indications: Patients requiring long-term invasive ventilatory support are those who have demonstrated an inability to be weaned completely from invasive ventilatory support or a progression of disease etiology that requires increasing ventilatory support. Conditions that meet these criteria may include, but are not limited to, ventilatory muscle disorders, alveolar hypoventilation syndrome, primary respiratory disorders, obstructive diseases, restrictive diseases, and cardiac disorders, including congenital anomalies.

Contraindications: Long-term invasive mechanical ventilation is contraindicated in the presence of a physiologically unstable medical condition requiring a higher level of care or resources than is available in the home. Indicators of a medical condition too unstable for the home and long-term care setting are FIO_2 requirement >0.40, PEEP >10 cm H_2O; need for continuous invasive monitoring in adult patients; lack of mature tracheostomy; patient's choice not to receive home mechanical ventilation; lack of an appropriate discharge plan; unsafe physical environment as determined by the patient's discharge planning team; presence of fire, health, or safety hazards including unsanitary conditions; inadequate basic utilities (such as heat, air conditioning, electricity); inadequate resources for care in the home; inability of ventilator-assisted individual to care for self if no caregiver is available; inadequate respite care for care givers; inadequate numbers of competent caregivers.

Assessment of need: Need is determined when indications are present and contraindications are absent, when continued need exists for higher level of services, and when frequent changes in the plan of care are not needed.

Assessment of outcome: At least the following aspects of patient management and condition should be evaluated periodically: implementation and adherence to the plan of care, quality of life, patient satisfaction, resource usage, growth and development in the pediatric patient, and unanticipated morbidity or mortality.

Monitoring: The frequency of monitoring should be determined by the ongoing individualized care plan and based on the patient's current medical condition. The ventilator settings, proper function of equipment, and patient's physical condition should be monitored and verified with each initiation of invasive ventilation to the patient, including altering the source of ventilation, as from one ventilator or resuscitation bag to another ventilator; with each ventilator setting change; on a regular basis as specified by individualized plan of care. All appropriately trained caregivers should follow the care plan and implement the monitoring that has been prescribed. These caregivers may operate, maintain, and monitor all equipment and perform all aspects of care after having been trained and evaluated on their level of knowledge for that equipment and the clinical response to each of the interventions. Lay caregivers should monitor the following regularly: patient's physical condition (respiratory rate, heart rate, color changes, chest excursion, diaphoresis, lethargy, blood pressure, body temperature), ventilator settings (the frequency at which alarms and settings are to be checked should be specified in the plan of care), peak pressures, preset tidal volume, frequency of ventilator breaths, verification of oxygen concentration setting, PEEP level, appropriate humidification of inspired gases, temperature of inspired gases, heat and moisture exchanger function, equipment function (appropriate configuration of ventilator circuit, alarm function, cleanliness of filters according to manufacturer's recommendation, battery power levels, overall condition of equipment), self-inflating manual resuscitator cleanliness and function. A practitioner should perform a thorough, comprehensive assessment of the patient and the patient-ventilator system on a regular basis as prescribed by the plan of care. The practitioner should implement, monitor, and assess results of other interventions as indicated by the clinical situation and anticipated in the care plan; pulse oximetry should be used in patients requiring a change in prescribed oxygen levels or in patients with a suspected change in condition; specimen collection (and analysis, as applicable) as prescribed by physician, including but not limited to sputum and blood work; cardiorespiratory monitoring (electrocardiogram, heart rate trending), pulmonary function testing, ventilator settings, exhaled tidal volume, analysis of fraction of inspired oxygen. Personnel are also responsible for maintaining interdisciplinary communication concerning the plan of care. Personnel should integrate respiratory plan of care into the patient's total care plan. Plan of care should include all aspects of patient's respiratory care and ongoing assessment and education of the caregivers involved.

American Association of Respiratory Care. Clinical practice guideline: Long-term invasive mechanical ventilation in the home. *Respir Care* 1995;40:1313.

Gilmartin[19] has reviewed the patient and family characteristics that are important predictors of the success of home mechanical ventilation. These are summarized in Table 18–7. It is important to note that medical criteria alone are insufficient for selection of patients for home ventilation. The patient's mental outlook, and that of the family and care providers, are of equal importance.

Thorough training of the primary caregiver is essential to good outcome. This process may be prolonged and frustrating for both the family and the caregiver. Those who provide the training should be chosen for their empathy and rapport with patients and families as well as their technical expertise. A small group of professionals committed to home care can provide the needed consistency and excellence. A general summary of the training needs of caregivers is provided in Table 18–8.

Patients discharged on home mechanical ventilation almost always require additional human resources for appropriate care. In some cases, only occasional help with bed-making and bathing is required. Sometimes, overnight care is needed to allow family members to sleep without interruption. A brief guide to determining the amount of assistance needed is provided in Table 18–9.

Finally, a thorough assessment of the home must be performed. An overview has already been presented, but home mechanical ventilation requires considerable attention to detail. This is especially true if the home ventilator patient is using a wheelchair for mobility. Discharge planners must also consider that professional caregivers may be in the home for all or part of the day, and the family's privacy may be compromised in small apartments or homes. An overview of home assessment is presented in Box 18–5.

The Home Ventilator

The ideal ventilator for home care is reliable, simple to operate, inexpensive, small, and portable. A variety of devices have been developed in an attempt to meet these criteria.[20] Some examples are illustrated in Figures 18–8, 18–9, and 18–10, and their operating characteristics are displayed in Tables 18–10 and 18–11. Most devices marketed for home mechanical ventilation use a piston to deliver a preset volume and are capable of being operated in the assist-control and control modes. Some are also capable of being used in a pressure-limited mode.

Home ventilators usually have an internal, rechargeable battery that can power the ventilator for up to 2 hours. When longer periods of time away from a source of electricity are anticipated, an external portable 12-volt battery can power the ventilator for up to 20 hours. To avoid depleting the battery, the patient should be encouraged to plug the unit into an electrical outlet whenever possible.

CARE OF THE HOME TRACHEOSTOMY PATIENT

Patients with tracheostomies and their caregivers in the home setting must be instructed in the purpose of the tube, methods for securing the tube in place, procedures for cleaning the inner cannula and changing the tube, procedures for tracheal suctioning, and management of cuff leak

Table • 18–7　PATIENT CHARACTERISTICS THAT MAY DETERMINE SUCCESS IN HOME VENTILATOR CARE

Ideal	Acceptable	Unacceptable
Individual Coping Style		
Optimistic	Optimistic	None
Motivated	Motivated	
Resourceful	Sense of humor	
Flexible		
Adaptable		
Sense of humor		
Directive		
Support Systems		
Close family and social supports	Social supports	Lack of family and social supports
Education		
College degree	Ability to learn	Altered mental status
Ability to learn	Mechanically astute	Unable to learn
Financial Resources		
Adequate personal assets	Adequate health insurance	Lack of personal assets
Optimal health insurance		Lack of health insurance
Medical Condition		
Stable neuromuscular disease	Stable neuromuscular or obstructive disease	Medically unstable
Adequate free time off ventilator	Limited or no time off ventilator	
No other illnesses		
Self-Care Ability		
Able to provide self-care and/or direct others	Able to provide self-care	Unable to care for self or direct others

Table • 18–8 SKILLS NEEDED BY PATIENT OR CARE GIVERS BEFORE DISCHARGE

Self-Care Techniques
Airway management
 Tracheostomy and stoma care
 Cuff care
 Tracheal suctioning
 Changing the tracheostomy tube
 Changing the tracheostomy ties
Chest physical therapy techniques
 Positioning
 Secretion clearance techniques
 Coughing
Medication administration
 Oral
 Inhaled
Bed-to-chair transfers
Feeding tube care
Indwelling catheter care
Implantable intravenous line care
Bowel care
Switching from the ventilator to weaning device

Equipment Maintenance
Ventilator
Humidifier
Suction machines
Battery and charger
Oxygen administration
Manual resuscitator
Troubleshooting for problems
Cleaning and disinfection

Emergency Measures
Ventilator failure
Power failure
Dislodged tracheostomy tube
Obstructed airway
Cuff leaks
Shortness of breath
Ventilator circuit problems
Infection
Falls
Bleeding
Cardiac arrest

Box • 18–5 ASSESSMENT OF THE VENTILATOR-DEPENDENT PATIENT'S HOME

Accessibility
☐ In and out of home
☐ Bathroom
☐ Kitchen
☐ Between rooms
☐ Wheelchair mobility
 ☐ Doorway width
 ☐ Thresholds
 ☐ Stairways
 ☐ Carpeting
Equipment
☐ Space
☐ Electrical power supply
 ☐ Amperage
 ☐ Grounded outlets
Environment
☐ Temperature
☐ Lighting
☐ Living space

emergencies. Most often, sterile technique is not required for routine suctioning in the home. Typically, one disposable catheter can be used throughout the day, with thorough rinsing with distilled sterile water between uses.

 Suction machines used by the home-bound patient can be electrically driven, stationary units (Fig. 18–11). Patients who are able to leave the home on occasion should have a portable battery-operated unit available (Fig. 18–12). Patients with tracheotomies have obvious difficulties in communication. Home care planning must take this into account and provide alternative methods of communication. This may include simple measures, such as providing paper and pens for writing. For patients unable to write, provide a board with written phrases or pictures to which the patient can point to communicate needs.

AEROSOL THERAPY

For most patients requiring administration of drugs to the airway, metered dose inhalers (MDIs) with holding chambers are preferred.[21] However, nebulizers are occasionally required when medications are not available in MDI form (eg, antibiotics) or when the patient or caregiver simply cannot master the use of an MDI with holding chambers.

Table • 18–9 PATIENT AND FAMILY CAPABILITIES AND THE SELECTION OF CAREGIVERS

Patient and Family Capabilities	Care Needs
Patient provides own care	Needs minimal or no help from family
Patient provides only minimal care but can direct others in care.	Needs maximal help from family or outside caregivers
Patient cannot perform any self-care.	Needs full support from family or caregivers
Family member is healthy and can provide all care.	Other family members will take on the responsibility to provide intermittent support
Family member is unable to provide any care, secondary to ill health.	Will need full-time support from professional or unskilled caregivers
Patient requires complex care.	Will need full-time professional care

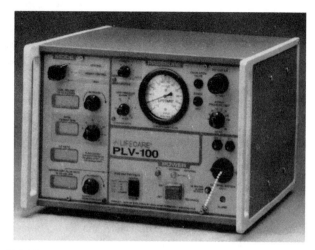

FIGURE 18–8 • One brand of home ventilator. (Courtesy of Lifecare, Intl., Inc., Westminster, CO.)

Use of a home nebulizer requires that the patient be thoroughly instructed in cleaning and reassembling the unit. Battery-powered units may be ideal for patients who occasionally require therapy outside of the home. An oxygen tank can be used to power a nebulizer as well, but may be discouraged unless the patient reliably returns oxygen to the prescribed setting after the treatment.

THE HOME CARE COMPANY

Regulation and Accreditation

Successful management of a home care company requires compliance with regulatory bodies and with systems for equipment maintenance and meticulous record keeping. The Joint Commission on Accreditation of Health Care Organiza-

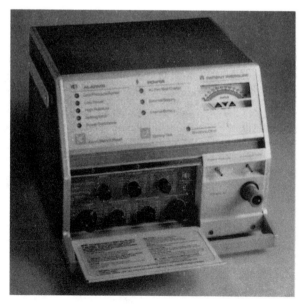

FIGURE 18–9 • Another common home ventilator. (Courtesy of Aequitron Medical, Inc., Minneapolis, MN.)

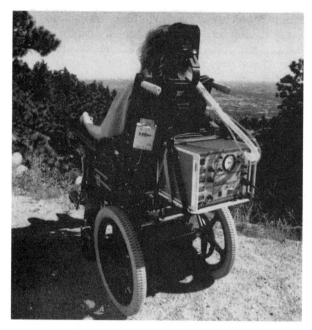

FIGURE 18–10 • Ventilator mounted to a wheelchair. (Courtesy of Lifecare, Intl., Inc., Westminster, CO.)

tions offers accreditation of home care agencies; this accreditation implies that the organization has met minimal standards in patient care, staff training, education, and safety.

In addition, home care companies are subject, directly or indirectly, to several federal laws and agencies. The federal Occupational Safety and Health Act (OSHA) guidelines mandate that all employers in the health care setting have an occupational exposure to blood-borne pathogens plan in place. The plan must address the following:

- Control of occupational exposure to hepatitis B, including offering vaccinations at no cost to high-risk employees
- Engineering and work practice controls to avoid exposure to infectious waste, including use of sharps containers, self-sheathing needles, and personal protective devices, such as gloves
- Control of occupational exposure to tuberculosis, including plans to identify high-risk patients and the provision of periodic tuberculosis testing

Because many home care companies transfill oxygen from bulk to more portable devices, they are considered "repackagers" of drugs and are required to comply with Food and Drug Administration (FDA) guidelines, including the following:

- Registering with the FDA as a drug repackager
- Training staff in what the FDA terms "current good manufacturing guidelines"
- Developing a written recall plan and tracking system
- Establishing a file of consumer complaints

The Safe Medical Devices Act also mandates that suppliers of medical equipment in the home develop a system to track

Table • 18–10 ALARM SYSTEMS OF POSITIVE-PRESSURE VENTILATORS

Alarms	Nellcor Puritan-Bennett 740	Aequitron Medical LP-6	Life Care PLV-100	Life Care PLV-102	Intermed Bear 33	Medimex ARF 1500E
High inspiratory pressure	Yes	Yes	Yes	Yes	Yes	Yes
Low inspiratory pressure	Yes	Yes	Yes†	Yes†	Yes	Yes
Apnea	Yes	Yes	Yes†	Yes†	Yes	No
Low battery	Yes	Yes	Yes‡	Yes‡	Yes	Yes
Inverse I : E ratio§	Yes	Yes‖	Yes	Yes	No	No
Ventilation malfunction	Yes	No	Yes	Yes	Yes	Yes
Low inspiratory flow	Yes	No	Yes	Yes	No	No
Reverse external battery connections	Yes	No	Yes	Yes	No	No
Microprocessor failure	Yes	No	Yes	Yes	Yes	No
Switch to battery	Yes	No	Yes	Yes	Yes	No
Power failure	Yes	No	Yes	Yes	No	No
Oxygen	Yes	No	No	Yes	No	No

†The low inspiratory pressure and the apnea alarms are actually combined.
‡Has separate alarms for low internal and low external batteries.
§I:E ratio =inspiratory/expiratory ratio.
‖Actually referred to as setting error, controls set outside machine limits. An inverse I:E ratio will not be delivered.

the location of all equipment deployed in the home in preparation for a government- or manufacturer-initiated recall.

The Department of Transportation regulates the transportation of potentially dangerous substances. Applicable regulations include the following:

- Use of approved drivers. This includes a biannual medical examination.
- Use of yellow flammable hazard signs when large quantities (more than 1000 lb) are transported
- Use of green (oxygen) hazard signs when smaller quantities are transported

Home Care Reimbursement

Most patients receiving home respiratory care are older than 65 years of age and are therefore covered by Medicare part B. The rules and regulations covering what Medicare will pay for home health services are developed by the Health Care Finance Authority (HCFA). In early 1998, HCFA cut the reimbursement rate for home oxygen therapy by 25% and plans to reduce compensation a further 10% in 1999. It is too early to evaluate the impact of this reduction on the availability of home oxygen therapy. However, it highlights the need for the RCP to serve as a cost-control consultant in the home respiratory care field.

Home Care Documentation

The Joint Commission for Accreditation of Health Care Organizations requires that the home care medical record have the following elements:

- A list of patient needs or problems based on patient assessment

Table • 18–11 NEGATIVE-PRESSURE GENERATORS

Ventilator	Mode	Rate	Maximum Negative Pressure (cm H$_2$O)	Maximum Positive Pressure (cm H$_2$O)	Power Failure Alarm	Low Pressure Alarm	I:E Ratio
33 CRE	Control	≤40	−50	No	No	No	Variable
33 CRX	Control	≤40	−60	No	No	No	Variable
33 CRA	Assistor	≤60	−50	No	No	No	Patient variable
Iron lung	Control	10–30	−60	—	—	—	1 : 1 (fixed)
Life Care 170C	Control	10–40	−60	+60	Yes	No	1 : 1.5 (fixed)
Nellcor Puritan Bennett Thompson Maxivent	Control	8–24	−70*	+70*	Yes	Yes	1 : 2 (fixed)

*The combined positive and absolute value of the negative pressure cannot exceed 70 cm H$_2$O.
I:E ratio, inspiration/expiration ratio.

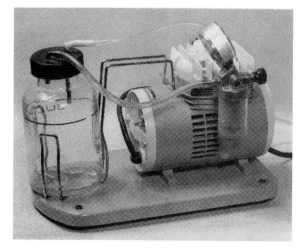

FIGURE 18–11 • Portable suction machine.

• A set of outcome-oriented goals based on the problems identified
• Actions taken to meet these goals

Such records serve as justification for agency charges and provide a means of quality assurance.

Use of Clinical Practice Guidelines

The development and use of clearly stated **clinical practice guidelines** (CPGs) assists home health care providers

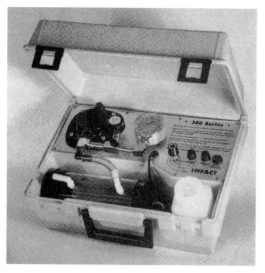

FIGURE 18–12 • Impact battery-operated suction machine. (Courtesy of Impact Medical, West Caldwell, NJ.)

to ensure that a specific level of quality is always maintained in defined groups of patients or for defined clinical procedures. The quality of services can be measured against clearly stated goals and objectives defined in the CPGs. Likewise, they can be used for staff education. CPGs should also delineate the responsibilities of all parties involved. CPGs developed by the American Association for Respiratory Care are reproduced or summarized throughout this chapter.

References

1. Pierson DJ. Controversies in home respiratory care: Conference summary. *Respir Care.* 1994;39:294–307.
2. Aaronson NK. Methodologic issues in addressing the quality of life of cancer patients. *Cancer.* 1991;67:844–850.
3. Jalowiec A. Issues in using multiple measures of quality of life. *Semin Oncol Nurs.* 1990;6:271–277.
4. Ferrans CE. Development of a quality of life index for patients with cancer. *Oncol Nurs Forum.* 1990;17(suppl 3):15–19.
5. Schumacher M, Olschewski M, Schulgen G. Assessment of a quality of life in clinical trials. *Stat Med.* 1991;10:1915–1930.
6. Strauss AL. *Chronic Illness and the Quality of Life.* St. Louis: CV Mosby; 1975.
7. Lorig K, Holman H, Sobel D, et al. *Living a Healthy Life With Chronic Conditions.* Palo Alto, CA: Bull Publishing; 1994.
8. Meichenbaum D, Turk DC. *Facilitating Treatment Adherence: A Practitioner's Guidebook.* New York: Plenum; 1987.
9. Joint Commission on Accreditation for Healthcare Organizations. *Comprehensive Accreditation Manual for Home Care 1997-1998.* Oakbrook Terrace, IL: JCAHO; 1996.
10. Doak CC, Doak LG, Root JH. *Teaching Patients With Low Literacy Skills.* Philadelphia: Lippincott-Raven; 1996.
11. Pepin JL, Barjhoux CE, Deschaux C, et al. Long-term oxygen therapy at home. *Chest.* 1996;109:1144–1150.
12. Silverman BG, Gross TP, Babish JD. Home oxygen therapy in medicare beneficiaries, 1991 and 1992. *Chest.* 1997;112:380–386.
13. Corden ZM, Bosley CM, Rees PJ, Cochrane GM. Home nebulizer therapy for patients with COPD. *Chest.* 1997;112:1278–1282.
14. Tu SP, McDonell MB, Spertus JA, et al. A new self-administered questionnaire to monitor health related quality of life in patients with COPD. *Chest.* 1997;112:614–622.
15. Kiely JL, McNicholas WT. Bed partners' assessment of nasal continuous positive airway pressure therapy in obstructive sleep apnea. *Chest.* 1997;111(5):1261–1265.
16. Petty TL, O'Donohue WJ. Further recommendations for prescribing, reimbursement, technology development and research in long term oxygen therapy. *Am J Respir Crit Care Med.* 1994;150:857.
17. Claman DM, Piper A, Sanders MH, et al. Nocturnal noninvasive positive pressure ventilatory assistance. *Chest.* 1996;110:1581–1588.
18. Hill NS. Complications of noninvasive positive pressure ventilation. *Respir Care.* 1997;42:432–441.
19. Gilmartin ME. Long term mechanical ventilation: Patient selection and discharge planning. *Respir Care.* 1991;36:205–216.
20. Kacmarek RM. Home mechanical ventilatory equipment. In: Branson RD, Hess DR, Chatburn RL, eds. *Respiratory Care Equipment.* Philadelphia: JB Lippincott; 1995.
21. O'Donohue WJ. Guidelines for the use of nebulizers in the home and at domiciliary sites. *Chest.* 1996;109:814–820.

Lippincott Credits

Chapter 3

Figures 3–4, 3–34ab: Burton GG, Hodgkin JE, and Ward JJ. *Respiratory Care: A Guide to Clinical Practice,* 4th Edition. Philadelphia: Lippincott-Raven Publishers, 1996.

Figures 3–6, 3–21, 3–23, 3–29, 3–30, 3–31, 3–39: Bullock BL. *Pathophysiology: Adaptations and Alterations in Function,* 4th Edition. Philadelphia: Lippincott-Raven Publishers, 1996; Figure 3-23: Braun HA, Cheney FW, Loehn CP. *Introduction to Respiratory Physiology,* 2nd Edition. Boston: Litttle, Brown and Company, 1980.

Figures 3–7, 3–8, 3–10, 3–11, 3–35, 3–36: Rosse C and Gaddum-Rosse P. *Hollinshead's Textbook of Anatomy,* 5th Edition. Philadelphia: Lippincott-Raven Publishers, 1997.

Figure 3–9: Chaffee EE and Lytle JM. *Basic Physiology and Anatomy,* 4th Edition. Philadelphia: J.B. Lippincott Company, 1980.

Figure 3–14: Crystal RG and West JB. *The Lung: Scientific Foundations.* New York: Raven Press, 1991.

Figures 3–17, 3–18, 3–25, 3–37, 3–44: Porth CM. *Pathophysiology: Concepts of Altered Health States,* 4th Edition. Philadelphia: J.B. Lippincott Company, 1994.

Figure 3–26: Snell RS. *Clinical Histology for Medical Students.* Boston: Little, Brown and Company, 1984.

Figure 3–32: Rhoades RA and Tanner GA. *Medical Physiology.* Boston: Little, Brown and Company, 1995.

Chapter 4

Figures 4–1, 4–4, 4–7: Miller WF, Scacci R, and Gast LR. *Laboratory Evaluation of Pulmonary Function.* Philadelphia: J.B. Lippincott Company, 1987.

Figure 4–3: Branson RD, Hess DR, and Chatburn RL. *Respiratory Care Equipment.* Philadelphia: J.B. Lippincott Company, 1995.

Figures 4–13, 4–14, 4–15, 4–16, 4–17, 4–31, 4–36, 4–37, 4–38, 4–39, 4–40, 4–41, 4–42, 4–43: Illustrations by Catherine M. Albert © Lippincott-Raven Publishers, 1999.

Figure 4–28: Aloan CA and Hill TV. *Respiratory Care of the Newborn and Child,* 2nd Edition. Philadelphia: Lippincott-Raven Publishers, 1997.

Chapter 5

Figures 5–2, 5–5, 5–11, 5–13, 5–19, 5–21, 5–22, 5–24, 5–28: Bullock BL. *Pathophysiology: Adaptations and Alterations in Function,* 4th Edition. Philadelphia: Lippincott-Raven Publishers, 1996.

Figures 5–3, 5–8: Porth CM. *Pathophysiology: Concepts of Altered Health States,* 5th Edition. Philadelphia: Lippincott-Raven Publishers, 1998.

Figures 5–10, 5–20, 5–23: Porth CM. ***Pathophysiology: Concepts of Altered Health States,*** 4th Edition. Philadelphia: J.B. Lippincott Company, 1994.

Chapter 6

Figures 6–2, 6–11, 6–12: Burton GG, Hodgkin JE, and Ward JJ. ***Respiratory Care: A Guide to Clinical Practice,*** 4th Edition. Philadelphia: Lippincott-Raven Publishers, 1996.

Figures 6–3, 6–4, 6–7, 6–8, 6–9, 6–10, 6–13, 6–14: Bates B, Bickley LS, and Hoekelman RA. ***A Guide to Physical Examination and History Taking,*** 6th Edition. Philadelphia: Lippincott-Raven Publishers, 1995.

Figures 6–5, 6–6: Matthews LR. ***Cardiopulmonary Anatomy and Physiology.*** Philadelphia: Lippincott-Raven Publishers, 1996.

Chapter 7

Figures 7–6, 7–7, 7–14, 7–15, 7–16, 7–17: Branson RD, Hess DR, and Chatburn RL. ***Respiratory Care Equipment.*** Philadelphia: J.B. Lippincott Company, 1995.

Chapter 8

Figure 8–1: Bullock BL. ***Pathophysiology: Adaptations and Alterations in Function,*** 4th Edition. Philadelphia: Lippincott-Raven Publishers, 1996.

Figure 8–6: Burton GG, Hodgkin JE, and Ward JJ. ***Respiratory Care: A Guide to Clinical Practice,*** 4th Edition. Philadelphia: Lippincott-Raven Publishers, 1996.

Chapter 9

Figures 9–1, 9–2, 9–3: McCall RE and Tankersley CM. ***Phlebotomy Essentials,*** 2nd Edition. Philadelphia: Lippincott-Raven Publishers, 1997.

Chapter 10

Figure 10–12ab: Current Status of Oxygen Therapy. *Problems in Respiratory Care* 1990;3:597, F2, 3. Philadelphia: J.B. Lippincott Company.

Figures 10–14, 10–18, 10–22, 10–24, 10–26: Branson RD, Hess DR, and Chatburn RL. ***Respiratory Care Equipment.*** Philadelphia: J.B. Lippincott Company, 1995.

Figures 10–20, 10–21(a–d), 10–31, 10–32, 10–33, 10–34, 10–35, 10–36, 10–37, 10–38, 10–39, 10–40, 10–41, 10–42ab, 10–43(a&b), 10–44(a&b), 10–45: Illustrations by Catherine M. Albert © Lippincott-Raven Publishers, 1999.

Figure 10–46: Burton GG, Hodgkin JE, and Ward JJ. ***Respiratory Care: A Guide to Clinical Practice,*** 4th Edition. Philadelphia: Lippincott-Raven Publishers, 1996.

Chapter 11

Figures 11–6(a–d), 11–7(a&b): Illustrations by Catherine M. Albert © Lippincott-Raven Publishers, 1999.

Chapter 12

Figures 12–3(a&b), 12–7(a&b): Illustrations by Catherine M. Albert © Lippincott-Raven Publishers, 1999.

Figure 12–18b: Burton GG, Hodgkins JE, and Ward JJ. ***Respiratory Care: A Guide to Clinical Practice,*** 4th Edition. Philadelphia: Lippincott-Raven Publishers, 1996.

Chapter 13

Figures 13–2(a–e), 13–3, 13–4, 13–6(a), 13–8(1–12), 13–10: Illustrations by Catherine M. Albert © Lippincott-Raven Publishers, 1999.

Figures 13–5, 13–11, 13–13, 13–14, 13–16a, 13–16b, 13–18, 13–19, 13–25, 13–26: Burton GG, Hodgkin JE, and Ward JJ. ***Respiratory Care: A Guide to Clinical Practice,*** 4th Edition. Philadelphia: Lippincott-Raven Publishers, 1996.

Chapter 14

Figures 14–3, 14–5(a&b), 14–8, 14–12, 14–13, 14–14(a–c), 14–15: Illustrations by Catherine M. Albert © Lippincott-Raven Publishers, 1999.

Figures 14–2, 14–4, 14–6, 14–9, 14–11, 14–20, 14–21: Burton GG, Hodgkin JE, and Ward JJ. ***Respiratory Care: A Guide to Clinical Practice,*** 4th Edition. Philadelphia: Lippincott-Raven Publishers, 1996.

Figures 14–18, 14–19: Branson RD, Hess DR, and Chatburn RL. ***Respiratory Care Equipment.*** Philadelphia: J.B. Lippincott Company, 1995.

Chapter 18

Figure 18–11: Branson RD, Hess DR, and Chatburn RL. ***Respiratory Care Equipment.*** Philadelphia: J.B. Lippincott Company, 1995.

INDEX

NOTE: Entries in bold face type indicate key terms. A *b* following a page number indicates boxed material, a *d* following a page number indicates a display, a *t* following a page number indicates tabular material, and an *f* following a page number indicates a figure. Drugs are listed under their generic names. When a drug trade name is listed, the reader is referred to the generic name.